TECHNIQUES IN DIAGNOSTIC IMAGING

Techniques in Diagnostic Imaging

EDITED BY

GRAHAM H. WHITEHOUSE

MB, BS(Lond), FRCP, FRCR, DMRD, AKC
Professor of Diagnostic Radiology
University of Liverpool

AND

BRIAN S. WORTHINGTON

BSc, MB, BS(Lond), FRCR, DMRD, LIMA
Professor of Diagnostic Radiology
University of Nottingham

THIRD EDITION

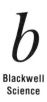

**Blackwell
Science**

© 1983, 1990, 1996 by
Blackwell Science Ltd
Editorial Offices:
Osney Mead, Oxford OX2 0EL
25 John Street, London WCIN 2BL
23 Ainslie Place, Edinburgh EH3 6AJ
238 Main Street, Cambridge
   Massachusetts 02142, USA
54 University Street, Carlton
   Victoria 3053, Australia

Other Editorial Offices:
Arnette Blackwell SA
  1, rue de Lille, 75007 Paris
  France

Blackwell Wissenschafts-Verlag GmbH
  Kurfürstendamm 57
  10707 Berlin, Germany

  Feldgasse 13, A-1238 Wien
  Austria

First published 1983
(under the title *Techniques in Diagnostic Radiology*)
Second edition 1990
Third edition 1996

Set by Setrite Typestters, Hong Kong
Printed and bound in Great Britain
by The Bath Press, Avon

DISTRIBUTORS

Marston Book Services Ltd
PO Box 87
Oxford OX2 0DT
(Orders: Tel: 01865 791155
        Fax: 01865 791927
        Telex: 837515)

North America
Blackwell Science, Inc.
238 Main Street
Cambridge, MA 02142
(Orders: Tel: 800 215-1000
         617 876-7000
         Fax: 617 492-5263)

Australia
Blackwell Science Pty Ltd
54 University Street
Carlton, Victoria 3053
(Orders: Tel: 03 9347-0300
         Fax: 03 9349-3016)

A catalogue record for this title
is available from the British Library

ISBN 0–86542–808–5 (BSL)
ISBN 0–86542–617–1 (International Edition)

Library of Congress
Cataloging-in-Publication Data

Techniques in diagnostic imaging / edited by G.H.
   Whitehouse and B.S. Worthington. — 3rd ed.
         p.   cm.
   Includes bibliographical references and index.
   ISBN 0–86542–808–5 (BSL)
   ISBN 0–86542–617–1 (International Edition)
   1. Diagnostic imaging.   I. Whitehouse, G.H.
   II. Worthington, B.S.
   [DNLM: 1. Diagnostic Imaging — methods.
WN   180   T255   1996]
RC78.7. D53T44   1996
616.07'54—dc20
DNLM/DLC
for Library of Congress

Contents

vi   *Contents*

List of Contributors

C. I. BARTRAM MB, BS(Lond) FRCP, FRCR, DMRD, *Consultant Radiologist, St Marks Hospital, London*

G. R. CHERRYMAN MB, ChB, FRCR, *Professor of Diagnostic Radiology, University of Leicester, Leicester*

J. F. COCKBURN MRCP, FRCR, FFRRCSI, *Senior Registrar in Radiology, Hammersmith Hospital, London*

J. O. M. C. CRAIG FRCSI, FRCS, FRCR, FFRRCSI (Hon), *Formerly Consultant Radiologist, St Mary's Hospital, London; Member of Council, Medical Protection Society*

P. DAWSON PhD, FRCP, FRCR, *Reader in Diagnostic Radiology, Hammersmith Hospital, London*

K. C. DEWBURY BSc, MB, BS(Lond), FRCR, DMRD, *Consultant Radiologist, Ultrasound Unit, Southampton University Hospital, Southampton*

R. DICK MB, BS(Sydney), FRCR, FRACR, *Consultant Radiologist, Royal Free Hospital, London*

A. F. EVANS MB, ChB (L'pool), FRCR, DMRD, *Consultant Radiologist, Whiston Hospital, Merseyside*

C. EVANS MB, BCh, FRCR *Consultant Radiologist, Cardiff Royal Infirmary, Cardiff*

C. D. R. FLOWER MA(Cantab), MB, BChir, FRCP Canada, FRCR, *Consultant Radiologist, Addenbrooke's Hospital, Cambridge*

A. H. FREEMAN MB, BS(Lond), FRCR, *Consultant Radiologist, Addenbrooke's Hospital, Cambridge*

S. J. GOLDING MB, BS(Lond), FRCR, *Clinical Director, The MRI Centre, John Radcliffe Hospital, Oxford*

R. G. GRAINGER MD, FRCP, DMRD, FRCR, FACR(Hon), FRACR(Hon), *Emeritus Professor of Radiology, University of Sheffield, Sheffield*

R. H. S. GREGSON BSc, MB, BS(Lond), FRCR, DMRD, *Consultant Radiologist, University Hospital, Queens Medical Centre, Nottingham*

A. P. HEMINGWAY MD(Lond), MRCP, FRCR, DMRD, *Senior Research Fellow in Diagnostic Radiology, Hammersmith Hospital, London*

K. LAKIN MA, DPhil, FRCR, *Senior Registrar in Radiology, Nuffield Orthopaedic Centre, Oxford*

R. K. LEVICK TD, MB, ChB(Wales), FRCP, FRCR, DMRD, *Formerly Consultant Radiologist, Sheffield Children's Hospital, Sheffield*

G. A. S. LLOYD MA, DM (Oxon), FRCR, DMRD, *Consultant Radiologist, Royal National ENT Hospital, London*

S. McGEE MB, BS, MRCP, FRCR, *Senior Registrar in Radiology, Cardiff Royal Infirmary, Cardiff*

M. V. MERRICK MA, BM, BCh(Oxon), MSc(Lond), FRCPE, FRCR, *Senior Consultant Nuclear Physician, Western General Hospital, Edinburgh*

A. R. MOODY MA, MRCP, FRCR, *Senior Lecturer in Diagnostic Radiology, University of Nottingham, Nottingham*

D. J. NOLAN MD, MB, BCh, BAO(NUI), MRCP, FRCR, DMRD, *Consultant Radiologist, John Radcliffe Hospital, Oxford*

S. OSTLERE MB, BS, MRCP, FRCR, *Consultant Radiologist, Nuffield Orthopaedic Centre, Oxford*

J. P. OWEN MB, BS(Newc), FRCR, DMRD, *Senior Lecturer in Diagnostic Radiology, University of Newcastle, Newcastle*

S. P. G. PADLEY BSc, MB, BS, MRCP, FRCR, *Consultant Radiologist, Chelsea and Westminster Hospital, London*

D. RICKARDS MRCS, LRCP, FRCR, *Consultant Radiologist, Middlesex Hospital, London*

E. J. ROEBUCK MB, BS(Lond), FRCR, DMRD, *Emeritus Consultant Radiologist, Queens Medical Centre, Nottingham*

C. ROOBOTTOM BSc, MB, ChB(Hon), MRCP, FRCR, *Lecturer, Bristol Royal Infirmary, Bristol*

N. J. D. SMITH MPhil, MSc, BDS, DDRRCR, *Professor of Dental Radiology, King's College Hospital Dental School, London*

S. L. SNOWDON, MB, ChB(L'pool), FFARCS, *Formerly Senior Lecturer in Anaesthesia, University of Liverpool, Liverpool*

A. SPRIGG MB, FRCR, DMRD, DCH, DRCOG, *Consultant Radiologist, Sheffield Children's Hospital, Sheffield*

H. L. WALTERS MB, ChB(Wales), FRCR, DMRD, *Consultant Radiologist, King's College Hospital, London*

G. H. WHITEHOUSE MB, BS(Lond), FRCP, FRCR, DMRD, AKC, *Professor of Diagnostic Radiology, University of Liverpool, Liverpool*

R. P. WILDE BSc (L'pool), BM, BCh(Oxon), MRCP, FRCR, *Consultant Radiologist, Bristol Royal Infirmary, Bristol*

D. J. WILSON MB, BS, BSc, MRCP, FRCR *Consultant Radiologist, Nuffield Orthopaedic Centre, Oxford*

B. S. WORTHINGTON BSc, MB, BS(Lond), FRCR, DMRD, LIMA *Professor of Diagnostic Radiology, University of Nottingham, Nottingham*

Preface to the Third Edition

In the preface to the second edition, published 6 years ago, we observed that the interrelationships of imaging modalities and radiological techniques had become increasingly complex since the first edition in 1983. This trend has continued and is reflected in the approach taken in the present edition to, for instance, the pancreas, the brain and spine, and the joints. Furthermore, the development and refinement of non-invasive imaging techniques has led to the decline and even elimination of several invasive procedures. It would be inappropriate, therefore, to discuss only the practical methods used to outline the body systems without describing these complementary imaging modalities, and the scope of the book has been extended to include isotope imaging and magnetic resonance imaging. Another change over the last decade has been the increasing application of interventional radiology as a natural extension to diagnostic procedures. While it would not be appropriate to describe interventional techniques in fine detail, commoner methods have been outlined in the text. This comprehensive approach, embracing imaging modalities and methods as well as principles of interventional radiology, matches the recent changes in the Part I FRCR syllabus. However, it is hoped that radiology trainees in many countries and training systems will find this book to be of help. It is also intended to be a source of reference to all who work in imaging departments, including radiographers in training.

We wish to express our profound gratitude to all the contributors. New contributors whom we welcome to this edition are Professor Cherryman, Drs Cockburn, Dawson, Evans, Lakin, McGee, Merrick, Moody, Ostlere, Padley, Rickards, Roobottom, Sprigg, Wilde and Wilson. Once again we are grateful to Mrs Joan Scott for her secretarial help in guiding the manuscript to its completed form. We also thank Julie Locke and Victoria Whitehouse for their help. It is a pleasure to acknowledge the continued support and expertise of Peter Saugman and the staff of Blackwell Science.

GRAHAM H. WHITEHOUSE
BRIAN S. WORTHINGTON

Preface to the First Edition

The scope and complexity of diagnostic imaging has greatly increased in recent years; with the development of interventional radiology, ultrasonography, radionuclide imaging, computed tomography and nuclear magnetic resonance. All these modalities have increased the knowledge demanded of trainee radiologists. It is necessary, however, for the trainee radiologist to be well versed in the practical radiological procedures which still have an important role in the day-to-day practice of diagnostic radiology. The common investigations, such as barium studies and intravenous urography, are performed by all general radiologists and should be carried out with the same scrupulous care as the esoteric angiograms performed by the experienced few.

It is intended that this book should fill a void in the radiological literature by providing a comprehensive and up-to-date compendium of practical radiological procedures. The increasing importance of an economical and rational approach to diagnostic imaging is reflected by the systematic elaboration of the indications and contraindications of each technique, and its relationship to other modalities. The risks of the procedure have to be weighed against the need for information and the patient's best interests. Modifications to the basic method are necessary in specific instances. This format has been followed for each body system, pathological consideration being raised only for the understanding of a particular technique. In some instances, as in the orbits and the breast, it has been deemed relevant to extend the description to cover plain radiography. The physical properties and chemical nature of contrast media, pertaining to their application, have been given detailed description. The role of the anaesthetist in the X-ray department, including the use of his skills in clinical measurement, has also merited consideration.

In essence, it is hoped that this book will be a useful guide to all radiologists, especially those in training, and will provide a convenient encapsulation of many facts which are otherwise disseminated throughout the radiological literature. We would envisage that it will also be a helpful reference source to radiographers as well as to radiologists.

We are indebted to the many contributors who have devoted time and effort to writing their sections, despite their many other commitments. Our gratitude is due to Miss Joan Doyle for preparing the manuscript. It is also a pleasure to acknowledge the consistent help and encouragement of Richard Zorab and the work of Bridget Cook of Blackwell Scientific Publications.

GRAHAM H. WHITEHOUSE
BRIAN S. WORTHINGTON

Section 1
Gastrointestinal Tract

1   Salivary Glands

N. J. D. SMITH

The term sialography appears to have been coined by the anatomist Anton Nuck in 1690 to describe the casts he made of the salivary glands by injecting wax into the ducts. It now describes the radiographic demonstration of the major salivary glands after the injection of contrast medium into the duct system.

The first recorded sialogram was made by Arcelin in 1912, using a contrast medium containing bismuth. Further development was delayed because of the inadequacy of this and other available contrast media. Following the development of iodized oil as a contrast medium, Uslenghi (1925) and Carlsten (1926) independently pioneered the routine clinical use of sialography. Subsequently, sialography has become a firmly established technique in the investigation of salivary gland disease (Ollerenshaw & Rose, 1951).

Indications

The presenting symptoms of disorders affecting the salivary glands are relatively few and include pain, swelling, which may be recurrent, xerostomia, bad taste and, rarely, sialorrhoea (Mason & Chisholm, 1975). Sialography should only be performed when the information derived from the examination may be of assistance in reaching a diagnosis or in the subsequent management of the patient. Indications for sialography include the following.

Suspected calculi

A sialogram is indicated in the presence of a salivary calculus in order to ascertain whether or not there is normal salivary gland tissue beyond it, when this information will alter the subsequent management of the case. Sialography also demonstrates whether or not a calcific opacity lies within the gland system.

Swelling

Sialography is indicated when there is unilateral or bilateral enlargement of the salivary glands for which the cause is unknown, or when there are recurrent episodes of swelling. In the presence of a suspected tumour mass, sialography may be indicated but computed tomography (CT) or magnetic resonance imaging (MRI) often give more diagnostic information.

Xerostomia

There are many causes of dry mouth resulting from conditions extrinsic to the glands and which exert their effect through either the salivary centre or the nervous pathways to the glands. When there is doubt, sialography is indicated to distinguish these conditions from intrinsic causes of xerostomia, which include Sjögren's syndrome.

Contraindications

The examination must not be performed in the presence of acute infection in the salivary glands. It is contraindicated in cases of known iodine allergy, but these are rare.

Basic technique

The basic requirements are relatively few and equipment should be readily available on a trolley during the examination (Fig. 1.1).

Probes

A set of graded probes is needed to explore and dilate the orifice of the salivary duct. The preference is for Liebreich's double-ended lacrimal probes,

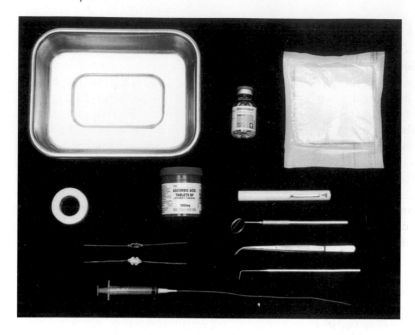

Fig. 1.1 Basic equipment should be readily available on a trolley during the examination.

which usually come in sets of four, graded 00/0, 1/2, 3/4 and 5/6. Only the two finer probes, 00/0 and 1/2, are required for sialography. Directional control of the probe is easily achieved by holding the flat portion at the centre of the instrument lightly between forefinger and thumb.

Cannula

It is best to introduce the contrast medium through a flexible cannula. A 30 cm Portex intravenous cannula with an outside diameter of 1.02 mm and a pink Luer connection is most suitable. The distal end of the cannula should then be drawn out to a fine-diameter tip. This is achieved by grasping the end of the cannula in a pair of Spencer Wells forceps at the same time holding the main part of the cannula firmly between finger and thumb near to the forceps and drawing out the intervening segment to a smaller diameter by giving a sharp tug on the forceps. The narrow part of the cannula is now cut with a sharp scalpel to produce a fine tip for insertion into the orifice after minimal dilatation. The thicker portion gives sufficient rigidity for the operator to handle the cannula and control the direction of movement (Fig. 1.2).

A variety of metal cannulae have been used in sialography, varying from blunted hypodermic needles to metal-tipped catheters. The Rabinov sialography catheter is obtainable in a sterile pack and is recommended. The danger of inadvertently piercing the duct wall, with subsequent extravasation of the contrast medium, is greater with a metal cannula than with a flexible cannula.

Syringe

A 2 ml disposable syringe is suitable since it is rare to use more than this volume of contrast medium.

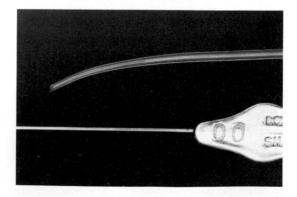

Fig. 1.2 The finely drawn out tip of a Portex cannula shown alongside a size 00 Liebreich's lacrimal probe.

Dental mirror

There should always be a good external light source. As it is sometimes difficult to illuminate the orifices of the submandibular ducts directly because of their position behind the lower incisor teeth, a dental mirror may be found useful to reflect light on to the floor of the mouth. The back of the mirror also prevents the tip of the tongue moving forward to cover the orifice.

Flexible examination light

As well as external illumination, an additional light source such as a Henleys medical doctor's diagnostic light, may be helpful when held close to the orifice of the duct by an assistant.

Gauze

Identification of the orifice of the salivary ducts is facilitated by a dry mucosa, particularly in the case of the submandibular duct where saliva pools in the floor of the mouth. Excess saliva can be easily removed by sterile gauze squares.

Stainless steel dish

As a result of reflex stimulation of the salivary glands, patients may sometimes produce excessive saliva, which may be collected in a suitable dish. During the later clearing stages, when contrast medium mixed with saliva is being passed into the mouth, the patient should be able to spit into a dish.

Plaster tape

A roll of sticking plaster or Micropore and scissors should be available to tape the syringe to the forehead at the end of the injection of contrast medium.

Lemon or ascorbic acid tablets

A slice of fresh lemon is the ideal way to produce reflex stimulation of saliva before taking clearing radiographs, although ascorbic acid tablets make an acceptable substitute.

Contrast medium

Either a water-soluble contrast medium, such as Omnipaque (350 mg iodine ml^{-1}), or the oil-based medium Lipiodol Ultrafluid is used in sialography. Oil-based media have the disadvantages of being more viscous and remaining *in situ* for many years should they be accidentally injected into the tissues surrounding the duct. A recent study by Nicholson (1990) of a prospective study of 60 patients undergoing sialography showed that there was little to choose between the two for duct opacification, but that side effects were both more common and more severe when the oil-based contrast medium was used.

Preliminary radiographs

Plain radiographs should be taken before embarking on sialography because a considerable proportion of salivary gland pathology is associated with opaque calculi within the glands themselves or their ducts, particularly in the submandibular gland (Fig. 1.3). The projections used for these preliminary radiographs are the same as those described later for sialography. In addition a dental film, placed in the buccal sulcus *outside* the upper molar teeth, will be found useful if a calculus is suspected near the orifice of the parotid duct.

Procedure

It is usual to carry out the procedure with the patient lying on an X-ray couch in the supine position.

Parotid gland

The orifice of the parotid duct (Stensen's duct) opens on to a small papilla on the inner surface of the cheek, approximately opposite the crown of the upper second molar tooth. The orifice itself cannot usually be identified by inspection alone. The inner surface of the cheek should first be dried with a gauze square and then the gland itself should be gently massaged by means of external pressure applied by the fingers just behind the posterior border of the ascending ramus of the mandible. This usually results in a bead of saliva becoming visible on the inner surface of the cheek where the duct opens into the mouth. In many

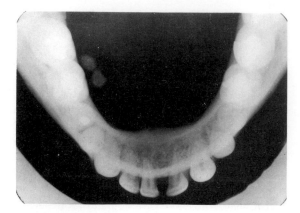

Fig. 1.3 A mandibular occlusal film showing two calculi in the right submandibular duct.

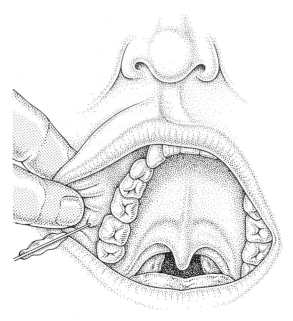

Fig. 1.4 A lacrimal probe inserted into the parotid duct. The cheek is pulled gently forwards and the probe is held parallel to the occlusal plane.

cases the opening of the orifice itself becomes visible at the same time. Gentle exploration with the finest probe should now follow and, once the orifice has been located, the probe should be inserted into it (Fig. 1.4). Resistance will be met after the probe has passed about 1 cm into the duct, because of the sharp bend where it penetrates the buccinator muscle in its passage across the anterior border of the masseter. On no account should any attempt be made to force the probe further along the duct.

The probe should be left in the duct for a minute or two in order to dilate the orifice. This probe should then be withdrawn and immediately replaced with the next largest size. The orifice is almost invariably visible for a few seconds after the probe has been withdrawn. Ideally, this procedure should be repeated until a size 2 Liebreich's probe is inserted into the duct. Sometimes this cannot be achieved, especially when a stricture is present, and in these cases an attempt must be made to cannulate the duct through a smaller opening.

It is a great help when changing probes to be able to pass the probe which has just been withdrawn to an assistant, who then replaces it with one of the next size. Constant observation of the orifices may therefore be maintained by the operator.

Once the orifice has been dilated sufficiently, the fine end of the cannula, which has been filled with contrast medium, is inserted into the duct and advanced until resistance is felt at the point where the duct turns to pierce the buccinator. The orifice usually closes around the wider portion of the

cannula, forming an effective seal, which prevents reflux of contrast medium into the mouth. The contrast medium should then be injected *tediously* slowly at a rate of approximately 0.2 ml min⁻¹. Between 0.5 and 0.75 ml of contrast medium should be sufficient to outline the duct system within a healthy gland, but more may be needed where there is gross dilatation of the duct or an abscess cavity. The injection is terminated either when 1 ml of contrast medium has been injected or as soon as the patient indicates discomfort by a prearranged signal. With the cannula still within the duct, the syringe barrel is taped to the contralateral side of the forehead, rather than in the mid-line where it may interfere with radiography. This produces a slight hydrostatic pressure of contrast medium and prevents premature emptying of the gland.

An oblique lateral radiograph should be taken at this time. If there is satisfactory filling of the gland, radiography should be completed as soon as possible. A small top-up of contrast medium is made just before each exposure. Where filling is inadequate, further contrast medium should be injected before taking a radiograph.

Posteroanterior (PA) and lateral radiographs should be taken, and may be complemented by an axial projection to show the portion of the gland which lies medial to the mandible. The basic PA view is an offset occipitofrontal projection, centring through the gland with the lower border of the ala of the ear making a good surface marking (Fig. 1.5). The traditional lateral projection is the 15° oblique lateral (Fig. 1.6), while an excellent alternative lateral view may be obtained with dental panoramic equipment (Fig. 1.7). If the patient is positioned about 2 cm further forward than is the case for a dental examination, then the region behind the posterior border of the mandible which contains the parotid gland will be in the tomographic cut (Pappas & Wallace, 1970; Azouz, 1978).

Submandibular gland

The orifice of each submandibular duct (Wharton's duct) is considerably more difficult to identify and cannulate than a parotid duct. The duct orifices open on to very flaccid papillae which lie on either side of the mid-line, in the lax tissues of the floor of the mouth behind the central incisor teeth (Fig. 1.8). In some patients, tongue thrusting via an almost involuntary reaction can make sialography very difficult. A dental mirror, as well as reflecting light, is invaluable in holding the tongue out of the way.

After drying the floor of the mouth with gauze squares, the position of the submandibular orifice is often identified by the expression of a few drops of saliva after external massage of the gland. This is achieved by forward pressure from the fingers just behind the angle of the mandible. Sometimes the orifice itself can be identified as it opens momentarily, but in other cases the position is only indicated by the formation of beads of saliva. Very gentle exploration by the finest lacrimal probe should identify the orifice. The probe should be steadied above the papilla, applying only slightly more pressure than is available from its own weight. Too much pressure merely depresses the mucosa in the floor of the mouth, making it harder to find the orifice. Once the orifice has been located, the probe may usually be inserted further than in the parotid duct. Thereafter the procedure is the same as that described for the parotid duct except that the cannula should be inserted further along the duct, since tongue movement can all too easily displace the cannula.

The usual projections are an oblique lateral (Fig. 1.9) and a true lateral, supplemented by a mandibular occlusal radiograph to show the course of the duct in the floor of the mouth. As in the case of the parotid gland, an excellent view is obtained by using dental panoramic equipment.

The submandibular gland is awkwardly placed for PA radiography and, in an attempt to overcome the

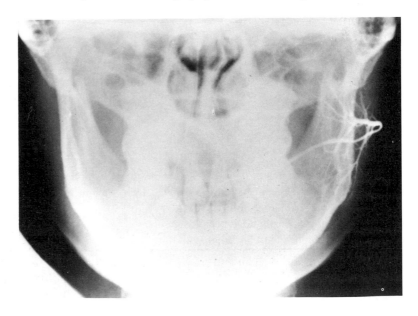

Fig. 1.5 A posteroanterior projection of a normal parotid sialogram.

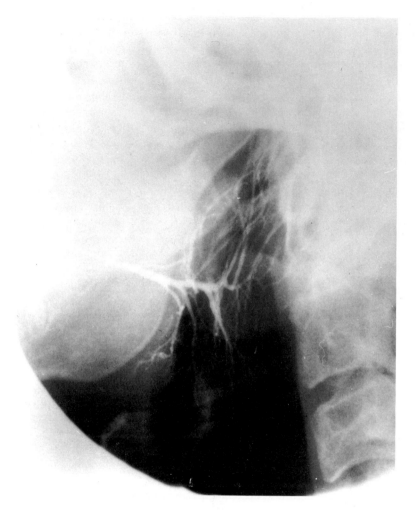

Fig. 1.6 The oblique lateral projection. This is the lateral view of the sialogram shown in Fig. 1.5.

superimpositions resulting from the anatomical position of the gland, Park and Bahn (1968) have recommended a submentovertical projection while an oblique AP projection was described by Hollender and Lindvall (1977).

Pain

Patients vary considerably in their assessment of the degree of discomfort experienced during sialography. The exploration that is sometimes necessary to discover the orifice of the gland, especially in the case of the submandibular gland, together with the slow injection, may be tedious and uncomfortable. The procedure, however, should not cause acute pain or distress.

Over-rapid injection with contrast medium often results in pain within the healthy gland. When the gland is diseased, especially when much glandular tissue has been destroyed, it often becomes relatively insensitive and for this reason it is unwise to place too much reliance on the onset of pain as the end-point for injection.

Pain appears to occur more readily with a water-soluble contrast medium than with an oil-based agent.

Clearing films

After the routine radiographs have been taken, it is possible to obtain a crude indication of the functional status of the gland after stimulating secretory activ-

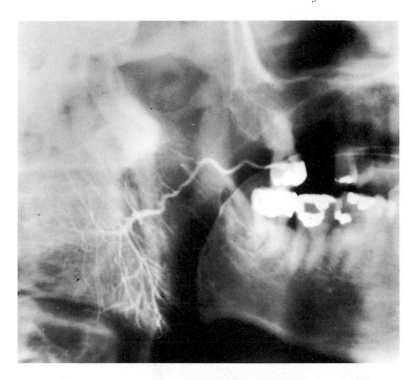

Fig. 1.7 Part of a dental panoramic tomogram (orthopantomograph). This view gives excellent visualization of both the parotid and the submandibular salivary glands.

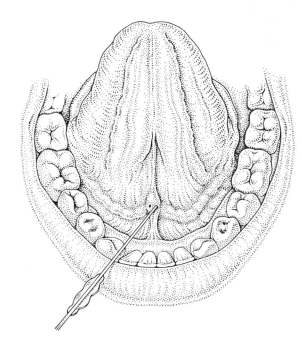

Fig. 1.8 The orifice of the submandibular duct is close to the mid-line. Initially, the probe should be nearly at right angles to the floor of the mouth but once it has been introduced into the duct it will be found to take a more oblique path.

ity. The cannula should be removed and the patient asked to suck a piece of lemon or an ascorbic acid tablet. After an interval of approximately 5 min one further radiograph is taken and, if normal secretory activity is present, no contrast medium will be seen.

Variations on basic technique

Hydrostatic sialography (Gullmo & Book-Henderstrom, 1958; Park & Mason, 1966) replaces the imprecise hand injection technique by gravity feed of the contrast medium through the cannula. Mason and Chisholm (1975) have shown that the secreting pressure of stimulated salivary gland lies between 54 and 76 cmH$_2$O. By raising an open reservoir of contrast medium to a height of between 70 and 90 cm above the orifice, the hydrostatic pressure from the contrast medium exceeds that exerted by the secreting gland and the medium then runs into the gland.

Another attempt to avoid excessive intraglandular pressure during sialography is the method of Ferguson *et al.* (1977), which uses a constant flow rate infusion pump connected to a pressure transducer in order to monitor the injection pressure.

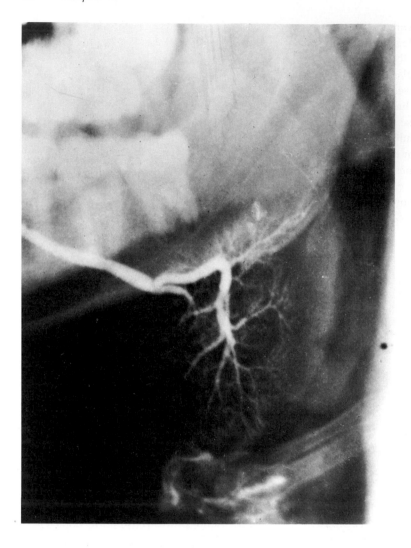

Fig. 1.9 A lateral oblique projection of a normal submandibular sialogram.

Subtraction sialography

The use of subtraction radiography in sialography is described by Liliequist and Welander (1969) and Buchignani and Shimkin (1971). This did not appear to have any significant advantage over routine radiographs. However, interest in this technique has been reawakened by the advent of digital subtraction imaging (DSI) and Buckenham *et al.* (1994) report the use of DSI in a series of 109 patients.

Complications

Serious complications are rare during sialography (Ansell, 1968). Glottic oedema in one case followed as an allergic reaction to iodine. The accidental injection of contrast medium into the tissues of the floor of the mouth is more of a hazard with oil-based media. Extravasated oil-based contrast media are not readily absorbed and may persist in the extrasalivary tissue for several years.

Relationship to other techniques

Radioisotope scanning

Isotope scanning of the salivary glands with ^{99m}Tc pertechnetate has been in use for some years (Gates

& Work, 1967; Harden *et al.*, 1967; Schmitt *et al.*, 1976). This isotope has very similar biological properties to the iodine ion, being taken from the blood stream and concentrated by the salivary glands. Its uptake following intravenous injection gives an indication of salivary gland function but is of limited use in the evaluation of salivary gland disease.

The lack of consistency in the results coupled with the limited resolution detract from the routine use of radioisotope scanning as an adjunct to sialography. The rare case of congenital absence of some or all of the major salivary glands may, however, be confirmed using this technique (Smith & Smith, 1977).

Computed tomography

CT has increasingly become the examination of choice in the investigation of masses in the region of the salivary glands. The use of CT with contrast enhancement (CT-sialography) is now well recognized and is of particular value in distinguishing between lesions within the deep pole of the parotid and those extrinsic pharyngeal masses which tend to compress and laterally displace the gland (Som & Biller, 1979; Rice *et al.*, 1980; Iko, 1984; Evers *et al.*, 1985).

Magnetic resonance imaging

There are a number of reports on the use of MRI for evaluating salivary disorders (Schaefer *et al.*, 1985; Lloyd & Phelps, 1986; Rice & Becker, 1987). More recent work has concentrated on the use of MRI for tissue characterization of salivary gland tumours (Tsushima *et al.*, 1994), and it appears that some progress is being made, particularly in the case of tumours containing myxoid tissue.

References

Ansell, G. (1968) A national survey of radiological complications: interim report. *Clin. Radiol.*, **19**, 175–91.

Arcelin, A. (1912) Radiographie d'un calcul salivaire de la glande sublinguale. *Lyon Med.*, **118**, 769–73.

Azouz, E.M. (1978) The panoramic view of sialography. *Radiology*, **127**(1), 267–8.

Buchignani, J.S. & Shimkin, P.M. (1971) Subtraction sialography: an improved and simplified technique. *Oral Surg.*, **37**, 828–30.

Buckenham, T.M., George C.D., McVicar D. & Moody A.R. (1994) Digital sialography: imaging and intervention. *Br. J. Radiol.*, **67**, 524–9.

Carlsten, D.B. (1926) Lipiolinjektion in den Ausfurhrungsgang der Speicheldrusen. *Acta Radiol.*, **6**, 221–3.

Evers, K., Zito, J.L., Fine, J. *et al.* (1985) CT sialography: utilising acinar filling. *Br. J. Radiol.*, **693**, 839–43.

Ferguson, M.M., Evans, A. & Mason, W.N. (1977) Continuous infusion pressure-monitored sialography. *Int. J. Oral Surg.*, **6**, 84–9.

Gates, G.A. & Work, W.P. (1967) Radioisotope scanning of the salivary glands. *Laryngoscope*, **77**, 861.

Gullmo, A. & Book-Henderstrom, E. (1958) A method of sialography. *Acta Radiol.*, **49**, 17–24.

Harden, R. McG., Hilditch, T.E., Kennedy, I. *et al.* (1967) Uptake and scanning of the salivary glands in man using pertechnetate ^{99m}Tc. *Clin. Sci.*, **32**, 49.

Hollender, L. & Lindvall, A.M. (1977) Sialographic technique. *Dentomaxillofacial Radiol.*, **6**, 34–40.

Iko, B.H. (1984) Computed tomography and sialography of chronic pyogenic parotitis. *Br. J. Radiol.*, **57**(684), 1083–90.

Liliequist, B. & Welander, U. (1969) Sialography — new application of the subtraction technique. *Acta Radiol. Diagn.*, **8**, 228–34.

Lloyd, G.A. & Phelps, P.D. (1986) The demonstration of tumours of the parapharyngeal space by magnetic resonance imaging. *Br. J. Radiol.*, **59**(703), 675–83.

Mason, D.K. & Chisholm, D.M. (1975) *Salivary Glands in Health and Disease*. WB Saunders, London.

Nicholson, D.A. (1990) Contrast media in sialography: a comparison of Lipiodol Ultra Fluid and Urografin 290. *Clin. Radiol.*, **42**, 423–26.

Ollerenshaw, R. & Rose, S. (1951) Radiological diagnosis of salivary gland disease. *Br. J. Radiol.*, **24**, 538–48.

Pappas, G.C. & Wallace, W.R. (1970) Panoramic sialography. *Dent. Radiog. Photog.*, **43**, 17–33.

Park, W.M. & Bahn, S.L. (1968) Sialography simplified. *Oral Surg.*, **26**(5), 728–35.

Park, W.M. & Mason D.K. (1966) Hydrostatic sialography. *Radiology*, **86**, 116–22.

Rice, D.H.Y. & Becker T. (1987) Magnetic resonance imaging of the salivary glands. A comparison with computed tomographic scanning. *Arch Otolaryngol.*, **113**(1), 78–80.

Rice, D.H., Mancuso, A.A. & Hanaffee, W.N. (1980) Computerized tomography with simultaneous sialography in evaluating parotid tumours. *Arch Otolaryngol.*, **106**, 472–3.

Schaefer, S.D., Maravilla, K.R., Close, L.G. *et al.* (1985) Evaluation of NMR versus CT for parotid masses: a preliminary report. *Laryngoscope*, **95**(8), 945–50.

Schmitt, G., Lehmann, G., Strotges, M.W. *et al.* (1976) The diagnostic value of sialography and scintigraphy in salivary gland disease. *Br. J. Radiol.*, **49**, 326–9.

Smith, N.J.D. & Smith, P.B. (1977) Congenital absence of major salivary glands. *Br. Dent. J.*, **142**, 259–60.

Som, P.B. & Biller, H.F. (1979) The combined computerised tomography sialogram. A technique to differentiate deep lobe parotid tumours from extraparotid pharyngo-maxillary space tumours. *Ann. Otol. Rhinol. Laryngol.*, **88**, 590–5.

Tsushima Y., Katsumoto M., Endo K., Aihara T. & Nakajima T. (1994) Characteristic bright signal of parotid pleomorphic adenomas on T2-weighted MR images with pathological correlation. *Clin. Radiol.*, **49**, 485–89.

Uslenghi, J.P. (1925) Nueva technica para la investigacion radiologica de las glandulas salivarias. *Rev. Soc. Argent. Radiol. Electrol.*, **1**, 4–16.

2   Oesophagus

A. H. FREEMAN

Barium swallow

This examination remains the mainstay in the investigation of possible oesophageal pathology. Although the history and clinical examination may be helpful in pointing the way to some oesophageal abnormalities, a barium swallow and/or endoscopy are almost always indicated in these cases.

As with the barium meal, double-contrast studies have become more popular in recent years and show fine mucosal detail to better advantage. There is, however, still a place for single-contrast studies, particularly when looking for oesophageal compression, displacement or disordered motility.

Indications

The prime symptom requiring oesophageal investigation is dysphagia. Other symptoms which may indicate oesophageal disease include heartburn, retrosternal pain, regurgitation, eructation and odynophagia, Odynophagia refers to pain when swallowing, as opposed to dysphagia, which is difficulty when swallowing. These symptoms may be manifestations of a number of pathological conditions, the most common of which are hiatus hernia and reflux oesophagitis with or without stricture formation. Carcinoma always has to be excluded and this can be particularly difficult in the presence of a stricture. In this situation, it is probably best to biopsy all oesophageal strictures as there is an increased risk of adenocarcinoma developing in association with columnar lining of the lower gullet.

Less common entities include motility disorders, such as achalasia and diffuse oesophageal spasm, as well as pressure and invasion from extrinsic lesions. The pharyngo-oesophageal junction is subject to its own problems, including Zenker's diverticulum, cricoid webs and cricopharyngeal achalasia.

Contraindications

The main contraindications to a barium swallow are situations where there is likely to be a leakage from the oesophagus into the mediastinum or pleural and peritoneal cavities. Aspiration into the bronchial tree is a relative contraindication.

There is conflicting evidence as to the seriousness of barium leakage into the mediastinum, because of its potential to stimulate a fibrotic reaction. James *et al.* (1975) pointed out that this effect may not be deleterious and that, in addition, the barium had a sterilizing effect on salivary flora, probably by a simple mechanical process. Barium, however, has another disadvantage in that it may remain loculated in the mediastinum and obscure follow-up studies for months or even years.

For these reasons it has been traditional practice to use a water-soluble contrast medium such as Gastrografin* when initially investigating a potential oesophageal leak. However, the detail obtained with these agents is not as good as with barium and the possibility of missing oesophageal lesions has been stressed (Foley *et al.* 1982).

The usual policy, therefore, is to start with a water-soluble contrast medium and, if this shows no major leakage, to follow it with barium. The latter may then demonstrate the small mucosal tears which can be missed when using Gastrografin. This policy also has the advantage that, if an oesophageal tear communicates with the pleural or peritoneal

---

* Gastrografin: sodium and meglumine diatrizoate together with a flavouring agent (Schering Health Care Ltd, Burgess Hill, West Sussex, UK).

cavity, excess barium in these cavities will be avoided. The presence of barium in serous cavities incites a marked inflammatory response which leads to fibrosis. In the peritoneal cavity, this fibrosis may be so marked as to cause bowel obstruction (Ansell & Wilkins, 1987), but is not such a serious complication as when there is leakage from a barium enema with the inevitable contamination by faecal material.

The main problem with using Gastrografin as a contrast agent occurs if there is any risk of aspiration into the bronchial tree. Aspiration of Gastrografin causes a very severe form of chemical pneumonitis and consequent acute pulmonary oedema. Gastrografin must therefore be avoided in this situation. If there is a risk of this happening then it is best to start with a non-ionic water-soluble contrast medium such as Gastromiro*, which causes no inflammatory change at all in the lung parenchyma (Bell *et al.*, 1987). If barium sulphate is aspired it does not incite a reaction in the bronchial tree and is usually coughed up without any sequelae. Large volumes, however, can give rise to severe respiratory embarrassment and even death (Ansell & Wilkins, 1987). It is therefore important to curtail the examination if modest amounts of barium are observed to be aspirated. The nature of the barium sulphate suspension will depend on whether a single- or double-contrast examination is to be performed. For a single-contrast study, a medium-density (100 w/v), low-viscosity barium is best and one of the ready-prepared suspensions, such as Baritop†, is ideal. This agent will also provide good double-contrast views of the oesophagus but, as the procedure is commonly performed in association with a double-contrast examination of the stomach, a higher density barium is used instead.

The latter is often a powder form of barium, for instance EZM HD‡, which is reconstituted to 250 w/v. Both single- and double-contrast studies will be performed on a standard fluoroscopic table with the facility to take spot films. A video or cine facility is

extremely useful and is mandatory for studying disorders of motility.

Single-contrast examination

Basic technique

The initial radiographs are taken with the table erect and the patient standing in the right anterior oblique (RAO) position. In this position the oesophagus is projected clear of the spine. It is customary to screen the first mouthful of contrast medium as it passes along the oesophagus, noting any gross lesion. Spot films are taken in this position, usually by splitting 24 × 30 or 35 × 35 cm films. At least two views should be taken to include the upper and middle thirds as well as the middle and lower thirds.

The single-contrast study is most appropriate for the demonstration of extrinsic displacement or disordered motility. If the former is suspected then posteroanterior (PA) and lateral chest radiographs are extremely useful at this stage to give an overall demonstration of anatomical relationships to the opacified oesophagus.

For motility disorders, a prone swallow is essential to assess oesophageal contraction in the absence of gravity. The table is therefore placed horizontal with the patient lying in the prone left posterior oblique (LPO) position. Barium is then swallowed via a straw and spot films are taken as it passes down the oesophagus. Particular attention is paid to the action of 'stripping' waves, which pass downwards and completely empty the oesophagus. Apart from demonstrating the motility, stripping waves are also helpful in showing the mucosal relief pattern of the oesophagus. It is unusual to miss significant pathology when the oesophagus contracts down completely throughout its length.

Although motility abnormalities can be illustrated on static film, they are best recorded by a cine or video facility.

Dynamic studies

These include cine (35 mm), video and 100 mm roll film as recording media. Each of these techniques has advantages and disadvantages. Cine can be run at a much higher frame speed than roll film but lacks clarity and involves a higher radiation dose. Video is cheap, allows an instant replay, but lacks a hard-copy facility.

The advantages of 100 mm roll film are that it is economical in price, low in radiation dose and allows hard-copy images of the stomach and duodenum as well.

Dynamic studies are used in two main situations: (i) in the assessment of motility disorders; and (ii) in the demonstration of the pharyngo-oesophageal junction. When recording motility disorders, a speed of 6–16 frames s^{-1} will suffice when using cine or roll film. This should be performed in the prone oblique position. It is important not to pan up and down the oesophagus when recording, but to image one section at a time. It is also important to record long enough to assess the passage of a complete bolus through the oesophagus and not just in short bursts.

The patient should be instructed to take a single bolus of barium at a time, as the motor activity of the oesophagus will be affected by a second bolus passing through the cricopharyngeus before distal contraction is complete. Demonstration of the pharyngo-oesophageal junction may be achieved on static film but is best recorded by a dynamic facility, because high dysphagia can be caused not only by anatomical abnormalities but also by subtle changes in neuromuscular incoordination. These can only be demonstrated on a dynamic examination using cine or video because of the higher frame speed of up to 56 frames s^{-1} (Ekberg, 1987). The patient swallows contrast medium in the erect position and true anteroposterior (AP) and lateral views are taken. It is important with the latter to include part of the oropharynx as well as the epiglottis and cricopharyngeal relaxation and closure of the laryngeal aditus. Minor abnormalities of function of the pharyngo-oesophageal segment can unquestionably cause dysphagia (Ekberg, 1987).

Cine or 100 mm roll film is also used to demonstrate the anatomy of this region if it proves difficult to obtain good views on static film.

Modification of basic technique

Most common motility disorders are relatively easy to diagnose, although the diagnosis of early achalasia can be very difficult and several manoeuvres are advocated for its confirmation. The diagnosis of early achalasia, before there is disordered motility without oesophageal dilation, is suggested by a positive test when the subcutaneous injection of methylcholine stimulates oesophageal contraction and causes chest pain. This test is usually performed in association with oesophageal manometry. In the later stages of achalasia, when there is hold-up at the cardia and oesophageal dilatation, the cardia can be stimulated to open by either giving the patient a hot-water drink or an injection of Buscopan (Berridge, 1975). The hot-water test is especially useful, with the cardia opening wide as soon as the hot water fills the oesophagus. These two tests are performed with the patient erect. Even with these tests, it may be impossible to make the difficult distinction of infiltrating carcinoma (Lawson & Dodds, 1976).

Double-contrast barium swallow

The majority of oesophageal diseases, apart from motility disorders, are best demonstrated by the double-contrast technique. This requires the intravenous injection of a hypotonic agent, such as Buscopan or glucagon, followed by a gas mixture as in double-contrast radiology of the stomach (see Chapter 3). The initial films are again taken with the patient erect and quickly swallowing a bolus of high-density barium. Although this will usually result in a very good demonstration of the mucosal pattern of the oesophagus, various other methods of introducing air have been advocated. These include simple measures such as making the patient swallow barium through a perforated tube so that air is swallowed as well, pinching the nose whilst swallowing, or using the slightly more complicated method of an insufflator with a two-way cup as advocated by Rossetti (1985). These are the most convenient and acceptable methods as the only other route is via a nasogastric tube, the passage of which can cause considerable discomfort.

Radiographs (usually split 24 × 30 or 35 × 35 cm) are exposed with the patient erect, in both the RAO and left anterior oblique (LAO) projections in order to show the body of the oesophagus. It is often helpful to turn the patient slightly whilst taking these radiographs, so that the oesophagus is viewed at different angles (Fig. 2.1).

The table is then placed in the horizontal position for a prone swallow, during which particular attention is paid to the gastro-oesophageal junction. The patient lies in the LPO position and drinks barium through a straw. Split 24 × 30 cm films are taken of the lower oesophagus and gastro-oesophageal junction as barium passes through this region and there is maximum distension. This is the best way to demonstrate a hiatus hernia and there is probably little indication to apply pressure on the abdomen to make the hernia more obvious. The other reason for obtaining views of the gastro-oesophageal junction at full distension is to measure its diameter, there being a close correlation between a wide hiatus and the presence of reflux. A diameter of more than

25 mm strongly suggests that reflux is occurring (Graziani *et al.*, 1983), even in the absence of a true hiatus hernia (Fig. 2.2).

There is controversy about the demonstration of frank gastro-oesophageal reflux. Failure to demonstrate reflux during a barium meal does not necessarily mean that it does not occur at other times. Equally, the demonstration of reflux during a barium meal need not be the cause of symptoms. The issue is further confused by 30–50% of patient with symptoms of gastro-oesophageal reflux having normal endoscopic appearances (De Meester, *et al.*, 1980). The usual practice is to attempt to demonstrate reflux by the physiological method and to note how freely it occurs. To demonstrate reflux, the patient is first

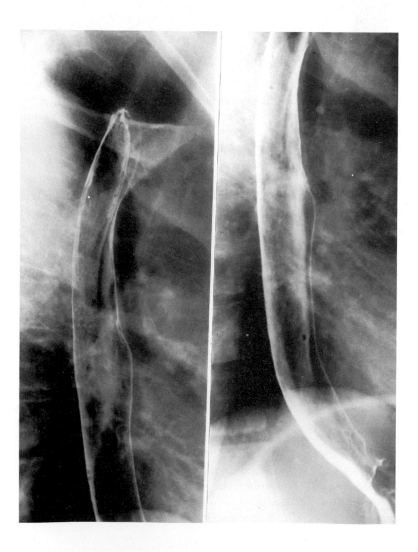

Fig. 2.1 Double-contrast view of the body of the oesophagus taken in the right anterior oblique position. Note the slight anterolateral bulge in the mid-oesophagus corresponding to the interaorticobronchial segments.

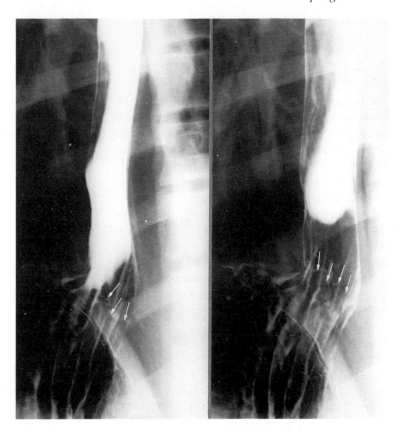

Fig. 2.2 Prone swallow taken in the left posterior oblique position to show the gastro-oesophageal junction. In this case the hiatal segment is wide and nearly the width of the distended body of the oesophagus. The 'Z' line or squamocolumnar junction can be faintly seen (arrows).

placed in the left decubitus position and is then turned supine. Barium has now accumulated in the fundus of the stomach. The patient is then slowly turned onto the right side whilst the gastro-oesophageal junction is continually observed under fluoroscopy. The barium in the fundus will pour over the cardia during this manoeuvre and reflux may be observed. It is preferable to have the table in a slightly head-down position and the manoeuvre is repeated several times to evaluate this area fully.

Some authors advocate the use of abdominal compression to help precipitate reflux and, using a double-contrast technique, have been able to demonstrate a high sensitivity and specificity for gastro-oesophageal reflux as a cause of chest pain (Sellar *et al.*, 1987).

As oesophageal symptoms may also be caused by pathology in the stomach and duodenum, a formal study of these organ is necessary in the prone, supine and erect positions.

A further specific examination is required if the patient's symptoms suggest disease in the upper oesophagus or pharyngo-oesophageal junction. Reference has already been made to the cine swallow of this area. Static radiographs should be taken and are of course essential if cine is not available. The table is again brought erect and straight AP and lateral views are taken during deglutition. This requires close coordination between radiologist and patient.

The best method is to position the fluoroscopic unit level with the patient's neck and then ask the patient to take a mouthful of barium and hold it until the command 'swallow'. In the mean time the cassette is brought across into the exposure position so that the radiologist is able to press the exposure button just as the bolus passes down the laryngopharynx and upper oesophagus. This can be judged by the upward movement of the larynx. It may require several attempts before catching the fully distended pharynx. Some patients are quite unable to cooperate and video is then a necessity. Static views obtained during a Valsalva manoeuvre will show a double-contrast effect in the distended pharynx.

Paediatric swallow

Whilst gastro-oesophageal reflux and its complications may be a cause of morbidity in infants and young children, this age group is subject to a number of specific oesophageal problems which are not encountered in the adult population. These include oesophageal atresia, tracheo-oesophageal fistula and vascular rings.

The diagnosis of oesophageal atresia can usually be confirmed by simply passing a nasogastric tube down the blind-ending upper pouch and taking a chest radiograph. Assuming there is a fistula from the bronchial tree to the distal segment of the oesophagus, there will be gas in the stomach and an estimate can thus be made of the length of the atretic segment.

The demonstration of tracheo-oesophageal fistula requires meticulous technique and either a cine or at least a rapid film capacity using a 100 mm camera. It is best performed with a nasogastric tube *in situ* and the child held in a face-down and horizontal position so that gravity may help fill the fistula. The table is kept in the erect position so that a horizontal lateral shoot-through beam may be used with the child either cradled or held on the table foot-rest. The tube is slowly withdrawn into the mid-oesophagus whilst contrast medium is injected and the whole procedure is continuously recorded. It is important not to overfill the oesophagus as some of the contrast medium may then be aspirated via the larynx, giving rise to diagnostic difficulties. The contrast medium used may be either Gastromiro or dilute barium sulphate. Neither of these in small doses will cause any hazard to the bronchial tree, but it is important not to overfill the bronchi and so cause respiratory embarrassment.

As with adults, Gastrografin is absolutely contra-indicated because it causes pneumonitis and acute pulmonary oedema on aspiration. It also presents an additional hazard to small children because of its hyperosmolar effect in the small intestine, which may severely dehydrate the child and even cause death.

Diagnosis of vascular rings requires that the oesophagus is maximally distended with barium. Radiographs taken in the true AP and lateral projec-

tions will then show the typical impression at the aortic arch level.

Bread barium swallow

Occasionally, it is helpful to give a solid component to the barium swallow if a stricture is suspected but cannot be adequately demonstrated or if there is a question about a motility disorder. This is usually in the form of a piece of bread which has been soaked with barium. The patient is then asked to swallow the whole morsel intact. This can give very useful information about localized non-distensibility or areas of poor contraction.

Relationship to other techniques

Plain films

PA and lateral chest radiographs are of value if there is any question of extrinsic compression or displacement of the oesophagus. Soft-tissue views of the neck are indicated if a foreign body has become lodged in the throat, particularly if it contains bone. There is otherwise little indication for plain films.

Computed tomography (CT)

CT is used in assessing the operability of oesophageal carcinoma. It gives very useful information about local spread and whether or not the tumour involves the aorta and other adjacent structures. CT can also define local lymph-node involvement, although this is probably now best achieved by endoscopic ultrasound. However, CT will give a good demonstration of the liver in regard to metastasis.

Magnetic resonance imaging (MRI)

Like CT, MRI gives excellent detail of the spatial relationships of the oesophagus, including the ability to produce coronal images (Fig. 2.3). Like CT, its major role so far has been in the assessment of oesophageal carcinoma, although to date its advantages in this respect appear to be marginal (Takashima *et al.*, 1991).

Endoscopy

Undoubtedly the widespread application of fibreoptic endoscopy has had a profound effect on the role of the barium swallow. Instruments are now very easy to pass and a diagnostic upper gastrointestinal endoscopy has a very low morbidity with an oesophageal perforation rate of 0.018% (Dawson & Cockel, 1981).

The ability to see the oesophageal mucosa and to perform biopsy and therapeutic techniques obviously gives endoscopy a major advantage over barium studies. However, there is still a role for the barium swallow. For example, it is notoriously difficult to localize dysphagia. A pharyngeal pouch has to be excluded in cases of high dysphagia, while the cricopharyngeal area is particularly difficult for the endoscopist. If a pouch is present the endoscope will almost certainly pass into its orifice, whereupon only gentle pressure is required to rupture the pouch wall with the subsequent risk of mediastinitis and even death. It is therefore mandatory in cases of high dysphagia to have a prior barium swallow to assess the anatomy. If the dysphagia is low retrosternal in site then it is likely to be due to an abnormality beyond 20–25 cm from the incisors. In this situation it is permissible to endoscope without a previous barium swallow, but confusion may arise at endoscopy if there is, for instance, an intrathoracic stomach or extrinsic pressure from, for instance, an ectatic descending aorta.

The barium swallow is especially valuable in cases of motility disorder. In achalasia, for instance, the barium examination will clearly demonstrate early disease and yet the endoscope will pass without hindrance straight into the stomach.

It is therefore appropriate to perform a barium swallow as the first examination in any patient suffering from suspected oesophageal disease. The two examinations are complementary, the barium swallow giving a good general assessment of the whole gullet and surrounding structures whilst endoscopy, with or without biopsy, gives the optimal demonstration of mucosal detail.

Endoscopic ultrasound

This is the best means of examing localized segments of the oesophageal wall. The apparatus consists of a modified oblique-viewing endoscope (Shorvon *et al.*, 1987). Although early ultrasound units comprised a mechanical sector-scan transducer mounted in an oil-filled chamber, linear array probes are the most popular variation at the present time. The probe is attached to a rubber bag containing water, so that acoustic contact can be maintained between the probe and the oesophageal wall. The endoscope functions in a normal fashion and contains biopsy and suction channels.

The disadvantage of the ultrasound endoscope is the rigid end, which is 4–5 cm long. As with normal endoscopy, the patient is sedated and lies on his or her left side. Orientation within the oesophagus is confirmed by direct vision as well as the distance from the incisor teeth. The local anatomy can then be clearly described by using landmarks such as the heart valves.

The technique gives intimate detail of all the coats of the oesophageal wall (Fig. 2.4) and can demonstrate spread of a tumour from the mucosal layer into the submucosa and muscle coats. It also clearly defines lymph-node involvement and appears to be the most sensitive test currently available for staging oesophageal cancer.

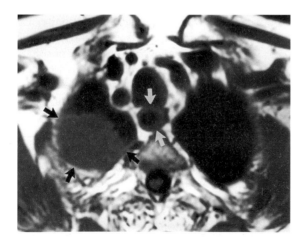

Fig. 2.3 T_1 weighted magnetic resonance image through the thorax delineating an air-filled oesophagus (white arrows). Note also the large carcinoma in the right lung (black arrows).

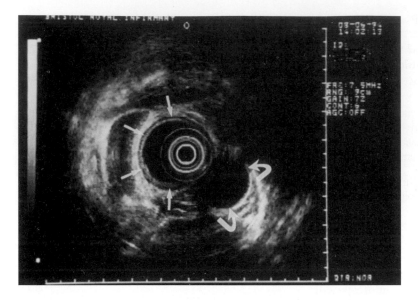

Fig. 2.4 Endoscopic ultrasound of the distal oesophagus clearly showing the oesophageal wall (white arrows) separated from the tip of the probe by a water-filled balloon. The aorta is marked by curved arrows. Courtesy of Dr J. Virjee, Bristol Royal Infirmary.

Manometry

This technique measures the intraluminal pressure within the oesophagus, using a multilumen tube through which water is perfused at a constant rate. Pressure changes are then transmitted through the fluid medium and are continuously recorded at different points in the oesophagus during slow withdrawal of the tip of the tube. The main role of manometry is in the investigation of oesophageal motility disorders and it is especially valuable in the diagnosis of early achalasia. Similarly, manometry may be helpful in the diagnosis of diffuse oesophageal spasm, a condition which presents with dysphagia and chest pain and may mimic coronary artery insufficiency.

Radionuclide imaging

This technique is increasingly being used to assess gastro-oesophageal reflux. The patient swallows a food mixture containing ^{99m}Tc sulphur colloid and then lies under a gamma camera. The procedure takes 10 min and episodes of gastro-oesophageal reflux can be recorded and correlated with any symptoms the patient might experience. In many centres an abdominal binder is used to raise intra-abdominal pressure and thus make reflux more obvious. This technique can also be used to assess oesophageal transit.

pH monitoring

This is usually regarded as the 'gold standard' when evaluating symptoms thought to be due to gastro-oesophageal reflux. The pH probe, which consists of a glass electrode, is passed down the oesophagus so that it lies about 5 cm above the gastro-oesophageal junction. Continuous measurement of pH is then recorded at this level. Episodes of reflux are marked by the pH falling as low as 1.5–2. This is usually followed by rapid clearing as oesophageal contraction empties the distal oesophagus. Originally, the patient was connected by wires to a monitor, so that recordings could be made only in a supine position. The procedure has been greatly simplified by the introduction of radio probes the signals of which are recorded by a monitor attached to the patient. A full 24-hour recording can then be made whilst the patient goes about his or her normal duties. In particular, the patient is able to eat and so subject the stomach to the normal physiological stimuli which might induce reflux.

The Bernstein test

This is a further test for evaluating gastro-oesophageal reflux. Dilute hydrochloric acid and sodium chloride are alternately instilled in the oesophagus. The test can be conducted as a double-blind trial and patient symptoms assessed. A positive response occurs when the hydrochloric acid induces symptoms similar to those caused by gastro-oesophageal reflux, although a negative test is of relatively little clinical value (Bernstein & Baker, 1958).

References

Ansell, G. & Wilkins, R.A. (1987) *Complications in Diagnostic Imaging*, 2nd edn. Blackwell Scientific Publications, Oxford.

Bell, K.E., McKinstry, C.S. & Mills, J.O.M. (1987) Iopamidol in the diagnosis of suspected upper gastro-intestinal perforation. *Clin. Radiol.*, **38**, 165–8.

Bernstein, L.M. & Baker, L.A. (1958) A clinical test for oesophagitis. *Gastroenterology*, **34**, 760–81.

Berridge, F.R. (1975) Lower oesophagus and gastrooesophageal junction. *In* Lodge, T. & Steiner, R.E. (eds) *Recent Advances in Radiology*, Vol. 5. Churchill Livingstone, London.

Dawson, J. & Cockel, R. (1981) Oesophageal perforation at fibre-optic gastroscopy. *Br. Med. J.*, **283**, 583.

De Meester, T.R., Wang, C.I., Wernely, J.A. *et al.* (1980) Technique, indications and clinical use of 24-hour pH monitoring. *J. Thorac. Cardiovasc. Surg.*, **79**, 656–70

Ekberg, O. (1987) Dysfunction of the pharyngo-oesophageal segment in patients with normal opening of the upper oesophageal sphincter: a cineradiographic study. *Br. J. Radiol.*, **60**, 637–44.

Foley, M.J., Ghahremani, G.G. & Rogers, L.F. (1982) Reappraisal of contrast media used to detect upper gastro-intestinal perforations. *Radiology*, **144**, 213–7.

Graziani, L., Dengigris, E., Pesaresi, A. *et al.* (1983) Reflux oesophagitis: radiographic-endoscopic correlation in 39 symptomatic cases. *Gastrointest. Radiol.*, **8**, 1–6.

James, A.E., Montali, R.J., Chafee, V. *et al.* (1975) Barium or Gastrografin: which contrast media for diagnosis of oesophageal tears? *Gastroenterology*, **68**, 1103–13.

Lawson, T.L. & Dodds, W.J. (1976) Infiltrating carcinoma simulating achalasia. *Gastrointest. Radiol.*, **1**, 245–48.

Rossetti, G. (1985) *Double Contrast Radiology of the Oesophagus*. Piccin Nuova Libraria, SPA, Padua, Italy.

Sellar, R.J., Decaestecker, J.S. & Heading, P.B. (1987) Barium radiology: a sensitive test for gastro-oesophageal reflux. *Clin. Radiol.*, **38**, 303–7.

Shorvon, P.J., Lees, W.R., Frost, R.A. & Cotton, P.B. (1987) Upper gastrointestinal endoscopic ultrasonography in gastroenterology. *Br. J. Radiol.*, **60**, 429–38.

Takashima, S., Takeuchi, N., Shiozaki, H. *et al.* (1991) Carcinoma of the oesophagus. CT versus MR imaging in determining resectability. *AJR*, **156**, 297–302.

Further reading

Gelfand, D.W. (1980) Complications of gastro-intestinal radiologic procedures. 1. Complications of routine fluoroscopic studies. *Gastrointest. Radiol.*, **5**, 293–315.

Hall, C.M. (1984) Non-invasive investigation of the gastrointestinal tract in neonates and infants. *Clin. Gastroenterol.*, **13**, 161–83.

3   Stomach and Duodenum

D. J. NOLAN

Plain radiographs are important in patients who present with symptoms or signs of acute abdominal disorders. Although the radiographic projections will depend on the presenting clinical problem, the essential radiographs are a supine abdomen and a view of the chest (Miller, 1973; Frimann-Dahl, 1974; Field, 1986). Good radiographic technique is essential. The lower edge of the supine radiograph is positioned at the level of the symphysis pubis and includes the hernial orifices. The chest radiograph is important as patients with lung or pleural disorders may present with abdominal pain. Additional horizontal radiographs may be required, including an upright and / or left, right and supine radiographs of the abdomen.

The mid-inspiratory upright chest and expiratory left lateral abdominal radiographs are best for demonstrating pneumoperitoneum (Miller *et al.*, 1980). As little as 1 ml of intraperitoneal air can be detected with good radiographic technique (Miller & Nelson, 1971). The patient should be in position for at least 10 min, so that the free air reaches the highest point before radiographs are obtained (Miller, 1973). The left lateral decubitus position allows air to escape freely from the stomach through a perforated duodenal or lesser-curve gastric ulcer, whereas in other positions gastric fluid and solid contents are likely to leak into the peritoneum (Frimann-Dahl, 1974). The left lateral decubitus radiograph should be exposed with a less penetrating technique than is usually employed in abdominal radiography, as air is likely to collect on the right border between the liver edge and the right wall of the abdomen and over the right ilium (Miller & Nelson, 1971).

The supine abdominal radiograph is the best projection for diagnosing intestinal obstruction (Hodges & Miller, 1955; Field *et al.*, 1985; Simpson *et al.*, 1985), although the upright or decubitus projection may provide useful information, particularly when the obstructed loops are filled with fluid.

The indications for plain radiographs are suspected perforation or rupture of an abdominal organ, intestinal obstruction or ileus, volvulus, acute colitis or toxic megacolon, acute conditions of the gallbladder and biliary tract, acute pancreatitis, urinary calculi or other acute conditions of the urinary tract, abscess, foreign body, appendix calculi or an abdominal aneurysm.

Barium examination

The double-contrast examination is now widely used as the barium technique of choice for demonstrating the stomach and duodenum, having largely replaced the conventional single-contrast method. Japanese radiologists originally refined the technique and have been routinely performing successful double-contrast studies of the stomach for about 40 years. The aim of the double-contrast method is to distend the stomach and duodenum with gas after coating the mucosa with a thin, even layer of barium. The lesions are seen *en face* and the size, shape and details of the margin can be accurately assessed. The radiological appearances closely resemble those of the resected specimen.

Mucosal views, compression radiography and the filling method were incorporated into the double-contrast examination by the Japanese radiologists. Op den Orth named the technique the 'biphasic' examination in order to emphasize the importance of incorporating conventional views when performing the double-contrast examination (Op den Orth & Ploem, 1977; Op den Orth, 1979). For optimum results, compression radiography and mucosal view of the anterior wall should be part of the examination routine.

Indications

The double-contrast barium meal is indicated in patients with dyspepsia, unexplained weight loss, anaemia, gastrointestinal bleeding or a palpable mass in the upper abdomen. A single-contrast barium examination without the use of hypotonic or effervescent agents is indicated in patients who present with vomiting due to a suspected obstructive lesion of the gastric antrum or duodenum.

Contraindications

Barium should not be given to patients with suspected perforation of the upper gastrointestinal tract. The presence of barium in the gastrointestinal tract may make it impossible to carry out satisfactory angiography and it should therefore not be used in patients who present with bleeding until the question of performing angiography has been fully considered.

Barium suspension

Barium suspensions suitable for double-contrast radiography may be of medium or high density and should be of low viscosity. Suitable concentrations include barium preparations already in suspension ranging from 82.5 to 100 w/v% (Op den Orth & Ploem, 1977; Nolan, 1980) or higher density barium suspensions (200–250 w/v%) which are prepared shortly before use by adding water to barium sulphate powder. The high-density barium suspensions do not always give a significantly better mucosal coating than those of medium density, because the local water supply has an effect on the performance of the latter (Miller & Skucas, 1977).

Gas

There are numerous ways of introducing gas into the stomach and duodenum for double-contrast examinations. Initially, nasogastric intubation was used (Shirakabe, 1971) but is unsuitable for routine use and has been superseded by effervescent agents in the form of powder, granules, tablets and aerated liquids. The 'bubbly barium' method (Pochaczevsky, 1973; Op den Orth & Ploem, 1977) is another satisfactory technique for introducing gas. Refrigerated barium is put in a soda-making dispenser and carbon dioxide cartridges are attached to the syphon, resulting in a slow release of gas into the barium.

Hypotonic agents

High-quality double-contrast studies are obtained by using smooth muscle relaxants to produce a state of hypotonia in the stomach and duodenum during the examination. Hyoscine butylbromide (Buscopan) and glucagon are widely used for this purpose.

Hyoscine butylbromide (Buscopan) is a quaternary ammonium synthesized from scopolamine (Ayre-Smith, 1976). It is a ganglion-blocking agent but, unlike scopolamine, has no central action. It causes only minor atropine-like side effects unless used in doses over 40 mg. Massive gastric dilatation is a rare complication. Contraindications to its use are prostatism, glaucoma, cardiac failure and angina pectoris. The dose normally used for the double-contrast examination — 20 mg i.v. — is unlikely to aggravate heart failure or angina or cause urinary retention. It has recently been suggested that the practice of enquiring about a history of glaucoma should be abandoned and instead give advice to seek urgent medical attention should eye pain or visual loss develop (Fink & Aylward, 1995). Buscopan produces transient loss of accommodation but vision should have returned to normal within 1 hour of the injection.

Glucagon, a straight-chain polypeptide derived from the islets of Langerhans, produces gastric and duodenal hypotonia. Nausea and vomiting may occur, but are rare with the dose used for double-contrast studies. Glucagon may produce severe hypertension in patients with phaeochromocytoma and is also contraindicated in insulinoma. Hypersensitivity reactions occur but are rare. A dose of 0.15 mg given i.v. at the beginning of the examination is adequate for the double-contrast examination. There may be a slight delay before the barium and gas pass through the pylorus when glucagon is used, with the advantage that radiographs of the stomach can normally be obtained before barium passes into the distal part of the duodenum and obscures part of the lower half of the stomach.

Examination technique

The aim of the double-contrast part of the examination is to obtain views of all parts of the stomach distended with gas. The mucosal surface should be outlined with an even coating of barium to show details of the mucosal pattern. Sufficient gas is used to put the gastric mucosa under slight tension so that lesions that lack distensibility, such as ulcers, ulcer scars and carcinomas, produce a clearly visible series of converging folds (Gelfand, 1975), making it possible to identify small lesions and any slight irregularity of the mucosa. It is essential that the method adopted is quick to perform and reproducible. The technique described here is similar to the methods of Shirakabe (1971) and Kreel *et al.* (1973).

The patient arrives in the department after fasting for at least 6 hours. A short history is taken and the patient is given an i.v. injection of 20 mg of Buscopan or 0.15 mg of glucagon. Effervescent granules or tab-

lets, sufficient to produce 300–400 ml of gas, are taken by the patient and washed down with a small amount, 5–10 ml, of water and 50 ml of barium suspension. With the table horizontal, the patient lies in the prone position and a radiograph of the mucosa of the anterior wall of the stomach is taken (Fig. 3.1). The patient drinks a further 100–150 ml of barium and turns once or preferably twice on to the right side and then on the left side before lying supine. A radiograph is taken of the whole stomach in this position (Figs 3.2a & 3.3) and shows the mucosal pattern of the body and antrum. The mucosa of the antrum and body is again washed with barium by rotating the patient as before and a view is obtained in the right anterior oblique (RAO) position to show the mucosal pattern of the antrum (Figs 3.2b & 3.4). A left anterior oblique (LAO) radiograph is taken to show the mucosal pattern of the fundus and upper body of the stomach (Figs 3.2c & 3.5). If the patient turns from the LAO to the supine position, about

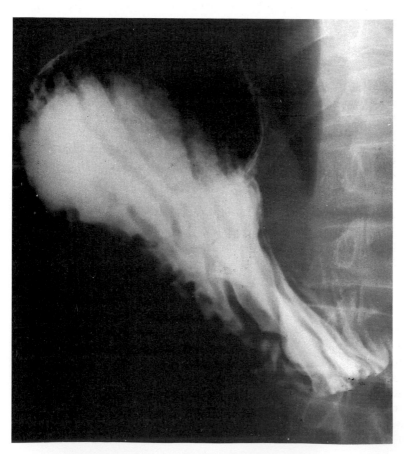

Fig. 3.1 Prone mucosal view showing the anterior wall of the stomach.

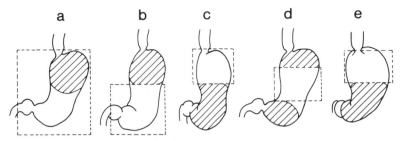

Fig. 3.2 Patient positions for double-contrast views of the stomach. The shaded area indicates the location of the barium. By collimating to the areas outlined by the rectangles, optimum double-contrast views of different parts of the stomach are obtained. (a) Supine view of the whole stomach taken immediately after the patient has been positioned on the right and left sides to show the body and proximal antrum. This is usually the only double-contrast radiograph that is taken to include the barium-filled part of the stomach. (b) Supine right anterior oblique to show the body and antrum. (c) Supine left anterior oblique to show the fundus and upper body. (d) Supine view to show the upper body taken after the patient has been positioned on the right side. (e) Supine left anterior oblique with the head of the table elevated 45° to show the fundus.

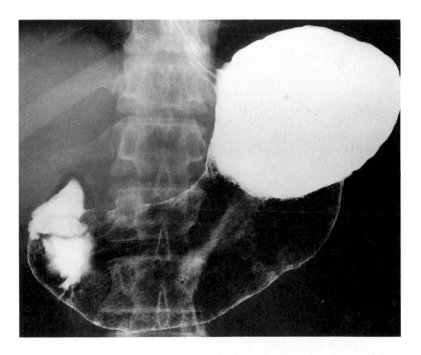

Fig. 3.3 Supine view showing the lower body and proximal antrum of the stomach outlined in double contrast.

half the barium remains in the antrum while the remainder passes to the fundus and a spot mucosal view of the upper body of the stomach is obtained (Figs 3.2d & 3.6). A double-contrast view of the fundus of the stomach is then taken with the patient in the supine LAO (Figs 3.2e & 3.7) or the prone left posterior oblique (LPO) position with the head of the table elevated to an angle of 45°. The patient is positioned on the right side before this view is taken, in order to empty barium from the fundus.

The table is then brought to the upright position and compression is applied. The anterior and posterior walls of the body and antrum of the stomach are compressed against the spine using a compression paddle or rubber ball (Fig. 3.8). Only a small segment of the stomach is compressed against the spine at one time. By rotating the patient into slightly different positions it is normally possible to compress most of the lower body and antrum of the stomach and the duodenal cap. Compression takes a very

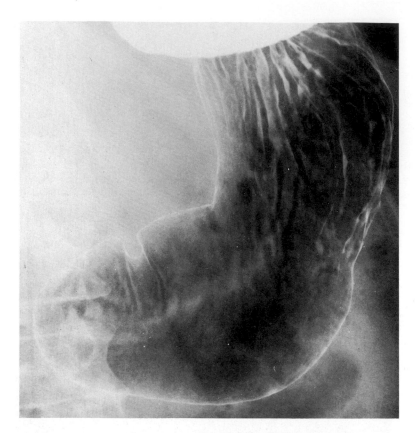

Fig. 3.4 Supine right anterior oblique double-contrast view of the antrum and body of the stomach.

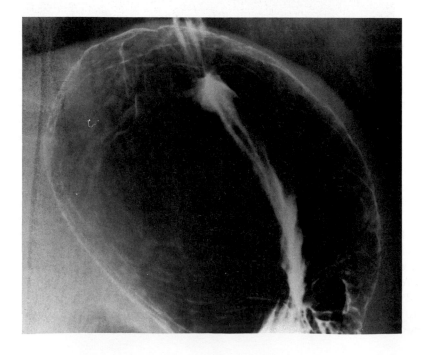

Fig. 3.5 Double-contrast view of the upper body and fundus of the stomach taken with the table horizontal and the left side raised.

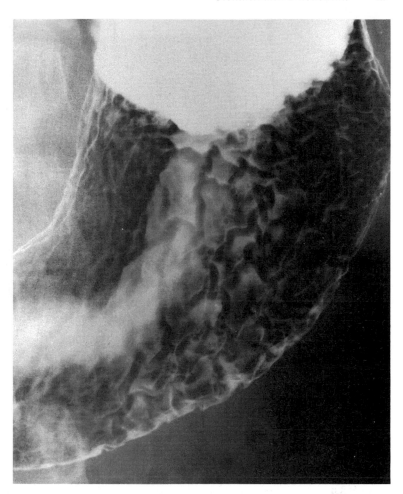

Fig. 3.6 Supine double-contrast view of the upper body of the stomach.

short time, about 30 s. Radiographs are taken only if an abnormal feature is recognized on fluoroscopy. Protuberant lesions are often shown best with compression. The areae gastricae can be identified on compression (Fig. 3.8), indicating how detailed information about the mucosal surface may be revealed at this stage of the examination. The lesser curve can also be viewed briefly at the same time to check that ulcers there are not overlooked.

Filled single-contrast views may be taken after the patient has taken a further 200 ml of dilute barium. These views are taken with the patient standing straight and in the RAO position. When the stomach has been examined using mucosal and double-contrast views as well as compression, it is unlikely that the filling method will yield any further information.

Anterior wall lesions are uncommon (Goldsmith *et al.*, 1976) and, when present, are normally detected during the standard double-contrast examination. The prone view and the compression parts of the technique are important in this respect. However, a double-contrast examination of the anterior wall of the stomach is occasionally indicated. Such a technique was described by Goldsmith *et al.* (1976) and involves the use of a small amount of barium suspension and gas. The patient is turned from side to side in the prone position. Radiographs are taken with the patient prone in a 15° head-down position with the right side elevated and a pad under the left side, in the prone horizontal position, and prone with the head of the table raised.

Radiographs of the duodenum are normally

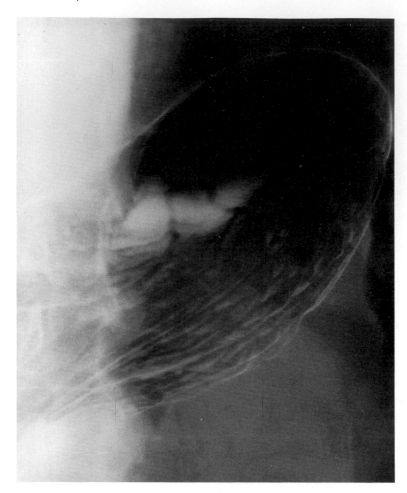

Fig. 3.7 Double-constrast view of the fundus of the stomach taken with the patient in the supine right anterior oblique position and with the head of the table elevated to an angle of 45°.

obtained when the table is horizontal, after the LAO view or the supine view showing the upper body of the stomach. Double-contrast views of the duodenal cap are taken with the patient in the RAO position. It may be necessary to elevate the head of the table slightly from the horizontal position in order to drain the barium from the apex of the cap into the second part of the duodenum. The patient is turned on the left side and then prone, sometimes with the left side raised a little, to obtain a double-contrast view of the anterior wall of the duodenal cap and the duodenal loop. Further spot radiographs of the duodenal cap may be taken with the patient standing.

Another method for obtaining good views of the duodenum is described by Stevenson *et al.* (1980). The patient is first turned on to the right side so that

barium fills the duodenum. Buscopan acts more quickly and reliably than glucagon because it relaxes the pylorus. The patient is then rotated to lie on the left, a pad is placed under the upper abdomen, and the patient is rolled forward to lie semiprone on the pad. The pad compresses the proximal antrum against the spine, the patient's respiration driving air from the distal antrum around the duodenal loop. A radiograph is taken either prone oblique, with the second part of the duodenum seen through the air-filled antrum, or prone, with the second part of the duodenum clear of the stomach. The patient is then turned supine and a supine RAO radiograph is taken (Fig. 3.9).

The stomach and duodenum should ideally be examined before the oesophagus, unless the patient presents with oesophageal symptoms, because the

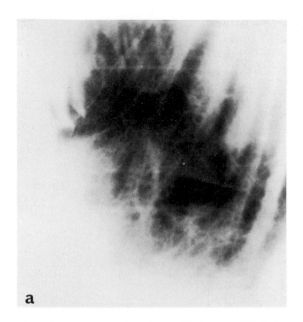

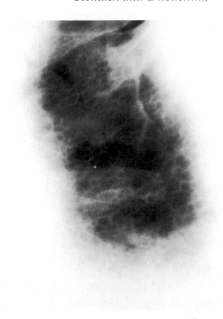

a

b

Fig. 3.8 Spot compression views of the barium-filled stomach showing the mucosal folds and the areae gastricae pattern. Reproduced with permission from Nolan (1983).

optimum amount of barium and gas is necessary to examine the stomach and duodenum. However, filled views of the oesophagus can be obtained when the second amount of barium is taken after the prone mucosal view. The barium should be taken by the patient through a drinking straw in the prone oblique position. Details of the technique used for examining the oesophagus are given in Chapter 2.

Some modifications to the double-contrast technique are necessary in patients who have had previous gastric surgery. A smaller quantity of barium is required initially in patients with a previous Billroth I partial gastrectomy, although further quantities of barium and effervescent agent may be necessary as barium and gas escape through the anastomosis into the small intestine. It is important to outline the afferent loop in patients with a Pólya or Billroth II type partial gastrectomy and this can be achieved by getting the patient to drink the barium suspension while lying on his or her right side with the head of the table slightly elevated (Op den Orth, 1977). When the barium has outlined the afferent loop the table is returned to the horizontal position. Normally, the gas passes into the afferent loop if the patient turns into the RAO position. Radiographs of the afferent loop are obtained in the supine RAO and prone positions.

Selective intubation of the afferent loop followed by injection of barium and air through the tube allows a detailed examination of the afferent loop.

Variations in basic technique

Patients who are not fit to stand while undergoing double-contrast studies may be examined in the horizontal position with relatively good results. A smaller amount of barium and effervescent agent is used in immobile elderly patients.

Hypotonic duodenography

The duodenum, as far as the ligament of Treitz, should be shown on at least one view during a routine double-contrast examination of the upper gastrointestinal tract. If the prime interest is the duodenal loop, hypotonic duodenography should be carried out as a separate study. Although it is possible to obtain good views of the duodenum in some cases by the tubeless method, intubation gives consistently better results. The amount of barium and air insufflation can be controlled and there is no overlying barium in the gastric antrum or jejunal loops (Eaton & Ferrucci, 1978).

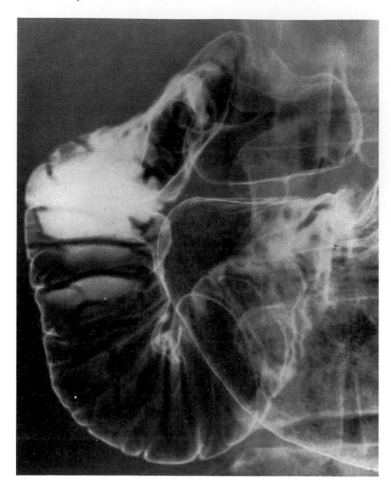

Fig. 3.9 A double-contrast view of the duodenal cap and loop taken with the patient in the supine right anterior oblique position.

The duodenal intubation technique is described in Chapter 4. The tip of the catheter is placed in the lower part of the descending duodenum and about 40 ml of barium suspension is injected. As the second part of the duodenum fills, a smooth muscle relaxant, such as 20 mg Buscopan or 0.25 mg glucagon, is injected i.v. Air is then injected through the catheter. The best projections for showing the duodenal loop are judged on fluoroscopy and are normally a supine RAO and a prone view with a pad under the right side. The proximal duodenum is often shown best with the head of the table elevated about 45–60°. Narrowed segments of duodenum are usually best demonstrated by the single-contrast barium column.

Hypotonic duodenography is indicated if routine studies have resulted in equivocal findings, when there is a suspicion of a primary lesion of the duodenum or in the investigation of obscure gastrointestinal bleeding.

Tubeless hypotonic duodenography is similar to the duodenal part of the double-contrast examination. A smaller amount of barium is used and the hypotonic agent is injected after the barium has outlined the duodenum.

Relationships to other diagnostic techniques

Barium studies versus endoscopy

Modern fibreoptic endoscopes are now widely used and make it possible to visualize, photograph and obtain aimed biopsy and cytology specimens from lesions in the upper gastrointestinal tract. When fibreoptic endoscopy was first introduced, many studies showed that it was superior to the single-contrast barium meal. Studies comparing the double-contrast examination and endoscopy, however, show that the double-contrast examination of the stomach is an accurate investigation (Laufer, 1976; Salter, 1977). The accuracy of both double-contrast barium studies and endoscopy depends on the experience and skill of the person performing the examination. The proper detection and diagnosis of lesions in the upper gastrointestinal tract is best achieved by close cooperation between the radiologist performing the double-contrast studies and the endoscopist (Scobie, 1970; Fevre *et al.*, 1976; Dekker & Op den Orth, 1977).

The double-contrast barium examination has a number of advantages over endoscopy: it is quick to perform and is safer and more comfortable for the patient. Each radiograph obtained provides an image of a large area of gastric and duodenal mucosa which may be retained as a permanent record available at any time for detailed review.

Computed tomography (CT)

CT is being used with increasing frequency for evaluation of disorders of the stomach and duodenum. Unsuspected abnormalities of the stomach or duodenum may be detected when CT scanning of the abdomen is performed in the investigation of unrelated abdominal disorders. The stomach should therefore be identified during abdominal scanning.

Gastric opacification with contrast medium is necessary to evaluate the stomach and to outline the extent of pathological processes in the upper abdomen (Megibow, 1986). A 1–4% suspension of barium sulphate or a 3–4% solution of water-soluble contrast medium is given orally before scanning commences. A smooth-muscle relaxant such as Buscopan or glucagon may be required to produce sufficient hypotonia and opacification when examining the duodenum.

Gas is proving to be an excellent contrast agent for CT of the stomach and is useful in selected cases when examining the duodenum (Megibow & Zerhouni, 1986). Effervescent granules dissolved in a small volume of water are ingested. The best results are achieved with an empty stomach and patients should therefore be fasted for 5–6 hours. The body, antrum and pyloric region are most distended with the patient in the supine position. The right-side-down decubitus is the best position for examining the fundus and oesophagogastric junction.

The main indication for performing CT of the stomach is staging and assessing the operability of gastric carcinoma and lymphoma. CT may also provide useful information about other mass lesions such as leiomyomata and gastric varices.

Ultrasound

Ultrasound has a very limited role to play in the investigation of gastric and duodenal disorders at the present time. The recognition of gastric wall thickening or a mass lesion may be helpful in directing further investigations to the stomach in patients referred for abdominal ultrasound with non-specific upper abdominal symptoms due to underlying gastric carcinoma. Abdominal ultrasound may be used to assess the spread of gastric carcinoma into adjacent viscera (Yek & Rabinowitz, 1981; Derchi *et al.*, 1983a,b).

Endoscopic ultrasound is a new technique using high-frequency, high-resolution, real-time ultrasound from within the gastrointestinal tract. The ultrasound probe is incorporated into the tip of a fibroscopic endoscope (Shorvon *et al.*, 1987). A rubber balloon attached to the tip and containing de-aerated water provides contact with the gastro-intestinal wall. The technique is proving to be a useful method for assessing the depth of invasion of the wall of the oesophagus or stomach by carcinoma. Metastatic involvement of lymph nodes may also be identified.

Radionuclide studies

Liquid and solid test meals containing radionuclides are ideal for studying the rates of gastric emptying. If a liquid meal is being studied, a chelate of ^{99m}Tc or ^{113m}In with diethylenetriamine penta-acetic acid (DTPA) is a suitable agent that is not absorbed in significant amounts and does not become attached to gastric mucus or mucosa (Heading *et al.*, 1971; Donovan & Harding, 1986). The effects of disorders of the stomach such as diabetic gastroparesis, gastric surgery and drugs on gastric emptying are best assessed using radionuclide-labelled solid meals.

Radionuclides that may be used for solid-meal labelling include [113m]In DTPA and ^{99m}Tc pertechnetate (Donovan & Harding, 1986).

Radionuclides can also be used to assess enterogastric reflux following gastric surgery (Tolin *et al.*, 1977).

Angiography

Selective visceral angiography may be invaluable in certain patients who present with acute bleeding from the upper gastrointestinal tract. There are two reasons for performing angiography in patients who present with acute bleeding: (i) to locate the site of bleeding; and (ii) to stop the bleeding by selective infusion of drugs or embolic material into the bleeding territory (Allison, 1980). Both applications apply in some cases, therapeutic embolization being particularly indicated when the patient is a poor operative or anaesthetic risk. The technique for performing selective visceral angiography is described in Chapter 8.

A bleeding site with a blood loss of 0.5–0.6 ml min[-1] or more should be shown on a technically satisfactory angiogram (Frey *et al.*, 1970). Coeliac axis and superior mesenteric angiography should be performed for acute upper gastrointestinal bleeding. When the bleeding point has been found, the haemorrhage may be controlled by the selective infusion of vasopressin (Athanasoulis *et al.*, 1974) or by the deliberate injection of embolic material (Allison, 1980), such as sterile absorbable gelatin sponge (Sterispon), lyophilized human dura mater (Lyodura), steel coils, acrylic polymers or detachable balloons.

Selective coeliac and superior mesenteric angiography is a useful diagnostic procedure in patients with intermittent acute bleeding. The angiogram should be performed during an episode of active bleeding to demonstrate the site of leakage of contrast medium (Allison, 1980). Angiography should not be performed if the bleeding has stopped; endoscopy or barium studies should be performed instead. Barium studies should not, however, be undertaken if there is a strong possibility of another acute bleed occurring within 2 days as the presence of residual barium in the intestine may then obscure the field for angiography.

Water-soluble contrast examinations

Plain abdominal radiographs are the initial diagnostic procedure in patients with suspected perforation of the stomach or duodenum. Water-soluble contrast agents should be used when perforation is still suspected but the plain radiographs fail to show the presence of free gas. The water-soluble contrast medium may be injected through a nasogastric tube directly into the stomach. Either the examination is conducted completely under fluoroscopic control or the contrast medium may be injected with the patient lying on the right side with a right decubitus radiograph being taken after a short interval. About 50 ml of contrast medium is usually adequate.

Studies using diatrizoate in the form of Gastrografin are frequently requested by clinicians. Gastrografin is more likely to produce local tissue reaction than other water-soluble contrast agents (Margulis, 1977). Therefore, Gastrografin should only be used for suspected perforation or an anastomotic leak in the stomach and duodenum when the patient takes the contrast medium by mouth. It is recommended that the term 'water-soluble contrast examination' should be adopted in place of the 'Gastrografin examination' so often requested by clinicians.

References

Allison, D.J. (1980) Gastrointestinal bleeding: radiological diagnosis. *Br. J. Hosp. Med.*, **23**, 358–65.

Athanasoulis, C.A., Baum, S. & Waltman, A.C. (1974) Control of acute gastric mucosal haemorrhage. *N. Engl. J. Med.*, **290**, 597–603.

Ayre-Smith, G. (1976) Hyoscine-*N*-butylbromide (Buscopan) as a duodenal relaxant in tubeless duodenography. *Acta Radiol. (Diagn.) (Stockh.)*, **17**, 701–13.

Dekker, W. & Op den Orth, J.O. (1977) Early gastric cancer. *Radiol. Clin. (Basel)*, **46**, 115–29.

Derchi, L.E., Biggi, E., Neumaier, C.E. & Cicio, G.R. (1983a) Ultrasonographic appearances of gastric cancer. *Br. J. Radiol.*, **56**, 365–70.

Derchi, L.E., Biggi, E., Rolland, G.A. *et al.* (1983b) Sonographic staging of gastric cancer. *AJR*, **140**, 273–6.

Donovan, I.A. & Harding, L.K. (1986) Gastric emptying. *In* Robinson, P.J.A. (ed.) *Nuclear Gastroenterology*, pp. 24–35. Churchill Livingstone, Edinburgh.

Eaton, S.B. & Ferrucci, J.T. (1978) Commentary. *Gastrointest. Radiol.*, **3**, 233–4.

Fevre, D.I., Green, P.H.R., Barratt, P.J. & Nagy, G.S. (1976)

Review of five cases of early gastric cancer. *Gut*, **17**, 41–7.

Field, S. (1986) The acute abdomen — the plain radiograph. *In* Grainger, R.G. & Allison, D.J. (eds) *Diagnostic Radiology: an Anglo-American Textbook of Organ Imaging*, pp. 719–42. Churchill Livingstone, Edinburgh.

Field, S., Guy P.J., Upsdell, S.M. & Scourfield, A.E. (1985) The erect abdominal radiograph in the acute abdomen: should its routine use be abandoned? *Br. Med. J.*, **290**, 1934–6.

Fink, A.M. & Aylward, G.W. (1995) Buscopan and glaucoma: a survey of current practice. *Clin. Radiol.*, **50**, 160–4.

Frey, C.F., Reuter, S.R. & Bookstein, J.J. (1970) Localization of gastrointestinal haemorrhage by selective angiography. *Surgery*, **67**, 548–55.

Frimann-Dahl, J. (1974) *Roentgen Examinations in Acute Abdominal Diseases*, 3rd edn. Charles C. Thomas, Springfield.

Gelfand, D.W. (1975) The double contrast upper gastrointestinal examination in the Japanese style. *Am. J. Gastroenterol.*, **63**, 216–20.

Goldsmith, M.R., Pane, R.E.., Poplack, W.E. *et al.* (1976) Evaluation of routine double contrast views of the anterior wall of the stomach. *AJR*, **126**, 1159–63.

Heading, R.C., Tothill, P., Laidlaw, A.J. & Shearman, D.J.C. (1971) An evaluation of indium DTPA chelate in the measurement of gastric emptying by scintiscanning. *Gut*, **12**, 611–15.

Hodges, P.C. & Miller, R.E. (1955) Intestinal obstruction. *AJR*, **74**, 1015–25.

Kreel, L., Herlinger, H. & Glanville, J. (1973) Technique of double contrast barium meal with examples of correlation with endoscopy. *Clin. Radiol.*, **24**, 307–14.

Laufer, I. (1976) An assessment of the accuracy of double contrast gastroduodenal radiology. *Gastroenterology*, **71**, 874–8.

Margulis, A.R. (1977) Water-soluble radiographic contrast agents in the gastrointestinal tract. *In* Miller, R.E. & Skucas, J. (eds) *Radiographic Contrast Agents*, pp. 169–88. University Park Press, Baltimore.

Megibow, A.J. (1986) Techniques of gastrointestinal computed tomography: classical techniques. *In* Megibow, A.J. & Balthazar, E.J. (eds) *Computed Tomography of the Gastrointestinal Tract*, pp. 1–14. CV Mosby, St Louis.

Megibow, A.J. & Zerhouni, E.A. (1986) Techniques of gastrointestinal computed tomography: air contrast techniques. *In* Megibow, A.J. & Balthazar, E.J. (eds) *Computed Tomography of the Gastrointestinal Tract*, pp. 14–31. CV Mosby, St Louis.

Miller, R.E. (1973) The technical approach to the acute abdomen. *Semin. Roentgenol.* 8, 267–79.

Miller, R.E. & Nelson, S.W. (1971) The roentgenologic demonstration of tiny amounts of free intraperitoneal gas: experimental and clinical studies. *AJR*, **112**, 574–85.

Miller, R.E. & Skucas, J. (eds) (1977) *Radiographic Contrast Agents*. University Park Press, Baltimore.

Miller, R.E., Becker, G.J. & Slabaugh, R.D. (1980) Detection of pneumoperitoneum: optimum body position and respiratory phase. *AJR*, **135**, 487–90.

Nolan, D.J. (1980) *The Double-contrast Barium Meal: a Radiological Atlas*. HM+M, Aylesbury.

Nolan, D.J. (1983) *Radiological Atlas of Gastrointestinal Disease*. John Wiley, Chichester.

Op den Orth, J.D. (1977) Tubeless hypotonic examination of the afferent loop of the Billroth II stomach. *Gastrointest. Radiol.*, **2**, 1–5.

Op den Orth, J.O. (1979) *The Standard Biphasic Contrast Examination of the Stomach*. Martinus Nijhoff, The Hague.

Op den Orth, J.O. & Ploem, S. (1977) The standard biphasic-contrast gastric series. *Radiology*, **122**, 530–2.

Pochaczevsky, R. (1973) 'Bubbly barium'. A carbonated cocktail for double contrast examination of the stomach. *Radiology*, **107**, 461–2.

Salter, R.H. (1977) X-ray negative dyspepsia. *Br. Med. J.*, **2**, 235–6.

Scobie, B.A. (1970) Early gastric carcinoma. *Australas. Radiol.*, **14**, 181–2.

Shirakabe, H. (1971) *Double Contrast Studies of the Stomach*. Bunkodo Company, Tokyo.

Shorvon, P.J., Lees, W.R., Frost, R.A. & Cotton, P.B. (1987) Upper gastrointestinal endoscopic ultrasonography in gastroenterology. *Br. J. Radiol.*, **60**, 429–38.

Simpson, A., Sandeman, D., Nixon, S.J. *et al.* (1985) The value of the erect abdominal radiograph in the diagnosis of intestinal obstruction. *Clin. Radiol.*, **36**, 41–2.

Stevenson, G.W., Somers, S. & Virjee, J. (1980) Routine double-contrast barium meal: appearance of the normal duodenal papillae. *Diagn. Imaging*, **49**, 6–14.

Tolin, R.D., Malmud, L.S., Stelzer, F. *et al.* (1977) Enterogastric reflux in normal subjects and patients with Billroth II gastroenterostomy. *Gastroenterology*, **77**, 1027–33.

Yek, H.C. & Rabinowitz, J.E. (1981) Ultrasound and computed tomography of gastric wall lesions. *Radiology*, **141**, 147–55.

Mosby, St Louis.

4   Small Intestine

D. J. NOLAN

There are a number of radiological techniques available for investigating the small intestine. For patients who present with acute symptoms and signs, plain radiographs of the abdomen and chest are the initial investigation. A barium examination is used to investigate the small intestine when symptoms present less acutely and it is the established method for the diagnosis and management of disorders of the small intestine. Water-soluble contrast agents have little practical value in the investigation of the small intestine. Selective superior mesenteric arteriography plays an important role in suspected small intestinal bleeding. Radionuclide scanning is also used for screening patients with suspected bleeding, detecting Meckel's diverticulum, and for assessing inflammatory bowel disease. Computed tomography (CT) may be useful for evaluating selected patients, for example in the management of complications of Crohn's disease, assessing the degree of spread of malignant neoplasms and in suspected intestinal infarction. CT is playing an increasing role in the investigation of small-intestinal obstruction. Ultrasound has a limited role in the small intestine but, as it is now an extensively used abdominal investigation, the ultrasonographer should be able to recognize normal and abnormal small-intestinal patterns.

Plain abdominal radiographs

Plain abdominal radiographs are indicated in patients with suspected obstruction, perforation or infarction of the small intestine.

Barium studies

Good quality barium studies are essential when investigating the small intestine. A variety of techniques are available but there is little agreement as to which should be used routinely.

The barium follow-through is the most widely used method, although duodenal intubation techniques are replacing it as the routine method in many centres. Excellent visualization is achieved when the barium is introduced through a tube directly into the small intestine. Sellink's method, using single-contrast dilute barium, is a quick and efficient duodenal intubation technique. Some radiologists prefer a double-contrast modification, giving an aqueous suspension of methylcellulose with the barium. Another double-contrast method, which uses barium and air, is popular in Japan and some centres in Europe.

In patients with small-intestinal obstruction, long intestinal tubes are used in some centres to decompress the distended intestine. When the tube has reached the site of obstruction and is no longer advancing, barium suspension injected through the tube may provide diagnostic information (Herlinger, 1978). The distal ileum can be evaluated by refluxing barium through the ileocaecal valve during barium enema examination or by performing a per oral pneumocolon examination of the ileocaecal region (Kellett *et al.*, 1977). In the 'complete reflux examination', dilute barium is refluxed through the ileocaecal valve in order to outline the small intestine (Miller, 1965). This technique is only very occasionally used as the information it provides is similar to that obtained with enteroclysis (small-bowel enema).

Barium follow-through

The indications for the barium follow-through examination will depend on whether or not it is routinely used in a particular department. If enteroclysis is the routine method, the barium follow-through will only be used for elderly patients with suspected jejunal diverticulosis who present with malabsorption, or in patients who are unwilling or in whom it is not possible to perform intubation.

The follow-through examination of the small intestine normally follows a barium examination of the oesophagus, stomach and duodenum but in some centres it is performed as a dedicated examination of the small intestine (Diner *et al.*, 1984). The patient ingests 500–600 ml of barium suspension of approximately 50% w/v. Large radiographs of the abdomen (43 × 35 cm) are taken at 30-min intervals while the barium progresses through the small intestine. The first radiograph is taken with the patient supine at the end of the barium meal, or about 15 min later, to show the proximal jejunum (Marshak & Lindner, 1976). Further radiographs are taken with the patient in the prone position. When the barium has reached the distal ileum, a pad is placed under the right iliac fossa in order to separate the loops of ileum. Spot compression views of the terminal ileum are also obtained.

The head of the barium column can normally take 2–6 hours to reach the terminal ileum and caecum, although ways have been found to speed up the barium as it passes through the small intestine. A dose of 20 mg metoclopramide — given i.v. after the barium meal has been completed (James & Hume, 1968) or orally beforehand (Kreel, 1970) — promotes gastric emptying and accelerates the barium through the small intestine. Adding sodium/meglumine diatrizoate (Gastrografin) to the barium also reduces transit time (Rosenquist, 1975). Other pharmacological agents which have been used include neostigmine (Marshak & Lindner, 1976), glucagon (Kreel, 1975), cholecystokinin (Parker & Beneventano, 1970) and ceruletide (Novak, 1980; Robbins *et al.*, 1980). Preliminary cleansing of the colon, as well as using 280 g or more of oral barium suspension, and placing the patient in the right lateral recumbent position are tips suggested by Nice (1963). Regardless of the means employed, the advantage of decreasing the transit time is offset by diminished anatomical detail, particularly in the terminal ileum (Robbins *et al.*, 1980).

Effervescent agents may be used to improve intestinal distension and give double-contrast views of the small intestine during the the follow-through examination (Fraser & Preston 1983; Griffiths *et al.*,

1993). Gas tablets, capable of releasing 750–1000 ml gas, are given to the patient when the head of the barium column has reached the terminal ileum. The gas passes through rapidly and fills the intestine.

Enteroclysis

Credit for the current interest and increasing use of duodenal intubation techniques for examining the small intestine is due to Sellink (1971, 1974). Sellink refined the enteroclysis technique, using a modification of the Bilbao–Dotter tube for the intubation and a precise dilution of the barium suspension. He found that the technique saved a considerable amount of time and yielded information which was far superior to that achieved with the barium follow-through. He suggested that the oral administration of barium contrast medium should be abandoned and replaced by enteroclysis as a routine technique (Sellink, 1974).

During enteroclysis the small intestine is distended with the barium suspension, making it easier to identify any morphological abnormality that may be present. Stenotic segments and even minimal narrowing can be identified (Theoni, 1987). Enteroclysis is a reliable technique. A recent study of ours showed it to have a sensitivity of 93.1% and a specificity of 96.9% (Dixon *et al.*, 1993). The technique is easy to learn and the radiologist can quickly become more skilled with enteroclysis than with the time-consuming repeated fluoroscopy that is necessary during the barium follow-through (Theoni, 1987).

Patient discomfort during the intubation and the potentially high dose of radiation during the procedure are the main disadvantages of the technique. Discomfort is minimized by intubating via the nasal route (Maglinte *et al.*, 1986) and using one of the newer small-bore catheters. The 10 French (F) gauge version of the Nolan catheter* (Nolan, 1979) is ideal for rapid duodenal intubation with minimum discomfort to the patient (Traill & Nolan, 1995). This catheter is based on Sellink's modification of the Bilbao–Dotter catheter (Bilbao *et al.*, 1967). Intubation of the duodenum can also be quickly and easily performed using the Merck† enteroclysis catheter

* William Cook Europe, Bjaeverskov, Denmark.
† E. Merck Pharmaceuticals, Alton, Hampshire, UK.

(Chippendale & Desai, 1989; Nicholson et al., 1989; Law & Longstaff, 1992).

A low patient radiation dose can be achieved during enteroclysis by using a low fluoroscopy current and rare earth screens or low-dose digital equipment. Hart et al. (1994) recently calculated patient radiation dose and found that the mean effective dose to the patient for enteroclysis was 1.5 mSv. The dose for barium meals was 0.9 mSv and barium enemas 2.8 mSv in the same room (Hart & Wall, 1994). The average dose for a routine CT scan of the abdomen is 7–8 mSv (Shrimpton et al., 1991).

Indications

Enteroclysis is indicated when disorders causing morphological changes in the small intestine are suspected, such as Crohn's disease, tuberculosis, neoplasms, radiation damage and ischaemia. The most common presenting features of these conditions are unexplained abdominal pain, diarrhoea and weight loss. Patients may present with unexplained anaemia or as an 'acute abdomen'. The examination is indicated in patients with recurrent bleeding from the alimentary tract when a full investigation of the upper gastrointestinal tract and colon has proved negative.

The technique can be most helpful in patients in whom the clinical findings are suggestive of small-intestinal obstruction but plain abdominal radiographs are either negative or do not give sufficient information about the site or cause of the obstruction. There is a certain reluctance to use barium in investigating an obstructed small intestine for fear that the barium will become impacted and cause a partial obstruction to become complete. Barium is not likely to become impacted because it will be diluted by small-intestinal fluid. In a retrospective review of 172 patients with proven small-intestinal obstruction, Miller and Brahme (1969) found no record of impaction of barium in the small or large intestine. Their findings confirmed the results of earlier studies when the effect of barium was assessed in obstructed animals (Donato et al., 1954; Nelson et al., 1963). Barium suspension is superior to water-soluble iodinated compounds in obstruction because of its greater density. It has fewer side effects, producing less vomiting and crampy abdominal pain.

Water-soluble compounds may cause dehydration and electrolyte imbalance.

Malabsorption is often quoted as an indication for barium study of the small intestine. Coeliac disease, one of the most common conditions causing malabsorption, is usually diagnosed by jejunal biopsy which should therefore be the initial diagnostic procedure. Barium examination of the small intestine should be reserved for those in whom jejunal biopsy is normal or patients with a suspected complication of coeliac disease such as lymphoma.

Contraindications

Barium is contraindicated if perforation of the small intestine is suspected. Gross disruption is usually recognized on clinical grounds and barium contrast studies are then deemed unnecessary. If a small leak is suspected, the ability of the barium study to demonstrate the site outweighs the theoretical consideration of toxicity due to leakage of barium (Freeark et al., 1968).

Technique

The enteroclysis technique outlined here is similar to Sellink's method and has previously been described in detail (Miller & Sellink, 1979; Sellink & Miller, 1982; Nolan & Cadman, 1987).

Preparation of the patient

It is necessary that the colon is clean so that the barium column can flow freely through the distal ileum into the caecum. A full caecum causes the flow of intestinal contents to be seriously retarded in the ileum (Nice, 1963). In order to achieve a clean colon a low-residue diet and cathartics are prescribed and fluids are encouraged on the day before the examination. The usual cathartic is 340 g of magnesium sulphate, but this is not given to patients with known Crohn's disease, severe diarrhoea, an ileostomy or a previous right hemicolectomy. Cleansing enemas are not performed because the cleansing fluid and faecal material may be washed into the distal ileum and retained there. The patient fasts overnight prior to the barium examination.

Duodenal intubation

The 10F Nolan catheter is made of radio-opaque polyvinyl chloride, measures 135 cm in length and has six side-holes at the distal closed end. A Teflon-coated guide wire, 1.65 mm in diameter and 135 cm long, acts as a stiffener inside the catheter as it passes through the stomach (Fig. 4.1).

Other modifications of the catheter are available. Maglinte (1984) recommends a catheter with a balloon near its tip that is inflated in the distal duodenum or proximal jejunum to prevent reflux of barium into the stomach. This is particularly useful in patients who have had previous gastric surgery and in whom reflux is likely to be a problem. Catheters of a smaller size, 7F, are available for use in children.

The procedure is explained to the patient. Anaesthetic gel is applied inside the patient's nostril and on to the catheter. Local anaesthesia is not applied to the throat because the application of topical anaesthesia itself usually causes more discomfort in the throat than the catheter. With the patient sitting,

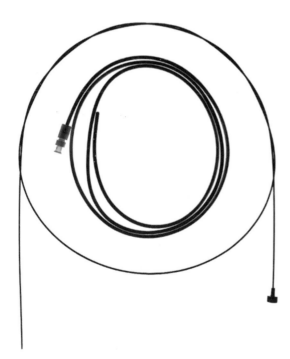

Fig. 4.1 The 10F catheter and guide wire used for duodenal intubation.

the catheter is introduced into the nostril and directed backwards and downwards. If there is difficulty advancing the catheter from the nasal cavity to the nasopharynx, the patient's head should be extended until the tip of the catheter has passed into the oropharynx. The catheter is then advanced further and swallowed by the patient. Swallowing the catheter is easier if the patient's neck is flexed, as this prevents the tip from passing into the trachea (R.E. Miller, personal communication). The catheter is advanced through the oesophagus and into the stomach until the tip is presumed to have reached the gastric antrum (Fig. 4.2a). The patient is placed supine on a fluoroscopic table so that the position of the catheter can be checked. The guide wire is then introduced into the external end of the catheter and advanced to within 3–4 cm of the distal end (Fig. 4.2b). The flexible tip of the catheter is advanced to the pylorus and is gently eased through the pyloric sphincter into the duodenum. The catheter continues to be advanced while the guide wire is gradually withdrawn so that its tip remains proximal to the pyloric sphincter (Figs 4.2c & 4.3). The catheter is advanced through the duodenum until its tip is positioned at the duodenojejunal flexure (ligament of Treitz) or 5–10 cm into the jejunum (Fig. 4.4).

There may be problems advancing the catheter through the stomach. It can pass up the greater curve and form a loop in the fundus (Fig. 4.2d), in which case the double-back manoeuvre is helpful (Maglinte *et al.*, 1982). This manoeuvre is performed by advancing the catheter further into the stomach so that it forms an extra loop, the apex of which is directed towards the pylorus (Fig. 4.2e). The guide wire is then introduced and advanced as far as the apex of the curve. It continues to be advanced and the catheter is slowly withdrawn so that the stiffer end of the catheter, with the guide wire inside, remains pointing towards the pylorus (Fig. 4.2f). This manoeuvre usually succeeds in bringing the tip of the catheter down from the fundus to a position in the gastric antrum. Other techniques that may be used to uncoil the catheter in the fundus include withdrawing and then rotating the catheter by applying torque (Figs. 4.2g & 4.2h), using a guide wire with an angled tip (Shipps *et al.*, 1979) or tilting the fluoroscopy table to the upright position. In patients with a transverse

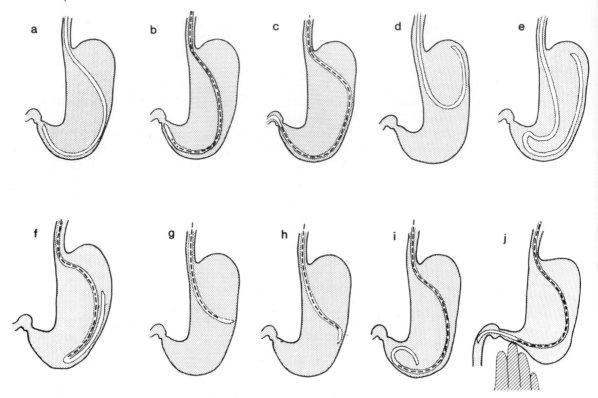

Fig. 4.2 Positions of the catheter and guide wire in the stomach during intubation. (a) After nasogastric intubation, the tip of the catheter lies in the gastric antrum. (b) The guide wire has been inserted into the catheter, to within 3–4 cm of the distal end. (c) As the catheter is advanced through the duodenum, the tip of the guide wire is maintained in position just proximal to the pylorus. (d) The catheter coiling in the fundus. (e) An extra loop of catheter has been advanced into the stomach and the apex of the loop is now directed towards the gastric antrum. (f) The guide wire is introduced and advanced to stiffen the proximal part of the catheter and maintain the apex of the loop in the gastric antrum as the catheter is withdrawn from the fundus. (g & h) The positions of the guide wire before and after applying torque to rotate the tip of the catheter and direct it downwards. (i) The catheter, having failed to pass into the duodenum, forms a loop in the gastric antrum. (j) Upward pressure on the greater curve aspect of the prepyloric gastric antrum facilitating entry of the catheter into the duodenum.

stomach, it may be easier to get the tip of the catheter to negotiate the fundus and pass along the lesser curve to the pylorus and into the duodenum (Fig. 4.5).

If the catheter forms a coil in the antrum (Fig. 4.2i) and fails to pass into the duodenum, it should be withdrawn a little and the guide wire advanced to uncoil the catheter and reposition it in the prepyloric gastric antrum (Fig. 4.2b). The patient is then positioned on their left side to allow air to collect in the antrum and duodenal bulb. A small volume of air, about 50–100 ml, may be injected to outline the anatomy and to stimulate peristalsis. The catheter will often pass easily from the stomach to the duode-

num when the patient is in the left lateral position (Ferrucci & Benedict, 1971; Nolan, 1979; Sellink & Miller, 1982). If there is persistent difficulty in passing the catheter into the duodenum, further attempts should be made with the patient in the right decubitus and/or prone positions. Applying upward pressure on the greater curve aspect of the distal antrum by the radiologist's lead-gloved hand, with the patient supine, while advancing the catheter gently at the same time (Fig. 4.2j) is another useful manoeuvre if difficulty is encountered in advancing the catheter into the duodenal bulb. A small amount of barium may be injected to demonstrate the normal anatomy

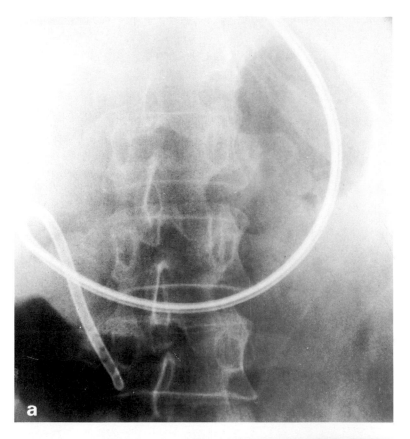

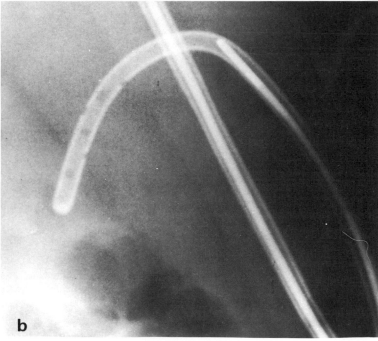

Fig. 4.3 (a) An anteroposterior view showing the tip of the catheter being passed through the duodenum. The guide wire is slowly withdrawn so that its tip lies in the catheter just proximal to the pylorus. (b) A lateral spot view.

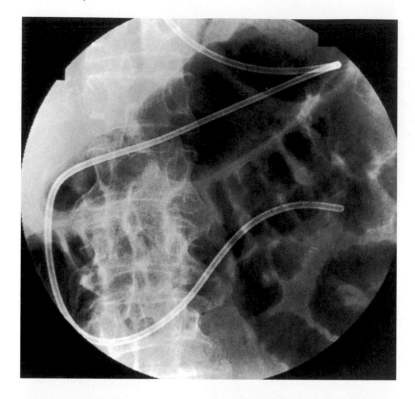

Fig. 4.4 The new 10F catheter in position with its tip positioned just distal to the ligament of Treitz. Reproduced with permission from Traill and Nolan (1995).

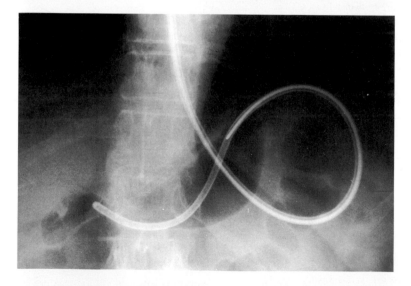

Fig. 4.5 The catheter has passed along the greater curve of the fundus before entering the gastric antrum.

and establish that no obstruction is preventing the catheter from passing into the duodenum.

It is usually possible to pass the catheter swiftly through the duodenum, but failure to advance may mean that the tip has become trapped in a duodenal diverticulum. Barium should be injected to define the anatomy and, if a diverticulum is present, the catheter should be withdrawn a little before advancing it past the diverticulum under fluoroscopic control.

The guide wire should not be allowed to pass through the distal 3 cm of the catheter except under fluoroscopic control, because it might pass through a side-hole in the catheter and possibly damage the wall of the stomach or duodenum. The radiation dose to the patient should be kept to a minimum by using a low fluoroscopy current, good collimation and short periods of intermittent fluoroscopy.

Infusion

The barium suspension may be injected using large syringes or an infusion pump. Previously, when using the 12F catheter, the barium suspension was infused under gravity from a plastic enema bag. An electric motor-driven infusion pump* (Abu-Yousef *et al.*, 1983; Maglinte & Miller, 1984) is now used as the small-bore 10F catheter is less satisfactory for a gravity infusion. The pump tubing is connected by a Portex connector† to the catheter.

It is important to use barium of the correct density. A dilute barium suspension, 20% wv, gives excellent results in adult patients and a more dilute suspension may be used in children. The barium suspension, which should be cool (5–15°), is infused at a rate of about 75 ml min^{-1} (Oudkerk, 1981). A fast infusion of barium may distend and paralyse the jejunum and result in delayed filling of the ileal loops. A slower infusion rate will not adequately distend the intestine. Usually 800–1200 ml of barium suspension is sufficient to reach the terminal ileum and outline the small intestine. It is important to maintain a steady flow of contrast medium during the examination, as any interruption can significantly delay the progress of the barium column through the intestine. Water may be infused to maintain the flow of contrast medium during the final stages of the radiographic examination.

Radiography

Intermittent fluoroscopy is performed while the barium column advances through the small intestine. Radiographs are taken at high kilovoltage (110–115 kV). The sequence of radiographic exposures will depend on the clinical presentation in any particular case. A radiograph of the proximal jejunum is normally taken after about 300 ml of barium suspension has been infused. A large-sized radiograph (35 × 35 cm) is taken when there is about 600 ml of barium suspension in the small intestine. A further large radiograph (35 × 35 cm) is taken after the contrast medium reaches the terminal ileum (Fig. 4.6a). Spot compression radiographs are taken of the pelvic loops of ileum, the terminal ileum (Fig. 4.6b) and any other segments of interest. In patients with an ileostomy, views of the ileum just proximal to the ileostomy and a lateral view of the ileostomy are taken (Kay & Nolan, 1988). Finally, a large radiograph (43 × 35 cm) is taken of the abdomen when the right half of the colon, as well as as the small intestine, is outlined with the contrast medium.

The radiographs should be developed immediately and reviewed so that any suspicious segments, not seen at fluoroscopy, can be evaluated further while the intestine is still distended

Compression

Compression is an extremely important part of the examination technique. A compression paddle or rubber ball should be used to separate overlapping loops of intestine. Small lesions such as strictures, neoplasms and Meckel's diverticulum are only demonstrated adequately on compression views. It may occasionally be necessary to turn the patient into an oblique or lateral position to obtain optimum views of a lesion. Loops of ileum can be elevated out of the pelvis by using rectal air insufflation to distend the sigmoid colon (Sellink & Miller, 1982).

Modifications of the basic technique

Contrast medium may reflux into the stomach, particularly in elderly patients or those with chronic obstruction. Balloon catheters are advocated as a way of preventing reflux (Fournier *et al.*, 1979; Maglinte, 1984). The peristaltic activity of the jejunum and the action of the pyloric sphincter prevent reflux into the stomach in the great majority of patients.

A double-contrast modification of the Sellink

---

* Renal Systems Inc., Minneapolis, Minnesota, USA.
† Portex Ltd, Hythe, Kent, UK.

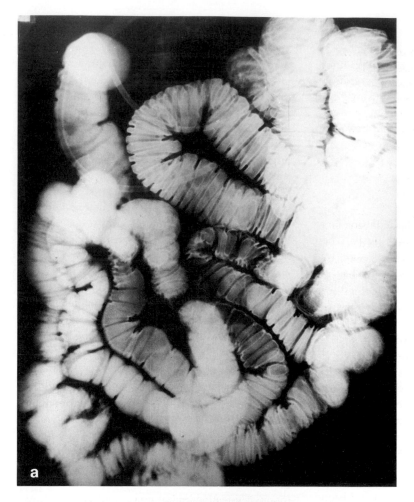

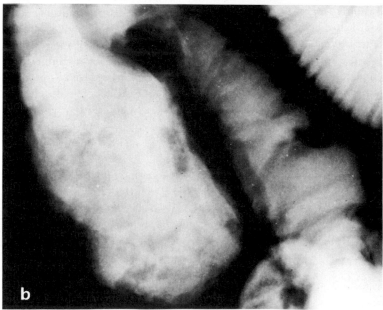

Fig. 4.6 Normal enteroclysis examination. (a) A radiograph showing the small intestine outlined with dilute barium. (b) A spot view of the terminal ileum.

method is advocated for routine use by Herlinger (1978), Vallance (1980), Antes & Lissner (1983) and Herlinger and Maglinte (1989), who recommend the injection of 200 ml of moderate-density barium suspension (85% w/v) through the catheter followed by 1–2 litres of a 0.5% aqueous suspension of methylcellulose. The barium column is pushed forward by the methylcellulose suspension, leaving a thin coating of barium to give a double-contrast outline to the small intestine. The mucosal detail of the normal intestine is excellent but diseased segments are better demonstrated by the barium at the head of the column than by the double-contrast produced by the combined barium and aqueous suspension of methylcellulose. Increased secretions from abnormal mucosa may prevent the thin layer of barium from remaining adherent to the wall of a diseased segment as the aqueous solution flows past. With the Sellink method, the dilute barium distends a diseased segment and it is not necessary for it to adhere to the mucosa to produce good visualization. The dilute barium technique is also easier and quicker to perform.

Ekberg (1977) prefers a double-contrast method using barium and air. Barium suspension (600 ml) is injected into the duodenum. When the column of barium has reached the caecum, air is injected to obtain a double-contrast outline of the small intestine; radiographs are then taken. The dilute barium suspension is superior to air for distending the intestine because air passes through the intestine very quickly and fails to distend narrowed segments adequately. Severe stenosis may be overlooked because overlapping ring shadows are not as obvious as a loop which is well filled with barium (Miller & Sellink, 1979). The air-contrast method will not demonstrate sinuses and fistulae as well as the dilute barium technique.

Small-intestinal intubation

There are a variety of catheters available for decompressing the distended intestine in patients with small-intestinal obstruction. The Miller–Abbott type (Miller & Abbott, 1934) is a double-lumen tube with a balloon at the tip. When the tip of the tube reaches the duodenum, the balloon is inflated with air. Peristaltic activity then carries the tube along the small intestine until it stops at the site of obstruction. Other catheters have a mercury-filled bag at the tip which is taken to the site of obstruction by peristalsis. When the catheter is arrested, barium suspension may be injected to outline the obstructing lesion. The barium suspension needs to be of low viscosity because of the length and small internal diameter of the lumen of the Miller–Abbott tube (Herlinger, 1978).

Reflux examination

Refluxing barium and air through the ileocaecal valve during routine double-contrast barium enema examination (Fig. 4.7) has been advocated as the radiological technique of choice for demonstrating the terminal ileum (Figiel & Figiel, 1964). The terminal ileum is frequently involved in patients with Crohn's disease and its delineation by partial reflux is very helpful in patients with suspected inflammatory bowel disease. The partial reflux technique, using single-contrast dilute barium suspension, is an excellent method for detecting recurrent disease in patients who have had a right hemicolectomy and ileocolic anastomosis for Crohn's disease. Other abnormalities, including neoplasms and Meckel's diverticulum, are also detectable on careful examination of the distal ileum when performing barium enemas. In ileostomy patients, barium suspension may be injected directly into the small intestine in a retrograde manner (Sanders & Ho, 1976; Zagoria *et al.*, 1986).

It is possible to demonstrate all the small intestine by refluxing barium from the colon into the terminal ileum, using a technique described by Miller (1965). The patient is prepared as for a double-contrast barium enema with a low-residue diet, increased fluid intake, laxatives and a cleansing enema. Preparation is omitted in patients with suspected intestinal obstruction. A single-contrast study of the colon is normally performed first, using a dilute barium suspension. With the patient supine, the barium is allowed to flow under fluoroscopic control through the terminal ileum in a retrograde direction initially to fill the ileum and then the jejunum. The flow is stopped when the barium column reaches the duodenum, or when 4500 ml of barium suspension has been infused. When the barium reaches the duodenum, a single large radiograph (43 × 35 cm) is exposed with the patient turned into the prone position. The barium is then drained off with the patient in

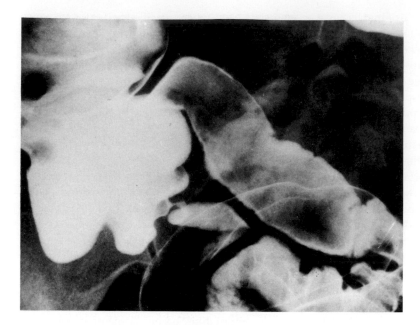

Fig. 4.7 Normal terminal ileum. A view obtained during a double-contrast barium enema examination.

the supine position and a further large radiograph is exposed. Fluoroscopy is then performed in order to detect any lesion of the small intestine. The patient is then sent to the toilet to void as much barium as possible, further prone and supine radiographs being taken immediately on return. The technique is particularly useful in the diagnosis of distal small-intestinal obstruction.

A large volume of barium suspension (2000–4500 ml) is required for this examination. Discomfort from the procedure may require analgesia. The ileocaecal valve is competent in some of these patients and a smooth muscle relaxant, such as 0.5 mg of glucagon or 20 mg hyoscine butylbromide (Buscopan), should be given i.v. to relax the valve and allow barium to flow into the terminal ileum. Failure to reflux barium through the ileocaecal valve occurred in only three out of 75 patients examined by Miller (1965).

Peroral pneumocolon examination of the ileocaecal region

Excellent visualization of the ileocaecal region is obtained by giving barium orally and introducing air per rectum when the barium is in the region of the terminal ileum and caecum (Kellett *et al.*, 1977; Fitzgerald *et al.*, 1985). The patient is prepared as for a double-contrast enema with a low-residue diet, increased fluid intake, laxatives and a cleansing enema. The progress of the barium is observed and air is introduced when the head of the column reaches the transverse colon. This air distends the caecum and terminal ileum. Radiographs are then taken (Fig. 4.8). Crohn's disease of the terminal ileum and carcinoma of the caecum are particularly well demonstrated by this technique.

Relationship to other diagnostic techniques

Angiography

The main indication for selective visceral angiography of the small intestine is to determine the cause of obscure gastrointestinal bleeding when barium studies of the upper gastrointestinal tract, small intestine and colon, as well as fibreoptic endoscopy, are negative. The small intestine may be the site of angiomatous malformations, small neoplasms or Meckel's diverticulum, all of which may present as anaemia or recurrent acute bleeding. Selective catheterization of the coeliac axis, superior mesenteric artery and inferior mesenteric artery may be necessary in the investigation of gastrointestinal bleeding (Allison, 1980).

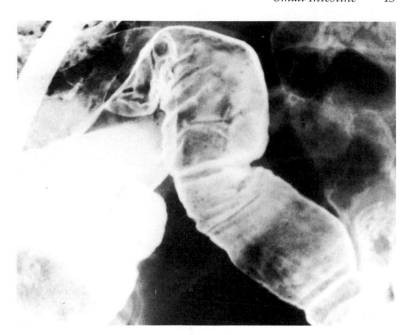

Fig. 4.8 Normal terminal ileum shown during a peroral pneumocolon examination of the ileocaecal region.

Radionuclide studies

Radionuclide scintigraphy is useful for screening patients with suspected intestinal bleeding, for detecting Meckel's diverticulum, and in the assessment of inflammatory bowel disease. The general anatomical location of bleeding may be identified and further investigations, such as barium studies or angiography, can then be performed to define the precise bleeding site. It is possible to establish the optimum time for performing angiography by using radionuclide scanning to demonstrate active bleeding (Baum, 1982). In the detection of bleeding, ^{51}Cr-tagged red cells (Ebaugh *et al.*, 1958), ^{99m}Tc-labelled albumin (Miskowiak *et al.*, 1977) and *in vivo* and *ex vivo* labelling of red cells with pyrophosphate have all been used. The two radionuclide tests that are currently recommended involve ^{99m}Tc sulphur colloid and red cells labelled with ^{99m}Tc by a modified *in vivo* technique (Baum, 1982). The ^{99m}Tc sulphur colloid is given as an i.v. injection (Alavi & Ring, 1981). A small amount of radionuclide extravasates at the bleeding point. This increases with each circulation, leaving more radionuclide deposited at the bleeding site. Meanwhile the radionuclide is also cleared from the circulating blood volume by the reticuloendothelial cells of the liver, spleen and bone

marrow. The site of active bleeding can be identified in 5–10 min. When extravasation is demonstrated, further images are taken to confirm the site of bleeding. If no bleeding is detected, images are taken of the upper abdomen to include the liver and spleen and a left anterior oblique projection is used to scan the splenic area, proximal small intestine and the left upper quadrant. The examination is extended for an additional 30–45 min if necessary. The technique is simple, non-invasive and remarkably sensitive, detecting bleeding rates of as low as 0.1 ml min^{-1} (Baum, 1982).

When red blood cells labelled with ^{99m}Tc by a modified *in vivo* technique are used, the red cells remain in the circulation and imaging may be repeated for up to 24 hours (McKusick *et al.*, 1981). The advantage is that extravasation may even be seen if bleeding is intermittent and not taking place at the time of the first scan. The method has two disadvantages (Baum, 1982): (i) if bleeding occurs and then stops, the radioactivity may have moved along the intestine so that the scan obtained later may show the activity at a different site; and (ii) the background activity remains high. Despite these disadvantages, ^{99m}Tc-labelled red cells are more accurate for detecting bleeding than ^{99m}Tc sulphur colloid, having a sensitivity of 93%, specificity of 95% and an overall accuracy of 94% in detecting and localizing gastrointestinal haemorrhage (Bunker *et al.*, 1984).

Meckel's diverticulum may be detected by radionuclide scanning using ^{99m}Tc pertechnetate (Conway, 1980). A dose of 100 μCi of ^{99m}Tc pertechnetate lb^{-1} (3.7 mBq kg^{-1}) is injected i.v. and images are taken at 5–10 min intervals for 45 min. The area of ectopic uptake is identified within the first 5–10 min of injection as an area of increased radionuclide activity in the lower abdomen, usually on the right side, which becomes more intense with time.

The technique is more accurate in the paediatric age group (Sfakianakis & Conway, 1981; Cooney *et al.*, 1982) but there is a high false negative rate in adults (Bartram & Amess, 1980; Spiller & Parkins, 1983; Schwartz & Lewis, 1984; Thompson *et al.*, 1984; Dixon & Nolan, 1987). The use of pentagastrin or cimetidine may reduce the number of false negative results (Petrokubi *et al.*, 1978; Treves *et al.*, 1978).

Inflammatory bowel disease can be imaged using ^{111}In-labelled leucocytes. The labelled leucocytes migrate to segments of active inflammation, enabling an estimation of the extent of the disease. The severity of the disease is related to the proportion of labelled leucocytes in the faeces (Buxton-Thomas *et al.*, 1984). The technique is particularly useful in Crohn's disease of the small intestine, mainly for detecting recurrence after previous resections and for assessing activity when following up patients with known disease (Saverymuttu *et al.*, 1983).

Ultrasound

Ultrasound has a limited role in the management of disorders of the small intestine and is only rarely used as the initial diagnostic procedure. Because ultrasound is widely used in the investigation of the abdomen, abnormalities of the small intestine are frequently encountered (Dubbins & Kurtz, 1984; Somers & Stevenson, 1994). It is therefore important for the ultrasonographer to recognize normal and abnormal patterns (Vecchioli *et al.*, 1994) so that appropriate follow-up investigations can be recommended. Small-intestinal obstruction may be diagnosed on ultrasound (Scheible & Goldberger, 1979). The valvulae conniventes are recognized when they project into the fluid-filled intestinal lumen (Scheible & Goldberger, 1979; Fleischer *et al.*, 1979). Neoplasms of the small intestine may be identified using a dedicated ultrasound technique (Bin *et al.*, 1992)

Ultrasound is a quick, non-invasive method for demonstrating thickening of the intestinal wall in patients with Crohn's disease and for assessing response to treatment (Holt & Samuel, 1979; Sonnenberg *et al.*, 1982; Dubbins, 1984).

Computed tomography

CT is useful for evaluating patients with certain disorders of the small intestine. Its main contribution is in the management of problems in patients with Crohn's disease (Goldberg *et al.*, 1983), assessing small-intestinal neoplasms (Hulnick, 1986) and in the diagnosis of intestinal infarction (Federle *et al.*, 1984; Smerud *et al.*, 1990). CT may provide important information about the extraluminal component of intestinal disorders, the relationship of adjacent organs and tissues and ancillary intra-abdominal findings (Hulnick, 1986). CT is proving useful for diagnosing small-intestinal obstruction and establishing the site and cause of obstruction (Frager *et al.*, 1994; Gazelle *et al.*, 1994).

Optimum opacification of the intestinal lumen is required for CT evaluation of the small intestine. Positive contrast opacification is achieved by oral administration of a dilute barium suspension (3–6% w/v) or a 2–3% concentration of iodinated water-soluble contrast medium. Barium suspension is normally preferred for routine CT scanning because it is palatable, unabsorbed by the intestine and does not have the irritant properties of water-soluble solutions (Megibow, 1986). Water-soluble contrast agents are indicated for blunt abdominal trauma, when scanning patients following abdominal surgery, in patients with suspected gastrointestinal perforation and as an intestinal marker for CT interventional procedures.

In general, more contrast medium results in more reliable intestinal opacification. A minimum of 750 ml is necessary, beginning at least 45 min before scanning and with approximately 250 ml being given 15 min before scanning commences (Hulnick, 1986). Enteric-coated time-release effervescent tablets administered orally may be used to outline the intestinal lumen with negative contrast (Megibow *et al.*, 1985). However, positive contrast opacification remains the method of choice (Hulnick, 1986).

References

Abu-Yousef, M.M., Benson, C.A., Lu, C.H. & Franken, E.A. (1983) Enteroclysis aided by an electric pump. *Radiology*, **147**, 268–9.

Alavi, A. & Ring, E.J. (1981) Localization of gastrointestinal bleeding: superiority of ⁹⁹ᵐTc sulphur colloid compared to angiography. *AJR*, **137**, 741–8.

Allison, D.J. (1980) Gastrointestinal bleeding: radiological diagnosis. *Br. J. Hosp. Med.*, **23**, 358–65.

Antes, G. & Lissner, J. (1983) Double-contrast small-bowel examination with barium and methylcellulose. *Radiology*, **148**, 37–40.

Bartram, C.I. & Amess, J.A. (1980) The diagnosis of Meckel's diverticulum by small bowel enema in the investigation of obscure intestinal bleeding. *Br. J. Surg.*, **67**, 417–18.

Baum, S. (1982) Angiography and the gastrointestinal bleeder. *Radiology*, **143**, 569–72.

Bilbao, M.K., Frische, L.H., Dotter, C.T. & Rosch, J. (1967) Hypotonic duodenography. *Radiology*, **89**, 438–43.

Bin, W., Jianguo, L. & Baowei, D. (1992) The sonographic appearances of small bowel tumours. *Clin. Radiol.*, **46**, 30–3.

Bunker, S.R., Lull, R.J., Tanasescu, D.U. *et al.* (1984) Scintigraphy of gastrointestinal haemorrhage: superiority of ⁹⁹ᵐTc red blood cells over ⁹⁹ᵐTc sulphur colloid. *AJR*, **143**, 543–8.

Buxton-Thomas, M.S., Dickinson, R.J., Maltby, P. *et al.* (1984) Evaluation of indium scintigraphy in patients with active inflammatory bowel disease. *Gut*, **25**, 1372–5.

Chippindale, A.J. & Desai, S. (1989) Experience with the Merck small bowel enema tube. *Clin. Radiol.*, **40**, 518-19.

Conway, J.J. (1980) Radionuclide diagnosis of Meckel's diverticulum. *Gastrointest. Radiol.*, **5**, 209–13.

Cooney, D.R., Duszynski, D.O., Camboa, E. *et al.* (1982) The abdominal technetium scan (a decade experience). *J. Ped. Surg.*, **17**, 611–19.

Diner, W.C., Hoskins, E.O. & Navab, F. (1984) Radiologic examination of the small intestine: review of 402 cases and discussion of indications and methods. *South. Med. J.*, **77**, 68–74.

Dixon, P.M. & Nolan, D.J. (1987) The diagnosis of Meckel's diverticulum: a continuing challenge. *Clin. Radiol.*, **38**, 615–19.

Dixon, P.M., Roulston, M.E. & Nolan, D.J. (1993) The small bowel enema: a 10-year review. *Clin. Radiol.*, **47**, 46–48.

Donato, H., Mayo, H.W. & Barr, L.H. (1954) The effect of peroral barium in partial obstruction of the small bowel. *Surgery*, **35**, 719–23.

Dubbins, P.A. (1984) Ultrasound demonstration of bowel wall thickness in inflammatory bowel disease. *Clin. Radiol.*, **35**, 227–31.

Dubbins, P.A. & Kurts, A.B. (1984) Normal and abnormal bowel. *In* Goldberg, B.B. (ed.) *Abdominal Ultrasound*, 2nd edn, pp. 287–305. New York, John Wiley.

Ebaugh, F.G. Jr, Clements, T.J., Rodnan, G. & Peterson, R.E. (1958) Quantitative measurement of gastrointestinal blood loss. The use of radioactive ⁵¹Cr in patients with gastrointestinal haemorrhage. *Am. J. Med.*, **25**, 169–81.

Ekberg, O. (1977) Double contrast examination of the small bowel. *Gastroint. Radiol.*, **1**, 349–53.

Federle, M.P., Chun, G., Jeffery, R.B. & Rayor, R. (1984) Computed tomography findings in bowel infarction. *AJR*, **142**, 91–5.

Ferrucci, J.T. Jr & Benedict, K.T. Jr (1971) Anticholinergic aided study of the gastrointestinal tract. *Radiol. Clin. N. Am.*, **9**, 23–39.

Figiel, L.S. & Figiel, S.J. (1964) Tumours of the terminal ileum. Diagnosis by retrograde filling during the barium enema study. *AJR*, **91**, 816–18.

Fitzgerald, E.J., Thompson, G.T., Somers, S.S. & Franic, S.F. (1985) Pneumocolon as an aid to small-bowel studies. *Clin. Radiol.*, **36**, 633–7.

Fleischer, A.C., Dowling, A.D., Weinstein, L. & Jones, A.E. (1979) Sonographic patterns of distended fluid filled bowel. *Radiology*, **133**, 681–5.

Fournier, A.M., Cave, P., Duval, J. *et al.* (1979) Double contrast small intestine examination...in 6 minutes. *J. Radiol. d'Electrol.*, **60**, 71–4.

Frager, D., Medwid, S.W., Baer, J.W. *et al.* (1994) CT of small bowel obstruction: value in establishing the diagnosis and determining the degree and cause. *AJR*, **162**, 37–41.

Fraser, G.M. & Preston, P.G. (1983) The small bowel barium follow-through enhanced with an oral effervescent agent. *Clin. Radiol.*, **34**, 673–9.

Freeark, R.J., Love, L. & Backer, R.J. (1968) An active diagnostic approach to blunt abdominal trauma. *Surg. Clin. N. Am.*, **48**, 97–109.

Gazelle, G.S., Goldberg, M.A., Wittenberg, J. *et al.* (1994) Efficacy of CT in distinguishing small-bowel obstruction from other causes of small-bowel dilatation. *AJR*, **162**, 43–7.

Goldberg, H.I., Gore, R.M., Margulis, A.R. *et al.* (1983) Computed tomography in the evaluation of Crohn's disease. *AJR*, **140**, 277–82.

Griffiths, P.D., Hufton, A.P. & Martin, D.F. (1993) The use of effervescent agents in the small bowel meal examination. *Clin. Radiol.*, **48**, 275–7.

Hart, D., Haggett, P.J., Boardman, P., Nolan, D.J. & Wall, B.F. (1994) Patient radiation doses from enteroclysis examinations. *Br. J. Radiol.*, **67**, 997–1000.

Hart, D. & Wall, B.F. (1994) Estimation of effective dose from dose–area product measurements for barium meals and barium enemas. *Br. J. Radiol.*, **67**, 485–9.

Herlinger, H. (1978) A modified technique for the double-contrast small bowel enema. *Gastrointest. Radiol.*, **3**, 201–7.

Herlinger, H. & Maglinte, D.D.T. (1989) The small bowel enema with methylcellulose. *In* Herlinger, H. & Maglinte, D.D.T. (eds) *Clinical Radiology of the Small Intestine*, pp. 119–37. WB Saunders, Philadelphia.

Holt, S. & Samuel, E. (1979) Grey scale ultrasound in Crohn's disease. *Gut*, **20**, 590–5.

Hulnick, D.H. (1986) Small intestine. *In* Megibow, A.J. & Balthazar, E.J. (eds) *Computed Tomography of the Gas-*

trointestinal Tract, pp. 217-78. CV Mosby, St Louis.

James, W.B. & Hume, R. (1968) Action of metoclopramide on gastric emptying and small bowel transit time. *Gut*, **9**, 203–5.

Kay, V.J. & Nolan, D.J. (1988) The small bowel enema in the patient with an ileostomy. *Clin. Radiol.*, **39**, 418–22.

Kellett, M.J., Zboralske, F.F. & Margulis, A.R. (1977) Peroral pneumocolon examination of ileocaecal region. *Gastrointest. Radiol.*, **1**, 361–5.

Kreel, L. (1970) The use of oral metoclopramide in the barium meal and follow-through examination. *Br. J. Radiol.*, **43**, 31–5.

Kreel, L. (1975) Pharmacoradiology in barium examinations with special reference to glucagon. *Br. J. Radiol.*, **48**, 691–703.

Law, R.L. & Longstaff, A.J. (1992) Technical report: a 'new' tube providing rapid insertion for the small bowel enema. *Clin. Radiol.*, **45**, 35–6.

McKusick, K.A., Froelich, J., Callahan, R.J. *et al.* (1981) ^{99m}Tc red blood cells for detection of gastrointestinal bleeding: experience with 80 patients. *AJR*, **137**, 1113–18.

Maglinte, D.D.T. (1984) Balloon enteroclysis catheter. *AJR*, **143**, 761–2.

Maglinte, D.D.T., Burney, B.T. & Miller, R.E. (1982) Technical factors for a more rapid enteroclysis. *AJR*, **138**, 588–91.

Maglinte, D.D.T., Lappas, J.C., Chernish, S.M. & Sellink, J.L. (1986) Intubation routes for enteroclysis. *Radiology*, **158**, 553–4.

Maglinte, D.D.T. & Miller, R.E. (1984) A comparison of pumps used for enteroclysis. *Radiology*, **152**, 815.

Marshak, R.H. & Lindner, A.E. (1976) *Radiology of the Small Intestine*. WB Saunders, Philadelphia.

Megibow, A.J. (1986) Stomach. *In* Megibow, A.J. & Balthazar, E.J. (eds) *Computed Tomography of the Gastrointestinal Tract*, pp. 99-174. CV Mosby, St Louis.

Megibow, A.J., Zerhouni, E, Hulnick, D.H. *et al.* (1985) Air contrast techniques in gastrointestinal computed tomography. *AJR*, **145**, 418.

Miller, R.E. (1965) Complete reflux small bowel examination. *Radiology*, **84**, 457–63.

Miller, R.E. & Brahme, F. (1969) Large amounts of orally administered barium for obstruction of the small intestine. *Surg. Gynecol. Obstet.*, **129**, 1185–8.

Miller, R.E. & Sellink, J.L. (1979) Enteroclysis: the small bowel enema. How to succeed and how to fail. *Gastrointest. Radiol.*, **4**, 469–83.

Miller, T.G. & Abbott, W.O. (1934) Intestinal intubation: a practical technique. *Am. J. Med. Sci.*, **187**, 595-9.

Miskowiak, J., Nielsen, S.L., Munk, O. & Anderson, B. (1977) Abdominal scintiphotography with ^{99m}technetium-labelled albumin in acute gastrointestinal bleeding. *Lancet*, **ii**, 852–4.

Nelson, S.W., Christoforidis, A.J. & Roenigk, W.J. (1963) Barium suspensions vs. water-soluble iodine compounds in the study of obstruction of the small bowel. An experimental study of physiologic characteristics and radiographic value. *Radiology*, **80**, 252–4.

Nice, C.M. (1963) Roentgenographic pattern and motility in small bowel studies. *Radiology*, **80**, 39–45.

Nicholson, D.A., Zammit-Maempel, I., Hughes, M. *et al.* (1989) The influence of type of tube and experience of the operator on performance of small bowel enema. *Br. J. Radiol.*, **62**, 447–9.

Nolan, D.J. (1979) Rapid duodenal and jejunal intubation. *Clin. Radiol.*, **30**, 183–5.

Nolan, D.J. & Cadman, P.J. (1987) The small bowel enema made easy. *Clin. Radiol.*, **38**, 295–301.

Novak, D. (1980) Acceleration of small intestine contrast study with ceruletide. *Gastrointest. Radiol.*, **5**, 61–5.

Oudkerk, M. (1981) *Infusion rate in enteroclysis*. Thesis, University of Leiden.

Parker, J.G. & Beneventano, T.C. (1970) Acceleration of small bowel contrast study by cholecystokinin. *Gastroenterology*, **58**, 679–84.

Petrokubi, R.J., Baum, S. & Rohrer, G.V. (1978) Cimetidine administration resulting in improved pertechnetate imaging of Meckel's diverticulum. *Clin. Nuc. Med.*, **3**, 385–8.

Robbins, A.H., Wetzner, S.M. & Landy, M.D. (1980) Ceruletide-assisted examinations of the small bowel. *AJR*, **134**, 343–7.

Rosenquist, C.J. (1975) Methods of acceleration of small intestinal radiographic examination. *West. J. Med.*, **122**, 320.

Sanders, D.E. & Ho, C.S. (1976) The small bowel enema: experience with 150 examinations. *AJR*, **127**, 743–51.

Saverymuttu, S.H., Peters, A.M., Hodgson, H.J. *et al.* (1983) ^{111}Indium leukocyte scanning in small-bowel Crohn's disease. *Gastrointest. Radiol.*, **8**, 157–61.

Scheible, W. & Goldberger, L.E. (1979) Diagnosis of small bowel obstruction: the contribution of diagnostic ultrasound. *AJR*, **133**, 685–8.

Schwartz, M.J. & Lewis, J.H. (1984) Meckel's diverticulum: pitfalls in scintigraphic detection in the adult. *Am. J. Gastroenterol.*, **79**, 611–18.

Sellink J.L. (1971) *Examination of the Small Intestine by Means of Duodenal Intubation*. Stenfert Kroese, Leiden.

Sellink, J.L. (1974) Radiologic examination of the small intestine by duodenal intubation. *Acta Radiol. Diagn.*, **15**, 318–22.

Sellink, J.L. & Miller, R.E. (1982) *Radiology of the Small Bowel: Technique and Atlas*. Martinus Nijhoff, The Hague.

Sfakianakis, G.N. & Conway, J.J. (1981) Detection of ectopic gastric mucosa in Meckel's diverticulum and in other aberrations by scintigraphy: I. Pathophysiology and 10-year clinical experience. *J. Nuc. Med.*, **22**, 647–54.

Shipps, F.C., Sayler, C.B., Egan, J.F. *et al.* (1979) Fluoroscopic placement of intestinal tubes. *Radiology*, **132**, 226–7.

Shrimpton, P.C., Jones, D.G., Hillier, M.C. *et al.* (1991) *Survey of CT Practice in the UK*. Part 2. *Dosimetric Aspects*. NRPB-R249. HMSO, London.

Smerud, M.J., Johnson, C.D. & Stephens, D.H. (1990) Diagnosis of bowel infarction: a comparison of plain films and CT scans in 23 cases. *AJR*, **154**, 99–103.

Somers, S. & Stevenson, G.W. (1994) the small bowel: anatomy and nontube examinations. *In* Freeny, P.C. & Stevenson, G.W. (eds) *Marggulis and Burhenne's Alimentary Tract Radiology*, pp. 512–32. CV Mosby, St. Louis.

Sonnenberg, A., Eckenbrecht, J., Peter, P. & Niederau, C. (1982) Detection of Crohn's disease by ultrasound. *Gastroenterology*, **83**, 430–4.

Spiller, R.C. & Parkins, R.A. (1983) Recurrent gastrointestinal bleeding of obscure origin: report of 17 cases and a guide to logical management. *Br. J. Surg.*, **70**, 489–93.

Thoeni, R.F. (1987) Radiography of the small bowel and enteroclysis: a perspective. *Invest. Radiol.*, **22**, 930–6.

Thompson, J.N., Hemingway, A.P., McPherson, G.A.D. *et al.* (1984) Obscure gastrointestinal haemorrhage of small-bowel origin. *Br. Med. J.*, **288**, 1663–5.

Traill, Z.C. & Nolan, D.J. (1995) Technical note: intubation times using a new enteroclysis tube. *Clin. Radiol.*, **50**, 339–40.

Treves, S., Grand, R.J. & Eraklis, A.J. (1978) Pentagastrin stimulation of technetium-99m uptake by ectopic gastric mucosa in a Meckel's diverticulum. *Radiology*, **128**, 711–12.

Vallance, R. (1980) An evaluation of the small bowel enema based on an analysis of 350 consecutive examinations. *Clin. Radiol.*, **31**, 227–32.

Vecchioli, A., De Franco, A., Maresca, G. & Gore, R.M. (1994) Cross-sectional imaging of the small intestine. *In* Gore, R.M., Levine, M.S. & Laufer, I. (eds) *Textbook of Gastrointestinal Radiology*, pp. 789-801. WB Saunders, Philadelphia.

Zagoria, R.J., Gelfand, D.W. & Ott, D.J. (1986) Retrograde examination of the small bowel in patients with an ileostomy. *Gastrointest. Radiol.*, **11**, 97–101.

5   Large Bowel

C. I. BARTRAM

The first radiographic examination of the colon is credited to Williams who, in 1901, used air as a contrast medium to outline the colon during fluoroscopy. Schüle later performed the first single-contrast enema, using an oily suspension of bismuth subnitrate. In 1910, Bachem and Guenter suggested replacing the rather toxic bismuth salts with barium sulphate. The first modern double-contrast barium enema (DCBE) with air insufflation was performed by Fischer in 1923, and later popularized by Welin, from Malmö, Sweden, in the 1960s.

In the 1990s, the large bowel may be imaged in a variety of ways. Luminal contrast agents demonstrate the mucosal surface and overall anatomical configuration of the bowel. The most detail is still obtained with barium sulphate suspensions, but ultrasonography (US), computed tomography (CT) and magnetic resonance imaging (MRI) can also show the mucosal surface when appropriate luminal contrast agents are used, and have the advantage of revealing mural and extramural detail. Also, i.v. contrast agents may be used to highlight blood flow through the bowel wall during CT and MRI, although angiography remains the examination of choice for small-vessel detail.

This chapter describes a practical approach to the DCBE which is still the most common primary examination of the large bowel. Some related examination techniques are discussed more briefly.

Luminal studies — barium enema

In many centres colonoscopy is challenging the DCBE as the first-line investigation of colonic disease. The prime disadvantage of DCBE, compared to the direct endoscopic view, is the absence of colour. Small vascular lesions and very early colitis may not be detected radiologically, as there is no surface irregularity to alter the mucosal coating, but will be obvious endoscopically from the colour change associated with the vascular component of the disease. Small polyps (less than 5 mm in diameter) are difficult to distinguish from faecal residue radiologically, whereas the distinction is again easily made by endoscopy, based on the obvious colour difference and the ability to wash off any residue. Radiology also has the advantages of safety, speed, ease, economy and the ability to demonstrate the caecum in almost all examinations. However, a consistently high standard is essential to maintain credibility in the competitive situation that exists today. It is common to find the examination undervalued by radiologists, yet properly performed it is a highly accurate method of diagnosing one of the most treatable cancers, as well as its precursor the adenomatous polyp.

The preferred method of examination is the DCBE. The single-contrast barium enema (SCBE) may be quicker and less demanding technically, but it does not give such a detailed view of the mucosa. It is not as accurate as the DCBE in detecting small polyps (5–10 mm) and early colitis. The ability to clearly 'see through' overlapping loops prevents larger lesions being obscured and is a further advantage of DCBE. Residue is also more difficult to distinguish from a polyp in SCBE. Fluoroscopy and compression are critical components of the SCBE, but remain important in the DCBE. The caecum, sigmoid and some of the transverse colon may be compressed, which can be very useful in confirming an intraluminal lesion (McLean & Bartram, 1985) as it will show as a negative filling defect in the barium pool.

Quality control of all aspects of the examination is the responsibility of the radiologist. An understanding of barium suspensions, bowel preparation, techniques of examination and the interrelationship between these, forms a basis for a smooth running and successful barium enema practice

Barium suspensions

Pure crystals of barium sulphate are formed by milling of the mined raw mineral barytes, precipitation with sulphuric acid, followed by washing and drying. The particle size can be varied from a uniform 0.6–1.4 µm, to much larger crystals in a more heterogeneous range of 4–50 µm. Barium enema suspensions use the smaller and more uniform particle size. The particles are coated with various agents to achieve several basic suspension characteristics.

1 Rapid flow.
2 Good mucosal adhesion.
3 Adequate radiographic density in a thin layer.
4 An even coating which remains plastic and does not crack.
5 The absence of artefact or foaming.

Barium preparations may be in powder form, requiring mixing with water for reconstitution, or in suspension. Suspensions have some technical advantages, as it is easier to add various additives to a suspension in order to manipulate its characteristics. The exact ingredients are trade secrets, as patents cannot be applied. Large organic molecules, such as gum arabic, pectin and methylcarboxycellulose may be added to coat the particles and control the characteristics of the suspension. Antifoaming agents may be incorporated into the suspension, or added when it is made up, to prevent bubble formation.

Viscosity is a measure of how easily the suspension flows. Apparent viscosity is the ratio of shear stress to rate of shear. Simple fluids have a constant viscosity. Plastic flow describes an increase in shear stress before flow starts. If this decreases at higher shear rates the liquid is said to be pseudoplastic. Thixotropy refers to variations in the shear stress with different rates of shear (Fig. 5.1). Barium suspensions show complex pseudoplastic and thixotropic behaviour. The terms 'thin' and 'thick' suspensions are often used but are imprecise. A suspension may be viscous and 'thick' but with a low barium content and so radiographically 'thin'. The flow characteristics of a suspension are not necessarily the same as its radiographic density. The double-contrast technique is really thin layer contrast radiography. The radiographic density of this layer is a product of its thickness and the barium content within the layer, which reflects the barium per cent weight/volume of the suspension.

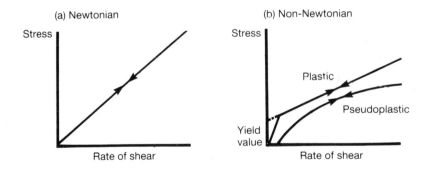

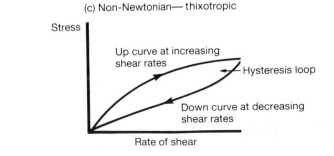

Fig. 5.1 Diagrams illustrating different types of viscosity behaviour. Stress 1 : 1 rate of shear plotted from a rotating viscometer. Reproduced with permission of *BJR* from Conry *et al.* (1978).

A sudden increase in both viscosity and thixotropy is evidence of flocculation. A change in surface charge leads to particles aggregating into irregular large clumps, with loss of normal flow and coating properties. The suspension breaks up, there is no mucosal adhesion, and definition is lost. Barium sulphate particles are amphoteric and will adsorb any charged molecule. Pure barium sulphate flocculates rapidly in the presence of large charged molecules, such as mucin. To combat this a strong negative charge is applied to the surface by adding large molecules with an overall negative charge, such as carboxymethylcellulose.

The requirements of the suspension vary according to the type of examination. The SCBE needs a low-density suspension of 12–20% w/v to achieve some 'see-through' effect. This places few demands on the suspension, mainly that it does not settle out or flocculate. Suspensions for DCBE are usually in the 60–110% w/v range, so that there will be sufficient radiographic density in a thin layer (about 0.2 mm thick) for fine mucosal detail to be visualized *en face*. The suspension must flow easily, so that it can be manipulated around the bowel, leaving a thin and even coating that does not flocculate and remains plastic when dried out. This occurs naturally during the examination as the colon reabsorbs water. Loss of plasticity results in a crazy paving effect (Fig. 5.2). Foaming should be minimal. Some bubble formation may occur during air insufflation (Fig. 5.3), but should disperse rapidly. Bubbles may persist if the film coating them is viscous. Colloids, such as mucinous glycoproteins, have a high surface viscosity and create quite stable foams. Antifoaming agents, such as dimethyl polysiloxane emulsion, may be added to destabilize formed bubbles. This must be done carefully, as too much or the wrong sort of antifoaming agent may have the converse effect and actually stabilize bubbles. If moisture is allowed to enter a powdered preparation, small gritty sand-like particles will form and precipitate out of suspension in the distal colon, forming very fine dense opacities within the mucosal coating (Fig. 5.4).

Bowel preparation

Bowel preparation is probably the least standardized

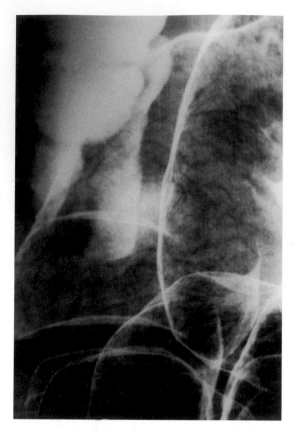

Fig. 5.2 Flaking due to loss of elasticity in the barium suspension.

part of the examination, although one of its most important aspects. Most regimens rely on a combination of dietary restriction, purgation and overhydration, with the possible addition of a cleansing water enema (Bartram, 1994).

A wide choice of laxatives is available. These are a heterogeneous group of compounds that act by altering intestinal electrolyte and fluid movement so that there is an increase in faecal water excretion, and/or by stimulating colonic motility.

Laxatives in common use include the following.
1 Castor oil (30 ml) which is cheap and, although unpleasant to take, is relatively gentle in effect. It has a dual action, being broken down in the small bowel into ricinoleic acid, which inhibits water reabsorption, and a mineral oil residue that probably has a direct motor action causing contractions in the distal small bowel and proximal colon.

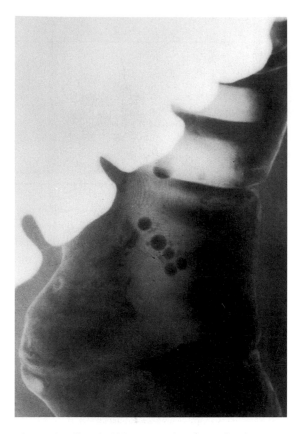

Fig. 5.3 Small air bubbles trapped in the surface layer.

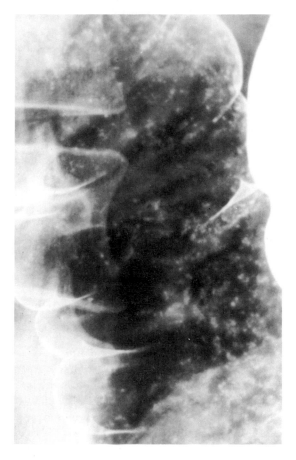

Fig. 5.4 Sand-like floccules of barium due to agglomeration of particles within a powder that have not been dispersed by mixing.

2 Bisacodyl (15–20 mg) is a contact laxative belonging to the polyphenolic group of compounds. It is hydrolysed by intestinal enzymes in the small and large bowel into desacetylbisacodyl, which has a direct motor action on the bowel, and also a slight secretory effect.

3 Magnesium citrate (5–10 g of equivalent magnesium oxide) is a saline type cathartic, which is more pleasant to take than magnesium sulphate. Magnesium and the sulphate or citrate radicles are poorly absorbed from the gut, leading to osmotic retention of fluid and increased peristalsis. There is also probably a more complex action through cholecystokinin release. There may also be a direct secretory component in the small bowel. A linear relationship between ingested magnesium, the stool levels of magnesium and faecal weight has been established. It is apparently contraindicated in renal failure, but in practice this is not a significant risk (L. Baker, 1993, personal communication). Care is

needed not to overdose small children. Two preparations are currently available in the UK:

(a) Picolax*(one sachet contains 10 mg of sodium picosulphate, 3.5 g of magnesium oxide and 12 g of citric acid) is a mixture of an osmotic and a contact laxative. Magnesium citrate is formed when the sachet is dissolved in water. Sodium picosulphate, a phenolester compound, is broken down by bacterial sulphatase enzymes in the large bowel into the same active metabolite as bisacodyl, desacetylbisacodyl. The difference is that its action is limited to the large bowel, as enzymatic activation only occurs there. It is therefore similar in action to the anthranoid glycosides, such as

* Ferring Ltd, Feltham, Middlesex, UK.

senna, although its activity is more uncertain, being dependent on the bacterial flora;

(b) Citramag* contains magnesium citrate equivalent to 5 g of magnesium oxide without any other additive.

4 Osmotically balanced, polyethylene glycol-based electrolyte solutions (Golytely†, Klean Prep‡) are effective and safe to use in situations such as active colitis, where other preparations would be contraindicated. The patient has to drink large volumes of fluid, up to 4 litres, which often causes nausea and possibly vomiting. These agents are preferred by colonoscopists for rapid bowel preparation. The bowel is left very wet, which is no hindrance to endoscopy but is so for an immediate barium enema.

Brown, in the early 1960s, developed a non-washout regimen using a combination of low-residue diet, overhydration, osmotic purgation and a contact laxative (Brown, 1961). His idea was to stop the intake of residue-producing foods, overhydrate the patient and then flush the bowel through with an osmotic purgative. When this process had finished, any residual particulate matter was cleared out by a contact laxative causing mass contractions in the large bowel. The process is both effective and well tolerated. A modification of Brown's method is given in Table 5.1. The manufacturer's protocol for Picolax is presented in Table 5.2, with modifications for children in Table 5.3. Oral lavage techniques (Table 5.4) using a proprietary balanced solution, provide a rapid intestinal flush. As this leaves the colon very wet, it must be given the day before.

Miller (1975) described a simple technique for administering cleansing water enemas: 1.5 litres of warm tap water is usually sufficient to fill the colon. The reservoir should be not more than 1 m above the patient to prevent rectal filling being too rapid. Rectal distension causes discomfort and leads to incontinence if sphincter tone is weak. The patient should be on their left side initially, turning prone and then onto the right side to fill the caecum. If the patient experiences any pain, the bag should be lowered below the table to allow fluid to drain out from the rectum. A disposable closed system is

* Bioglan Laboratories, Hitchin, Hertford, UK.
† Braintree Laboratories, Braintree, Massachusetts, USA.
‡ Norgine Ltd, Oxford, UK.

Table 5.1 A modified version of Brown's method of bowel cleansing

Day before barium enema
Clear fluids only from noon
One full glass (225 ml) water every hour (1–9 p.m.)
300 ml of cold magnesium citrate (equivalent to 4 g of magnesium oxide) at 5 p.m.
Four (5 mg) tablets of bisacodyl at bedtime

Day of barium enema
Nil by mouth after midnight
Bisacodyl suppository inserted on waking

essential for this. When the colon has been filled, the patient is sent to the toilet to evacuate as completely as possible. Cleansing enemas guarantee an absolutely clean colon, but are seldom used in the UK. The technique, however, still has some use as it is possible to clean out the colon even if the patient has not taken any laxative, or if the preparation has been incomplete for any reason.

Special care must be taken with diabetic patients. How far the standard regimen needs modifying depends on how the diabetes is treated. If controlled by diet alone, the standard regimen is followed with diabetic low-calorie drinks used for fluid intake. Patients on oral hypoglycaemic agents and dietary therapy should take their diabetic tablets as normal the day before, using fruit juice or Lucozade to provide a balanced carbohydrate fluid intake. No medication should be taken until after the examination, when the patient can eat a light meal. Patients on insulin should take their normal insulin on the day before, covering the required carbohydrate intake with fruit juice, milk or cordial. The morning insulin dose must be omitted on the day of the examinations, with half the normal morning dose given when the examination is over and taken with a light meal. Diabetics should be given an early morning appointment to avoid prolonged starvation.

The main side effect of Picolax preparation is headache. This is not associated with dehydration and is not influenced by any fluid regimen (Lawrance *et al.*, 1994).

Female patients should be warned that diarrhoea may interfere with the absorption of oral contraceptives. Although the contraceptive should still be taken, other types of contraceptive precaution should be used for the rest of the cycle.

Table 5.2 Manufacturer's recommendations for Picolax

Day before barium enema

Before breakfast (not later than 8 a.m.) take the first sachet of Picolax

Breakfast limited to one boiled egg, one slice of white bread with honey (not jam or marmalade), one cup of tea or coffee with sugar and milk as required

Lunch is a small portion of grilled or poached fish/chicken with a little cooked rice, plain yoghurt, clear jelly or junket. No potatotes/vegetables or fruit. One cup of tea or coffee without milk, but sweetened if desired

At 4 p.m. take the second sachet of Picolax

For supper (7–9 p.m.) no solid food but clear soup or meat extract drinks

Drink plenty of clear fluids throughout the day. Continue to take fluids until bowel movements have ceased. Drink as much as is required to satisfy thirst

Day of barium enema

Clear fluids only

N.B. Patients should be warned that when Picolax is added to water an exothermic reaction occurs. Only a little water should be added to the powder at first. When this has cooled after about 5 min it should be diluted with 150 ml of water and drunk. Frequent bowel movements start within 3 hours.

Table 5.3 Bowel preparation for children (modification of the Picolax schedule). As for adults, give two doses of Picolax, but the amount of each sachet is adjusted according to age

1–3 years	25% sachet
4–6 years	50% sachet
7–12 years	75% sachet
Over 12 years	one sachet

Table 5.4 Balanced oral lavage. From Fitzsimons *et al.* (1987)

Day before barium enema

Clear fluids only from noon

2 p.m. four tablets (5 mg) of bisacodyl taken with 300 ml water

5 p.m. lavage started at about 1 litre hour^{-1} continuing for a maximum of 4 litres or until rectal effluent clear

Day of barium enema

Nil by mouth after midnight

Relationship between method of bowel preparation and DCBE

The use of cleansing water enemas has a deleterious effect on mucosal coating. A delay of at least 45 min before DCBE allows for reabsorption of retained fluid (Lee & Bartram, 1990). However, the barium suspension needs to be more viscous to cope with any fluid and the thicker coating may obscure fine mucosal detail. Oral lavage preparations have the same problem, unless given the day before. The Brown method leaves a dry colon, ideal for barium studies. Less viscous suspensions may be used, which are easier to manipulate around the colon. The coating will be thinner, without any excess fluid/mucus interface, and so may be more detailed. It has been suggested that only non-washout preparations will show the fine mucosal detail of the innominate groove pattern (Matsuura *et al.*, 1977).

Magnesium preparations leave an excess of electropositive ions in the mucus. These will neutralize the electronegative charge of the barium suspension, increasing its viscosity and causing a 'gel' effect. In moderation this improves coating and is generally beneficial as it allows the use of a slightly less viscous suspension, which flows more rapidly and is easier to handle yet maintains good coating. However, there is variation in the dryness of the colon and in the amount of magnesium retained in the mucus. If sufficient to cause flocculation, the mucosal layer becomes very thick, does not flow easily and coats unevenly. About 200 ml of water must be added to the suspension to offset this effect.

System for administration

The closed disposable system (Fig. 5.5) has the following advantages:

1 There is no possibility of cross-infection.

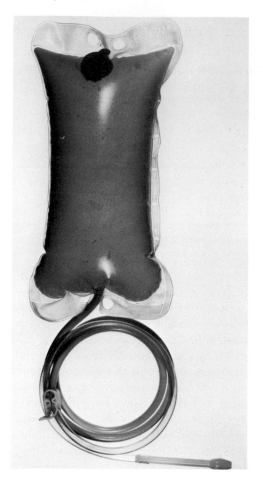

Fig. 5.5 Disposable system for barium enema. The bag contains sufficient barium for a single or doublecontrast examination and may be distended with air or carbon dioxide, or an enema tip with side-arm and inflator used. The E-Z-EM 520 bag is illustrated (E-Z-EM Ltd). Similar system also available from Smith & Nephew (Cambridge, UK).

2 Rectal drainage may be performed whenever required.

3 The bag, either that containing the barium or a separate one, may be inflated with carbon dioxide instead of air. A simple method is to connect a special pressure reducing valve* to a compressed carbon dioxide bottle (Bartram, 1989) and inflate the bag directly. Carbon dioxide is absorbed much more rapidly than nitrogen from the gut. The degree of dis-

---

* Cat. No. 6018: regulator with pin index for carbon dioxide, Unit 14, Station Field, Kidlington, Oxford, UK.

comfort during the examination is of course unaffected by the gas used, but persisting abdominal distension and pain is significantly less with carbon dioxide. Most workers strongly recommend the use of carbon dioxide (Taylor & Beckly, 1991).

Single-contrast barium enema

Indications

1 Uncooperative, very debilitated or immobile patient.
2 Evaluation of acute obstruction or volvulus.
3 Reduction of intussusception.
4 To show the configuration of the colon.
5 Where only gross pathology is to be excluded.

Contraindications

1 Peritonitis, free intraperitoneal air.
2 Allergy to barium suspensions.
3 Where there is any risk of perforation such as acute appendicitis, diverticulitis or fistula. A water-soluble contrast agent must be used in these situations.

Technique

A 15–20% w/v barium suspension is run in slowly, with careful observation of the barium column during fluoroscopy. Where possible — i.e. in the sigmoid, parts of the descending, transverse and ascending colons, and caecum — compression either manually with a lead glove, a prone compression paddle or a spoon is applied. A spot radiograph is taken of any filling defect or mural abnormality. Routine spot views of the sigmoid, flexures and caecum, followed by a straight prone overhead of the abdomen, one with 30° caudal angulation for the sigmoid and a lateral view of the rectum, complete the series. Excess barium is then drained back into the bag, the enema tip removed and the patient sent to the toilet. A prone post-evacuation film is optional.

Double-contrast barium enema

Indications

1 Preferred method for routine examination.

2 High-risk patient — i.e. rectal bleeding, previous history of carcinoma or polyp, family history of colorectal cancer or polyposis.
3 Diarrhoea, ?colitis.

Contraindications

1 As for any barium enema (see above).
2 If it takes two people to get the patient onto the table, only a limited study will be possible and it may be preferable to plan an SCBE from the onset (Scholz, 1993).

Technique

The objective must be to obtain clear double-contrast images of every part of the large bowel. To achieve this some basic principles must be followed, although it is possible to vary many aspects of the examination.

An i.v. smooth muscle relaxant — 20 mg of hyoscine butylbromide (Buscopan) or 0.5–1 mg of glucagon — should always be given, but the exact timing of the dose is a matter of preference. Several problems may be encountered if a relaxant is not used. Magnesium citrate/bisacodyl bowel preparations induce considerable colonic spasm, particularly in the sigmoid, which will prevent the barium column moving proximally. If filling is then continued, the rectum will become overdistended and anal incontinence is likely. A crinkled mucosal pattern, also common after Picolax bowel preparation, is due to persisting contraction of the muscularis mucosae and is abolished by an i.v. smooth muscle relaxant. Although satisfactory distension may be achieved during screening, the higher colonic tone often results in sudden contractions of large segments of the bowel. If an overhead series is taken, the bowel may be contracted in several views, and repeat radiographs are then necessary.

An advantage of the higher colonic tone is that the colon is narrower during filling and less barium will be needed to fill the bowel. There will then be less to drain and the higher tone may also facilitate drainage. Sometimes a mass contraction will be induced and empty the colon almost completely, so that it has to be refilled. The options are to give the smooth muscle relaxant initially, or after rectal drainage before gas insufflation. Filling, avoiding incontinence and drainage are more predictable when the relaxant has been given. It practice it is simpler to inject 20 mg of hyoscine butylbromide i.v. routinely at the beginning of the examination.

It is easier to insert the enema tip with the patient prone. Large prolapsed haemorrhoids may cause problems. If there is any difficulty or pain on inserting the enema tip, the gloved finger should be used to locate the anal canal and then guide in the well-lubricated enema tip.

Barium may be run in with the patient prone or in the left lateral position. The bag should be 1–1.2 m above the patient. Never overdistend the rectum. Screen intermittently to check the progress of the barium column. Scholz (1993) describes a 'descending and pointing' sign where the levators fatigue, the pelvic floor descends, and barium points as it surrounds the enema tip in the anal canal. Incontinence is then imminent. When this sign is seen, stop the infusion immediately and lower the bag to the floor with the tube unclamped to allow the rectum to drain. Encourage the patient to squeeze their buttocks together to prevent leakage as barium is run in. Lower the bag intermittently to allow the patient to rest. If there is still difficulty in retaining barium, or the anal tone is obviously very poor, use a balloon catheter (Fig. 5.6). It is a good idea to run a little barium into the rectum before inflating the balloon. Screen quickly when inflating the balloon to check that the balloon is only touching and is not distending the rectal wall. This will avoid any complication from inflation in a pathologically narrowed rectum. Never inflate above the manufacturer's recommendation. An alternative method of dealing with incontinence is to put shoulder rests in position and tilt the patient very steeply head down. The rectum will not then become distended as gravity will ensure that the barium flows down through the colon, rather than back up and out of the anus. It is possible to fill the colon in this position, even when there is a total lack of anal tone. Redundant sigmoid loops may be compressed by an obese abdomen in the prone position. In some patients barium may therefore run in faster in the left lateral position. Filling should be continued until barium flows around the splenic flexure and into the transverse colon.

At the end of filling, bring the head of the table up

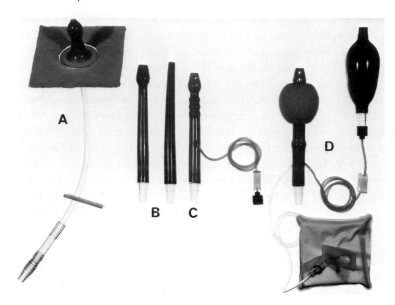

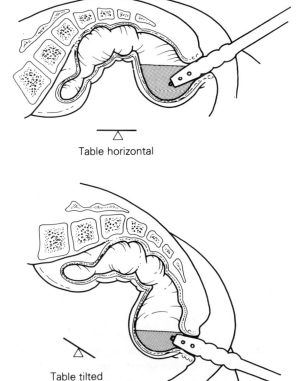

Fig. 5.6 Selection of disposable enema tips (E-Z-EM Ltd). A, Colostomy tip with adhesive pad; B, standard tips with different ends; C, tip with airline; and D, a self-retaining catheter with balloon and square plastic inflator to limit balloon distension, and side-arm with bulb inflator fitted.

30° with the patient prone and lower the bag to allow drainage. This is the optimum position in which to drain the rectum completely (Fig. 5.7).

It is then preferable to take a series of spot radiographs of the rectosigmoid area before the caecum fills. Digital imaging or 100 mm cut film incur only a small radiation penalty. These may be the only views where the sigmoid is not overlapped. The usual problem is clearing barium pools from a redundant sigmoid colon. In most cases turning the patient onto the left side, insufflating gas, rotating the patient prone, then back onto the left side, and finally supine will clear the entire sigmoid (Dobranski *et al.*, 1990). Some sigmoid configurations require the patient to be turned onto the right side from the supine. A right anterior oblique (RAO) view of the opened out sigmoid loop, followed by a left lateral view of the rectosigmoid should be taken. The patient is then turned prone again and the left side elevated slightly for a left posterior oblique (LPO) view. Gas insufflation prior to each view ensures good distension.

The bag may then be lowered with the tube unclamped so that the rectum drains, while the colon is screened quickly to check the progress of the main barium column. Insufflate some gas to see if more of the distal barium column can be pushed around the splenic flexure. It if does not move out of the descending colon, turn the patient onto the left side, insufflate, then turn the patient prone again.

Table horizontal

Table tilted

Fig. 5.7 The rectum drains completely only when the patient is prone with the head elevated. Reproduced with permission of *Radiology* from Miller and Peterson (1978).

With some splenic flexure configurations it may be necessary to turn the patient supine and onto the right side to get the tail end of the column around the flexure. Once this has been achieved, bring the head of the table up. This traps barium in the transverse colon, preventing it from running back around the splenic flexure, and moves the column forward into the most dependent mid-part of the transverse colon (Fig. 5.8). This in turn helps with the next manoeuvre.

Filling the proximal colon should not be attempted until the transverse colon is about two-thirds full. The column must then be manipulated around the hepatic flexure. The hepatic flexure runs anteroposteriorly (AP), so that in the prone position (Fig. 5.9), barium would have to go uphill to go around it. If this is attempted gas will just bubble through the column and overdistend the caecum, but the barium will not move into the ascending colon. The flexure must be made dependent by turning the patient onto the right side. Insufflation will help push more barium around the flexure. The patient may have to be screened and turned further onto their back to find the critical angle where barium cascades around the flexure. In some patients there is a double loop to the hepatic flexure, and to get barium around the last loop it may be necessary to turn the patient onto the left side. Putting the head of the table down about 10° will help prevent the column running back into the transverse colon during this manoeuvre. Once sufficient barium has entered the proximal part of the ascending colon, the head of the table should again be elevated to trap it there. The patient is then turned prone to fill the caecum. The caecum runs anteriorly and is dependent in the prone position (see Figs 5.8 & 5.9).

By the time the proximal colon has been filled, the colon is usually quite well distended with gas. Once the lumen has become distended by gas, the suspension flows along the dependent wall. Large areas of non-dependent wall in the proximal colon are therefore not coated by the initial manoeuvres to fill the caecum. To ensure a uniform coating, the patient should be turned twice: from prone to right side down, to supine, to left side down and prone again, i.e. clockwise. It may then be necessary to refill the caecum by turning onto the right side, bringing the patient's head up and then turning prone again. The final rectal drainage and gas insufflation is then performed.

There are several points worth remembering during the barium filling and gas distension phases of a DCBE.

1 The rectum is the part of the colon most sensitive to distension.

2 Drain the rectum as frequently as possible. Lower the bag and leave the tube unclamped when turning the patient. This allows the rectum to drain, making the patient more comfortable, and removing as much barium from the distal colon as possible.

3 The barium column cannot be pushed uphill. Gas insufflation will help move the column along the bowel or around loops if these are made dependent, so that the gas is on top of the barium. Once the colon is distended with air, only gravity will cause the barium column to move around loops. Use screening to observe the movement of the barium column with changes in the position of the patient and then plan how to move the column around any redundant loop.

4 To obtain good double-contrast views of the caecum, first turn the patient onto the left side so that barium flows back into the transverse colon while gas rises up to distend the proximal colon. If necessary insufflate further. Roll the patient over a little onto their front to empty barium around the flexure, then roll them back for a good double-contrast view of the ascending colon. The caecum may still contain a barium pool or be overlapped by the sigmoid. Turn the patient onto their right side. Barium tends to pool between the medial wall of the caecum and the ileocaecal valve, so that the pool will drain away only on turning onto the left side. A little compression to the abdominal wall will push the sigmoid medially. Screen to find the best position for a double-contrast view of the caecal pole.

5 Patients with limited mobility will have to turn onto the right side at least once. Once the caecum is filled, it may not be possible to rotate the patient completely to coat the proximal colon evenly. Instead, gently roll the patient onto the left side and then back onto the right side. It is better to overfill the colon a little, until the column in the transverse colon passes the spine, as excess barium is less of a problem in DCBE than poor coating.

6 Avoid insufflation with the patient supine. The ileocaecal valve is then dependent, as it arises from the medial posterolateral wall in most cases, so that

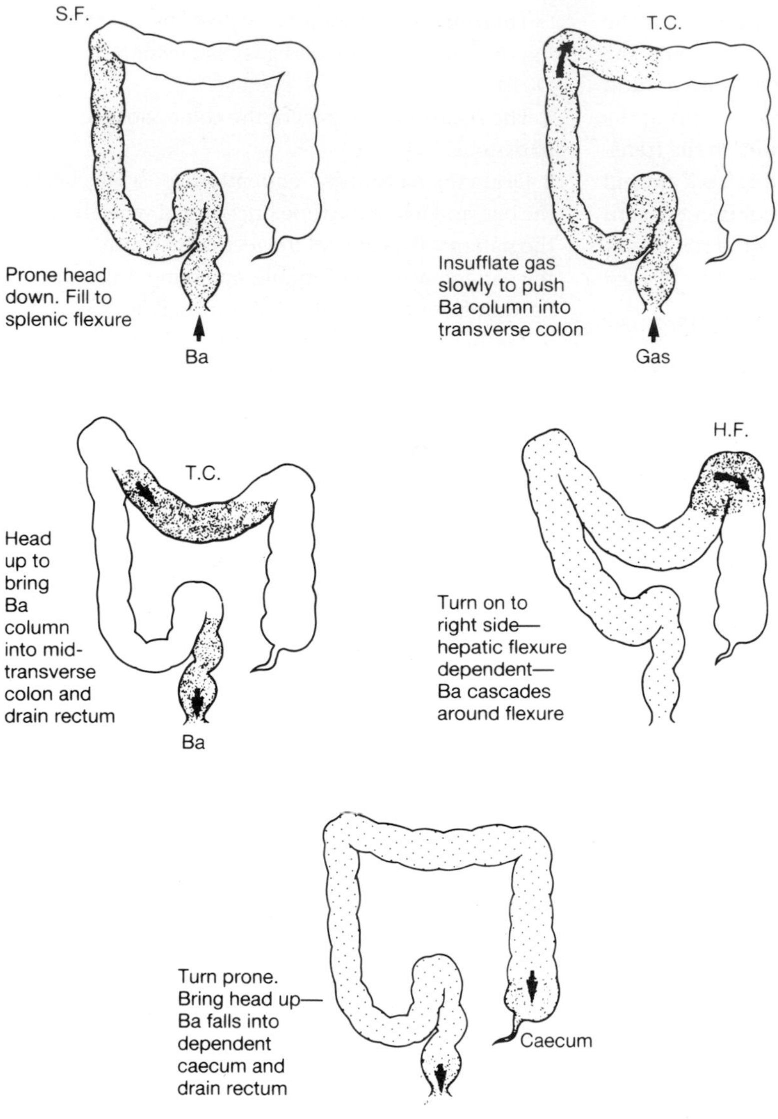

S.F.

Prone head down. Fill to splenic flexure

Ba

T.C.

Insufflate gas slowly to push Ba column into transverse colon

Gas

T.C.

Head up to bring Ba column into mid-transverse colon and drain rectum

Ba

H.F.

Turn on to right side— hepatic flexure dependent— Ba cascades around flexure

Turn prone. Bring head up— Ba falls into dependent caecum and drain rectum

Caecum

Fig. 5.8 Diagrammatic representation of the principles of manipulating the barium column and gas insufflation during the double-contrast barium enema. Ba, barium; HF, hepatic flexure; SF, sigmoid flexure; TC, transverse colon.

pooled barium in the caecum will then reflux into the ileum. When the patient is prone, the valve will not be dependent and only gas will reflux into the small bowel, which does not matter.

7 If there is significant difficulty in filling the bowel, usually due to redundant loops, dilute the suspension by adding 500–700 ml of water. Then run in the diluted suspension with the head of the table down and the patient prone.

8 If there is still spasm after one dose of i.v. smooth muscle relaxant, give another. Otherwise, there

may be a mass contraction when films are taken.

9 Prone compression with the pneumatic paddle is still a useful part of a DCBE examination. Compression is used in diverticular disease of the sigmoid, to separate small-bowel loops, or to confirm an intraluminal lesion in the caecum.

Value of a preliminary plain radiograph

To minimize film costs and radiation this is no longer recommended unless there is a clinical suspicion of

Fig. 5.9 Diagram showing the configuration of the large bowel in the prone position, as seen from a lateral view. The rectum runs uphill in the curve of the sacrum. From the splenic flexure the colon runs downhill to its most dependent part in the mid-transverse colon. It then runs almost vertically up to the hepatic flexure. Note that the caecum is more anterior to the hepatic flexure, which is why it fills when made dependent in the prone position. Reproduced with permission of *AJR* from Miller (1979).

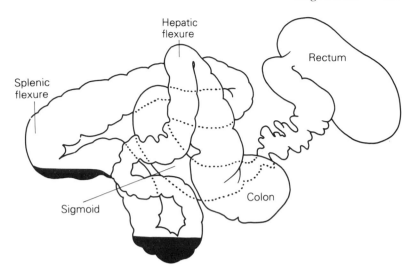

renal calculus, bowel obstruction, perforation or toxic megacolon.

A plain abdominal radiograph is often taken if there is uncertainty about the efficacy of bowel preparation. The rationale is that if residue is present the examination should be postponed and further bowel preparation arranged. Providing it is established that the patient has actually taken the preparation, there may well be a cause for the faecal retention, most commonly a partially obstructing carcinoma. It might be dangerous to give more bowel preparation and better to perform a limited examination to see if an obstructing lesion is present or not. Clinical judgement in such situations should decide the more appropriate course of action.

Radiographic views

The standard St Mark's examination relies on overhead radiographs (Table 5.5 & Fig. 5.10). Spot radiographs are taken of any lesion seen on screening where it is judged that this might be difficult to see on the routine radiographic series; compression views of the sigmoid and caecum are taken as necessary to separate overlapping loops. Remote control units have the added advantage of tube angulation. Petersen and Miller (1978) considered that about 35° of caudal tube angulation for a 15° RAO and 45° LPO were optimum angulations for the sigmoid. With a remote control unit it is simple to find the most appropriate angle. A series of views using a remote

control unit without any decubitus view have been recommended by Gelfand *et al.* (1991) (Table 5.6). Spot radiographs with digital imaging involve a reduction of radiation dosage of about one-third compared to rare earth screen combinations, so that a few more views can be taken while still keeping a lower overall dose. A typical mixed set of views with digital imaging is given in Table 5.7.

The decubitus views with horizontal beam are a useful combination. Except in the erect position one is always looking down onto the gas/barium interface of any barium pool. With the decubitus and erect views one looks across this interface, often revealing double-contrast views of parts not seen in any other projection. An important technical point with decubitus views is to use a grid/film holder. It is essential that the grid is at right angles to the table to prevent grid cut-off. In practice this is impossible without a dedicated fixing device. Another error is concentrating on the flexures in these views. The rectum should always be included. It does not matter that the flexures are not included, as these will be clearly seen on the erect views. A dished top table makes it very difficult to take decubitus views and is not recommended for barium work. A wedge filter is useful to compensate for the obese abdomen (De Lacey *et al.*, 1978).

A prone cross table view of the rectum gives a good double-contrast view of the rectum (Niizuma & Kobayashi, 1977), but this should be seen in the decubitus films. There is often a barium fluid level

Table 5.5 St Mark's Hospital overhead radiograph series. Tube distance, 110 cm; Kodak rare earth screens, regular speed; Lysholm Schonander parallel grid type N30, ratio 6.5 : 1

View	Radiograph size (mm)	Centring	Patient position	Tube position	Kilovoltage
Prone	35 × 43	2.5 cm below level of iliac crests in mid-line	Prone	Angled 30° caudally	90
Left lateral pelvis	30 × 40	3 cm below iliac crests in mid-line	Left lateral	Vertical	125
Right posterior oblique	35 × 43	2.5 cm to left of mid-line, 2.5 cm below level of iliac crests	Supine turned 30° to right	Vertical	95
Left posterior oblique	35 × 43	2.5 cm to right of mid-line, 2.5 cm below level of iliac crests	Supine turned 30° to left	Vertical	95
Posteroanterior decubitus	30 × 40	2.5 cm below iliac crests to mid-line of grid down	Left side down	Horizontal	80–85
Anteropositerior decubitus	30 × 40	2.5 cm below iliac crests to mid-line of grid	Right side down	Horizontal	80–85
Anteroposterior erect	35 × 43	Mid-line 2.5 cm above iliac crests	Standing	Horizontal	110

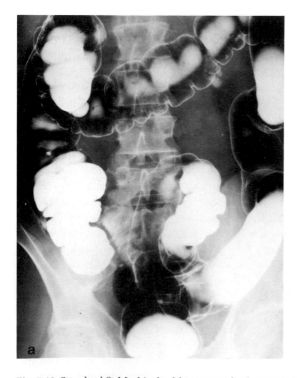 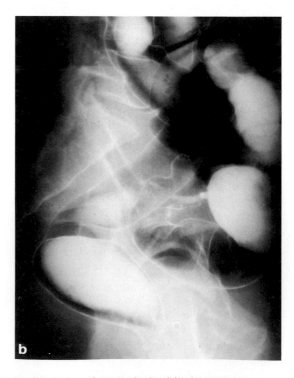

Fig. 5.10 Standard St Mark's double-contrast barium enema series: (a) prone with vertical tube, (b) left lateral pelvis.

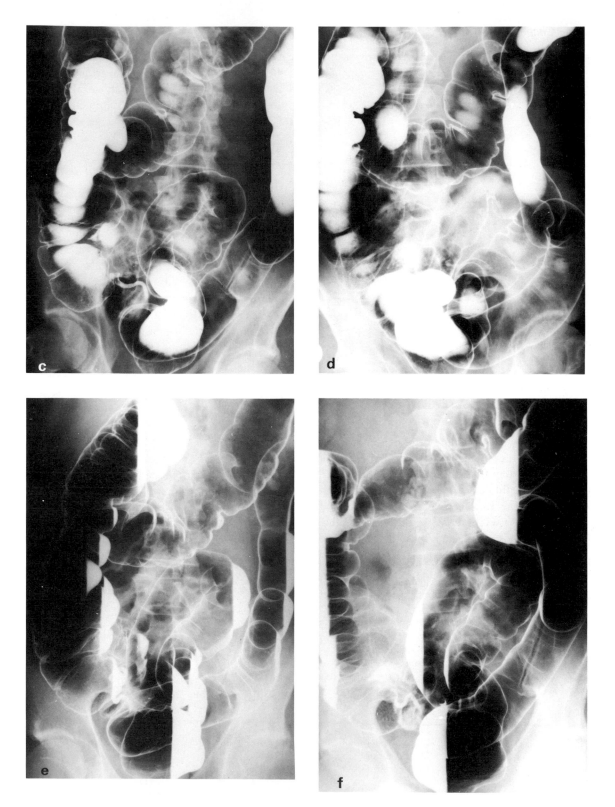

Fig. 5.10 *Continued.* (c) Supine right posterior oblique, (d) supine left posterior oblique, (e) posteroanterior decubitus with horizontal beam and left side down, (f) anteroposterior decubitus with horizontal beam and right side down.

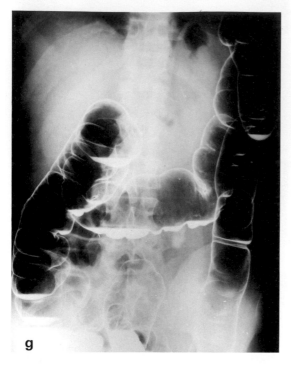

g

Fig. 5.10 *Continued.* (g) Erect.

in the rectosigmoid, which is a difficult segment to visualize. This will be shown on the lateral pelvic view, provided the rectosigmoid has been drained adequately. If this has been performed correctly, a prone cross table will not usually add much to the combination of spot films and decubitus views.

A post-evacuation radiograph is of no value in the DCBE. If an area requires further investigation, spot views with more barium/gas should be taken as required. If the DCBE quality is poor, supplement with an SCBE examination.

Variations on basic technique

'Sigmoid flush'

This is used in patients with severe diverticular disease to improve visualization of the affected bowel. 500–700 ml of dilute barium suspension is run in at the end of a standard DCBE, and spot radiographs taken of the filled sigmoid and descending colon. The numerous rings formed in DCBE are easier to interpret in SCBE. The dense barium adheres to the mucosa, while the dilute suspension gives a see-through effect that is said to improve imaging in up to 75% of cases (Lappas *et al.*, 1988).

Colostomy enema

A non-wash-out bowel preparation is strongly advised in patients with a colostomy. They must be warned to expect a large stomal output.

A standard suspension may be used, the problem being how to administer it. The safest way is to use either a proprietary colostomy tip (see Fig. 5.6) or to construct a similar device from a Foley catheter (Goldstein & Miller, 1976). First cut the balloon of a

Table 5.6 Remote control table — no decubitus radiography. From Gelfand *et al.* (1991)

Area of interest	Patient position	Radiograph size (cm)	Table position
Sigmoid*	Prone	24 × 30	Horizontal
Rectum	Right lateral	24 × 30	
Sigmoid*	Supine	24 × 30	
	Turn patient twice to coat colon thoroughly		
Entire colon	Straight	35 × 43	Upright
Hepatic flexure	Turn to left	24 × 30	
Splenic flexure	Turn to right	24 × 30	
Entire colon	Prone	35 × 43	Horizontal
	Right posterior oblique	35 × 43	
	Left posterior oblique	35 × 43	
	Left posterior oblique	35 × 43	
Caecum	Supine	24 × 30	Head down 20°

* Tube may be angled to obtain the best view of the sigmoid.

Table 5.7 Sequence of manoeuvres and spot radiographs with digital imaging or 100 mm camera

Action	Spot radiographs
Smooth muscle relaxant (i.v.)	
Patient prone, fill with barium to transverse colon	
Head up 30°, drain rectum	
Turn onto left side, then prone, left side, and supine insufflating gas	Supine right anterior oblique Lateral rectum
Turn prone	Prone left posterior oblique
Check transverse colon filling. If less than half filled, turn left side to prone with gas insufflation, or left side to supine to right side to move barium column around splenic flexure	
Turn onto right side to fill ascending colon, bring head up to trap and turn prone to fill caecum	
Supine — turn twice clockwise	
Turn onto right side, bring table upright, insufflate to distend flexures	Erect views of hepatic and splenic flexures, turning to open out flexure
Table flat, patient supine, check gas distension	Transverse colon
Bring left side up	Descending colon
Turn onto right side to maximize double-contrast view of ascending colon and clear barium	Ascending colon
Supine left anterior oblique view of caecum with compression	Caecum

Overhead radiographs
Right and left decubitus views with horizontal beam
Prone with 30° caudal angulation
Left lateral pelvis or prone cross table with horizontal beam if spot views inadequate

Foley catheter, and then fit an infant bottle feeding nipple over this, having cut a suitably sized hole in the end. The catheter is advanced for about 15 cm through the nipple and is then inserted into the stoma until the nipple acts as a bung in the stoma. Some gauze swabs, with a central cut, are placed around the nipple and the patient's hand is used to hold this in place. The suspension is run in through the main tube and gas is introduced through the side-arm.

An alternative is gently to insert the balloon of a 16F Foley catheter into the colostomy and inflate the balloon with 10 ml of air. Stop inflating immediately if resistance is felt or the patient experiences pain. There is a theoretical risk of rupturing any prestomal stricture. However, the Foley balloon is still pliable when distended with only this amount of air. It is a good idea to examine the colostomy first with the gloved finger in order to ascertain if there is any fixed narrowing. Having used the same system for ileostomy enemas, the author has not encountered any difficulty. The seal from the distended balloon inside the stoma is much more effective. This technique may also be used with the patient's bag *in situ*. A small hole cut in the bag allows catheter access, so that any spillage is contained within the bag.

The colon should be filled to the mid-transverse colon, the patient turned onto the right side and gas insufflated. Screen and rotate the patient to manipulate the column around the hepatic flexure, then bring the head up to trap it in the ascending colon.

Stand the patient completely upright to move the column into the caecum. Next return the table to the horizontal and turn the patient from side to side to improve coating. It is usually impractical to turn the patient prone. The catheter is then spigoted and a series of spot radiographs taken, supplemented by two decubitus views.

'Instant' barium enema

The instant enema was developed by Young (1963) to show the extent and severity of known colitis, where the upper extent was not visible on sigmoidoscopy. No bowel preparation is required as residue does not accumulate in a segment of active colitis. It is therefore possible to run in a little barium, distend the bowel with gas and take just a few radiographs to map out the colitis. The technique works best in ulcerative colitis where the disease is in continuity, but gives acceptable results in Crohn's colitis, particularly with advanced disease (Patel & Bartram, 1993). Bowel preparation may be distressing for colitics and possibly dangerous. Osmotic balanced solutions are recommended for colitics where bowel preparation is required, for example to exclude malignancy, as there is no systematic disturbance from these agents.

A preliminary plain radiograph is recommended to exclude toxic megacolon or perforation, which are absolute contraindications to an instant enema. In an acute attack, the plain radiograph may give sufficient information on the extent and severity of the colitis, so that a contrast examination is unnecessary.

It is helpful to give an i.v. smooth muscle relaxant, as colitics often have considerable spasm during filling. The colon should be filled until either residue is encountered or the transverse colon is reached. The rectum is then drained and gas is very gently insufflated, turning the patient as required. A prone radiograph is often all that is required. A lateral pelvic view will show the size of the rectum, and an erect radiograph the flexures and transverse colon in double contrast (Fig. 5.11). There is little advantage in taking more than three views. The examination is designed to answer a clinical problem with the minimum of disturbance and danger to the patient.

Based on the experience at St Mark's Hospital of more than 8500 examinations, there is no evidence that an instant enema causes any deterioration in the colitis. Balloon catheters are contraindicated. Retention of barium proximal to active colitis is common and of no clinical effect.

Water-soluble contrast enema

A water-soluble contrast medium is indicated where there is risk of peritoneal contamination, or where its lower viscosity than barium may be an advantage. Any agent may be used, such as Urografin 150 or Gastrografin*. Gastrografin is isotonic at 1 : 5 dilution with water, but contrast is then too low. It is used normally at a 1 : 3 dilution for the colon. This is still hypertonic, small volumes causing diarrhoea. Giving more than 750 ml should be avoided. In children non-ionic agents are much safer and the added expense is justified.

Anastomoses may be examined on about the tenth day to exclude leaks (Shorthouse *et al.*, 1982). It is safer to use a 16F Foley catheter than a rigid rectal enema tip, particularly if there is a low anastomosis. A 16F is an easy push fit over the tubing of a disposable bag for the contrast medium. The balloon must not be inflated. Contrast medium is run in and two radiographs, a supine (Fig. 5.12) and a lateral, are taken of the distended anastomosis. A small track or pouch indicates a leak into a sealed cavity around the anatomosis. If there is free intraperitoneal spread, immediately cease running in contrast medium and drain as much as possible to minimize peritoneal contamination (Fig. 5.13).

A water-soluble contrast enema may differentiate large bowel obstruction from pseudo-obstruction (Chapman *et al.*, 1992); 500 ml of dilute Gastrografin or Urografin 150 is usually sufficient. Oblique views of the sigmoid loop, an angled and straight prone with appropriate spot radiographs, are recommended. Buscopan 20 mg i.v. should be given when an obstruction is encountered, in order to make absolutely sure it is not due to spasm. As much contrast medium as possible is drained out at the end of the study and the referring physician asked to ensure that the patient is kept well hydrated.

Narrow fistulae may be difficult to see and a more concentrated Gastrografin with a 1 : 2 dilution is rec-

*Schering Health Care Ltd, Burgess Hill, West Sussex, UK.

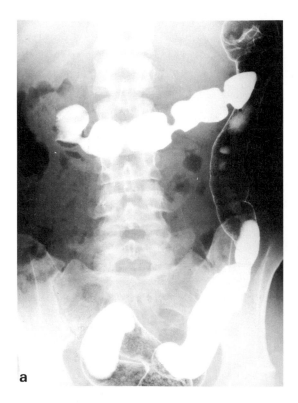

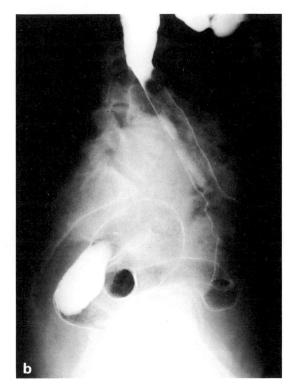

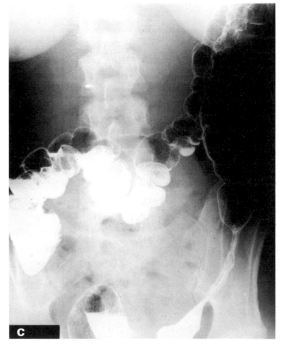

Fig. 5.11 Instant enema in ulcerative colitis extending into the mid-transverse colon. (a) Prone view with faecal residue extending into the transverse colon. Granular mucosa can be seen in double contrast in the descending colon. (b) Left lateral view of the pelvis showing a narrowed rectosigmoid. (c) Erect view with double contrast of the flexures and transverse colon.

ommended. For rectosigmoid fistulae this should be run in slowly with the patient screened in the lateral position. Spot radiographs must be taken immediately the fistula is seen, otherwise it may be obscured by filling of the other viscus (i.e. vagina, small bowel or bladder).

If a plain abdominal radiograph in chronic constipation shows gross faecal retention, bowel preparation should not be attempted and a water-soluble contrast enema performed to outline the configuration of the distal large bowel. This will exclude any obstructing lesion and distinguish Hirschsprung's disease from megarectum.

Complications

These may be related to preparation, contrast agents

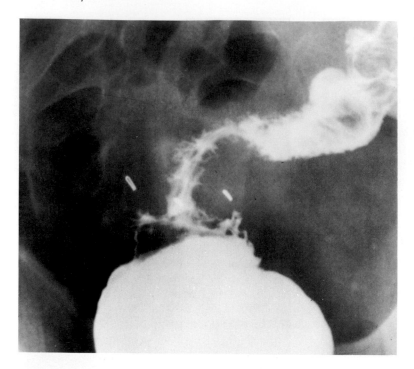

Fig. 5.12 Water-soluble contrast enema of an intact anastomosis (marked by a metal clip).

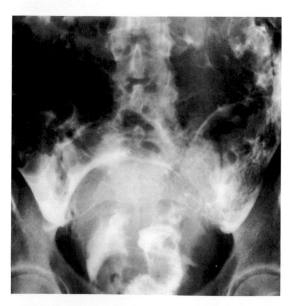

Fig. 5.13 Water-soluble contrast enema with gross disruption of a low rectal anastomosis leading to free peritoneal spillage of contrast.

and pharmacological agents, as well as trauma to the bowel.

During bowel preparation, electrolyte disturbance may result in cardiac failure or arrhythmia and may be compounded by the presence of renal failure. Water intoxication is a possible complication of a cleansing water enema if the patient has become very dehydrated or if a large volume of enema is given to a small child. Detergent or soap enemas should not be used, as these interfere with mucosal coating and may cause a caustic colitis. Colonic obstruction with perforation may result from residue impacting in a stricture and high intracolonic pressures generated by the purgative exceeding the integrity of the bowel wall.

Buscopan given i.v. produces a dry mouth and about 10% suffer with blurred near vision, which only lasts about 20 min (Skucas, 1994). Tachycardia may result in hypertension if the patient is receiving ß-blockers. Acute glaucoma is precipitated only in the rarer closed angle type of glaucoma. The risk of using Buscopan in patients with glaucoma is overemphasized. The main contraindications to its use are cardiac failure and arrhythmia.

Sensitivity reactions to the barium suspension are fortunately very rare. Anaphylactic reactions to latex balloon catheters have been reported. This is no longer a problem since the introduction of silicon rubber balloons (Gelfand, 1991). Balloon catheters are much more dangerous than standard enema tips. They may cause local trauma to the rectum and allow greater pressures to be generated in the colon (Nelson *et al.*, 1979). The bursting pressures of normal colon are approximately 81 mmHg for the caecum and 169 mmHg for the sigmoid. If the bowel wall is weakened by disease, it may rupture at a much lower pressure. A perforation rate of 1 in 12 000 is quoted for barium enemas (Gelfand, 1980), with very variable mortality figures. The figure for St Mark's Hospital is less than one in 25 000, and this low perforation rate is almost certainly because balloon catheters have never been used.

Perforation may be intra- or extraperitoneal. Intraperitoneal perforation is more common. Perforation may not be immediately obvious during screening and is sometimes not diagnosed until delayed radiographs are taken. Intraperitoneal perforation (Fig. 5.14) results in a massive serosal fluid exudate with hypovolaemia, which may be compounded by Gram-negative endotoxic shock. Immediate treatment with antibiotics, fluid replacement and peritoneal lavage is essential. The perforated segment may be stitched over or excised and protected by a temporary colostomy. Particles of barium sulphate remaining in the peritoneal cavity will cause a foreign-body reaction with the formation of dense adhesions.

Perforations may contain only gas, barium or both. Extraperitoneal perforation of gas may track retroperitoneally, causing retroperitoneal emphysema (Fig. 5.15). Symptoms from extraperitoneal perforation may be delayed until an abscess develops. Barium retention within the bowel wall from an intramural perforation creates a barium granuloma. These may develop into polypoid masses and be mistaken for malignant tumours. Barium crystals in the lesion are anisotropic in polarized light, and the diagnosis is easily proved on histology. Granulomas may also ulcerate, causing small perirectal abscesses.

Venous intravasation is fortunately very rare. Gas may be seen in the portal vein and intrahepatic divisions. The reticuloendothelial cells of the liver and spleen will filter out most of the barium, resulting in a hyperdense liver on CT, with figures of 138 Hounsfield units reported (Zaler *et al.*, 1993). Should barium enter

the systemic circulation, pulmonary embolism will result and carries a very high mortality.

Inadvertent insertion of the enema tip or balloon into the vagina may lacerate the vagina and cause bleeding, intra- or extraperitoneal perforation, systemic venous embolism, or peritoneal contamination from spillover secondary to a barium hysterosalpingogram (Carlsen *et al.*, 1992).

Transient bacteraemia may occur during any instrumentation or distension of the colon. DCBE is not a high-risk procedure, but antibiotic cover is recommended in patients with prosthetic heart valves or who are at risk from endocarditis for any reason. Gentamicin 80 mg and ampicillin 500 mg i.v. immediately prior to the examination provides adequate cover.

Patients with cardiac disease may have ST changes on electrocardiogram (ECG) during barium enema and can develop arrhythmias. Care in maintaining electrolyte balance in bowel preparation and using glucagon (not Buscopan) when there is a pre-existing arrhythmia will help prevent any major problem.

Balloon catheters are the major cause of perforation and should be used with care only when there is a significant risk of incontinence. If the balloon expands asymmetrically, it may impale the enema tip into the rectal wall and lacerate the mucosa (Nelson *et al.*, 1979). Overdistension of the balloon may rupture the rectum. It is important to use properly designed balloons and to inflate them only to the manufacturers' recommended volume. The balloon should act as a bung in the ampulla, occluding the weakened anal sphincters, not in the rectum. Rectal distension invokes the rectoanal reflex which lowers anal tone. Excessive balloon distension is therefore not only very dangerous, but is also likely to make the patient more incontinent.

Balloon catheters should never be used where the rectum is abnormal, as in colitis, following radiation therapy or where there is a low anastomosis. Much greater pressure can be generated in the colon when insufflating with a balloon catheter *in situ*. If there is any focal weakness in the bowel wall, as from ulceration in colitis or from diverticulitis, perforation may occur at relatively low pressures. The standard enema tips provide a natural safety valve which prevents overdistension. The proof of the safety of the DCBE without balloon catheters is reflected by the much lower incidence of perforation at St Mark's

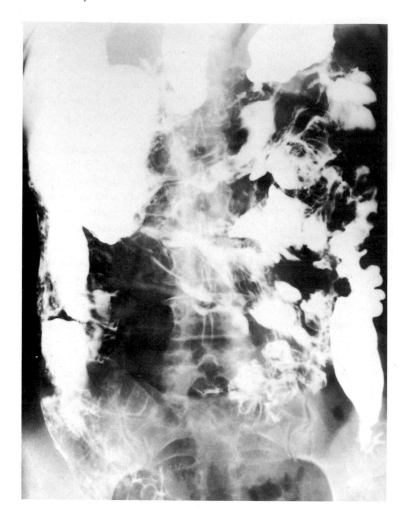

Fig. 5.14 Intraperitoneal perforation during a colostomy enema, due to rupture of a diverticular abscess at the splenic flexure. Barium has spread throughout the peritoneal cavity with large collections in the lesser sac and right subphrenic and subhepatic spaces.

Hospital, where they have never been used. Balloon catheters are implicated in almost all reports of perforation.

After rectal biopsy, a 7-day interval before barium enema is advised to allow mucosal regrowth over the biopsy site. The risk, however, is slight. Any decision to perform an examination immediately after biopsy should be made in conjunction with the clinician. Colonoscopic biopsies, except for the 'jumbo' type, are superficial and no delay is required.

Barium will take several days to clear completely after a DCBE. Proximal retention of barium for a number of days after an instant enema is common when there is severely active distal colitis, but does not seem to be of clinical significance. If the patient becomes obstructed after a barium enema, barium fluid levels indicate that the suspension has remained fluid and is not contributing to the obstruction.

Most water-soluble contrast agents used in the colon are hypertonic and will draw in fluid. This can be dangerous when the contrast medium becomes trapped proximal to an obstruction. Gross distension of the proximal segment leading to perforation has been reported. A sudden reduction in circulating blood volume might be critical in a small child and, as mentioned above, non-ionic media are indicated to prevent this.

Relationship of the barium enema to other investigations

If a patient is to have both the small and large intestines examined, the small bowel should be studied

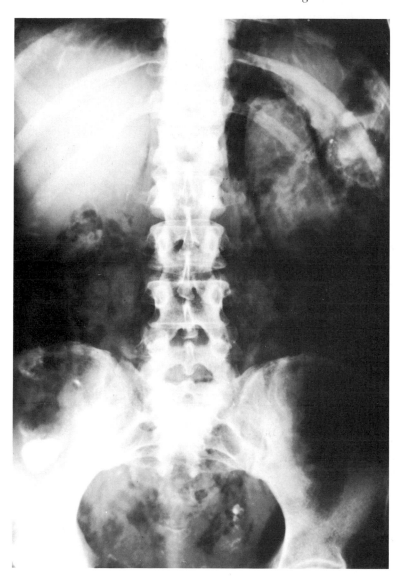

Fig. 5.15 Retroperitoneal emphysema following sigmoidoscopy and rectal biopsy.

first. The stomach and small bowel will be clear of barium within a few hours. Standard bowel preparation should be adequate to clear the barium from the colon. Both examinations may then be completed within a 48-hour period. If the barium enema is performed first, the patient will either have to wait several days until all the barium has cleared from the colon or have further purgation. This will not only inconvenience the patient, but adds to the time needed to perform both examinations.

The prepared bowel is an ideal setting for abdominal ultrasound, as there is no residue and the bowel is not usually gassy. It is therefore simple to combine it with a DCBE. Bowel preparation is not standard prior to CT or MRI and, if these are performed after a DCBE, the patient will require further bowel preparation. In water-soluble contrast enemas, the contrast medium is too high a density for CT and may be retained for several days, so that some mild bowel preparation may still be required prior to CT.

Rigid sigmoidoscopy reaches only as far as the distal sigmoid colon. Flexible sigmoidoscopy is becoming more routine and can be used to examine the entire sigmoid, often up to the splenic flexure. This complements the DCBE, which is least accurate in the sigmoid. Flexible sigmoidoscopy with a modified DCBE, limiting the number of radiographs as the sigmoid has already been examined, has been shown to be an accurate method to screen for colonic neoplasia (Hough *et al.*, 1994).

Total colonoscopy is technically difficult in 25%, and the caecum is reached in only 75% of studies outside specialized centres. In many centres a common reason for DCBE referral is incomplete colonoscopy. This may be performed at a later date, but it is possible to perform a DCBE after endoscopy, following a short delay to allow the patient to recover from any sedation. If a decision to proceed to DCBE is made, the endoscopist should arrange to have as much gas and retained fluid sucked out as possible. If any small polyps have been diathermied, these may leave small artefacts (Bartram & Hall-Craggs, 1987). The decision to proceed to DCBE after the removal of any larger polyp should be the responsibility of the endoscopist.

Cross-sectional imaging of the large bowel

The normal colonic wall may be visualized on transabdominal sonography with graded compression, but is more clearly demarcated by distending the bowel with water (Walter *et al.*, 1993). The bowel wall may be precisely detailed on CT with gas distension after bowel preparation. Routinely, 2% oral and rectal contrast medium is given without bowel preparation. Water or 12.5% fat emulsions have been used for negative contrast of the bowel lumen in CT to highlight post-contrast enhancement of the wall. Various contrast agents have also been tried with MRI to obtain either a high or a low luminal signal.

Functional assessment of the large bowel

Transit studies assess the time taken for markers to pass through the large bowel and are used to diagnose slow transit constipation. The simplest method is to cut up a radio-opaque catheter into 20 short

2–4 mm segments. The patient swallows these at breakfast time. A plain abdominal film is taken 120 hours later to show how many remain — normal is less than five; more than five implies slow transit. During the study period the patient should eat normally but not take any laxative. The examination may be refined by using three different shapes (20 of each), given on days 1, 2 and 3, with a radiograph taken on day 6. There should be less than four of marker type A, less than six of marker type B and less than 12 of marker type C left. An excess of any type of marker is taken to indicate slow transit (Evans *et al.*, 1992). This makes allowance for any bowel action. With only one set of markers, a bowel action early in the study period might clear the markers, although the overall bowel frequency and transit were abnormal during the time of examination.

Evacuation proctography, 'videoproctography' or 'defaecography' as the examination may be called, is a test of voluntary rectal evacuation. The rectum is prepared, either by full bowel preparation or glycerine suppositories, and filled with a thick barium paste. This may be prepared by mixing barium with potato starch, using oesophageal creams or specially formulated pastes. Bladder syringes are filled with the paste, carefully inserted via the anal canal and the contrast medium injected into the rectum. A minimum of 120 ml is used. The patient then sits sideways in the screening unit, on a special commode placed on the foot-rest with the table upright. The commode must incorporate some added filtration (equivalent to 4 mm of copper) to prevent screen flare out (Bartram *et al.*, 1988). A video recording is made of fluoroscopy of the rectum at rest, some recommend during pelvic floor contraction and straining (Shorvon *et al.*, 1989), then during evacuation of the rectal paste.

References

Bartram, C.I. (1989) Technical note: a simple method for using carbon dioxide during double contrast barium enema. *Clin. Radiol.*, **40**, 318.

Bartram, C.I. (1994) Bowel preparation — principles and practice. *Clin. Radiol.*, **49**, 365–7.

Bartram, C.I. & Hall-Craggs, M.A. (1987) Interventional colorectal endoscopic procedures: residual lesions on follow-up double contrast barium enema study. *Radiology*, **162**, 835–8.

Bartram, C.I., Turnbull, G.K. & Lennard-Jones, J.E. (1988) Evacuation proctography: an investigation of rectal expulsion in 20 subjects without defaecatory disturbance. *Gastrointest. Radiol.*, **13**, 72–80.

Brown, G.R. (1961) A new approach to colon preparation for barium enema: preliminary report. *Univ. Mich. Med. Bull.*, **27**, 225–30.

Carlsen, S.E., Thumond, A.S., Scanlen, R.M. & Patton, P.E. (1992) Inadvertent barium hysterosalpingography. *AJR*, **159**, 547–9.

Chapman, A.H., McNamara, M. & Porter, G. (1992) The acute contrast enema in suspected large bowel obstruction: value and technique. *Clin. Radiol.*, **46**, 273–8.

Conry, B.G., Jones, S. & Bartram, C.I. (1978) The effect of oral magnesium-containing bowel preparation agents on mucosal coating of barium sulphate suspensions. *Br. J. Radiol.*, **60**, 1215–19.

De Lacey, G., Wignall, B. & Ambrose, J. (1978) The double contrast barium enema: improvements to lateral decubitus views including the use of a wedge filter. *Clin. Radiol.*, **29**, 197–9.

Dobranowski, J., Stringer, D.A., Somers, S. & Stevenson, G.W. (1990) *Procedures in Gastrointestinal Radiology.* Springer Verlag, New York.

Evans, R.C., Kamm, M.A., Hinton, J.M. & Lennard-Jones, J.E. (1992) The normal range and a simple diagram for recording whole gut transit time. *Int. J. Colorect. Dis.*, **7**, 15–17.

Fitzsimons, P., Shorvon, P., Frost, R.A. & Stevenson, G.W. (1987) A comparison of Golytely and standard preparation for barium enema. *J. Can Assoc. Radiol.*, **38**, 109–12.

Gelfand, D.W. (1980) Complications of gastrointestinal radiologic procedures: I. Complications of routine fluoroscopic studies. *Gastrointest. Radiol.*, **5**, 293–7.

Gelfand, D.W. (1991) Barium enemas, latex balloons and anaphylactic reactions. *AJR*, **156**, 1–2.

Gelfand, D.W., Chen, Y.M. & Ott, D.J. (1991) Radiologic detection of colonic neoplasms: benefits of a system analysis approach. *AJR*, **156**, 303–6.

Goldstein, H.M. & Miller, R.E. (1976) Air contrast colon examination in patients with colostomies. *AJR*, **127**, 607–9.

Hough, D.M., Malone, D.E., Rawlinson, J. *et al.* (1994) Colon cancer detection: an algorithm using endoscopy and barium enema. *Clin. Radiol.*, **49**, 170–5.

Lappas, J.C., Maglinte, D.T., Kopecky, K.K., Cockerill, E.M. & Lehman, G.A. (1988) Diverticular disease: imaging with post-double-contrast sigmoid flush. *Radiology*, **168**, 35–7.

Lawrance, J.A.L., Massoud, T.F., Creasy, T.S., Shatwell, W.,

Mason, A. & Nolan, D.J. (1994) Colonic preparation with Picolax: patient tolerance and approaches to fluid replacement. *Clin. Radiol.*, **49**, 35–37.

Lee, S.H. & Bartram, C.I. (1990), Determining the minimal interval between cleansing water enema and double-contrast barium enema examination. *Clin. Radiol.*, **41**, 331–2.

Matsuura, K., Nakata, H., Takeda, N. *et al.* (1977) Innominate lines of the colon. *Radiology.*, **123**, 41–4.

McLean, A. & Bartram, C.I. (1985) Prone compression with the pneumatic paddle during barium studies. *Clin. Radiol.*, **36**, 213–15.

Miller, R.E. (1975) The cleansing enema. *Radiology*, **117**, 483.

Miller, R.E. (1979) Solution for the 'air block' problem during fluoroscopy. *AJR*, **132**, 1020–1.

Miller, R.E. & Peterson, G.H. (1978) Drainage of the rectum: a simple manoeuvre to improve the accuracy of colon examinations. *Radiology*, **128**, 506–7.

Nelson, J.A., Daniels, A.U. & Dodds, W.J. (1979) Rectal balloons: complications, causes, and recommendations. *Invest. Radiol.*, **14**, 48–59.

Niizuma, S. & Kobayashi, S. (1977) Rectosigmoid double contrast examination in the prone position with a horizontal beam. *AJR*, **128**, 591–3.

Patel, U. & Bartram, C.I. (1993) Utility of the instant (unprepared) enema in Crohn's colitis. *Clin. Radiol.*, **47**, 351–4.

Peterson, G.H. & Miller, R.E. (1978) The barium enema: a reassessment towards perfection. *Radiology*, **128**, 315–20.

Scholz, F.J. (1993) How to do a perfect, comfortable air-contrast enema. In *22nd meeting of the Society of Gastrointestinal Radiologists, Scottsdale.*

Shorthouse, A.J., Bartram, C.I., Eyers, A.A. & Thomson, J.P.S. (1982) The water soluble contrast enema after rectal anastomosis. *Br. J. Surg.*, **69**, 714–17.

Shorvon, P.J., McHugh, S., Diamant, N.E., Somers, S.E. & Stevenson, G.W. (1989) Defecography in normal volunteers: results and implications. *Gut*, **30**, 1737–49.

Skucas, J. (1994) The use of antispasmodic drugs during barium enema. *AJR*, **162**, 1323–5.

Taylor, P.N. & Beckly, D.E. (1991) Use of air in double contrast barium enema — is it still acceptable? *Clin. Radiol.*, **44**, 183–5.

Walter, D.F., Govil, S., William, R.R., Bhargava, N. & Chandy G. (1993) Colonic sonography: preliminary observations. *Clin. Radiol.*, **47**, 200–4.

Young, A.C. (1963) The instant barium enema in proctocolitis. *Proc. Roy. Soc. Med.*, **56**, 491–4.

Zaler, A.H., Warren, R.E. & Burnstein, M.J. (1993) Venous intravasation of barium: CT findings. *J. Comp. Assist. Tomogr.*, **17**, 813–15.

6   Biliary Tract

J. P. OWEN

Oral cholecystography (OCG)

In 1910 Abel and Rowntree reported that several phenolphthalein compounds were mainly excreted by the liver and appeared in the gallbladder some hours after ingestion (Abel & Rowntree, 1910). Based on these studies, the first successful cholecystogram was performed in 1923 by Graham and Cole on a fasting dog following the injection of tetrabromophenolphthalein (Graham & Cole, 1924).

Indications

OCG was traditionally used as a first-line investigation when the clinical history and examination suggested non-acute gallbladder disease. Ultrasound (US) has largely replaced its role for the initial diagnosis of the presence of gallstones but the OCG is probably the best initial test for determining the number and size of gallstones, cystic duct patency and gallbladder wall pathology (Maglinte *et al.*, 1991). There is a role for OCG in the work-up of patients for non-surgical gallstone treatments such as oral dissolution therapy, direct contact solvent dissolution therapy and extracorporeal shock-wave lithotripsy (Plaisier *et al.*, 1994).

Contraindications

OCG is contraindicated in the following:
1 Pregnancy.
2 Patients in combined hepatic and renal failure.
3 Known hypersensitivity to iodine.
4 Less than 14 days after an i.v. cholangiogram.
5 Acute cholecystitis.
Since the major pathways for elimination of the oral media are liver and kidney, the simultaneous failure of both organs is a recipe for potential disaster.

The reasons for avoiding the 14-day period be-tween OCG and an i.v. cholangiogram will be covered below (p. 81).

Regarding failure of gallbladder opacification in acute cholecystitis, Lasser (1966) showed that *Escherichia coli* deconjugated the conjugated contrast medium in the gallbladder and that the unconjugated contrast medium was rapidly reabsorbed by the gallbladder because of its lipid solubility.

There is a decreased likelihood of the examination being successful when there is elevation of the serum bilirubin, or elevation of the liver alkaline phosphatase even when there is a normal serum bilirubin level. These biochemical parameters may indicate hepatocyte dysfunction, the handling of the contrast medium by the liver depending on intact liver cells (Owen *et al.*, 1980).

Contrast media (Tables 6.1 & 6.2)

OCG media are tri-iodinated benzoic acid derivatives with iodine atoms at positions 2, 4 and 6, and incompletely substituted with a vacancy at position 5 on the nucleus (Fig. 6.1). In this respect they differ from the completely substituted water-soluble urographic agents. The incomplete substitution with the vacant position causes the media to be bound to protein. Mudge (1980) showed that the oral agent iopanoic acid was reversibly bound to human serum albumin at separate binding sites. Protein binding reduces the glomerular filtration and causes preferential excretion by the liver.

OCG media are absorbed via the small-intestinal mucosa but have variable rates of absorption. In the case of iopanoic acid, which has high lipid solubility but low aqueous solubility, absorption is probably by non-ionic diffusion. The aqueous solubility and hence absorption of iopanoic acid is increased by lowering the hydrogen ion concentration, which increases the degree of ionization (Taketa *et al.*, 1972),

Table 6.1. The metabolic pathway of oral cholecystographic media

Site	Activity	Solubility
Basic contrast medium		Iopanoic acid — predominantly lipid with weak aqueous solubility; other oral agents are also lipid-soluble but have greater aqueous solubility than iopanoic acid
Duodenum	To portal vein by non-ionic diffusion Absorption influenced by: (i) physical state of the contrast medium; (ii) pH in bowel lumen; and (iii) presence of bile salts: affects iopanoic acid absorption only	
Portal vein	Binding to serum albumin	No information about bound moiety
Hepatocytes	Albumen bond broken Contrast medium enters hepatocytes by a rate-limiting active transport mechanism	
	Conjugation with glucoronic acid To bile via an active-transport mechanism	Glucoronide conjugate is water-soluble
Bile-ducts	Transport to gallbladder	Water-soluble
Gallbladder	Reabsorption of water, hence concentration of contrast medium in bile	Water-soluble
Fate of contrast medium	Excretion of unabsorbed contrast medium in faeces	Lipid-soluble
	Deconjugation and enterohepatic circulation	Lipid-soluble
	Excretion of conjugate in faeces	Water-soluble
	Excretion of conjugate in urine	Water-soluble

and by increasing the bile salt flow (Goldberger *et al.*, 1974) particularly the taurocholate excretion (Berk *et al.*, 1980). Conversely, the more water-soluble oral media, such as sodium tyropanoate and sodium ipodate, have no such dependence on bile salts (Berk *et al.*, 1977).

The physical state of the oral media in the bowel is also important in determining the rate of absorption. The acid-precipitated sodium salt of iopanoic acid, which has small crystals, is more soluble and more readily absorbed than commercially available iopanoic acid, which has larger crystals and a smaller surface to weight ratio (Goldberger *et al.*, 1974).

The molecules of contrast media are bound to the portal blood plasma albumin (Lasser, 1966) although some unbound contrast medium may be temporarily stored in fat, blood, muscle and other organs including the liver (Dunn & Berk, 1972). Cholecystographic media are removed from the blood by the liver via a rate-limiting active-transport process and undergo conjugation with glucuronic acid in the hepatocytes, whence they are actively transported into the bile (Lasser, 1966). The active-transport mechanism is overloaded by excessive contrast medium so that, above a threshold value, increasing the rate of administration of the contrast medium produces no significant change in its biliary excretion rate. However, increasing the total dosage of the contrast

Table 6.2 Oral cholecystographic media

Generic name	UK trade name	Molecular weight of salt	Iodine content of salt (%)	Preparation	Iodine content of preparation
Currently available in UK (1995)					
Iopanoic acid	Telepaque (Sanofi-Winthrop Ltd)	571	66.7	Tablets containing 500 mg iopanoic acid	2.0 g from six tablets
Sodium ipodate	Biloptin (Schering Health Care Ltd)	620	61.4	Capsules containing 500 mg sodium ipodate	1.84 g from six capsules
Calcium ipodate	Solubiloptin (Schering Health Care Ltd)	1234	61.7	Sachet containing 3 g calcium ipodate	1.85 g from one sachet
Formerly marketed in UK					
Iopanoic acid	Cistobil (E. Merck Pharmaceuticals)	571	66.7	—	—
Iocetamic acid	Cholebrin (Napp Laboratories)	614	62.0	—	—
Iopronic acid	Bilimiro (E. Merck Pharmaceuticals)	673	56.6	—	—

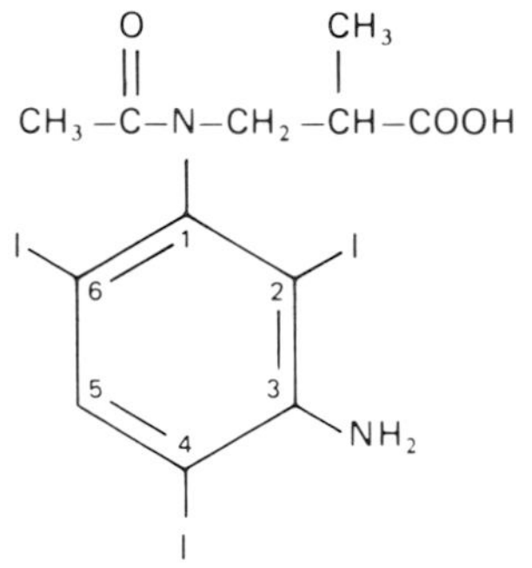

O   CH₃
‖ |
CH₃ –C–N–CH₂ –CH–COOH

Fig. 6.1 Iocetamic acid (Cholebrin) — a typical oral cholecystographic agent. Note the incomplete substitution at position 5 on the nucleus.

medium does increase the biliary iodine concentrations of some media, such as iopanoic acid, sodium tyropanoate and sodium ipodate, but not iopronic acid (Amberg *et al.*, 1980). Increased doses of iopronic acid and sodium ipodate were usually associated with increased biliary excretion rates, the effect being less marked with iopanoic acid and sodium tyropanoate. The glucuronide conjugates are less lipid-soluble than the free acid, which prevents them from being reabsorbed via the bile-ducts and gallbladder.

The time from oral administration of ipodate to peak concentration in the bile-ducts in humans is about 3 hours, within a range of 1–5 hours (Sperber & Sperber, 1971). In the non-inflamed gallbladder, the glucuronide conjugate is concentrated by reabsorption of water from the bile. The time from duodenal absorption to maximum concentration of the conjugate in the gallbladder is 14–19 hours. The optimal time to radiograph patients following oral administration of the contrast medium is, therefore, at 3 hours for the bile-ducts and 14–19 hours for the gallbladder. In practice, this is usually achieved by giving a divided dose of the contrast medium at 3 and 14 hours before the radiographic examination.

The urinary excretion of a standard dose of oral contrast media in humans is very variable: 10–45% for iopanoate and 21–57% for ipodate (McChesney, 1971). False urinary tests for albumin have been recorded after the administration of OCG agents (Samen, 1962).

The non-absorbed contrast medium and the excreted conjugates are both excreted in faeces. Some of the conjugate may be deconjugated by intestinal organisms, being reconverted into the lipid-soluble free contrast medium with some enterohepatic recirculation.

Patient preparation

There is some controversy regarding dietary preparation for OCG. Bile salts are important in promoting the intestinal absorption of iopanoic acid by a postulated allosteric interaction between the bile salts and the carrier for iopanoic acid (Berk *et al.*, 1974). This suggests that stimulating gallbladder emptying by the ingestion of a meal rich in fat, before the iopanoic acid is taken, would increase the amount of bile salt in the intestinal lumen and thus enhance absorption of the contrast medium. No such dependence on bile salts was found with the more water-soluble agents, sodium tyropanoate and sodium ipodate (Berk *et al.*, 1977). On this evidence, a high-fat diet prior to the examination should improve gallbladder visualization with iopanoic acid but not with other, more water-soluble, agents. Loeb *et al.* (1978) confirmed that iopanoic acid absorption was enhanced when given with a meal containing protein and fat but was impaired when administered to fasting volunteers. Most manufacturers recommend a restricted fat intake on the evening before the oral examination, in line with an early clinical study (Whitehouse, 1956) but subsequent series have failed to show any benefits for dietary restriction of fat (Parkin, 1973).

Patients are often instructed to drink at least 0.5–1 litre of water after ingestion of the contrast medium, the rationale being to prevent nephrotoxicity from the uricosuric actions of the OCG agents (Mudge, 1971).

It is advisable to stop smoking before radiological investigations of the biliary tract, in order that the response of the biliary tract to nicotine cannot interfere with contrast opacification. Since nicotine is capable of activating both the parasympathetic and sympathetic parts of the autonomic nervous system, it is likely that it has variable effects on the tone and motility of the gallbladder and sphincteric contraction. Cigarette smoking reduces biliary secretion but increases biliary flow into the duodenum (Koehler *et al.*, 1947).

Normal radiographic technique (Hodgson, 1970; Bryan, 1979)

There should be a radiographic table with an overcouch tube, an undercouch and vertical Bucky, and a facility for tomography. An oblique position projects the gallbladder clear of the spine. There are two methods.
1 Left anterior oblique (LAO), with the patient prome and the right side raised off the table with 20° of obliquity. The centring point is 7.5 cm to the right of the L3 spinous process and 2.5 cm cephalad to the level of the lower costal margin.
2 Right posterior oblique (RPO), with the patient supine and left side raised off the table with 10° of obliquity. Occasionally, greater obliquity is required in order to project the bile-ducts clear of the spine. The centring point is 7.5 cm to the right of L3 and 4.5 cm cephalad.

A low kilovoltage is preferred for maximum soft-tissue differentiation. For a person of average build, using a fast film/screen combination, typical factors are 65–75 kV, 100 mA and 0.2 s.

A short exposure time and the use of compression bands gives a sharp radiographic image. The radiographs should include an area bounded laterally by the tissues of the flank, medially by the lumbar spine, superiorly by the dome of the diaphragm and inferiorly by the right iliac crest.

While some have suggested that the control radiograph may not be essential, others have found that 6% of opaque calculi would be missed if this film were omitted (Twomey *et al.*, 1983).

Giving the contrast medium

The contrast medium is given orally in two divided doses of 3 g each. The first dose is taken about 14 hours before the radiographic examination and should be in a concentrated glucoronated form in the gallbladder at the time of the radiographic study. The second dose, taken 3–4 hours before the examination, should be in a non-concentrated form in the bile-ducts at the time of the examination.

Radiographic examination after contrast medium

1 Prone oblique view as for preliminary film (Fig. 6.2a).
2 An erect radiograph (Fig. 6.2b) in one of the following positions:
   (a) in the LAO position with the abdomen towards the cassette and the right side raised away from the cassette, centring to the right of the spine about 5 cm below the centring point for the prone oblique projections;
   (b) the erect RPO position with the patient's back towards the cassette and the left side raised from the cassette, centring to the left of the spine about 5 cm below the centring point for the prone oblique projection.

The right lateral decubitus view is useful if the gallbladder is obscured by bowel gas on the prone or erect radiographs. The patient lies on the right side facing a vertical film, with centring for the posteroanterior (PA) projection to the right of the L2 or L3 vertebrae. An alternative method is to fluoroscope the gallbladder in the erect position and take spot radiographs.

A recent report suggests that imaging using computed radiography (photostimulable phosphor plate) greatly improves the diagnostic accuracy of the technique over film/screen combinations (Srivastava *et al.*, 1991).

Fatty meal

A further, coned, supine oblique radiograph of the gallbladder area is taken 30–60 min after the oral ingestion of a proprietary fatty emulsion such as Prosparol (Fig. 6.2c). The fatty meal invokes the action of endogenous cholecystokinin liberated from the duodenal mucosa. Its main values are as follows:
1 To evaluate gallbladder contractility.
2 To detect small filling defects such as stones or polyps.
3 To visualize the cystic and common ducts in greater detail.

Assessment of gallbladder contractility using ultrasound (US) following i.m. Ceruletide, a synthetic decapeptide with a chemical composition and pharmacological mode of action similar to cholecystokinin, is as reliable as OCG assessment following a fatty meal (Muraca *et al.*, 1994).

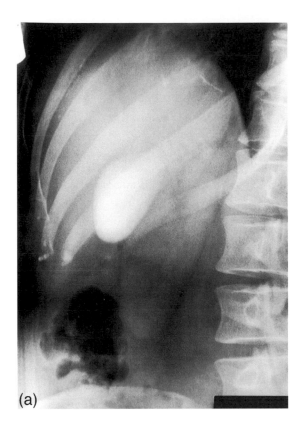

(a)

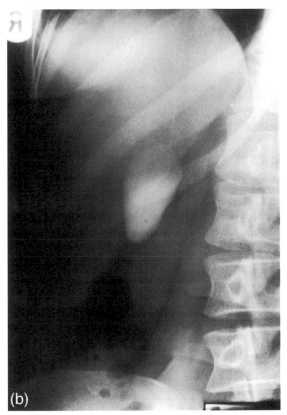

(b)

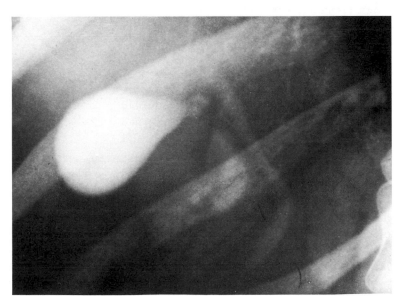

Fig. 6.2 Oral cholecystogram:
(a) prone oblique radiograph;
(b) erect position; (c) response of
gallbladder to oral fat.   (c)

The non-opacifying gallbladder

The causes of failure to opacify the gallbladder include the following:

1 Failure of the patient to take the contrast medium.

2 Failure to absorb the contrast medium in the presence of upper alimentary tract obstruction, such as in oesophageal stricture and pyloric stenosis; in duodenal disease, e.g. Crohn's disease and lymphoma; post-surgery, for example after ileal resection; and with acute diarrhoea.

3 Failure to transport the contrast medium. A low serum albumin would be a theoretical possibility.

4 Failure to conjugate the contrast medium, for example when there is hepatocyte dysfunction.

5 Failure to excrete the contrast medium into the bile, namely a failure of active transport.

6 Failure of the contrast medium to reach the gallbladder in cases of cystic or hepatic duct obstruction.

7 Failure of the gallbladder to function, as in severe chronic cholecystitis.

If liver function is normal, the degree of gall bladder opacification is inversely related to the severity of the chronic cholecystitis (Owen *et al.*, 1980b). In practice, the level of serum bilirubin above which the examination is unlikely to succeed is 2 mg% (34 µmol l^{-1}).

Variation of technique for failure to opacify the gallbladder

When the gallbladder is not visible after a conventional 6 g dose of oral contrast medium, a further 6 g of contrast medium is given in two 3 g doses and the patient returns for further radiographs the next day. The object is to almost saturate the active transport mechanism in the hepatocytes without exceeding the threshold level. Any further contrast medium would then be merely excreted by the kidneys, which could prove fatal in patients with a low creatinine clearance. If the conventional radiographs still fail to demonstrate the gallbladder, three further procedures may help.

1 A full-size abdominal radiograph in case the gallbladder has an ectopic situation.

2 Tomography. Linear or circular tomography are the movements of choice. Tomography is performed in the prone oblique position. Cuts should be taken at 0.5 or 1 cm intervals from 7–8 cm and may occasionally have to be as low as 4 cm in the obese. The potentials of the technique have been exhausted if there is failure of these manoeuvres.

3 Ultrasonography (see p. 95).

Complications (Ansell, 1978)

1 Minor side effects occur in 50% of cases and include nausea, vomiting, diarrhoea, headaches, abdominal pain, dysuria, dizziness and urticaria.

2 Hypotension and collapse in a few cases.

3 Myocardial infarction or cardiac arrest is a very rare complication.

4 A minor elevation of serum creatinine is a common occurrence.

5 The protein-bound iodine is elevated for up to 3 months. A few cases of thyrotoxicosis have been attributed to the procedure.

References

Abel, J.J. & Rowntree, L.G. (1910) On the pharmacological action of some phthaleins and their derivatives with especial reference to their behaviour as purgatives. *J. Pharmacol. Exp. Ther.*, **1**, 231–64.

Amberg, J.R., Thompson, W.M. & Goldberger, L. (1980) Factors in the intestinal absorption of oral cholecystopaques. *Invest. Radiol.*, **15**(Suppl.), S136–S141.

Ansell, G. (1978) Complications of X-ray investigations. In Davies, D.M. (ed.) *Adverse Drug Reaction Research Unit Bulletin*. Shotley Bridge General Hospital.

Berk, R.N., Barnhart, J.L. & Goldberger, L.E. (1980) The enhancement of iopanoate excretion by taurocholate. *Invest. Radiol.*, **15**(Suppl.), S116–S121.

Berk, R.N., Goldberger, L.E. & Loeb, P.M. (1974) The role of bile salts in the hepatic excretion of iopanoic acid. *Invest. Radiol.*, **9**, 7–15.

Berk, R.N., Loeb, P.M., Cobo-Frankel, A. *et al.* (1977) The biliary and urinary excretion of sodium tyropanoate and sodium ipodate in dogs: pharmacokinetics, influence of bile salts and choleric effects with comparison to iopanoic acid. *Invest. Radiol.*, **12**, 85.

Bryan, G.J. (1979), *Diagnostic Radiography*, 3rd edn., pp. 278–81. Churchill Livingstone, Edinburgh.

Dunn, C.R. & Berk, R.N. (1972) The pharmaco-kinetics of Telepaque metabolism: the relation of blood concentration and bile flow to the rate of hepatic excretion. *AJR*, **114**, 758–66.

Goldberger, L.E., Berk, R.N., Lang, J.H. *et al.* (1974) Biopharmaceutical factors influencing intestinal absorption of iopanoic acid. *Invest. Radiol.*, **9**, 16–23.

Graham, E. & Cole, W. (1924) Roentgenologic examination

of the gall bladder. *JAMA, 82*, 613–14.

Hodgson, J.R. (1970) The technical aspects of cholecystography. *Radiol. Clin. N. Am.,* 8(1), 85–97.

Koehler, A.E., Hill, E. & Marsh, N. (1947) The effect of cigarette smoking on malnutrition and digestion. *Gastroenterology,* **8**, 208–12.

Lasser, E.C. (1966) The pharmacodynamics of biliary contrast media. *Radiol. Clin. N. Am.,* 4(3), 511–19.

Loeb, P.M., Berk, R.N. & Janes, J.O. (1978) The effect of fasting on gall bladder opacification during oral cholecystography: a controlled study in normal volunteers. *Radiology,* **126**, 395–401.

Maglinte, D.D.T., Torres, W.E. & Laufer, I. (1991) Oral cholecystography in contemporary gallstone imaging: A review. *Radiology,* **178**, 49–58.

McChesney, E.W. (1971) *Routes and Rates of Excretion of Radio-contrast Agents.* Pergamon Press, Oxford.

Mudge, G.H. (1971) Uricosuric action of cholecystographic agents. *N. Engl. J. Med.,* **284**, 929–33.

Mudge, G.H. (1980) Cholecystographic agents and drug binding to plasma albumin. *Invest. Radiol.,* **15**, S102–S108.

Muraca, M., Cianci, V., Miconi, L. *et al.* (1994) Ultrasonic evaluation of gallbladder emptying with Ceruletide: comparison to oral cholecystography with fatty meal. *Abdom. Imaging,* **19**, 235–8.

Owen, J.P., Keir, M.J., Lavelle, M.I. *et al.* (1980a) Alkaline phosphatase and the oral cholecystogram. *Br. J. Radiol.,* **53**, 605–6.

Owen, J.P., McCarthy, J. & Makepeace, D. *et al.* (1980b) Chronic cholecystitis and the oral cholecystogram. *Clin. Radiol.,* **31**, 671–4.

Parkin, G.J.S. (1973) Dietary preparation for oral cholecystography — a critical reappraisal. *Br. J. Radiol.,* **47**, 452–3.

Plaisier, P.W., Brakel, K., ver der Hul, R.L. *et al.* (1994) Radiographic features of oral cholecystograms of 448 symptomatic gallstone patients: implications for nonsurgical therapy. *Eur. J. Radiol.,* **18**, 57–60.

Samen, F.J. (1962) Considerations of cholecystographic contrast media. *AJR,* **88**, 797–802.

Sperber, I. & Sperber, G. (1971) *Hepatic Excretion of Radiocontrast Agents.* Pergamon Press, Oxford.

Srivastava, D.N., Kulshrestha, A., Gujral, R.B. *et al.* (1991) Oral cholecystography: comparison of conventional screen-film with photostimulable imaging plate radiographs. *Gastrointest. Radiol.,* **16**, 49–52.

Taketa, R.M., Berk, R.N. & Lang, J.H. (1972) The effect of pH on the intestinal absorption of Telepaque. *AJR,* **114**, 767–72.

Twomey, B., de Lacey, G. & Gajjar, B. (1983) The plain radiograph in oral cholecystography: should it be abandoned? *Br. J. Radiol.,* **56**, 99–100.

Whitehouse, W.M. (1956) Re-evaluation of the fat free preparatory meal in Telepaque cholecystography. *AJR,* **76**, 21–3.

Intravenous cholangiography (IVC)

Indications

A declining role for IVC was predicted in the first edition of this book and experience has borne this out. In many countries, it has been superseded by US, percutaneous transhepatic cholangiography, endoscopic retrograde cholangiography, computed tomography (CT) or cholescintigraphy.

A description of this technique is included for the benefit of centres in which alternative methods are not available but also for the few occasions in which it may still be required by other hospitals.

The indications, in the absence of alternatives, are: (i) simultaneous failure of both oral cholecystography and real-time US; (ii) suspected common bile-duct disease in non-icteric patients; and (iii) post-cholecystectomy biliary symptoms.

Recent reports have advocated the routine or selective use of IVC in the work-up of patients for laparoscopic cholecystectomy (Joyce *et al.,* 1991; Scott-Coombes & Thompson, 1991). These opinions, however, are not universally accepted (Dawson *et al.,* 1993; Patel *et al.,* 1993).

Contraindications

Absolute contraindications are pregnancy, known iodine sensitivity and combined hepatic and renal failure. IVC should not be performed within 14 days of an OCG. The administration of the IVC agent meglumine iodipamide 24 hours after an OCG agent dramatically increased the incidence of adverse side effects, with 14% having severe reactions which included severe hypotension (Finby & Blasberg, 1964). Furthermore, there was a sharp reduction in the number of diagnostic cholangiograms by the competition in the liver for the active-transport mechanism, with consequent retention of the i.v. medium in the vascular compartment (Moss *et al.,* 1973).

Contrast media (Tables 6.3 & 6.4)

IVC agents are 'coupled compounds' consisting of two substituted benzoic acids linked by a difunctional radical (Fig. 6.3). Each molecule contains six iodine atoms and two available vacant binding sites.

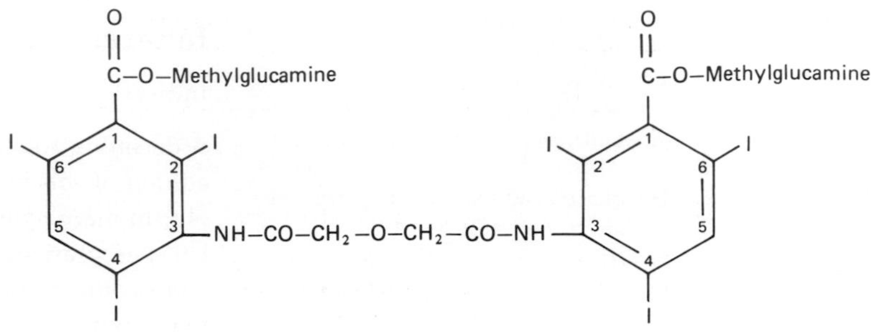

Fig. 6.3 Ioglycamide (Biligram) — a typical i.v. cholangiographic agent. Note the two vacant binding sites at position 5 on the nuclei.

They are highly ionized in solution and have a low lipid solubility with a high aqueous solubility which renders them suitable for i.v. injection but not for oral administration (Table 6.3). The two vacant binding sites also cause cholangiographic media to be protein-bound and this is a source of their toxicity (Lasser *et al.*, 1962). There is evidence that plasma albumin binding itself decreases the hepatic uptake of IVC agents, so that selective liver uptake is a complex process. The mechanism of liver uptake may be due to binding to hepatic cytoplasmic proteins, but the evidence is not conclusive (Sokoloff *et al.*, 1973).

IVC agents do not undergo glucuronization on passage through the hepatocytes, but their excretion into bile is by an active-transport mechanism similar to that of OCG agents. The IVC agents are also choleretic and stimulate water flow across the bile canaliculus without increasing bile salt excretion. The formation of bile occurs in two phases.

1 Canalicular bile flow, in which most of the water and organic materials are excreted.

2 Ductular bile flow, which adds water and inorganic ions.

The choleric effect is predominantly canalicular in origin and is accompanied by the stimulation of bicarbonate secretion (Barnhart *et al.*, 1980). The active-transport mechanism and cholalesis impose limits on the degree of opacification of the duct system which is obtained by increasing the administered dose of contrast medium. A list of available media is given in Table 6.4.

Infusion or bolus injection?

There are two main methods of IVC: (i) bolus injection over about 5–10 min; and (ii) slow i.v. infusion for 30–60 min. The fundamental principles which underlie the excretion of cholangiographic media by the liver are as follows:

1 The excretion of contrast medium by the liver is an active carrier-mediated transport process proceeding against a large concentration gradient.

2 This excretion is limited by a transport maximum.

3 The concentration of contrast medium in bile depends on the rate of excretion, the choleresis which is stimulated and the basal bile flow.

Iodipamide given in bolus injection produces higher plasma concentrations and greater renal excretion but less total biliary excretion than an equal amount infused over a longer period of time (Loeb *et al.*, 1975). In basic terms, in the case of a bolus injection, if too much contrast medium is injected too quickly into the system, then the liver is overwhelmed and the contrast medium is excreted by the kidneys. However, increasing the dose of contrast medium by i.v. infusion improves the quality of the resulting image but only up to a maximum for the contrast medium, after which no further improvement is possible.

The available evidence indicates that an infusion technique is preferable to bolus injection. Adequate information regarding the optimal rate of infusion is only available for ioglycamide. The transport maximum for ioglycamide is about 30 mg min^{-1} (Fuchs & Preisig, 1975). Optimal concentrations of iodine in the bile-duct are obtainable if ioglycamide is infused for 1 hour at a rate of about 4 mg kg^{-1} min^{-1} (Bell *et al.*, 1978). Significantly fewer side effects are induced by the infusion technique as compared with bolus injection.

Influence of liver function

Because cholangiographic contrast agents and biliru-

Table 6.3 The metabolic pathway of the i.v. cholangiographic media

Pathway	Activity	Solubility
The basic contrast media		Predominantly water-soluble and highly ionized (weak lipid-solubility)
i.v. administration	Strong binding to serum albumin	No information available about bound moiety
Hepatocytes	Albumen bond broken Contrast medium enters hepatocytes	Water-soluble
	To bile in an unchanged form by an active carrier-mediated transport system against a large concentration gradient and limited by a transport maximum	Water-soluble
Bile-ducts	Transport to gallbladder	Water-soluble
Gallbladder	Reabsorption of water and hence concentration of contrast in bile	Water-soluble
Fate of contrast media	Excretion of the bile-transported contrast in faeces Excretion of contrast in urine	Water-soluble

bin are excreted by the same transport mechanism, elevation of serum bilirubin is associated with a diminution in the biliary concentration of contrast media.

Normal radiographic technique

Patients should be in a fasting state, but well hydrated to reduce the nephrotoxicity of the contrast medium. An initial prone LAO control radiograph of the gallbladder area at low voltage (50–60 kV) is taken before the administration of contrast medium. If the LAO projection is not possible, an alternative is the supine RPO. The centring point is 7.5 cm to the right of the spinous processes and 2.5–3 cm cephalad to the level of the lower costal margin (Bryan, 1979).

A further prone oblique radiograph of the gallbladder area is taken 30 min after bolus injection or at the end of infusion. Linear tomography is performed if the duct system is not clearly shown on the first radiograph (Fig. 6.4). The technique is identical to that outlined on p. 80, with the exception that the cuts are usually taken from 8 to 12 cm. Zonography is preferred by some workers (Bryan, 1979).

The radiographic examination is continued at 30-min intervals for up to 2 hours after administration of the contrast medium in order to obtain gallbladder opacification. If the gallbladder is visualized, a prone radiograph is taken to show the gallbladder fundus, a supine radiograph for the neck of the gallbladder and Hartmann's pouch, and an erect radiograph to demonstrate the presence of gallstones.

Modification of the technique

Several reports describe the use of spiral CT after IVC for the three-dimensional surface reconstruction of the gallbladder and bile ducts (Vock *et al.*, 1989; Klein *et al.*, 1993).

Complications

Deaths attributed to the technique are said to occur once in every 5000 examinations. This is approximately eight times the risk of death from i.v. urography. The toxic effects of the IVC media may be related to their property of pseudocholinesterase inhibition (Lasser, 1966). Hepatotoxicity and renal failure have followed a high dose of the contrast agents (Craft & Swales, 1967; Stillman, 1974). The nephrotoxicity may be due to the uricosuric action and patients should therefore be adequately

Table 6.4 Media for i.v. cholangiography

Generic name	UK trade name	Molecular weight	Iodine content of salt (%)	Preparations	Iodine content mg ml⁻¹	Iodine content Per ampoule or bottle (g)	Viscosity (Cp) 20°C	Viscosity 37°C	Osmolality at 37°C (mol kg⁻¹ water)
Currently available in UK (1995)									
Meglumine iotroxate (formerly iotroxinate)	Biliscopin infusion (Schering Health Care Ltd)	1606	47.4	10.5% solution in 100 ml vials	50	5.0	1.3	0.9	0.28
Formerly marketed in UK									
Meglumine iodipamide	Biligrafin and Biligrafin Forte (Schering Health Care Ltd)	1530	49.8						
Meglumine ioglycamate	Biligram (Schering Health Care Ltd)	1518.1	50.2	35% solution in 30 ml ampoules	176	5.3	2.9	1.8	0.45
	Biligram infusion (Schering Health Care Ltd)	1518.1	50.2	17% solution in 100 ml vials	85	8.5	1.6	1.0	0.25
Meglumine iotroxate	Biliscopin (Schering Health Care Ltd)	1606	47.4	38% solution in 30 ml ampoules	180	5.4	3.5	2.1	0.55
Meglumine iodoxamate	Endobil (E. Merck Pharmaceuticals)	1678	45						

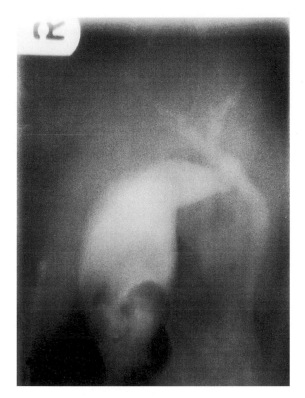

Fig. 6.4 Tomographic cut at 9 cm showing improved resolution of the hepatic ducts and distal common bile-duct.

hydrated for the examination (Mudge, 1971; Sargent *et al.*, 1973). Renal failure has occurred in patients with myelomatosis.

References

Barnhart, J.L., Berk, R.N. & Combes, B. (1980) Changes in bile flow and composition induced by radiographic contrast materials. *Invest. Radiol.*, **15**, S124–S131.

Bell, G.D., Frank, J. & Fayadh, M. (1978) Ioglycamide (Biligram) studies in man — radiological opacification of the bile duct. A comparison of a number of different methods. *Br. J. Radiol.*, **51**, 191–5.

Bryan, G.J. (1979) *Diagnostic Radiography*, 3rd edn, pp. 278–81. Churchill Livingstone, Edinburgh.

Craft, I.L. & Swales, J.D. (1967) Renal failure after cholangiography. *Br. Med. J.*, **2**, 736–8.

Dawson, P., Adam, A. & Benjamin, I.S. (1993) Editorial — Intravenous cholangiography revisited. *Clin. Radiol.*, **47**, 223–25.

Finby, N. & Blasberg, G. (1964) A note on the blocking of hepatic excretion during cholangiographic study. *Gastroenterology*, **46**, 276–7.

Fuchs, W.A. & Preisig, R. (1975) Prolonged drip-infusion cholangiography. *Br. J. Radiol.*, **48**, 539–44.

Joyce, W.P., Keane, R., Burke, G.J. *et al.* (1991) Identification of bile duct stones in patients undergoing laparoscopic cholecystectomy. *Br. J. Surg.*, **78**, 1174–6.

Klein, H.-M., Wein, B., Truong, S. *et al.* (1993) Computed tomographic cholangiography using spiral scanning and 3D image processing. *Br. J. Radiol.*, **66**, 762–7.

Lasser, E.C. (1966) The pharmacodynamics of biliary contrast media. *Radiol. Clin. N. Am.*, **4**(3), 511–19.

Lasser, E.C., Farr, R.S., Fujimagari, T. *et al.* (1962) The significance of protein binding of contrast media in roentgen diagnosis. *AJR*, **87**, 338–60.

Loeb, P.M., Berk, R.N., Fled, G.D. *et al.* (1975) Biliary excretion of iodipamide. *Gastroenterology*, **68**, 554–62.

Moss, A.A., Nelson, J. & Amberg, J. (1973) Intravenous cholangiography. *AJR*, **117**, 406–11.

Mudge, G.H. (1971) Uricosuric action of cholecystographic agents. *N. Engl. J. Med.*, **284**, 929–33.

Patel, J.C., McInnes, G.C., Bagley, J.S. *et al* (1993) The role of intravenous cholangiography in pre-operative assessment for laparoscopic cholecystectomy. *BJR*, **66**, 1125–7.

Sargent, E.N., Barbour, B.H., Espinosa, N. *et al.* (1973) Evaluation of renal function following double dose infusion intravenous cholangiography. *AJR*, **117**, 412–18.

Scott-Coombes, D. & Thompson, J.N. (1991) Bile duct stones and laparoscopic cholecystectomy. *Br. Med. J.*, **303**, 1281–2.

Sokoloff, J., Berk, R.N., Lang, J.H. *et al.* (1973) The role of Y and Z hepatic proteins in the excretion of radiographic contrast materials. *Radiology*, **106**, 519–23.

Stillman, A.E. (1974) Hepatotoxic reaction to iodipamide meglumine injection. *JAMA*, **228**(11), 1420–1.

Vock, P., Jung, H. & Kalender, W. (1989) Single breathhold spiral volumetric CT of the hepato-biliary system. *Radiology*, **173**, 377.

Peroperative cholangiography (POC)

In 1932, Mirizzi performed the first cholangiogram on an operating table. The POC technique was soon widely employed although it was not universally accepted in the UK for many years (Schulenberg, 1966). POC is one of the most neglected and badly executed radiological investigations. It can lead to diagnostic failures when conducted without scrupulous attention to detail. Ductal stones are overlooked in 3–10% of patients undergoing common duct exploration, mostly due to poor operative cholangiographic technique (Burhenne, 1976).

The importance of the radiologist in the interpretation of the results has been well illustrated (Derodra *et al.*, 1992).

Indications

There has been much discussion as to whether POC should be performed routinely or selectively. The advent of laparoscopic cholecystectomy has served only to intensify the debate. Arguments in favour of routine POC are as follows.

1 Unsuspected duct stones are found in 1–14% of patients (Levine *et al.*, 1983; Shively *et al.*, 1990).

2 It assists in the demonstration of bile-duct anatomy and reduces the incidence of bile-duct damage (Phillips, 1993).

3 A negative result is highly accurate and prevents unnecessary duct exploration (Levine *et al.*, 1983)

Arguments against routine use are as follows.

1 A negligible proportion of retained stones actually cause further trouble (Bogokowsky *et al.*, 1987).

2 False positive studies lead to unnecessary duct explorations and increased morbidity (Levine *et al.*, 1983).

3 The information required can be supplied by other techniques such as endoscopic retrograde cholangio-pancreatographic (ERCP) examination or preoperative ultrasound (Gillams *et al.*, 1992; Barkun *et al.*, 1993).

Attempts have been made to define criteria for the selective use of POC in conventional 'open' cholecystectomy (Taylor *et al.*, 1983; Wilson *et al.*, 1986; Pasquale & Nauta, 1989; Hauer-Jensen *et al.*, 1991; Huguier *et al.*, 1991; Pace *et al.*, 1992; Murison *et al.*, 1993) and in laparoscopic cholecystectomy (Barkun *et al.*, 1993; Clair *et al.*, 1993). Studies relating to open cholecystectomy may also be used as guidelines to indications for cholangiography at laparoscopic cholecystectomy (Corder *et al.*, 1992).

The following summarizes the criteria identified.

1 A dilated or abnormal common bile-duct at surgery or a dilated common bile-duct on preoperative imaging.

2 Older patients.

3 Dilated cystic duct.

4 Increased numbers of gallbladder stones.

5 History of jaundice.

6 History of pancreatitis.

7 History of cholangitis.

8 Elevated serum alkaline phosphatase or bilirubin in previous 6 months.

9 History of acute of chronic cholecystitis.

Contraindications

Known hypersensitivity to the contrast medium is a contraindication.

Technique

Few radiologists enter the operating theatre during the performance of POC, the control of which is therefore left to the surgeon and radiographer. Only a few operating theatres have dedicated X-ray units and generators, most examinations having to be performed with mobile generators of 100–300 mA capacity and either portable Bucky units or fine stationary grids. A sterile cover should be fastened over the tube housing to prevent accidental contact with the operating field.

There are a number of cassette tunnels available which allow the radiographic cassettes to be slid easily under the patient. Some operating tables themselves have a space in which to place a cassette. In many situations none of these aids is available. When a grid is required, it should be positioned with the grid lines running at right angles to the long axis of the patient's abdomen.

The description that follows relates to the technique for open cholecystectomy but a short account of the laparoscopic modification is appended.

Ideally, contrast examinations should be performed both before and after duct exploration. The pre-exploratory examination is performed by cannulation of the cystic duct with a thin polythene catheter and the post-exploratory examination usually via a T-tube catheter placed in the common duct. One author describes a method in which contrast medium is introduced into the gallbladder by a specially designed cannula (Tinckler, 1991).

It is essential to remove all surgical instruments from the operating field, to exclude leaks in the injection system, to irrigate the system with saline, and to ensure that no air bubbles are introduced into the system. The injection tubing must be of sufficient length to exclude the operator's hands from the primary X-ray beam.

The patient lies supine on the table and the gallbladder area should be over the film (Fig. 6.5). The choice of water-soluble contrast medium is critical, as too great an iodine content will obscure small

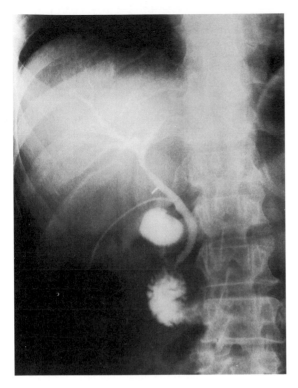

Fig. 6.5 Normal peroperative cholangiogram. There is a vascular clip at the origin of the cystic duct following cholecystectomy. Some contrast medium has entered the duodenum and refluxed into the duodenal cap.

stones. Hypaque 25% is the preferred contrast agent and at least 20 ml is drawn into the syringe. The contrast medium should be warmed to body temperature. The room should be cleared of all non-essential personnel during contrast injection and those remaining should be protected by either lead aprons or mobile lead screens. Before injecting, the patient should be tilted 20° obliquely to the right in order to project the common duct off the spine. The surgeon should indicate when he or she is commencing the injection and the anaesthetist suspends the patient's respiration during exposure of the radiograph. Fractionating the contrast injection and taking radiographs with each fraction is recommended, for example at 3, 5–8 and 12 ml (LeQuesne, 1960). A single 10 ml injection should be avoided as this could obscure the terminal portion of the duct and any small filling defects.

The radiographs should be processed immediately and interpreted by a radiologist, who may require further radiographs. It is very important that the surgeon prevents air bubbles by careful prefilling of the syringe and injection tube and that the duct system is delineated before operative manipulation, which may cause duct spasm.

An additional method which sometimes removes the need for patient rotation is 'contact cholangiography'. A small dental occlusal film, contained in a sterile polythene wrapping, is placed by the surgeon behind the duodenum. The X-ray beam is coned to the area of the film and an exposure is made during contrast injection.

A normal pre-exploratory cholangiogram should show a duct not exceeding 12 mm in diameter, free flow of contrast medium into the duodenum on all radiographs with the terminal narrow segment of the duct shown on at least one radiograph, an absence of filling defects and no excess retrograde filling of the hepatic ducts (LeQuesne, 1960).

Occassionally, spasm of the sphincter of Oddi mimics a distal common duct stone (Mujahed & Evans, 1972). This effect is abolished by the use of a smooth muscle relaxant such as glucagon (Ferrucci *et al.*, 1976).

Modification of technique for laparoscopic cholecystectomy

Laparoscopic cholecystectomy is performed under general anaesthesia. Following insufflation of carbon dioxide gas into the peritoneum, four small incisions (ports) are made in the anterior abdominal wall. An incision is placed just above the umbilicus and allows access for the laparoscope. The other three incisions are placed in an oblique line in the right subcostal region and kept patent by cannulas for later passage of surgical instruments.

Two cannulation techniques have been described for POC.
1 *Cystic duct cannulation* (Berci *et al.*, 1991; Balachandran *et al.*, 1992; Campenhout *et al.*, 1993; Clair *et al.*, 1993). The general principles are:
   (a) The cystic duct is dissected free and clipped close to its junction with the gallbladder.
   (b) A small incision is made in the cystic duct.
   (c) A catheter is inserted via the incision. A specially designed cholangiographic fixation clamp

(cholangioclamp) is available*. This device has a hollow channel for passage of a catheter and mobile jaws which when closed will keep the catheter in position with a water-tight seal. Catheters should be 4 or 5F gauge. The choice of catheters has included flexible ureteric catheters, tapered ERCP cannulae and paediatric feeding tubes.

(d) Imaging. Hypaque at 30–50% dilation has been suggested by some authors in volumes up to 30 ml. Some use fluoroscopy with spot radiographs (Berci *et al.*, 1991) but others use spot radiographs only. One group advocates an initial injection of a small volume of contrast (3–5 ml) followed by i.m. glucagon if there is no flow into the duodenum and i.v. morphine sulphate if the proximal intrahepatic ducts were not shown (Soper & Dunnegan, 1992).

2 *Gallbladder cannulation.* A post-procedural tubogram via a gallbladder drainage catheter has been recommended (Gillams *et al.* 1992).

Complications

These are few but include bile-duct rupture and septicaemia. There is a theoretical risk of pancreatitis from reflux of contrast medium into the pancreatic duct.

References

Balachandran, S., Goodman, P., Saydjari, R. *et al.* (1992) Operative cholangiography in patients undergoing laparoscopic cholecystectomy: unique radiographic findings. *AJR*, **159**, 65–7.

Barkun, J.S., Fried, G.M., Barkun, A.N. *et al.* (1993) Cholecystectomy without operative cholangiography. *Ann. Surg.*, **218**(3), 371–9.

Berci, G., Sackier, J.M. & Paz-Partlow, M. (1991) Routine or selected intraoperative cholangiography during laparoscopic cholecystectomy? *Am J. Surg.*, **161**, 355–60.

Bogokowsky, H., Slutzki, S. & Zaidenstein, L. (1987) Selective operative cholangiography. *Surg. Gynecol. Obstet.*, **164**, 124–6.

Burhenne, J.H. (1976) Non-operative extraction of stones from the bile ducts. *In Roentgenology of the Gall Bladder and Biliary Tract.* Grune & Stratton, London.

Campenhout, I., Prosmanne, O., Gagner, M. *et al.* (1993) Routine operative cholangiography during laparoscopic cholecystectomy. *AJR*, **160**, 1209–11.

Clair, D.G., Carr-Locke, D.L., Becker, J.M. *et al.* (1993) Routine cholangiography is not warranted during laparoscopic cholecystectomy. *Arch. Surg.*, **128**, 551–5.

Corder, A.P., Scott, S.D. & Johnson, C.D. (1992) Place of routine operative cholangiography at cholecystectomy. *Br. J. Surg.*, **79**, 945–7.

Derodra, J.K., Jackson, A.R. & Prout, W.G. (1992) Quality and interpretation of operative cholangiography in a district general hospital. *J. Roy. Coll. Surg. Edin.*, **37**, 241–3.

Ferrucci, J.T., Wittenberg, J., Stone, L.B. *et al.* (1976) Hypotonic cholangiography with glucagon. *Radiology*, **118**, 466–7.

Gillams, A., Cheslyn-Curtis, S., Russell, R.C.G. *et al.* (1992) Can cholangiography be safety abandoned in laparoscopic cholecystectomy? *Ann. Roy. Coll. Surg. Engl.*, **74**, 248–51.

Hauer-Jensen, M., Karesen, R., Nygaard, K. *et al.* (1991) Prospective randomized study of routine intraoperative cholangiography during open cholecystectomy: long-term follow-up and multivariate analysis of predictors of choledocholithiasis. *Surgery*, **113**(3), 318–23.

Huguier, M., Bornet, P., Charpak, Y. *et al.* (1991) Selective contraindications based on multivariate analysis for operative cholangiography in biliary lithiasis. *Surg. Gynecol. Obstet.*, **172**, 470–4.

LeQuesne, L.P. (1960) Discussion of cholangiography. *Proc. Roy. Soc. Med.*, **53**, 851–60.

Levine, S.B. Lerner, H.J., Leifer, E.D. *et al.* (1983) Intraoperative cholangiography. A review of indications and analysis of age-sex groups. *Ann. Surg.*, **198**, 692–7.

Mirizzi, P.L. (1932) La colangiografia durante las operaciones de las vias biliares. *Bol. Soc. Argent. Cirurg. Buenos Aires*, **16**, 1133–61.

Mujahed, Z. & Evans, A. (1972) Pseudocalculus defect in cholangiography. *AJR*, **116**, 337–41.

Murison, M.S.C., Gartell, P.C. & McGinn, F.P. (1993) Does selective peroperative cholangiography result in missed common bile duct stones? *J. Roy. Coll. Surg. Edin.*, **38**, 220–4.

Pace, B.W., Cosgrove, J., Breuer, B. *et al.* (1992) Intraoperative cholangiography revisited. *Arch. Surg.*, **127**, 448–50.

Pasquale, M.D. & Nauta, R.J. (1989) Selective vs. routine use of intraoperative cholangiography. *Arch. Surg.*, **124**, 1041–2.

Phillips, E.H. (1993) Routine versus selective intraoperative cholangiography. *Am J. Surg.*, **165**, 505–7.

Schulenberg, C.A.R. (1966) *Operative Cholangiography.* Butterworth, London.

Shively, E.H., Wieman, J., Adams, A.L. *et al.* (1990) Operative cholangiography. *Am.J. Surg.*, **159**, 380–5.

Soper, N.J. & Dunnegan, D.L. (1992) Routine versus selective intra-operative cholangiography during laparoscopic cholecystectomy. *World J. Surg.*, **16**, 1133–40.

Taylor, T.V., Torrance, B. & Rimmer, S. (1983) Operative cholangiography: is there a statistical alternative? *Am. J. Surg.*, **145**, 640–3.

Tinckler, L. (1991) Transcholecystic operative cholangiography: an alternative technique. *Ann. Roy. Coll. Surg. Engl.*, **73**, 39–43.

Wilson, T.G., Hall, J.C. & Watts, J.M. (1986) Is operative cholangiography always necessary? *Br. J. Surg.*, **73**, 637–40.

* Karl Storz, Endoscopy America, Culver City, California, USA.

Postoperative cholangiography (T-tube cholangiography)

Following explorations of the common bile-duct, a drainage tube is usually left *in situ* in the common duct to promote bile drainage. A contrast examination via this drainage tube is performed 7–10 days after the operation.

Indications

Postoperative T-tube cholangiography allows an assessment of the intra- and extrahepatic ducts prior to removal of the T-tube.

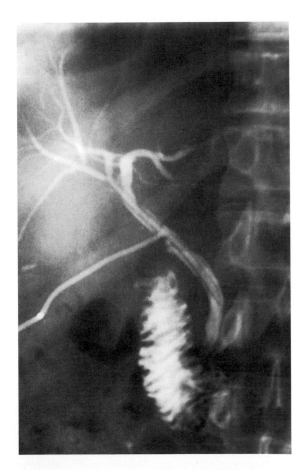

Fig. 6.6 Normal postoperative T-tube cholangiogram — some contrast medium has refluxed into the pancreatic duct.

Contraindications

Known hypersensitivity to the contrast medium.

Technique

Postoperative cholangiography is performed by a radiologist in the X-ray department on a fluoroscopic unit with an undercouch tube.

A control radiograph of the gallbladder area is a prerequisite. A clamp is temporarily applied to the T-tube. Patients should be warned that they may experience some discomfort in the right hypochondrium during the injection of contrast medium, especially when there is obstruction of the duct system. A small needle is inserted into the tube proximal to the clamp, followed by the aspiration of air bubbles and bile. Contrast medium, for instance Hypaque 25%, is warmed to body temperature and is injected, spot radiographs being taken in varying degrees of obliquity (Fig. 6.6).

These radiographs are processed immediately and assessed by the radiologist. If the duct system contains any translucencies which may be due to air bubbles, there are some helpful manoeuvres.

1 Air bubbles will rise upwards when the patient is brought into a semierect position.

2 The patient may be turned on to his or her right side in the head-down position, and 50 ml of saline forcefully injected into the tube, the cholangiogram being repeated when the patient is turned onto their back.

The 'pseudocalculus' phenomenon due to sphincteric spasm is occasionally seen in postoperative cholangiography, the appropriate technique for dealing with this situation being the same as that outlined on p. 87.

Complications

Duct rupture and septicaemia are rare complications.

Modifications of the basic technique

It is still possible to overlook residual calculi in the biliary tract despite a meticulous surgical and POC technique. Second surgical operations to remove retained stones are complicated by a higher morbidity and mortality than the primary surgical procedure. Non-operative techniques for the removal of these stones offer an alternative to surgery.

Stones can be extracted using specially designed forceps introduced along the tract left by the post-operative T-tube (Mazzariello, 1970). Other methods for removing retained calculi have employed irrigation with saline, aspiration by catheters and the use of antispasmodics (Lamis *et al.*, 1969). A Dormia ureteric basket may be used to grasp the retained stones (Burhenne, 1973). The optimum time for the technique is not less than 4 weeks, and preferably about 5 weeks, after initial biliary surgery (Burhenne, 1974). A prerequisite is the use of an indwelling T-tube catheter of not less than 16F, the sinus tracks from smaller catheters being too narrow to permit instrumentation. Localization of the stones by T-tube cholangiography precedes removal of the T-tube. Catheterization of the sinus track is usually possible for at least 48 hours after T-tube removal. A steerable catheter* is then guided through the sinus track and its tip is advanced beyond the retained stone. The Dormia basket is then fed through the lumen of the steerable catheter and the catheter is withdrawn. The basket is opened and slowly withdrawn until it engages the stone, which is then extracted through the sinus track. Stones of more than 10 mm in diameter usually require fragmentation either by forceful traction of the open basket into the proximal part of the sinus track or by closure of the basket within the duct system (Burhenne, 1974).

In the hands of experienced operators the success rate of the technique is as high as 96% but as low as 58% in centres treating only a few patients (Burhenne, 1974; Mason, 1980). Complications include the creation of false sinus passages, septicaemia, vagal stimulation with shock, and pancreatitis.

Another option for percutaneous stone extraction is T-tube tract fibreoptic choledochoscopy, first described by Sherman *et al.* (1975). The overall success rate ranges from 85 to 100%. The technique is performed about 3.5 weeks after initial surgery, under sterile conditions with i.v. sedation and prophylactic antibiotic cover (Hieken & Birkett, 1992). The T-tube is removed and the choledochoscope is passed down the tract under direct vision. Choledochoscopes have an irrigating/instrument channel through which a variety of accessories such as wire baskets and grasping forceps can be introduced to remove the stones. Complications include transient fever, abdominal discomfort, asymptomatic hyperamylasaemia, overt pancreatitis, perforation of the T-tube tract, bleeding, haemobilia and fistula formation.

References

Berci, G. (1989) Intraoperative and postoperative biliary endoscopy (choledochoscopy). *Surg. Clin. N. Am.*, **69**, 1275–86.

Burhenne, H.J. (1973) Non-operative retained biliary tract stone extraction. *AJR*, **117**, 388–99.

Burhenne, H.J. (1974) The techniques of biliary duct stone extraction. *Radiology*, **113**, 567–72.

Hieken, T.J. & Birkett, D.H. (1992) Postoperative T-Tube tract choledochoscopy. *Am. J. Surg.*, **163**, 28–31.

Lamis, P.A., Letton, A.H. & Wilson, J.P. (1969) Retained common duct stones: a new non-operative technique for treatment. *Surgery*, **66**, 291–6.

Mason, R. (1980) Percutaneous extraction of retained gallstones via the T-tube track — British experience of 131 cases. *Clin. Radiol.*, **31**, 497–9.

Mazzariello, R. (1970) Removal of residual biliary tract calculi without reoperation. *Surgery*, **67**, 566–73.

Sherman, H.I., Margeson, R.C. & Davis, R.C. Jr (1975) Postoperative retained choledocholithiasis: percutaneous endoscopic extraction. *Gastroenterology*, **68**, 1024.

Percutaneous transhepatic cholangiography (PTC)

The first PTC is credited to Huard and Do Xuan Hop (1937), who introduced Lipiodol into the biliary tree. Carter and Saypol (1952) described an anterior percutaneous approach into the left lobe of the liver using a No. 17 spinal needle in a case of obstructive jaundice. Prioton *et al.* (1960) used a posterior approach to direct the needle into the extraperitoneal segment of the liver in an attempt to contain any resultant leakage of bile.

These methods did not meet with universal acclaim and most operators preferred an anterior subcostal approach using a 20 gauge steel needle over which was drawn a flexible polyethylene tube (George *et al.*, 1965; Mujahed & Evans, 1966). In the

---

* Medi-Tech Inc., Watertown, Massachusetts, USA.

1960s and early 1970s PTC was restricted to the immediate preoperative period because of the risks of bile leakage, haemorrhage and septicaemia (Zinberg *et al.*, 1965; Machado, 1971).

In 1974, Kunio Okuda, working in Chiba University Hospital, Japan, reported his experience with a fine 23F flexible needle, subsequently known as the 'Chiba needle' (Okuda *et al.*, 1974). The Chiba needle technique has now replaced other methods. The principal advantages of the Chiba needle over the older sheathed needle are due to its flexibility and narrow calibre.

Indications

PTC is used to distinguish intrahepatic cholestasis from extrahepatic obstruction and to determine the site and, if possible, the nature of an extrahepatic biliary duct obstruction. It is the gold standard for patients with bile-duct strictures where it is more valuable than ERCP (Lillemoe *et al.*, 1990).

Contraindications

Strong contraindications to PTC are coagulation problems, for example a platelet count of less than $100 \times 10^9 \, l^{-1}$ (100 000 mm^{-3}) and a prothrombin time of less than 60% of the control value, biliary infection, hypersensitivity to contrast medium, severe heart disease and a respiratory problem which renders the patient unable to hold his or her breath.

Okuda *et al.* (1974) also included as contraindications a poor general condition of the patient, extreme jaundice, ascites and anaemia. They also considered that PTC should not be performed immediately after a severe attack of abdominal pain.

Technique

The Chiba needle is made of flexible stainless steel and is 15 cm in length, with outer and inner diameters of 0.7 and 0.5 mm, respectively, and a bevel angle of 30°. The procedure is usually performed under local anaesthesia, except in very young children and uncooperative adults. Patients may require sedation but it is unwise to administer any drugs in the presence of liver failure. The choice of sedative should be discussed with the referring clinician be-

fore the procedure. It is preferable to starve the patient.

If the patient is suspected of having a biliary obstruction, it is important to give a suitable antibiotic, such as i.v. gentamicin 120 mg, in order to prevent an ascending cholangitis. Some authors give antibiotic cover to all their patients (Okuda *et al.*, 1974; Jain *et al.*, 1977). Others point out that premedication with antibiotics will not necessarily prevent septicaemia (Dooley *et al.*, 1984) and advocate that, if a Gram stain or culture of bile taken at the time of the PTC is positive and/or bile-duct obstruction is present, antibiotics should be continued until sepsis has been treated or obstruction relieved. It is essential to check the prothrombin time and platelet count and to screen the patient for hepatitis B surface (Australia) antigen before commencing the procedure. Parenteral vitamin K is given in some centres to all jaundiced patients (Fraser *et al.*, 1978).

The examination is performed on a fluoroscopy unit with image intensification and facilities for spot radiographs with both supine and horizontal X-ray beams. The subject lies supine on the fluoroscopy table. It is worthwhile screening the upper abdomen to locate the inferior hepatic border during suspended respiration. A supine control radiograph of the right hypochondrium is sometimes recommended, centring in the mid-clavicular line 2.5–5 cm above the lower costal margin (Bryan, 1979).

The skin surface of the lower right chest and right hypochondrium is cleaned with a suitable antiseptic solution and sterile drapes are placed over the surrounding area. The skin and subcutaneous tissues down to the liver capsule are infiltrated with 1% lignocaine. A small incision is made in the skin at the optimum puncture site as determined by preliminary screening, usually in the mid-axillary line of the right 7th or 8th intercostal space. The needle is inserted parallel to the plane of the table and advanced during suspended respiration through the right lobe of the liver on a line above the gallbladder and the junction of the right and left hepatic ducts. The point to which the needle tip is inserted may be determined by placing a metal marker on the skin over the xiphisternum and using this as a guide (Fraser *et al.*, 1978), or by introducing a duodenal tube and aiming at the mid-point on the vertical line drawn from the vertex of the tube to the diaphragm (Okuda *et al.*, 1974). In practice, it has been found satisfactory to introduce the needle until it is judged to have reached the level of the right border of the spine (Jain *et al.*, 1977). The patient does not need to maintain suspended respiration, because of the flexible needle. A 20 ml syringe is filled with 300 mg iodine ml⁻¹ contrast medium and is connected via a long plastic anaesthetic extension set to the needle, thus avoiding irradiation to the hands of the operator. Approximately 0.5 ml of contrast medium is injected via the needle under the screen control. Injection into the hepatic blood vessels leads to instantaneous clearing of the contrast medium, while entry into a lymphatic vessel shows a slower but complete clearing of contrast medium. A persisting curvilinear collection of contrast medium is seen if the needle tip lies in the subcapsular space of the liver. The injection of contrast medium into the biliary tree leads to slow centrifugal flow and the persistent delineation of a short section of the duct system (Fig. 6.7).

If a biliary radicle has not been cannulated, the needle is withdrawn in increments of 0.5–1 cm with further small injections of contrast medium. An alternative method is to withdraw the needle whilst continually injecting the contrast medium (Fraser *et al.*, 1978). Up to 10 or even 20 needle passes may be made (Fraser *et al.*, 1978; Lintott, 1985). The incidence of complications is not related to the number of attempts made (Harbin *et al.*, 1980).

While the biliary tract may be delineated via the Chiba needle in patients who do not have dilated intrahepatic ducts, the failure of the technique in itself casts doubt on the diagnosis of bile-duct obstruction and a subsequent surgically treatable lesion. In a successful puncture, at least 20 ml of contrast medium should be injected before removal of the needle.

Some authors recommend suction and removal of bile with replacement of an equal volume of contrast medium in those cases with a dilated and obstructed

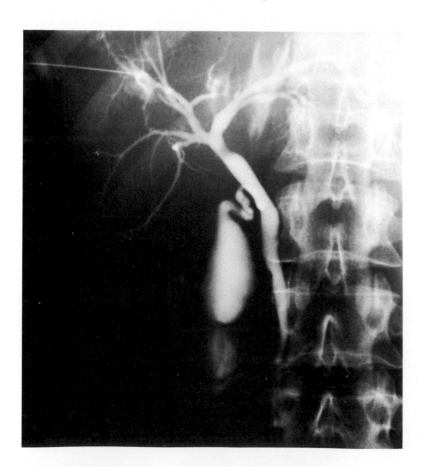

Fig. 6.7 Normal percutaneous transhepatic cholangiogram. There is filling of the gallbladder cystic duct. Some subcapsular contrast medium overlies the left hepatic duct.

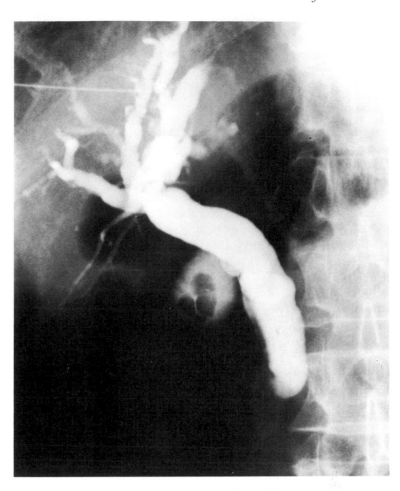

Fig. 6.8 Percutaneous transhepatic cholangiogram of a 74-year-old man with weight loss and jaundice. The intrahepatic ducts and common bile-duct are dilated and the common bile-duct is totally occluded distally. Note the incidental finding of gallstones in the gallbladder. Pathology — carcinoma of the pancreas.

biliary system (Fig. 6.8), but this may not be possible with the small-gauge needle. The injection site is sealed with collodion and covered with a light sterile dressing.

Radiographs are immediately taken in the anteroposterior (AP), lateral and oblique projections. The patient then lies on the left side to promote drainage of the bile-ducts, further radiographs being taken up to 2 hours after the procedure. These delayed radiographs are very useful in demonstrating the gallbladder and the site of common bile-duct obstruction. Erect radiographs are particularly helpful in demonstrating the point of obstruction because the dilated common bile-duct is frequently bowed anteriorly, which impairs its complete delineation in the supine position.

If extravasation of contrast medium has occurred into the liver parenchyma or in the subcapsular space of the liver, a delayed radiograph often shows reabsorption to have occurred and permits an unobscured view of the biliary ducts and gallbladder.

The patient should remain in bed and be carefully monitored for pulse, blood pressure and temperature, and the wound inspected regularly for at least 24 hours.

Complications

The most common complications are a leakage of bile into the peritoneal cavity, intraperitoneal haemorrhage and septicaemia. Other reported complications include hypotension and the formation of a blood–bile fistula. The incidence of serious complications is 3.1% and the mortality 0.1%, comparable with ERCP at 3 and 0.15%, respectively (Bilbao *et al.*, 1976; Harbin *et al.*, 1980). While the attendant risks of the procedure are small, and routine laparotomy is not indicated, the procedure should *never* be performed if surgical help is not immediately available.

Modifications of the basic technique

The diagnostic technique has been modified to provide biliary drainage in cases of obstructive jaundice. This may be a temporary measure to aid surgical management and diminish the incidence of postoperative complications, in particular renal failure. Permanent biliary drainage is used when surgery is contraindicated or to give palliation. The drainage procedure is preceded by PTC. Ultrasound guidance may improve the selectivity of the PTC procedure (Lameris *et al.*, 1990).

External biliary drainage

A biplane screening facility is especially helpful. The needle is inserted horizontally 1 cm posterior or 1 cm anterior to the PTC puncture to enter respectively the right or left hepatic ducts (Nakayama *et al.*, 1978). The sheathed needle, which was used for PTC in the past (Dooley *et al.*, 1979), and a 17 gauge steel needle with mandril have been used to enter the biliary tract prior to drainage (Nakayama *et al.*, 1978). A guide wire is then advanced along the Teflon sheath or steel needle into the bile-duct. A catheter is then inserted over the guide wire, which is then removed, and is secured to the skin surface. Long-term external drainage is complicated by cholangitis and by water, electrolyte and bile salt loss.

Combined internal/external biliary drainage (Ferrucci *et al.*, 1980)

A special rotary torque-control guide wire, with a curved right-angle memory tip, is passed through the biliary obstruction and into the duodenum. A catheter is then inserted over the guide wire until its tip lies in the duodenal lumen, followed by removal of the guide wire. Occlusion of the catheter is prevented by numerous side-holes, situated proximal and distal to the obstruction, over the distal 10–12 cm of the catheter. A pigtail configuration to the catheter provides anchorage in the duodenum. The catheter is allowed to drain externally for the first 3–4 days, following which the catheter is clamped and bile drains into the duodenum.

Internal biliary drainage (Burcharth *et al.*, 1979; Dooley *et al.* 1981)

This is provided by the insertion of a permanent endoprosthesis (stent) into the lumen of a stricture, following a percutaneous transhepatic puncture. Some stents are made of polyethylene or Teflon, and are 10–25 cm in length with an internal diameter of 1.5–3 mm, and multiple side-holes. Self-expanding, metallic stents are now available (Coons, 1989).

Following percutaneous transhepatic insertion of a guide wire, the stent is pushed through the obstruction by an introducer catheter so that its ends lie proximal to the obstruction and in the duodenum (Burcharth *et al.*, 1979). Bile is drained externally via a catheter for a few days after the procedure. The presence of ductal calculi is a contraindication to stent insertion. Recorded complications include cholangitis, local wound abscess, biliary peritonitis, external bile fistulae and bleeding.

Stents may also be placed in the biliary tract by the endoscopic route but in about 11% of cases this is technically impossible (Speer *et al.*, 1987). A combined percutaneous and endoscopic procedure has been developed for use in such cases (Hunt *et al.*, 1993). A guide wire is introduced by PTC and advanced across the stricture into the duodenum. The stent is then inserted over the guide wire by conventional endoscopic techniques (Seigel & Snardy, 1986).

Percutaneous balloon dilatation of benign bile duct strictures (Lillemoe *et al.*, 1990)

Following percutaneous transhepatic puncture, a guide wire is passed through the stricture under fluoroscopic control. The stricture is dilated using angioplasty ballon catheters. A transhepatic stent is left *in situ* to permit repeat cholangiography, repeat dilatations and also to maintain patency of the lumen during healing. The procedure is usually quite painful and may require general anaesthesia. Complications are frequent.

References

Bilbao, M.K., Dotter, C.T., Lee, T.G. *et al.* (1976) Complications of endoscopic retrograde cholangiography (ERCP). A study of 10 000 cases. *Gastroenterology*, **70**, 314–20.

Bryan, G.J. (1979) *Diagnostic Radiography*, 3rd edn. Churchill, Livingstone, Edinburgh.

Burcharth, F., Jenson, L.I. & Oleson, K. (1979) Endoprosthesis for internal drainage of the biliary tract. *Gastroenterology*, **77**, 133–7.

Carter, F.R. & Saypol, G.M. (1952) Transabdominal cholangiography. *JAMA*, **148**, 253–5.

Coons, H. (1989) Self-expanding stainless steel biliary stents. *Radiology*, **170**, 979–983.

Dooley, J.S., Dick, R. & Irving, D. (1981) Relief of bile duct obstruction by the percutaneous transhepatic insertion of an endoprosthesis. *Clin. Radiol.*, **32**, 162–72.

Dooley, J.S., Dick, R., Olney, J. *et al.* (1979) Non-surgical treatment of biliary obstruction. *Lancet* , **ii**, 1040–4.

Dooley, J.S., Hamilton-Miller, J.M.T., Brumfitt, W. *et al.* (1984) Antibiotics in the treatment of biliary infection. *Gut*, **25**, 988–98.

Ferrucci, J.T., Mueller, P.R. & Harbin, W.P. (1980) Percutaneous transhepatic biliary drainage. *Radiology*, **135**, 1–13.

Fraser, G.M., Cruikshank, J.G., Sumerling, M.D. *et al.* (1978) Percutaneous transhepatic cholangiography with the Chiba needle. *Clin. Radiol.*, **29**, 101–12.

George, P., Young, W.B., Walker, J.G. *et al.* (1965) The value of percutaneous cholangiography. *Br. J. Surg.*, **52**, 779–83.

Harbin, W.P., Mueller, P.R. & Ferucci, J.T. (1980) Transhepatic cholangiography: complications and use patterns of the fine needle technique. *Radiology*, **135**, 15–22.

Huard, P. & Do Xuan Hop (1937) La ponction transhepatique des canaux biliares. *Bul. Soc. Med. Chir. Indochine*, **15**, 1090–100.

Hunt, J.B., Sayer, J.M., Jacyna, M. *et al.* (1993) Combined percutaneous transhepatic and endoscopic placement of biliary stents. *Surg. Oncol.*, **1993**, 293–8.

Jain, S., Long, R.G. & Scott, J. (1977) Percutaneous transhepatic cholangiography using the 'Chiba' needle — 80 cases. *Br. J. Radiol.*, **50**, 175–80.

Lameris, J.S., Hesselink, E.J., van Leeuwan, P.A. *et al.* (1990) Ultrasound-guided percutaneous transhepatic cholangiography and drainage in patients with hilar cholangiocarcinoma. *Sem. Liver Dis.*, **10**(2), 121–5.

Lillemoe, K.D., Pitt, H.A. & Cameron, J.L. (1990) Postoperative bile duct strictures. *Surg. Clin. N. Am.*, **70**(6), 1355–80.

Lintott, D.J. (1985) Percutaneous transhepatic cholangiography. *Clin Gastroenterol.*, **14**(2), 373–85.

Machado, A.L. (1971) Percutaneous transhepatic cholangiography. *Br. J. Surg.*, **58**, 616–24.

Mujahed, Z. & Evans, J.A. (1966) Percutaneous transhepatic cholangiography. *Radiol. Clin. North Am.*, **4**(3), 535–45.

Nakayama, T., Ideda, A & Okuda, K. (1978) Percutaneous transhepatic drainage of the biliary tract. *Gastroenterology*, **74**, 554–9.

Okuda, K., Tanikawa, K. & Emura, T. (1974) Non-surgical percutaneous transhepatic cholangiography diagnosis: significance in medical problems of the liver. *Am. J. Dig. Dis.*, **19**, 21–35.

Prioton, J.B., Vialla, M. & Pous, J.G. (1960) Nouvelle technique de cholangiographie trans-parieto-hepatique. *J. Radiol. Electrol.*, **41**, 205.

Seigel, J.H. & Snardy, H. (1986) The significance of endoscopically placed prostheses in the management of biliary obstruction due to carcinoma of the pancreas — results of non-operative decompression in 277 patients. *Am. J. Gastroenterol.*, **81**, 634–41.

Speer, A.G., Cotton, P.B. & Russell, R.C.G. (1987) Randomised trial of endoscopic versus percutaneous stent insertion in malignant obstructive jaundice. *Lancet*, **ii**, 57–62.

Zinberg, SS., Berk, J.E. & Plasencia, H. (1965) Percutaneous transhepatic cholangiography: its use and limitations. *Am. J. Dig. Dis.*, **10**, 154–69.

Relationship of radiological investigations of the biliary tract to each other and to other techniques

Investigation of suspected gallbladder disease

The principal techniques for imaging the gallbladder are OCG and US. In the early 1980s several authorities were sounding the death-knell of the OCG (Ferrucci *et al.*, 1981; Berk *et al.*, 1983). Since the first edition of this book in 1983 the number of agents marketed in the UK (see Table 6.2) has diminished from six to only one. Whilst there has, in general, been a steady decline in the use of OCG the advent of non-surgical treatments for gallstones has stimulated a resurgence.

Gallstones

In relation to gallbladder stones there are two relevant practical issues, *detection* (stones present or absent) and *selection* (for non-surgical treatments).

Detection

Eighty per cent of gallstones are radiolucent and therefore only 20% will be visible on plain radiographs (Maglinte *et al.*, 1991).

Table 6.5 Oral cholecystography in the detection of gallstones

Author/year	Total cases	Sensitivity (%)	Specificity (%)	Overall accuracy (%)	Predictive value of abnormal positive study (%)	Predictive value of normal negative study (%)
Baker & Hodgson, 1960	1207	99.5	97	98.5	98	99
Alderson, 1960	315	95	100	96	100	71
Bartrum *et al.*, 1977	200	68	100	94	100	93
Crade *et al.*, 1978	92	100	100	100	100	100
Krook *et al.*, 1980	177	95.5	100	98	100	97
Detwiler *et al.*, 1980	76	82	50	79	93	25
Totals and mean % values	2067	90	91	94	99	81

Table 6.6 Ultrasound in the detection of gallstones

Author/year	Total cases	Sensitivity (%)	Specificity (%)	Overall accuracy (%)	Predictive value of abnormal positive study (%)	Predictive value of normal negative study (%)
Cooperberg & Burhenne, 1980	313	98	98	95.5	99.6	90
Krook *et al.*, 1980	163	91	99	97.5	98	94
Lee *et al.*, 1980	133	96	91	92	97	88
Walker, 1981	142	95	88.5	79	97	82
Han-Liang *et al.*, 1990	283	93.5	86.5	91.5	94.5	84.5
Walker *et al.*, 1992	128	97.5	50	94	96	62.5
Totals and mean % values	751	95	94	91	98	88.5

Table 6.5 presents studies in which OCG has been used for the detection of gallbladder stones. For the purposes of this meta-analysis non-diagnostic studies were defined as examinations in which the gallbladder failed to opacify. The sensitivity and specificity are around 90% whilst the negative predictive value is about 83%.

Table 6.6 reviews studies in which real-time US has been used for the detection of gallbladder stones. It shows that the technique is more sensitive than OCG but in other respects is not very different, including a negative predictive value of about 84%. CT was claimed to detect nearly 80% of all gallstones in a study which used either US or surgery as the gold standard (Barakos *et al.*, 1987). The role of CT in the evaluation of gallstones is considered in the next subsection.

Preliminary studies of the gallbladder using magnetic resonance imaging (MRI) suggested that it could be applied to the evaluation of gallbladder function and anatomy (Hricak *et al.* 1983). Gallstones were detected in 20 of 23 patients in one study (McCarthy *et al.*, 1986).

Preoperative evaluation of common bile-duct stones (choledocholithiasis) by US has given widely differing results. Studies have indicated sensitivities of 25–29% and specificities of 89–91% (Gross *et al.*, 1983; Laing, 1983). A study by Cronan (1986) recorded a sensitivity of 55% whilst Laing *et al.* (1984) claimed an enhanced sensitivity of 75% which they attributed to scanning the intrapancreatic portion of the bile-duct in a transverse fashion with the patient in the erect position. A more recent large study claimed a sensitivity of 75%, specificity of 83% and overall accuracy of 80% in choledocholithiasis (Dong & Chen, 1987), the improved results being attributed to technical manoeuvres including filling the duodenum and gastric antrum with water, scanning after a fatty meal and changing the patient's position during scanning.

Peroperative US is increasingly being used as an

alternative to peroperative cholangiography for the detection of common bile-duct stones during both conventional and laparoscopic cholecystectomy. Mechanical sector scanners or linear arrays have been employed for 'open' surgery (Orda *et al.*, 1994) and endoscopic US probes for the laparoscopic technique (Rothlin *et al.*, 1994). Early reports of endoscopic US at laparoscopic cholecystectomy claim sensitivities of over 90%.

Hepatobiliary scintigraphy has demonstrated absent or delayed bowel visualization or dilated ducts in patients with surgically proven bile duct calculi (Colletti *et al.*, 1986) but the technique is not usually capable of visualizing the individual calculi.

Studies with CT showed correct predictions of common duct stones in 76–90% of cases (Jeffrey *et al.*, 1983; Baron, 1987). Cholesterol stones were the ones most likely to be missed.

Selection

The non-surgical treatments currently available for gallstones are as follows:

1 Oral dissolution using either chenodeoxycholic acid (CDCA) or ursodeoxycholic acid (UDCA).

2 Direct contact dissolution using methyl-*tert*-butyl ether (MTBE).

3 Extracorporeal shock-wave lithotripsy (ESWL) or tunable dye lasers.

Essential prerequisities for all these treatments are gallbladder contractility and cystic duct patency, which may be assessed by either OCG or US following a fatty meal or a cholecystokinin analogue (Beswick *et al.*, 1991).

In the selection of patients for non-surgical treatments the following factors relating to gallstones are important:

1 Size. *In vivo* US was correct in up to 75% and OCG correct in up to 51% (Torres *et al.*, 1991; Brakel *et al.*, 1992).

2 Number. *In vivo* studies showed US correct in 57–74% and OCG correct in 65–80%.

3 Composition. The success rate of these treatments is related to the chemical composition and morphology of the stones, those with a high-cholesterol and low-calcium content being most susceptible to non-surgical treatments.

CT is the technique most commonly used to evaluate the chemical composition and morphology of gallstones. At a practical, clinical level there is evidence that measurements of CT attenuation are helpful in selecting patients most suited to non-surgical gallstone treatments (Caroli *et al.*, 1992; Walters *et al.*, 1992). However, there is some contoversy regarding the use of CT for predicting gallstone composition. (Baron, 1991; Brink & Ferrucci, 1991).

Acute cholecystitis (AC)

Acute right upper quadrant abdominal pain is a common clinical problem with a large differential diagnosis. In the biliary tract there is a need to differentiate between acute infective cholecystitis and biliary colic, although these two conditions may coexist.

AC occurs with or without associated gallstones in a ratio of 9 : 1. The trend towards early surgery in patients with AC, in order to prevent complications, requires prompt and accurate diagnosis.

The US diagnosis of AC is a complex issue based upon a plurality of ultrasonic signs such as gallstones, gallbladder wall thickening, wall sonolucency, pericholecystic fluid, intramural gas, lack of response to cholecystokinin, gallbladder distension and local tenderness to the US probe (sonographic Murphy sign) (Fink-Bennett *et al.*, 1985).

Table 6.7 looks at the role of US using multiple diagnostic criteria which appear to improve the specificity and negative predictive values but diminish the overall accuracy and positive predictive rates.

The diagnosis of AC by hepatobiliary scintigraphy depends upon the demonstration of cystic duct obstruction, which is inferred from failure to image the gallbladder between 1 and 4 hours post-injection whilst visualizing the common bile duct. Using these criteria, meta-analysis of studies using ^{99m}Tc hepatobiliary scintigraphy in acute cholecystitis shows a high sensitivity of 96%, a modest specificity of 84% and an overall accuracy of 89% with a high negative predictive value (94%) but a modest positive predictive value (81.5%). The reason for the low positive predictive values was the high incidence (59%) of chronic cholecystitis in the patients with false positive studies.

Table 6.7 Ultrasound in acute cholecystitis. Criterion for a positive study — multiple parameters

Author/year	Total cases	Non-diagnostic cases	Sensitivity (%)	Specificity (%)	Overall accuracy (%)	Predictive value of abnormal positive study (%)	Predictive value of normal negative study (%)
Shuman *et al.*, 1982	75	1	91	69	76	57	95
Samuels *et al.*, 1983	194	4	97	64	70.5	39.5	99
Gill *et al.*, 1985	47	0	91	92	91.5	91	92
Totals and mean % values	316	5	93	75	79	62.5	95

Table 6.8 Value of ultrasound in differentiating surgical from medical jaundice. Crierion for a positive study — dilated bile-ducts

Author/year	Total cases	Non-diagnostic cases	Sensitivity (%)	Specificity (%)	Overall accuracy (%)	Predictive value of abnormal positive study (%)	Predictive value of normal negative study (%)
Malini & Sabel, 1977	35	0	88	78	86	92	70
Neiman & Mintzer, 1977	30	1	89	82	86	89	82
Taylor & Rosenfield 1977	150	0	100	93	97	94	100
Behan & Kazam, 1978	101	0	93	100	96	100	92
Scott *et al.*, 1980	25	3	67	90	77	89	69
Trought *et al.*, 1980	45	1	93	93	93	96	87.5
Bondestam *et al.*, 1981	49	0	72	84	80	72	84
Baron *et al.*, 1982	64	5	95	86	91.5	92	90.5
Zeman *et al.*, 1984	125	0	78	87	82	86	79
Lieberman & Krishnamurthy, 1986	32	0	63	100	78	100	65
Totals and mean % values	656	10	84	89	87	91	82

On current evidence, hepatobiliary scintigraphy is a more reliable technique than real-time US for the diagnosis of AC. US is often more readily available and gives additional information that hepatobiliary scintigraphy cannot provide.

There are promising reports of the role of radionuclide labelled leucocytes (^{111}In or ^{99m}Tc HMPOA) for the demonstration of the inflamed gallbladder wall in AC (Lantto *et al.*, 1991; Fink-Bennett *et al.*, 1991). The CT diagnosis of AC is based, like US, on a combination of signs including a thickened, nodular or poorly defined gall-bladder wall, pericholecystic fluid collections, infiltration of the pericholecystic fat, subserosal oedema (halo), intramural gas, perforation, sloughed mucosa, gallbladder luminal distension, hyperdense bile or calculi (Kane *et al.*, 1983; Blankenberg *et al.*, 1991).

In very ill patients, considered unsuitable for major surgery, percutaneous transhepatic cannulation and drainage of the gallbladder contents (cholecystostomy) may be life-saving. The technique may be performed under US guidance and the patient preparation is similar to that for PTC. The biliary tract may also be demonstrated by injection of contrast medium during the procedure.

Regarding the use of MRI in the diagnosis of AC, liver/gallbladder signal intensity ratios on T_1 weighted imaging may distinguish AC from chronic cholecystitis and normal gallbladders (Pu, 1994).

Investigation of cholestatic jaundice

The differentiation must be made between intrahepatic cholestasis and extrahepatic obstruction.

Table 6.9 Ultrasound in obstructive jaundice — evaluation of site and cause of obstruction

Author/year	Total cases	Site of obstruction		Cause of obstruction	
		n	% correct	*n*	% correct
Koenigsberg *et al.*, 1979	32	30	94	25	78
Wild *et al.*, 1980	46	27	58	13	28
Dalla Palma *et al.*, 1982	85	77	91	63	74
Gibbons *et al.*, 1983	93	31	33	27	29
Honickman *et al.*, 1983	62	17	27	15	24
Gibson *et al.*, 1986	65	57	88	—	—
Laing *et al.*, 1986	110	78	71	101	92
Dixit *et al.*, 1993	169	78	46	93	55
Totals and mean % values	662	395	60	—	54

Table 6.10 Chiba needle percutaneous transhepatic cholangiography in obstructive jaundice — evaluation of site and cause of obstruction

Author/year	Total cases	Site of obstruction		Cause of obstruction	
		n	% correct	*n*	% correct
Koenigsberg *et al.*, 1979	28	27	96	25	89
Wild *et al.*, 1980	46	42	91	29	63
Owen, 1980	56	50	89	37	71
Dalla Palma *et al.*, 1982	85	84	99	76	89
Gibson *et al.*, 1986	111	102	92	97	87
Dixit *et al.*, 1993	79	78	99	61	77
Totals and mean % values	405	383	94.5	325	80

Ultrasound

The diagnosis of duct dilatation by US requires an ability to distinguish intrahepatic bile-ducts from other intrahepatic structures and an accurate knowledge of the range of normal duct measurements. Cooperberg *et al.* (1980) showed that common hepatic duct diameters greater than 4 mm indicate extrahepatic obstruction (sensitivity 99%, specificity 87%). Deitch (1981) concluded that extrahepatic obstruction was present with a common duct in excess of 10 mm or intrahepatic ducts larger than 5 mm. He also noted that obstruction could be excluded if the common duct was less than 8 mm and the intrahepatic ducts less than 4 mm. Absent duct dilation has been found in the presence of obstructive jaundice (Thomas & Zornoza, 1980).

Table 6.8 presents the value of US in distinguishing dilated from non-dilated bile-ducts in patients with jaundice. The technique is fairly reliable for this purpose though the sensitivity (84%) and negative predictive values (82%) are modest. Table 6.9 present the role of US in patients with obstructive jaundice. It is only able to define the site of obstruction in 60% and the cause in 54% of cases.

Chiba needle PTC

Table 6.10 presents the role of Chiba needle PTC in patients with obstructive jaundice. It is very successful at delineating the site of obstruction (94.5%) but less successful at predicting the cause (80%). Both these figures are considerably better than the comparable results from US.

Table 6.11 Computed tomography in differentiating surgical from medical jaundice. Criterion for a positive study — multiple parameters

Author/year	Total cases	Sensitivity (%)	Specificity (%)	Overall accuracy (%)	Predictive value of abnormal positive study (%)	Predictive value of normal negative study (%)
Havrilla *et al.*, 1977	44	96	90.5	93	92	95
Levitt *et al.*, 1977	65	88	95.5	91	97	81
Fawcitt *et al.*, 1978	23	93	89	91	93	89
Goldberg *et al.*, 1978	23	83	100	87	100	62.5
Morris *et al.*, 1978	41	72	94	80.5	95	68
Baron *et al.*, 1982*	64	97.5	95	92	97.5	95
Totals and mean % values	260	88	94	89	96	82

* Only proven cases.

Table 6.12 Computed tomography in obstructive jaundice — evaluation of site and cause of obstruction

Author/year	Total cases	Site of obstruction		Cause of obstruction	
		n	% correct	*n*	% correct
Havrilla *et al.*, 1977	25	22	88	17	68
Fawcitt *et al.*, 1978	14	13	93	11	79
Morris *et al.*, 1978	25	15	60	18	72
Pedrosa *et al.*, 1981	67	65	97	63	94
Baron *et al.*, 1982	40	35	87.5	33	82.5
Gibson *et al.*, 1986	51	46	90	32	63
Totals and mean % values	222	196	88	174	78

Endoscopic retrograde cholangiopancreatography

Papillary (vaterian) cannulation is successful in 84% of procedures. The yield of positive diagnostic studies, which includes information from endoscopy, approaches 76%. In the total population of jaundiced patients examined by ERCP, 14.6% have non-obstructed bile ducts and will perhaps be spared further surgery.

Computed tomography

Table 6.11 show the value of CT in distinguishing extrahepatic (surgical) obstruction from medical causes of jaundice. The technique is extremely reliable in this respect, faltering only in its negative pre-

dictive values (82%). Table 6.12 assesses CT in patients with obstructive jaundice. It is able to determine the site of obstruction in 88% and the cause in 78%. It is less good than PTC for determining site but as good for predicting cause. It is considerably better than US in both respects.

Hepatobiliary scintigraphy

Using ^{99m}Tc HIDA, the bile-ducts, gallbladder and proximal jejunum can be visualized within 30 min of injection (Rosenthall *et al.*, 1978). Using [99m] Tc di-isopropyl IDA the biliary tract is identified between 10 and 30 min post-injection with maximum activity at 45 min (Klingensmith *et al.*, 1981).

Duct dilation and delayed or absent small bowel activity are the most reliable signs of extrahepatic obstruction (Rosenthall *et al.*, 1978). Successful examinations have been recorded with serum bilirubins up to 250 µmol l⁻¹ (Oster-Jorgensen *et al.*, 1979) but the success of the procedure declines as the serum bilirubin rises (Scott *et al.*, 1980).

The performance of hepatobiliary scintigraphy in differentiating extrahepatic (surgical) obstruction from medical causes of jaundice is the worst of all the imaging techniques in this respect. The sensitivity is 75% while specificity, overall accuracy and positive predictive value are all 77% with a negative predictive value of 74%.

Choice of imaging techniques in jaundiced patients

In comparing non-invasive imaging techniques in differentiating surgical (extrahepatic obstruction) from medical causes of jaundice, the rank order for procedural reliability is: first CT (see Table 6.11); second US (see Table 6.8); and third hepatobiliary scintigraphy. CT is only marginally better than US in respect of sensitivity, specificity and positive predictive values. Both CT and US are considerably better than scintigraphy in all the measured parameters. Scintigraphy should probably be abandoned for this purpose.

In comparing non-invasive techniques in their ability to determine the site or cause of biliary obstruction, only CT and US are considered. CT outstrips US in both diagnoses (see Tables 6.9 & 6.12). In addition, CT may distinguish benign from malignant obstructions (Baron *et al.*, 1983).

The two invasive proceedures, PTC and ERCP, have the additional capability of acting as the therapeutic tools for stent placement, sphincterotomy or external biliary drainage. Indeed, the need for intervention may outweigh all other factors in the choice of imaging procedure. It has been possible to compare PTC with US and CT in their ability to determine the site or cause of biliary obstruction. In these respects the rank orders are as follows: first PTC (see Table 6.10); second CT (see Table 6.12); and third US (see Table 6.9). PTC succeeds over CT only in respect of defining the site of obstruction. Both PTC and CT are vastly superior to US with both diagnoses.

Investigation of peroperative and postoperative patients

In addition to peroperative cholangiography surgeons may use rigid or flexible choledochoscopes and intraoperative US. Choledochoscopy is increasingly being used for the safe removal of retained gallstones (Menzies & Motson, 1992). Operative sonography for common bile-duct stones has been considered to be as reliable as peroperative cholangiography (Siegel *et al.*, 1982).

In the immediate postoperative phase T-tube cholangiography has an important and probably unique role.

Patients who have previously had biliary surgery may cause diagnostic problems. Bile-duct dilatation often persists in the absence of obstruction. US cannot reliably diagnose or exclude bile-duct stones in postcholecystectomy patients. However, it does demonstrate residual fluid collections after laparoscopic cholecystectomy.

Hepatobiliary scintigraphy is used for demonstrating bile leaks and the patency of biliary enteric anastomoses.

ERCP may be difficult or impossible in some postsurgical patients with jaundice, who may require investigation by PTC as the first-line invasive imaging procedure.

New horizons in hepatobiliary imaging

There is growing interest in three-dimensional imaging of the biliary tract. Klein *et al.* (1993) have reported on the use of volumetric CT ('spiral CT') following administration of an i.v. cholangiographic agent. Gillams *et al.* (1994) have used three-dimensional post-processing of two-dimensional CT data sets following i.v. low-osmolar monomeric contrast in patients with biliary obstruction.

There are several promising reports of the use of contrast-enhanced Fourier-acquired steady-state (CE-FAST) gradient echo MRI with maximum intensity projection (MIP) post-processing three-dimensional reconstructions of the biliary tract in patients with biliary obstruction (Morimoto *et al.*, 1992). There are also a number of developments in the search for an ideal biliary-tract specific MRI contrast agent using complexes with paramagnetic ions such as iron, manganese and gadolinium (Muetterties *et al.*, 1991; Rummeny *et al.*, 1991; Schuhmann-Giampieri *et al.*, 1992; Schmiedl *et al.*, 1993).

References

Alderson, D.A. (1960) The reliability of Telepaque cholecystography. *Br. J. Surg.*, **47**(206), 655–8.

Baker, H.L. & Hodgson, J.R. (1960) Further studies on the accuracy of oral cholecystography. *Radiology*, **74**, 239–45.

Barakos, J.A., Ralls, P.W. & Lapin, S.A. (1987) Cholelithiasis: evaluation with CT. *Radiology*, **162**, 415–18.

Baron, R.L. (1987) Common bile duct stones: reassessment of criteria for CT diagnosis. *Radiology*, **162**, 419–24.

Baron, R.L. (1991) Role of CT in characterizing gallstones: An unsettled issue. *Radiology*, **178**(3), 635–6.

Baron, R.L., Stanley, R.J. & Lee, J.K.T. (1982) A prospective comparison of the evaluation of biliary obstruction using computed tomography and ultrasonography. *Radiology*, **145**, 91–8.

Baron, R.L., Stanley, R.J. & Lee, J.K.T. (1983) Computed tomographic features of biliary obstruction. *AJR*, **140**, 1173–8.

Bartrum, R.J. Jr., Crow, H.C. & Foote, S.R. (1977) Ultrasonic and radiographic cholecystography. *N. Engl. J. Med.*, **296**, 538–41.

Behan, M. & Kazam, E. (1978) Sonography of the common bile duct: value of the right anterior oblique view. *AJR*, **130**, 701–9.

Berk, R.N., Leopold, G.R. & Fordtran, J.S. (1983) Imaging of the gallbladder. *Adv. Intern. Med.*, **28**, 387–408.

Beswick, J.S., Hughes, P.M. & Martin, D.F. (1991) Ultrasonic evaluation of gallbladder function prior to non-surgical treatment of gallstones. *Br. J. Radiol.*, **64**, 321–3.

Blankenberg, F.., Wirth, R., Jeffrey R.B. Jr *et al.* (1991) Computed tomography as an adjunct to ultrasound in the diagnosis of acute acalculous cholecystitis. *Gastrointest. Radiol.*, **16**, 149–53.

Bondestam, S., Taavitsainen, M., Jappinen, S. *et al.* (1981) Ultrasound examination and cholescintigraphy in cholestasis. *Acta Radiol. Diag.*, **22**, 421–6.

Brakel, K., Lameris, J.S., Nijs, H.G.T. *et al.* (1992) Accuracy of ultrasound and oral cholecystography in assessing the number and size of gallstones: implications for non-surgical therapy. *Br. J. Radiol.*, **65**, 779–83.

Brink, J.A. & Ferrucci, J.T. (1991) Use of CT for predicting gallstone composition; a dissenting view. *Radiology* **178**, 633–4.

Caroli, A., Del Favero, G., Di Mario, F. *et al.* (1992) Computed tomography in predicting gall stone solubility: a prospective trial. *Gut*, **33**, 698–700.

Colletti, P.M., Ralls, P.W. & Lapin, S.A. (1986) Hepatobiliary imaging in choledocholithiasis: a comparison with ultrasound. *Clin. Nuc. Med.*, **ii**, 482–6.

Cooperberg, P.L. & Burhenne, H.J. (1980) Real-time ultrasonography: diagnostic technique of choice in calculous gallbladder disease. *N. Engl. J. Med.*, **302**, 1277–9.

Cooperberg, P.L., Li, D. & Wong, P. (1980) Accuracy of common hepatic duct size in the evaluation of extrahepatic biliary obstruction. *Radiology*, **135**, 141–4.

Crade, M., Taylor, K.J.W., Rosenfield, A.T. *et al.* (1978) Surgical and pathologic correlation of cholecystosonography and cholecystography. *Am. J. Roentgenol.*, **131**, 227–9.

Cronan, J.J. (1986) US diagnosis of choledocholithiasis: a reappraisal. *Radiology*, **161**, 133–4.

Dalla Palma, L., Maffessanti, M. & Bazzocchi, M. (1982) Combined use of ultrasonography and transhepatic percutaneous cholangiography in obstructive jaundice. *Eur. J. Radiol.*, **2**, 281–9.

Deitch, E.A. (1981) The reliability and clinical limitations of sonographic scanning of the biliary ducts. *Ann. Surg.*, **194**, 167–70.

Detwiler, R.P., Kim, D.S. & Longerbeam, J.K. (1980) Ultrasonography and oral cholecystography: a comparison of their use in the diagnosis of gallbladder disease. *Arch. Surg.*, **115**, 1096–8.

Dixit, V.K., Jain, A.K., Agrawal, A.K. *et al.* (1993) Obstructive jaundice: a diagnostic appraisal. *JAPI*, **41**(4), 200–2.

Dong, B. & Chen, M. (1987) Improved sonographic visualization of choledocholithiasis. *J. Clin. Ultrasound*, **15**, 185–90.

Fawcitt, R.A., Forbes, W.S.C. & Isherwood, I. (1978) Computed tomographic scanning in liver disease. *Clin. Radiol.*, **29**, 251–4.

Ferrucci, J.T., Fordtran, J.S. & Cooperberg, P.L. (1981) The radiological diagnosis of gallbladder disease: an imaging symposium. *Radiology*, **141**, 49–56.

Fink-Bennett, D., Clarke, K., Tsai, D. *et al.* (1991) Indium-111-leukocyte imaging in acute cholecystitis. *J. Nucl. Med.*, **32**, 803–4.

Fink-Bennett, D., Freitas, J.E. & Ripley, S.D. (1985) The sensitivity of hepatobiliary imaging and real-time ultrasonography in the detection of acute cholecystitis. *Arch. Surg.*, **120**, 904–6.

Gibbons, C.P., Griffiths, G.J. & Cormack, A. (1983) The role of percutaneous transhepatic cholangiography and grey-scale ultrasound in the investigation and treatment of bile duct obstruction. *Br. J. Surg.*, **70**, 494–6.

Gibson, R.N., Yeung, E. & Thompson, J.N. (1986) Bile duct obstruction: radiologic evaluation of level, cause, and tumour resectability. *Radiology*, **160**, 43–7.

Gill, P.T., Dillon, E., Leahy, A.L. *et al.* (1985) Ultrasonography, HIDA scintigraphy or both in the diagnosis of acute cholecystitis. *Br. J. Surg.*, **72**, 267–8.

Gillams, A., Gardener, J., Richards, R. *et al.* (1994) Three-dimensional computed tomography cholangiography: a new technique for biliary tract imaging. *Br. J. Radiol.*, **67**, 445–8.

Goldberg, H.I., Filly, R.A. & Korobkin, M. (1978) Capability of CT body scanning and ultrasonography to demonstrate the status of the biliary ductal system in patients with jaundice. *Radiology*, **129**, 731–7.

Gross, B.H., Harter, L.P. & Gore, R.M. (1983) Ultrasonic evaluation of common bile duct stones: prospective comparison with endoscopic retrograde cholangiopancreatography. *Radiology*, **146**, 471–4.

Han-Liang, Y., Zheng-Zhi, L. & Yi-Guo, S. (1990) Reliability of ultrasonography in diagnosis of biliary lithiasis. *Chinese Med. J.*, **103**(8), 638–41.

Havrilla, T.R., Haaga, J.R. & Alfidi, R.J. (1977) Computed tomography and obstructive biliary disease. *AJR*, **128**, 765–8.

Honickman, S.P., Mueller, P.R. & Wittenberg, J. (1983) Ultrasound in obstructive jaundice: prospective evaluation of site and cause. *Radiology*, **147**, 511–15.

Hricak, H., Filly, R.A. & Margulis, A.R. (1983) Work in progress: nuclear magnetic resonance imaging of the gallbladder. *Radiology*, **147**, 481–4.

Jeffrey, R.B., Federe, M.P. & Laing, F.C. (1983) Computed tomography of choledocholithiasis. *AJR*, **140**, 1179–83.

Kane, R.A., Costello, P. & Duszlak, E. (1983) Computed tomography in acute cholecystitis: new observations. *AJR*, **141**, 697–701.

Klein, H.-M., Wein, B., Truong, S. *et al.* (1993) Computed tomographic cholangiography using spiral scanning and 3D image processing. *Br. J. Radiol.*, **66**, 762–7.

Klingensmith, W.C., Spitzer, V.M., Fritzberg, A.R. *et al.* (1981) The normal fasting and postpandrial diisopropyl IDA Tc^{99m} hepatobiliary study. *Radiology*, **141**, 771–6.

Koenigsberg, M., Wiener, S.N. & Walzer, A. (1979) The accuracy of sonography in the differential diagnosis of obstructive jaundice: a comparison with cholangiography. *Radiology*, **133**, 157–65.

Krook, P.M., Allen, F.H. & Bush, W.H. (1980) Comparison of real-time cholecystosonography and oral cholecystography. *Radiology*, **135**, 145–8.

Laing, F.C. (1983) Diagnostic evaluation of patients with suspected cholecystitis: CT and ultrasonography in the acutely ill patient. *Radiol. Clin. N. Am.*, **21**(3), 477–93.

Laing, F.C., Jeffrey, R.B. & Wing, V.W. (1984) Improved visualization of choledocholithiasis by sonography. *AJR*, **143**, 949–52.

Laing, F.C., Jeffrey, R.B. & Wing, V.W. (1986) Biliary dilatation: defining the level and cause by real-time US. *Radiology*, **160**, 39–42.

Lantto E., Jarvi, K., Laitinen, R. *et al.* (1991) Scintigraphy with ^{99m}Tc-HMPAO labelled leukocytes in acute cholecystitis. *Acta Radiol.*, **32**, 359–62.

Lee, J.K.T., Melson, G.L. & Koehler, R.E. (1980) Cholecystosonography: accuracy, pitfalls and unusual findings. *Am. J. Surg.*, **139**, 223–8.

Levitt, R.G., Sage, S.S. & Stanley, R.J. (1977) Accuracy of computed tomography of the liver and biliary tract. *Radiology*, **124**, 123–8.

Lieberman, D.A. & Krishnamurthy, G.T. (1986) Intrahepatic versus extrahepatic cholestasis. *Gastroenterology*, **90**, 734–43.

Maglinte, D.D.T., Torres, W.E. & Laufer, I. (1991) Oral cholecystography in contemporary gallstone imaging: a review. *Radiology*, **178**, 49–58.

Malini, S. & Sabel, J. (1977) Ultrasonography in obstructive jaundice. *Radiology*, **123**, 429–33.

McCarthy, S., Hricak, H., Cohen, M. *et al.* (1986) Cholecystitis: detection with MR imaging. *Radiology*, **158**, 333–6.

Menzies, D. & Motson, R.W. (1992) Operative common bile duct imaging by operative cholangiography and flexible choledochoscopy. *Br. J. Surg.*, **79**, 815–17.

Morimoto, K., Shimoi, M., Shirakawa, T. *et al.* (1992) Biliary obstruction: evaluation with three-dimensional MR cholangiography. *Radiology*, **183**, 578–80.

Morris, A.I., Fawcitt, R.A. & Wood, R. (1978) Computed tomography, ultrasound and cholestatic jaundice. *Gut*, **19**, 685–8.

Muetterties, K.A., Hoener, B.-A., Engelstad, B.L. *et al.* (1991) Ferrioxamine B derivatives as hepatobiliary contrast agents for magnetic resonance imaging. *MR Med.*, **22**, 88–100.

Neiman, H.L. & Mintzer, R.A. (1977) Accuracy of biliary duct ultrasound: comparison with cholangiography. *AJR*, **129**, 979–82.

Orda, R., Sayfan, J., Strauss, S. *et al.* (1994) Intra-operative ultrasonography as a routine screening procedure in biliary surgery. *Hepato-Gastroenterol.* **41**, 61–4.

Oster-Jorgensen, E., Pedersen, S.A. & Schoubye, J. (1979) Hepatobiliary scintigraphy with ^{99}Tcm-HIDA in patients with jaundice. *Acta Radiol. Diagn.*, **20**, 299–310.

Owen, J.P. (1980) Analysis of the signs of common bile duct obstruction at percutaneous transhepatic cholangiography. *Clin. Radiol.*, **31**, 271–6.

Pedrosa, C.S., Casanova, R. & Rodriguez, R. (1981) Computed tomography in obstructive jaundice: Part 1 and 2. *Radiology*, **139**, 627–45.

Pu, Y., Yamamoto, F., Igimi, I. *et al.* (1994) A comparative study of usefulness of magnetic resonance imaging in the diagnosis of acute cholecystitis. *J. Gastroenterol.*, **29**, 192–8.

Rosenthall, L., Shaffer, E. A. & Lisbona, R. (1978) Diagnosis of hepatobiliary disease by ^{99m}Tc-HIDA cholescintigraphy. *Radiology*, **126**, 467–74.

Rothlin, M.A., Schlumpf, R. & Largiader, F. (1994) Laparoscopic sonography — an alternative to routine intraoperative cholangiography? *Arch. Surg.*, **129**, 694–700.

Rummeny, E., Ehrenheim, C., Gehl, H.B. *et al.* (1991) Manganese-DPDP as a hepatobiliary contrast agent in the magnetic resonance imaging of liver tumors. *Invest. Radiol.*, **26** (Suppl. 1), S142–S155.

Samuels, B.I., Freitas, J.E. & Bree, R.L. (1983) A comparison of radionuclide hepatobiliary imaging and real-time ultrasound for the detection of acute cholecystitis. *Radiology*, **147**, 207–10.

Schmiedl, U.P., Nelson, J.A., Robinson, D.H. *et al.* (1993) Pharmaceutical properties, biodistribution, and imaging characteristics of manganese-mesoporphyrin — a potential hepatobiliary contrast agent for magnetic resonance imaging. *Invest. Radiol.*, **28**(10), 925–32.

Schuhmann-Giampieri, G., Schmitt-Willich, H., Press, W.-R. *et al.* (1992) Preclinical evaluation of Gd-EOB-DTPA as a contrast agent in MR imaging of the hepatobiliary system. *Radiology*, **183**, 59–64.

Scott, B.B., Evans, J.A. Unsworth, J. (1980) The initial investigation of jaundice in a district general hospital: a study of ultrasonography and hepatobiliary scintigraphy. *Br. J. Radiol.*, **53**, 557–62.

Shuman, W.P., Mack, L.A. & Rudd, T.G. (1982) Evaluation of acute right upper quadrant pain: sonography and 99mTc-PIPIDA cholescintigraphy. *AJR*, **139**, 61–4.

Siegel, B., Coelho, J.C.U. & Nyhus, L.M. (1982) Comparison of cholangiography and ultrasonography in the operative screening of the common bile duct. *World J. Surg.*, **6**, 440–4.

Taylor, K.J.W. & Rosenfield, A.T. (1977) Grey-scale ultrasonography in the differential diagnosis of jaundice. *Arch. Surg.*, **112**, 820–5.

Thomas, J.L. & Zornoza, J. (1980) Obstructive jaundice in the absence of sonographic biliary dilatation. *Gastrointest. Radiol.*, **5**, 357–60.

Torres, W.E., Baumgartner, B.R., Todd-Jones, M. *et al.* (1991)

Comparison ultrasonography and oral cholecystography in biliary lithotripsy. *Invest. Radiol.*, **26**(7), 633–5.

Trought, W.S., Morgan, C.C., Jackson, D.C. *et al.* (1980) Evaluation of the biliary tree; a comparison of percutaneous transhepatic cholangiography and ultransonography. *South Med. J.*, **73**, 1592–3.

Walker, J., Chalmers, R.T.A. & Allan, P.L. (1992) An audit of ultrasound diagnosis of gallbladder calculi. *Br. J. Radiol.*, **65**, 581–4.

Walker, T.M. (1981) Ultrasound of the gallbladder: experience in a district hospital. *Br. Med. J.*, **282**, 145–6

Walters, J.R.F., Hood, K.A., Gleeson, D. *et al.* (1992) Combination therapy with oral ursodeoxycholic and chenodeoxycholic acids: pretreatment computed tomography of the gall bladder improves gall stone dissolution efficacy. *Gut*, **33**, 375–80.

Wild, S.R., Cruikshank, J.G., Fraser, G.M. *et al.* (1980) Grey-scale ultrasonography and percutaneous transhepatic cholangiography in biliary tract disease. *Br. Med. J.*, **281**, 1524–6.

Zeman, R.K., Lee, C. & Jaffe, M.H. (1984) Hepatobiliary scintigraphy and sonography in early biliary obstruction. *Radiology*, **153**, 793–8.

7   Pancreas

A. F. EVANS

The pancreas has always been a difficult organ to visualize accurately. It is only relatively recently that the 'newer' imaging techniques have made routine pancreatic imaging possible. Meticulous technique has to be applied in order to maximize the potential of the current imaging modalities. The wide variation in local expertise and availability of imaging equipment has meant that none of the techniques have clearly established themselves as superior in assessing all the various aspects of pancreatic disease. However, first-line investigations in patients with suspected pancreatic disease are described and their relationship to other diagnostic techniques assessed.

Ultrasound

Transabdominal ultrasound

This is the most widely used technique for pancreatic imaging (Figs 7.1 & 7.2). It is inexpensive, non-invasive and there is generally a high level of expertise available. Every imaging department has access to modern ultrasound equipment.

Preparation

Patient preparation is minimal for ultrasound imaging. It is usual to fast the patient for 6 hours prior to the examination as this allows gallbladder visualization which is usually performed concurrently. The prior ingestion of fluid into the stomach is advocated by some to provide an acoustic window for the pancreas. Ultrasound is generally well tolerated by patients. Acoustic coupling is applied to the skin. Real-time scanning is performed using a variety of transducers: sector, linear or curvilinear depending on operator preference. Sector probes have an advantage in the upper abdomen of being

versatile and allowing good visualization of the pancreas via a small anterior access. Bowel gas and intra-abdominal fat are a constant threat to adequate visualization of the intra-abdominal organs, unlike with computed tomography (CT) which relies on fat planes to delineate the pancreas and associated structures. Most scans are carried out with the patient lying supine. Scanning the patient in an erect or sitting position or positioning the patient obliquely will often allow better access to the pancreas by displacing the gas-containing bowel loops. A 5 mHz is usually the optimal size probe, although some prefer 3.5 mHz in visualizing the pancreas and biliary tree.

The anatomical markers of the superior mesenteric artery and the splenic vein are used to identify and delineate the pancreas. The immobile patient can be scanned in the bed. Postoperative scanning may be problematic if there are wound dressings, sutures or drainage bags on the anterior abdominal wall. However, it is usually possible to move the patient into a particular position to allow pancreatic imaging. The sensitivity of transabdominal ultrasound is limited by overlapping bowel gas which may completely obscure the pancreas in conditions such as ileus. Transabdominal ultrasound should always be the first imaging technique of choice before proceeding to other more time-consuming and expensive methods of imaging the pancreas.

Endoscopic ultrasound

At present this technique is not widely available. A small ultrasound transducer is built into the endoscope so that the pancreas can be visualized through the stomach wall with the transducer in very close proximity to the pancreas. Lesions as small as 5 mm have been identified. This technique is a highly sensitive and specific method for localizing

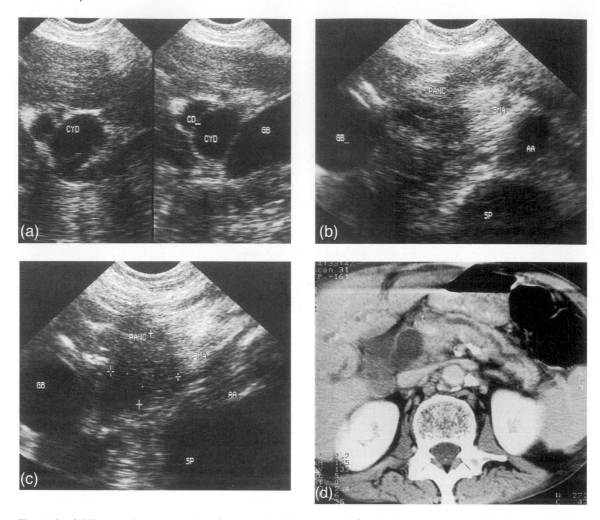

Fig. 7.1 (a–c) Ultrasound — cross-sectional images; 26 × 27 mm mass in head of pancreas causing dilated common duct, cystic duct and gallbladder. AA, abdominal aorta; CD, common bile-duct; CYD, cystic duct; GB, gallbladder; PANC, pancreas; SMA, superior mesenteric artery. (d) Computed tomography scan showing dilated common bile-duct, dilated pancreatic duct and mass in head of pancreas.

pancreatic endocrine tumours, once the clinical and laboratory diagnosis has been established (Glover *et al.*, 1992).

Intraoperative ultrasound

This may be used as an adjunct to the examination of the pancreas at surgery. Probes of 7.5 or 10 mHz are used. The role of this technique seems at present to be limited to defining the configuration of the pancreas or a small intrapancreatic mass such as an endocrine tumour during surgery, to localize the lesion and help assess operability (Gianello *et al.*, 1988).

Computed tomography

CT has revolutionized imaging of the pancreas, providing highly accurate visualization of both

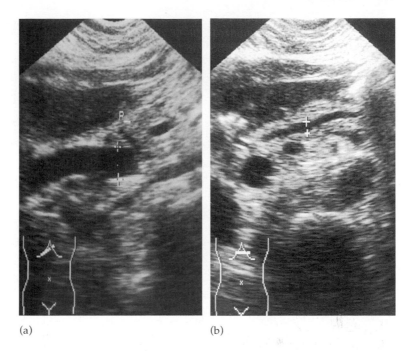

Fig. 7.2 Ultrasound —
carcinoma of ampulla of Vater:
(a) oblique image shows common
bile-duct dilated to 17 mm; (b) axial
image — pancreatic duct dilated to
6 mm.

(a)　　　　　　　　　　　(b)

anatomical and pathological changes within the gland (Fig. 7.3).

Preparation

Starvation for 6 hours is routine. Oral contrast medium is administered in order to opacify the stomach, duodenum and small bowel. The gastric contents and small bowel have attenuation values almost identical to soft tissue and may mimic mass lesions. Gastrografin diluted down to 2% is a suitable oral contrast agent, although similar agents including dilute barium preparations are used. Higher concentrations should be avoided as they produce artefact on the scan. It is the author's practice to give the patient 300–400 ml of 2% Gastrografin orally 30 min prior to the scan and to supplement this with 100–150 ml 5 min before the examination.

Examination technique

Most patients are scanned supine. If they are in pain, for example due to pancreatitis, they may be more comfortable with a support behind the knees. Movement artefact can be minimized by scanning during suspended respiration. It is essential to examine the patient in the same phase of respiration.

Antiperistaltic agents are seldom required, due to the speed of modern scanners. The choice of slice thickness depends on the machine used. The author's routine is to perform 10 mm contiguous slices to locate the pancreas, including the whole liver, especially if pancreatic neoplasm is suspected.

A 'dynamic' contrast enhanced scan is then performed. A non-ionic contrast agent minimizes patient discomfort and consequent movement: 50 ml are injected at a rate of 1 ml s^{-1} and a further 50 ml (the second phase) at the rate of 0.5 ml s^{-1}. The pancreas is 'targeted' and scanning commenced after the initial phase of the injection. If there is obvious pathology on the unenhanced scan, 10 mm slices are routine. Otherwise 2–5 mm contiguous slices are obtained, especially if small lesions such as endocrine tumours are being looked for. Dynamic scanning is especially useful in detecting areas of hypoperfusion in acute pancreatitis. CT scanning is now the procedure of choice in imaging acute pancreatitis.

CT examination should be performed under the direct supervision of the radiologist so that the routine technique can be altered if necessary. Spiral CT

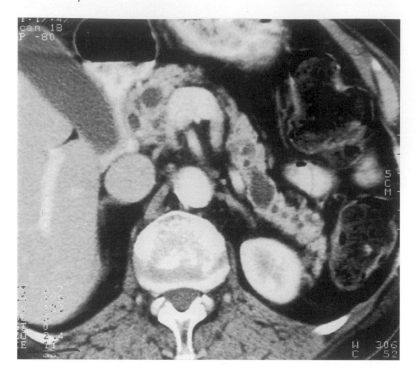

Fig. 7.3 Dynamic targeted computed tomography scan. Carcinoma of head of pancreas. Mass in head of pancreas; dilated common bile-duct; ectatic pancreatic duct.

scanning allows the pancreas to be scanned in a single breath-hold, resulting in sharper images and reducing motion artefact. There is also superior vascular opacification, which is useful in detecting small masses.

Acute pancreatitis

Patients with clinically mild pancreatitis in whom the diagnosis is secure do not require imaging as long as they respond appropriately to conservative management. In patients with clinically severe pancreatitis early CT should be performed to evaluate the extent and nature of local complications. If radiographic changes are mild and the patient responds to conservative treatment, no further imaging is required. If the patient fails to respond or worsens, follow-up CT is indicated to exclude delayed complications.

Patients whose initial CT shows severe pancreatitis or peripancreatic inflammatory changes require serial CT to assess resolution. If at any time during the progress of the illness there is clinical suspicion of infection, percutaneous fine-needle aspiration of the affected site is indicated. The decision to

intervene, whether for infection (abscess formation) or sterile (pseudocyst formation) complications, must be made on clinical grounds. CT can be very helpful in choosing the appropriate means of intervention (Freeney, 1992).

Chronic pancreatitis

CT can be accurate in the diagnosis of chronic pancreatitis. Parenchymal and ductal changes indicative of chronic pancreatitis can be identified.

Pancreatic carcinoma

In the diagnosis of pancreatic masses, CT is currently the imaging technique of choice. However, the imaging strategy for staging once a tumour has been found remains controversial. A recent survey of pancreatic carcinoma from Scandinavia (Bakkevold *et al.*, 1992) revealed that CT performs well in the diagnosis of pancreatic masses as compared to other imaging modalities (Table 7.1).

There is disagreement as to whether or not angiography is needed to detect vascular involvement. In some hands, CT angiography is as accurate

Table 7.1 Relative sensitivities of imaging methods for diagnosing pancreatic carcinoma. From Bakkevold *et al.* (1992)

Method	Sensitivity (%)
Endoscopic retrograde cholangiopancreatography	79
Computed tomography	75
Ultrasound	57
Fine-needle aspiration	86 (performed in 27%)
Angiography	43 (performed in 18% to assess operability)

as mesenteric angiography. Using spiral CT with volume acquisition in a single breath-hold and three-dimensional post-processing, high resolution images can be obtained of the vascular anatomy within the pancreatic bed. These allow very accurate assessment of venous and arterial encasement in pancreatic carcinoma (Lu & Krasny, 1994). Work in progress suggests that these new methods of data aquisition and manipulation will rapidly proceed to allow optimal visualization of pancreatic vessels by this non-invasive route.

Endoscopic retrograde cholangiopancreatography (ERCP)

ERCP was first performed in Japan 25 years ago (Oi *et al.*, 1969) The widespread use of endoscopy in recent years has allowed an ERCP service to be offered in most UK hospitals. Usually performed by an endoscopist in the imaging department with the close cooperation of the radiologist, ERCP is seldom performed without other complementary imaging techniques which are usually essential in optimizing patient management. It is the role of the radiologist to interpret these and correlate them with other imaging techniques. Contraindications to ERCP include oesophageal stenosis, gastric outlet obstruction, thoracic aortic aneurysm and severe pulmonary disease. ERCP should be avoided in patients known to be hypersensitive to contrast media and should not be performed within 4 weeks of an episode of acute pancreatitis or in the presence of pseudocyst.

Technique

The examination is performed in the X-ray department (Bauerle *et al.*, 1972) under fluoroscopic control. Starvation for 6 hours is routine. A chest radiograph is inspected in elderly patients to exclude a thoracic aortic aneurysm. Some would advocate a prior barium study in symptomatic patients to assess the oesophagus and the gastric outlet. The endoscopy is usually performed in the left lateral position. This allows the stomach and duodenum to be inspected prior to identifying the ampulla of Vater. Once cannulation has been obtained, 1–2 ml of contrast medium is injected under fluoroscopic control. Non-ionic contrast medium is associated with less pain and less hyperamylasaemia (Osnes *et al.* 1975). However, another study (Makela & Dean, 1986) has shown that hyperamylasaemia is a complication of minor importance following ERCP and unlikely to be reduced by the use of low-osmolar contrast media. Following successful cannulation, a slow injection of contrast medium is made under fluoroscopic vision. Radiographs are obtained when the duct is delineated to its tail (Fig. 7.4). The injection is stopped when the lateral branches of the duct are seen or when the patient complains of pain. The patient is then turned as necessary in order to obtain the optimum view of the duct and prevent the endoscope obscuring ductal detail. Further views of the pancreatic duct can be obtained in the prone oblique and anteroposterior (AP) positions. Patients who have had previous gastric surgery will usually present problems for the endoscopist and it may be impossible to cannulate the duodenum.

Selective duct cannulation allows pure pancreatic juice to be collected for biochemical and cytological analysis (Enco *et al.*, 1974; Hatfield *et al.*, 1976). Seifert *et al.* (1977) have described intraductal biopsy of the pancreatic duct.

Complications

The hazards of ERCP include those of upper gas-

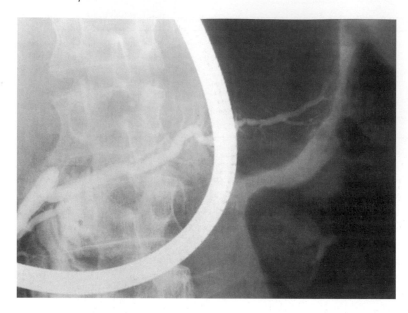

Fig. 7.4 Endoscopic retrograde cholangiopancreatography — pancreatic duct filled to the tail with side-duct filling.

trointestinal endoscopy, such as inhalation, perforation of the oesophagus and the risk of cross-infection. Bilbao *et al.* (1976) reported a 3% incidence of complications and a 0.15% mortality rate in a survey of 10 000 cases. Asymptomatic elevation of serum amylase has been reported (Cotton *et al.*, 1972). Acute pancreatitis is the most significant complication of ERCP, occurring in approximately 1% of patients (Silvis *et al.*, 1974; Bilbao *et al.*, 1976). The illness is generally not severe, although at least one fatality has resulted (Ammann *et al.*, 1973) and pseudocyst has been reported. The risk of pancreatitis is low in experienced hands and if the injection into the duct is terminated as soon as the branch ducts are visualized (Fig. 7.5). Pancreatic sepsis has followed pancreatography. It is now agreed that pseudocysts, if found at ERCP, should not be completely filled and the cyst should be drained within 24 hours of opacification.

ERCP is of great value in assessing pancreatic disease and is the gold standard in the diagnosis of chronic pancreatitis. High resolution CT, although of great value, has limitations. The Cambridge classification (Sarner & Cotton, 1984, expanded by Gyr *et al.*, 1984) is helpful in assessing pancreatograms. Success rates of the order of 93% have been recorded using this system in establishing this difficult diagnosis (Jones *et al.*, 1988). Despite the improving reso-

lution of CT, ERCP combined with ultrasound remains the current method of choice.

Pancreatic carcinoma is usually diagnosed by abdominal ultrasound and/or CT. ERCP is generally reserved for equivocal cases but has a high sensitivity and specificity in expert hands (Shalel, 1986).

Magnetic resonace imaging (MRI)

The application of MRI to imaging of the pancreas has not been widely used so far, in part owing to limited magnet time and to problems with resolution. As problems in obtaining high-resolution images free of artefact are overcome, with techniques such as respiratory motion artefact suppression, spatial presaturation and frequency-specific fat suppression, MRI will become a more widely used technique.

The technique used will largely depend on the type of magnet available but fat suppression T_1 weighted images should provide optimal pancreatic parenchymal images. T_2 weighted images should provide intrapancreatic detail with visualization of the pancreatic duct, common bile-duct and fluid collections such as pseudocysts in and adjacent to the pancreas (Fig. 7.6). Conventional spin-echo techniques may suffice, but Turbo spin echo will give higher resolution images. (Semelka & Simm, 1991).

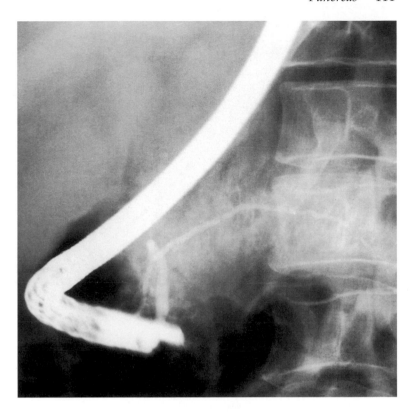

Fig. 7.5 Endoscopic retrograde cholangiopancreatography — overfilling has produced a faint pancreatogram.

Acute pancreatitis

At present MRI offers no significant advantage over CT scanning. T_2 weighted sequences and dynamic gadolinium–diethylenetriaminepenta-acetic acid (GdDTPA)-enhanced gradient echo images show similar detail to enhanced CT. Intrapancreatic gas loculi are a problem with MRI and are better appreciated with CT. It can be difficult to distinguish fluid-filled bowel loops from abnormal fluid collections using MRI, although bowel labelling agents may be of help in this situation (Tark *et al.*, 1991). The patient with acute pancreatitis, who is often ill and restless, is usually easier to monitor during CT than in a magnet. However, the new 'open-sided' magnets should overcome these difficulties.

Chronic pancreatitis

At the present time, MRI has no advantages over other imaging modalities in assessing chronic pancreatitis. The relative inability to visualize intrapancreatic

calcification works against its current use. CT in combination with ERCP remains the current gold standard in the imaging of chronic pancreatitis.

Carcinoma of the pancreas

No particular advantage is gained using MRI compared with CT in imaging pancreatic carcinoma.

Endocrine pancreatic tumours

MRI is the technique of choice for the location of small pancreatic endocrine tumours. Gd-enhanced T_1 weighted images can diagnose endocrine tumours such as gastrinomas and insulinomas as small as 5 mm in size. Pancreatic endocrine tumours should currently be imaged using preoperative MRI with intraoperative ultrasound assessment.

Isotope scanning

Radionuclide imaging is not usually a first-line

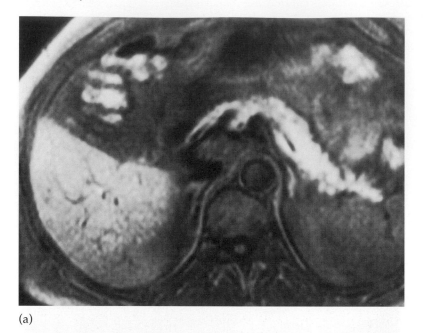

(a)

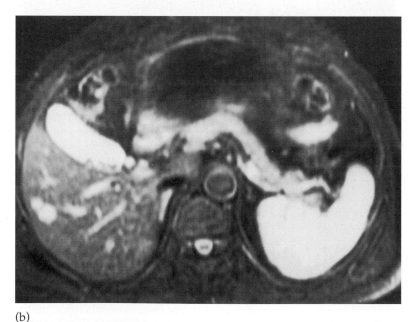

(b)

Fig. 7.6 Axial magnetic resonance images at the level of the body of the pancreas: (a) T_1 weighted image; (b) T_2 weighted image.

imaging technique in assessing pancreatic disease but has a role in problem-solving. The use of radiolabelled monoclonal antibodies has been delayed and is not yet available clinically. There is a role for radionuclide imaging in assessing pancreatic transplants. Pancreatic transplant is becoming more common and

a relatively non-invasive rapid evaluation of the vascular graft patency and function is available using ^{99}Tc HMPOA imaging.

Receptor scintigraphy with ^{111}In pentetreotide is a method of localizing endocrine pancreatic tumours if they express somastostatin receptors. It suffers from

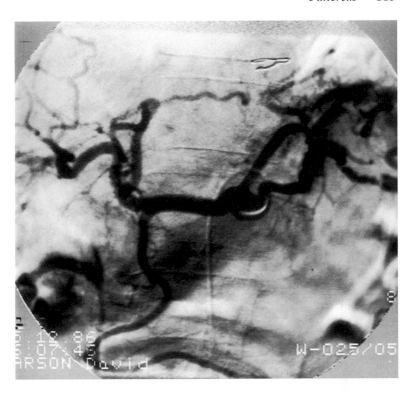

Fig. 7.7 Digital subtraction angiogram — coeliac axis injection. Encasement of splenic artery due to carcinoma of body of pancreas.

a low sensitivity but may be extremely useful in patients with widespread disease (Becker *et al.*, 1991).

Angiography

With the advent of cross-sectional imaging, the use of angiography in pancreatic disease has diminished. Some surgeons still make use of preoperative angiography in assessing the operability of pancreatic carcinoma (Fig. 7.7). However, enhanced dynamic CT can now replace this, thus avoiding the hazards of mesenteric angiography. Angiography has been very useful in localizing pancreatic endocrine tumours (Fig. 7.8). Selective injections into the coeliac axis and superior mesenteric arteries demonstrate the arterial anatomy of the pancreas and its portal venous drainage. Superselective studies are usually required to offer the best opportunity of visualization of these small enhancing lesions. The use of the digital subtraction technique is ideal for the more selective studies. The reported sensitivity of these techniques is as high as 90%. However, lesions may be missed on angiography because they are too small. False positives may result due to misinterpretation of a 'blush'

in a normal segment of adjacent normal bowel or spleen.

Percutaneous biopsy

Percutaneous aspiration for cytology can be applied to pancreatic lesions using either ultrasound or CT guidance. Fine needles of 20–23 gauge can be readily visualized when the needle tip is positioned accurately. Local anaesthetic infiltration of the skin at a selected site in the anterior abdominal wall is followed by insertion of the needle to the desired depth and angle. This is a relatively quick and inexpensive technique. It is almost totally free of complications.

CT, being less rapid in interventional procedures, is generally reserved for those cases where visualization of the pancreas is poor at ultrasound, due to overlying bowel contents.

Percutaneous pancreatography

This technique (Chong *et al.*, 1992) has been described as complementary procedure to imaging of the pancreas in chronic pancreatitis. A fine needle is passed

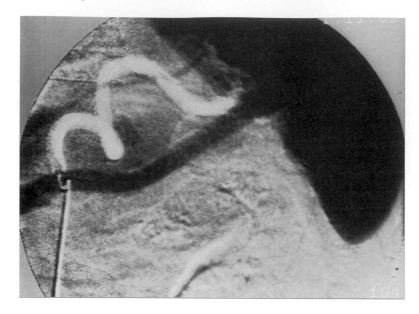

Fig. 7.8 Digital subtraction angiogram — splenic artery injection shows 'blush' in insulinoma of body of pancreas, not visible on computed tomography.

into the pancreatic duct under ultrasound guidance, allowing opacification of the pancreatic duct with contrast medium. Percutaneous pancreatography has been advocated in cases of failed ERCP. However, this is not recommended as a first-line diagnostic technique.

Percutaneous drainage

Drainage of pancreatic pseudocysts or abscesses can be performed under CT or ultrasound guidance. The initial steps of the technique are as for biopsy. Simple aspiration to dryness may be obtained for small lesions through a fine needle. Larger collections are likely to recur and require indwelling catheter drainage. Catheter insertion should be preceded by inserting a fine aspirating needle to ensure that the contents of the lesion are fluid. This allows specimen collection for bacteriological or biochemical analysis. Using large needle and catheter systems, it is possible to pass a catheter in one manoeuvre into the fluid collection. The draining catheter is fixed to the skin and allowed to drain. Following-up imaging is performed when drainage ceases to determine if any residual fluid persists and either removal of the catheter or further aspiration can be applied as appropriate.

Conclusion

Ultrasound remains the most readily available and least expensive of the imaging techniques used in the detection of pancreatic disease. If ultrasound fails or is inconclusive, CT should be performed. Patients with an inconclusive abnormality on ultrasound or CT should undergo ERCP. Even when ultrasound and CT appear normal, there is a strong indication to perform ERCP if the clinical suspicion of pancreatic carcinoma remains. CT is superior to angiography in assessing vascular involvement by tumour. Percutaneous biopsy is an important technique for confirming pancreatic carcinoma. MRI is the method of choice for localizing small pancreatic endocrine tumours. Because pancreatic imaging is fraught with difficulty, the various imaging techniques should be thought of as complementary and it will usually be necessary to use more than one technique to establish a diagnosis.

References

Ammann, R.W., Deyhle, P. & Butikofer, E. (1973) Fatal necrotising pancreatitis after per oral cholangiography. *Gastoenterology*, **64**, 320–3.

Bakkevold, K.E., Arnesjo, B. & Kambestad, B. (1992) Carcinoma of the pancreas and papilla of Vater: presenting symptoms, signs and diagnosis related to tumour site (Norwegian Pancreatic Cancer Trial). *Scand. J Gastroenterol.*, **27** (4), 317–25.

Bauerle, H. Grassman, P.H., Classen, M. *et al.* (1972) The use of radiographic techniques in gastroenterology. *Electromedica*, **4**, 109–16.

Becker, W., Marienhagens, J. *et al.* (1991) Octreotide scintigraphy localises somastatin receptor-positive islet cell carcinomas. *Eur. J. Nucl. Med.*, **18** (11), 924–7.

Bilbao, M.K., Dotter, C.T., Lee, T.G. *et al.* (1976) Complications of endoscopic retrograde cholangiopancreatography — a study of 10 000 cases. *Gastroenterology*, **70**, 314–20.

Chong, W.K., Theis, B., Russel, R.C. *et al.* (1992) Utrasound guided percutaneous pancreatography: an essential tool for imaging pancreatitis. *Radiographics*, **12**(1), 79–90.

Cotton, P.B., Salmon, P.R., Blumgart, L.H. *et al.* (1972) Cannulation of the papilla of Vater by endoscopy and retrograde pancreatography ERCP. *Gut*, **13**, 1014–25.

Enco, Y., Morris, T. Tanua, M. *et al.* (1974) Cytodiagnosis of pancreatic tumours by aspiration under direct vision, using a fibrescope. *Gastroenterology*, **67**, 944–9.

Freeney, P.C. (1992) Radiology of the pancreas. *Curr. Opin. Radiol.*, **4**(3), 53–4.

Gianello, P., Gigot, J.F., Berthet, F. *et al.* (1988) Pre- and intraoperative localisation of insulinomas: report of 22 observations. *World J. Surg.*, **12**, 389–97.

Glover, J.R., Shennon, P.J. & Lees, W.R. (1992) Endoscopic ultrasound for localisation of islet cell tumours. *Gut*, **33**(1), 108–10.

Gyr, K.E., Singe, M.V. & Serles, H. (1984) Pancreatitis; concepts and classification. *International Congress Series No. 624*, p. 239. Excerpta Medica, Amsterdam.

Hatfield, A.R., Smitties, A., Wilkens, R. & Lein, J. (1976) Assessment of endoscopic retrograde cholangiopancreatography (ERCP) and pure pancreatic juice cytology in patients with pancreatic disease. *Gut*, **17**, 14–21.

Jones, S.N., Lees, W.R. & Frost, R.A. (1988) Diagnosis and grading of chronic pancreatitis by morphological criteria directed by ultrasound and pancreatography. *Clin. Radiol.*, **39**, 43–8.

Lu, D.S. & Krasny, R.M. (1994) Pancreatic cancer staging yields to spiral technique. *Diagn. Imag. Int.*, Nov. 22 (Suppl.), 19.

Makela, P. & Dean, P.B. (1986) The frequency of hyperamylasaemia after ERCP with Diatrizoate and Iohexol. *Eur. J. Radiol.*, **6**, 303.

Oi, I., Takemoto, T. & Kondo, T. (1969) Fibreduodenoscopy: direct observation of the ampulla of Vater. *Endoscopy*, **1**, 101–5.

Osnes, M., Serck-Hansen, A. & Myren, J. (1975) Endoscopic retrograde brush cytology of the biliary and pancreatic ducts. *Scand. J. Gastroenterol.*, **10**, 829–31.

Sarner, M. & Cotton, P.B. (1984) Classification of pancreatitis. *Gut*, **25**, 756–9.

Seifert, E., Urakami, Y. & Elster, K. (1977) Duodenoscopic biopsy of the biliary and pancreatic ducts. *Endoscopy*, **9**, 154–61.

Shalel, S. (1986) Endoscopic diagnosis and therapeutic approach to pancreatic cancer. *Front. Gastroint. Res.*, **12**, 208–12.

Semelka, R.C. & Simm, F.C. (1991) MRI of the pancreas at high field strength: comparison of six sequences. *J. Comput. Assist. Tomogr.*, **15**, 966–71.

Silvis, S.E., Nebel, O., Rogers, G. *et al.* (1974) Endoscopic complications — results of 1974 Meeting of the American Society of Gastrointestinal Endoscopy Survey. *JAMA*, **235**, 928–30.

Tark, R.P., Li, K.C. *et al.* (1991) Enteric MRI contrast agents: comparative study of five potential agents. *MRI*, **9**(4), 559.

Section 2
Cardiovascular System

8   Arteriography

R. H. S. GREGSON

Diagnostic arteriography has its origins mainly in Europe, particularly in Portugal where Moniz performed the first carotid arteriogram in 1927 and Dos Santos described abdominal and lumbar aortography in 1929. However, Berberich had already performed the first brachial arteriogram in 1923 in Germany and Brooks the first femoral arteriogram in 1924 in the USA. Farinas, also in the USA, subsequently described catheter aortography in 1941, but it was not until 1953, when Seldinger (1953) in Sweden described percutaneous catheterization of the femoral artery, that modern diagnostic arteriography really became generally used in medicine.

Indications

Arteriography is one of the more invasive radiological procedures and produces an element of discomfort and a degree of risk to the patient. However, these have been greatly reduced in the last few years by technological advances in angiographic apparatus, catheterization equipment and contrast medium biochemistry, as well as the development of experience and expertise by the vascular radiological team (Halpern, 1964).

The indications for arteriography include (i) the assessment of the obliterative and aneurysmal types of arterial disease; (ii) the investigation of malignant tumours; (iii) the localization of the site of haemorrhage from any organ or system; and (iv) the delineation of arteriovenous malformations. The most common indications are undoubtedly peripheral vascular disease, ischaemic heart disease and cerebrovascular disease.

Contraindications

There are probably no absolute contraindications to arteriography, as even a patient who has had a previous reaction to contrast medium has only about a 15% risk of a similar reaction occurring again. (Shehadi, 1982). If arteriography is critical to the management of this type of patient, it can be performed under corticosteroid cover using a different type of non-ionic contrast medium. If similar diagnostic information can be obtained by ultrasound, radionuclide imaging, computed tomography (CT) or magnetic resonance imaging (MRI), then it is obviously prudent to use one of these investigations.

The relative contraindications to arteriography include severe hypertension with a diastolic blood pressure over 120 mmHg, cardiac failure, hepatic failure, renal failure, severe anaemia, thyrotoxicosis and dehydration. These medical conditions should be treated before angiography. Oral anticoagulant therapy should ideally be discontinued 3 days before the procedure, but for patients with clotting disorders the arteriography can be performed using the smaller 4 French (F) gauge catheters under cover of fresh frozen or platelet-rich plasma. Arteriography carries more risk in the paediatric and geriatric age groups and should be avoided in early pregnancy.

A particular arterial puncture site may also be contraindicated by the presence of an aneurysm, a stenosis or occlusion of the underlying artery, a synthetic graft in the artery, local scar formation or infection in the soft tissues overlying the artery.

Angiography room

Arteriography should be carried out in a specialized angiography room which must be large enough to contain the generator, fluoroscopy system, catheterization table, computers and contrast medium pressure injector. There should also be an electrocardiogram (ECG) monitor, arterial pressure monitor, pulse oximeter, defibrillator, emergency resuscitation trolley, anaesthetic trolley, emergency drug cupboard, a selected range of catheterization equipment, film-viewing facilities and washing facilities for aseptic technique. Waiting and recovery areas, as well as the main catheterization equipment store room, should be adjacent to the angiography room.

A three-phase high-capacity generator is required to produce about 1000 mA in order to obtain the short exposure times necessary for rapid sequence filming. The high-resolution fluoroscopy system consists of the X-ray tube with a high-speed rotating tungsten anode and a 0.3–1.2 mm² focal spot, image intensifier with a 15–40 cm input screen and dual high-resolution television monitors. The ideal fluoroscopy system is mounted in a rotating C-arm with craniocaudal angulation providing multiplanar imaging facilities without the need to move the patient. The catheterization table, on which the patient lies, has a floating top for multidirectional movement. A stepping horizontal movement facility in the table is useful for lower limb angiography. A vertical movement facility is necessary for magnification angiography, while a tilting facility is helpful for breathless patients and non-vascular interventional procedures. A biplane fluoroscopy system simplifies interventional procedures requiring needle-tip localization, but is really a luxury.

For state-of-the-art angiography a digital vascular imaging (DVI) system is added to the fluoroscopy system for computerized subtraction of the digitized pre-contrast image from the post-contrast image, with additional computerized processing of this subtracted image as required (see Chapter 12). If this is not available single-plane filming using a standard large 35 × 35 cm Puck film changer (up to 4 radiographs s⁻¹) with rare earth screens can be used. A smaller 24 × 30 cm Puck film changer is also available. Simultaneous biplane radiography may be useful in cardiac and neuroangiography, whereas cine fluorography/angiography using 35 mm film with up to 50 frames s⁻¹ is essential for cardiac angiography. Spot film photofluorography/angiography using 105 mm cut or roll film is useful in paediatric and neuroangiography, the former having the additional advantage of a low patient radiation dose and the latter a low film cost. A video tape-recording system is used, in conjunction with either the high-resolution fluoroscopy system or cine fluorography, for temporary storage and immediate replay of the image. A pressure injector is required to inject contrast medium through a catheter delivering the variable volumes (up to 100 ml) and flow rates (up to 30 ml s⁻¹) of contrast medium necessary for the different types of arteriography. A punched card or computer program is used to coordinate the injection of contrast medium, the filming sequence and table movement (Levin & Dunham, 1982).

The vascular radiologist, radiographers, nurses and technicians need to be experienced and able to work as a team in order to produce a high-quality diagnostic angiogram with the minimum of risk to the patient. All staff working in the angiography room should wear a lead apron with a lead equivalent of 0.25–0.5 mm and a whole-body radiation dose monitor and have been immunized against hepatitis B virus. Staff working directly with the patient can also wear a thyroid shield, lead glasses, peripheral radiation dose monitors and a visor to protect against eye splashes.

Arterial catheterization equipment

The vascular radiologist needs a good working knowledge of the large variety of catheterization equipment available, although the essential requirements for percutaneous catheterization of an artery are simply a needle, guide wire and catheter.

Needles

A selection of needles used for percutaneous arterial catheterization is shown in Fig. 8.1. The most commonly used needles are in two parts, with an 18 gauge thin-walled outer cannula which is about 8 cm long. The tip of the cannula can be blunt and square, or sharp and bevelled. The blunt square-ended cannula is used with either a sharp-angled or pencil-point stylette and the sharp bevel-ended cannula has a matching angled stylette. The cannula usually has a flange at the hub connection to make handling easier, but simple one-part needles are also available. The cannula may also have an outer Teflon sheath. The 18 gauge cannula or needle accepts the standard 0.89 mm (0.035 in.) or 0.97 mm (0.038 in.) guide wires. A 19 gauge needle is available for day-case angiography. A 20 gauge system, using smaller guide wires, is recommended for paediatric angiography.

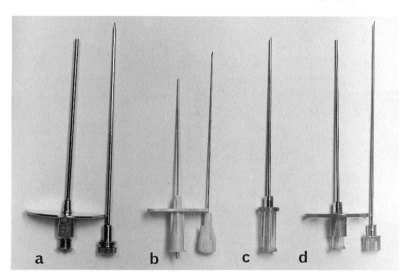

Fig. 8.1 Needles used for percutaneous arterial catheterization. (a) An 18 gauge thin-wall metal cannula 8 cm long with pencil-point stylette. (b) A 20 gauge thin-wall cannula 6 cm long with angled stylette for paediatric use (disposable). (c) An 18 gauge thin-wall cannula 8 cm long without stylette for venous puncture in digital subtraction angiography (disposable). (d) An 18 gauge thin-wall cannula 8 cm long for adult patients (disposable).

Guide wires

A selection of guide wires used for percutaneous arterial catheterization is shown in Fig. 8.2. The guide wire is used during the insertion of the catheter at the start of the procedure and during positioning and exchange of the catheter during the procedure, but not usually during the removal of the catheter at the end of the procedure.

The function of the guide wire is to guide the catheter through the skin and soft tissues at the puncture site, through the arterial wall and into the lumen of the artery, the walls of which may be tortuous or irregular due to vascular disease.

A guide wire consists of two inner stainless steel straight wires with an outer stainless steel wire tightly coiled around them. One of the central wires runs the whole length of the guide wire to prevent fracture. The other central wire tapers and terminates near the tip of the guide wire to produce a soft flexible tip at one end and a hard stiff tip at the other end.

The guide wires most commonly used are 150 cm long, with a diameter of 0.89 mm (0.035 in.) and are coated with Teflon to reduce friction. Guide wires with a diameter of 0.97 mm (0.038 in.) for easier handling and guide wires coated with benzylkonium heparin to reduce thrombus formation are also available. The flexible tip can be either straight or J-shaped and is usually 5 cm long, but may be up to 10–15 cm. The radius of curvature of the J-shaped tips varies between 1.5 and 15 mm, with 3 mm being the most useful.

Specialist guide wires with a hydrophilic coating and a steerable facility for difficult manipulations, a heavy duty core for added stiffness, a movable core for variable stiffness and shape, a central lumen for injections, as well as extra length (200 or 260 cm) for catheter exchanges are also available. Guide wires with a diameter of 0.53 mm (0.021 in.) or 0.64 mm (0.025 in.) are recommended for paediatric angiography.

Catheters

The catheter delivers the contrast medium into the arterial lumen at a particular site in the arterial tree. A selection of catheters used for percutaneous arterial catheterization is shown in Fig. 8.3. A catheter consists of a thin-walled polyurethane or polyethylene tube with a tapered tip and a Luer-Lok connection at the hub. Nylon and Teflon catheters are also available, as are catheters made from mixtures of these plastics. The catheters contain barium, bismuth or lead salts to make them radio-opaque. The different catheter materials have particular qualities — polyethylene catheters are softer than the stiffer polyurethane catheters, which have better torque control. Polyurethane catheters have a higher coefficient of friction than polyethylene catheters and have to be used with Teflon-coated guide wires.

The catheters most commonly used are 4 or 5F

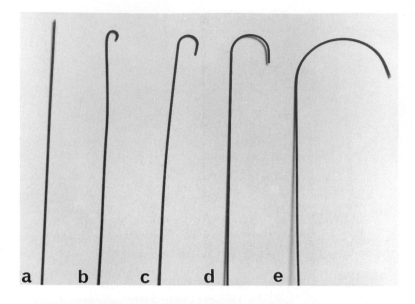

Fig. 8.2 Guide wires used for percutaneous arterial catheterization. (a) Straight guide wire for patients without vascular disease. (b) A 1.5 mm J-shaped tip guide wire for digital vascular imaging. (c) A 3 mm J-shaped tip guide wire for patients with vascular disease. (d) A 6 mm J-shaped tip guide wire for translumbar aortography. (e) A 15 mm J-shaped tip guide wire for patients with vascular disease.

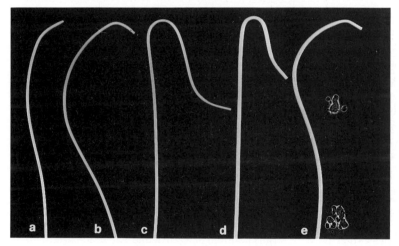

Fig. 8.3 Catheters used for selective arteriography of branches of abdominal aorta. (a) A 5F curved catheter for multipurpose use in paediatric patients. (b) A 5F cobra-shaped catheter for renal and mesenteric arteriography in adult patients. (c) A 5F sidewinder-shaped catheter for mesenteric and renal arteriography in adult patients. (d) A 7F sidewinder-shaped catheter for easier manipulation in tortuous arteries. (e) A 7F cobra-shaped catheter for easier manipulation in tortuous arteries.

gauge, 60–100 cm in length, and have a lumen which accepts the standard 0.89 mm (0.035 in.) guide wire (see above). Larger 6 or 7F catheters with 0.97 mm (0.038 in.) guide wires for easier handling and catheters coated with heparin to reduce thrombus formation are also available. The tapered tip of the catheter has an end-hole with no side-holes for superselective arteriography, an end-hole with two side-holes for selective arteriography or an end-hole with about 10 side-holes for aortography. There are four basic catheter shapes — straight or pig-tail for aortography, and single or double curve for selective arteriography (Rosch & Grollman, 1969). The maximum flow rate through a catheter mainly depends upon the inner lumen and the length of the catheter, but also upon the number of side-holes, whose main function is to increase stability. 4F catheters are available for day-case angiography (Dyet *et al.*, 1990) and 3F catheters are recommended for paediatric angiography.

Dilators help insertion of the larger 6–8F catheters in obese patients or patients with scars at the site of arterial puncture. They are about 15 cm long, have a smooth tapered tip, and are made of Teflon, which has a very low coefficient of friction but extra stiffness.

Introducer sheaths, which can have a side-arm for flushing heparinized saline around the catheter (Fig. 8.4), are also available for multiple catheter exchanges.

Contrast media

Contrast media for angiography should have a high radiographic density, a low osmolality, a low viscosity, a very low toxicity and rapid excretion.

Non-ionic contrast media such as iopamidol (Niopam), iohexol (Omnipaque), iopramide (Ultravist) and ioversol (Optiray) are the contrast media of choice for angiography, because their osmolality is lower than that of ionic contrast media. However, even their lower osmolality is greater than that of plasma, although iodixanol (Visipaque), which is a dimer, is isotonic. The low-osmolar contrast medium

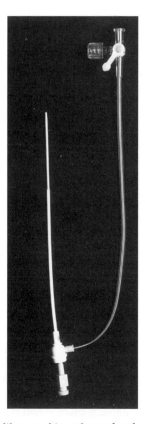

Fig. 8.4 A 5F dilator and introducer sheath with a side-arm for flushing.

ioxaglate (Hexabrix), which is a mono-acid dimer, is a very acceptable alternative contrast medium because of its low cost in comparison to the non-ionic contrast media. The high-osmolar ionic contrast media such as metrizoate (Triosil), iothalamate (Conray) and diatrizoate (Urografin and Hypaque) with their sodium or methylglucamine salts are no longer recommended for arteriography.

Aortography should be performed using a contrast medium containing 350–370 mg iodine ml^{-1}. In selective arteriography a contrast medium containing 300 mg iodine ml^{-1} is usually sufficient. Contrast media should be warmed to body temperature before injection to reduce their high viscosity. The total volume of contrast medium used during an examination should not normally exceed 4–5 ml kg^{-1}: that is, up to 350 ml in the average 70 kg person, although doses over 500 ml are occasionally used. This restriction is particularly important in paediatric angiography. Contrast media are considered in more detail in Chapter 30. Carbon dioxide gas has also been used as a contrast medium in the lower limb arteries in patients who have had a previous reaction to liquid contrast media, in conjunction with a digital imaging system (Hawkins, 1982).

Patient assessment and preparation

Arteriography is usually performed as an in-patient procedure and the patient will therefore require a 24–48 hour hospital admission, although it can be done as a day-case procedure.

Ideally the patient is admitted to hospital the day before arteriography, so that he or she can be examined and a history taken regarding previous intravascular contrast medium investigations and current drug treatment. Oral anticoagulant therapy should have been discontinued 3 days before admission. An examination is performed with particular reference to the femoral pulses, peripheral pulses in the legs and arms, pulse rate and rhythm as well as blood pressure. The following laboratory investigations should also be done as part of the preangiographic assessment of the patient: (i) haemoglobin level, platelet count, blood urea and electrolytes in all patients; (ii) clotting studies in patients on anticoagulants or with a coagulation defect; (iii) blood sugar in diabetic patients; and (iv) ECG in patients with vascular disease. Testing for sickle cell disease, Australia antigen or human immunodeficiency virus (HIV) is only performed in at-risk patients. The haemoglobin level should be at least 10 g dl⁻¹, platelet count over 100 000 and INR less than 1.4.

It is important for the vascular radiologist to visit the patient on the ward the day before the procedure, although this is not always possible in emergency referrals. The value of this preangiographic visit is to explain to the patient in general terms what the procedure involves, why it is necessary and what the potential risks are. Any questions can then be answered and the informed consent for the procedure obtained. The radiologist will examine the proposed puncture site, usually the femoral artery, for a palpable pulse, scars or local skin infection. The medical, nursing and portering staff on the ward should be informed of the planned time for the procedure. Both groins should be shaved and the patient should not eat any solid food for at least 6 hours before the procedure, although liquids should be encouraged up to 2 hours before the procedure to prevent dehydration, unless a general anaesthetic is required.

Premedication 1 hour before the procedure with oral temazepam 10–20 mg and i.m. papaveretum (Omnopon) 5–10 mg is useful for most patients, but for particularly anxious patients i.v. midazolam 2–5 mg can be given just prior to the procedure.

Patients who have had a previous major reaction to i.v. contrast media should receive corticosteroid cover for the procedure. Those who are at risk of developing subacute bacterial endocarditis should receive antibiotic cover for the procedure. Diabetic patients should not receive their morning dose of insulin or oral hypoglycaemic treatment.

Patient after-care and follow-up

Following the procedure, the patient returns to the ward for 12–24 hours' bed rest and observation of the puncture site for haemorrhage or haematoma formation. The pulse and blood pressure are recorded every 15 min for 1 hour, hourly for 4 hours and 4 hourly up to 12–24 hours. It is also important for the vascular radiologist to visit the patient again on the ward that evening or the day after the procedure to check that there have been no complications prior to discharge from hospital. The observation time for day-case or out-patient angiography is reduced to 1–4 hours (Dyet *et al.*, 1990).

Arterial catheterization technique

The common femoral artery is technically the most suitable and the most widely used vessel for arterial catheterization by the Seldinger technique (Fig. 8.5) because it is a large artery close to the skin surface. It is comfortable for the patient and gives access to the aorta and all its branches, including those in the head and neck, upper and lower limbs and the left ventricle. The femoral route has the lowest incidence of local complications. However, vascular disease in the iliac or femoral artery, a synthetic graft, scar tissue or skin sepsis in the groin may prevent the use of a particular common femoral artery. Vascular disease in the aorta or both iliac arteries may prevent the use of either common femoral artery. The alternative sites for arterial catheterization include the brachial and axillary arteries, the abdominal aorta and occasionally the popliteal, carotid or subclavian arteries. The most recent alternative is the development of i.v. DVI which only requires good venous access, via the median cubital, basilic or cephalic veins in the arm or the femoral vein in the leg.

Femoral artery

With the patient lying supine on the angiography table, both femoral pulses and the peripheral pulses in the lower limbs are again checked by the radiologist. Control radiographs of the appropriate area are performed by the radiographer to check the exposure factors. The stronger of the two femoral pulses is chosen for arterial catheterization. If the pulses are equal, the right femoral artery is usally easier to catheterize for a right-handed angiographer standing on the patient's right side, although catheterization of the femoral artery on the opposite side to the symptoms is recommended in patients with vascular disease. The vascular radiologist scrubs and puts on a sterile gown and gloves. The patient's groin is cleansed with a skin disinfectant such as 0.5–1% chlorhexidine solution. The patient is draped with sterile covers, apart from the proposed puncture site and head. General anaesthesia is recommended for

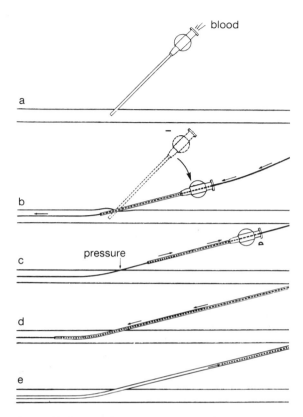

Fig. 8.5 Technique of percutaneous arterial catheterization. (a) Tip of cannula well positioned in the lumen of the artery with good backflow of blood. (b) Flexible end of guide wire advanced through cannula and positioned in the aorta. (c) Cannula removed over guide wire with digital compression over puncture site in artery preventing bleeding. (d) Catheter advanced over guide wire and positioned in the aorta. (e) Guide wire removed from catheter after tip positioned in the aorta or artery with good backflow of blood.

paediatric angiography and some embolization procedures.

The equipment on the sterile is trolley is checked. The guide wires and catheters are flushed with heparinized saline. The femoral artery is palpated in the groin with the index and middle fingers of the left hand. Then, 0.5–1 ml of local anaesthetic is injected through a small needle in order to raise a small wheal in the skin 1 cm below the groin crease in an average patient, but in or above the crease in an obese patient. Using a larger needle, a further 5 ml of 1% xylocaine or lignocaine is then infiltrated through the soft tissues around the artery at the site

of maximum pulsation. A 2 mm incision is made with the tip of a scalpel blade at the skin entry point. A thin-walled 18-gauge arterial cannula is then advanced at an angle of 30–45° through the soft tissues into the artery at the point of maximum pulsation, which will be about 2–4 cm below the inguinal ligament. It is usually possible to feel the tip of the needle in contact with the anterior arterial wall in a slim patient with a normal artery and then to stab it cleanly through into the arterial lumen. In an obese patient with a diseased artery, it may be necessary to thrust the needle tip through both the anterior and posterior walls and then withdraw it back into the arterial lumen. The central stylette is then removed and the cannula withdrawn until a strong pulsatile flow indicates a good intraluminal position. A weak flow of blood requires adjustment of the tip of the cannula and no flow indicates an initial failure. Repeated failure can be avoided by localizing the artery either by fluoroscopic screening over the medial third of the femoral head or by duplex ultrasound. A special needle containing a Doppler crystal is also available.

When there is a good backflow of blood, a 0.89 mm (0.035 in.) Teflon-coated guide wire with a 3 mm J-tip is inserted through the cannula into the femoral artery lumen, up the iliac artery and into the aorta if no resistance is met. The cannula is then removed over the guide wire whilst the arterial puncture site is compressed to prevent bleeding. The 5F catheter is then introduced over the guide wire and, after positioning its tip in the aorta, the guide wire is then removed. After adjustment, the position of the tip of the catheter can be checked with a test injection of 5 ml of contrast medium by hand under fluoroscopic control. The catheter is then flushed with 20 ml of heparinized saline (5000 U of heparin in 1 litre of normal saline) before the main injection of contrast medium from the pressure injector.

The use of larger 7F catheters requires the introduction of a 7F dilator over the guide wire prior to the insertion of the catheter. A 5F dilator may also be required when using a 5F catheter in an obese patient. Resistance to the advancement of the guide wire in an artery should not be overcome by force, but instead requires gentle manipulation under fluoroscopic control or even a test injection of contrast medium through the catheter to identify the problem — usually an atherosclerotic plaque or a tortuous artery.

During the procedure, the catheter should be flushed frequently with 5 ml boluses of heparinized saline by hand or with a continuous flushing pressure bag system, which can also be used for pressure monitoring. The patient generally receives about 250–500 U of heparin during the procedure. Systemic heparinization with 2500–5000 U of heparin intra-arterially through the catheter is essential during angioplasty procedures, but is not usually necessary during diagnostic arteriography. Heparin has a half-life of 6 hours and reversal of its anticoagulant effect with 10 mg of protamine sulphate for every 1000 U of heparin is rarely necessary.

The catheter is removed at the end of the procedure, while firm pressure with three fingers is applied over the arterial puncture site above the skin puncture site. This manual pressure should be maintained for 5–20 min, or occasionally even longer, to prevent the formation of a haematoma, without completely obliterating the femoral pulse. The compression time is prolonged with the use of larger catheters, in hypertensive patients and in those on anticoagulants. The skin puncture site can either be left exposed to the air or covered with a small plaster, as pressure bandages do not usually prevent bleeding from the puncture site. Compression devices are also available. The common or superficial femoral arteries can also be catheterized in an antegrade caudal direction, as opposed to the normal retrograde cranial direction, for angioplasty and other interventional procedures.

Axillary artery

The axillary artery has a smaller calibre than the common femoral artery but, as it lies even closer to the skin surface, is quite easy to catheterize, although this procedure is less comfortable for the patient. The axillary artery also lies close to the brachial plexus, making transaxillary catheterization a potentially risky procedure.

Catheterization of the left axillary artery gives access to the descending thoracic and abdominal aorta and the lower limbs. Catheterization of the right axillary artery gives access to the ascending aorta, head and neck, and left ventricle. The incidence of complications associated with transaxillary arteriography

is 3.3%, compared to only 1.7% in transfemoral arteriography (Hessel *et al.*, 1981). Because of the higher incidence of arterial complications, the axillary route should only be used when the transfemoral route is not available and there is no i.v. DVI facility.

The technique of axillary artery catheterization is similar to that described above for femoral artery catheterization. The patient lies supine on the angiography table with the arm abducted to 90° at the shoulder and flexed to 135° at the elbow and with the hand behind the head. The peripheral pulses in the arms are checked by the radiologist. The left axillary artery is usually safer for catheterization. The axillary artery is palpated in the axilla and catheterized at a point about 1 cm lateral to the axillary fold, over the neck of the humerus. A 0.89 mm (0.035 in.) Teflon-coated guide wire with a 15 cm long straight flexible tip and a 4 or 5F catheter is recommended. A 5F dilator and sheath system can be used prior to the insertion of the catheter (McIvor & Rhymer, 1992).

Brachial artery

The brachial artery has a much smaller calibre than the axillary artery. Although it can be catheterized percutaneously in the upper arm, the brachial artery is usually catheterized after direct minor surgical exposure in the cubital fossa.

The technique is similar to that described above for axillary artery catheterization. The patient lies on the angiography table with the arm abducted to 90° at the shoulder and extended to 180° at the elbow. The forearm and hand are held in supination or external rotation. The brachial artery is palpated above the cubital fossa and catheterized at the point of maximum pulsation. A 5F dilator and sheath system can be used prior to the insertion of the catheter (Gaines & Reidy, 1986). The brachial artery can also be catheterized in an antegrade caudal direction.

Abdominal aorta

Despite its situation in the retroperitoneum anterior to the lumbar spine, it is easy to puncture or catheterize the abdominal aorta although the procedure is less comfortable for the patient. The close relationship of the abdominal aorta to many abdominal organs increases the risk of the procedure. Puncture or catheterization of the lower abdominal aorta only gives access to the lower limbs (Stocks *et al.*, 1969).

The incidence of complications associated with translumbar aortography is 2.9%, compared with 1.7% for transfemoral arteriography (Hessel *et al.*, 1981). This route should only be used when the transfemoral route is not available and there is no i.v. DVI facility. Translumbar aortography is therefore performed infrequently.

The technique of direct puncture of the abdominal aorta is similar in principle to that described above for femoral artery catheterization. It is often performed under general anaesthesia although it can also be done under local anaesthesia. The patient lies prone on the angiography table. The abdominal aorta cannot be palpated through the left loin, but a small wheal of local anaesthetic is raised in the skin about 10–12 cm or a hand's breadth, lateral to the mid-line above the iliac crest and below the costal margin. A further 10 ml of local anaesthetic is then infiltrated through the soft tissues around the aorta, using the 22 cm 18 gauge translumbar needle–sheath assembly, which is advanced at an angle of 45–60° into the aorta at the L3 level for a low puncture. It is usually possible to feel the tip of the needle in contact with the posterolateral aortic wall and then to stab cleanly into the aortic lumen. The central stylette is then removed and a strong pulsatile flow indicates a good intraluminal position, which should be checked with a test injection of 5 ml of contrast medium by hand under fluoroscopic control. A weak flow of blood requires adjustment of the tip of the needle and no flow indicates an initial failure. The tip of the needle sheath or short catheter can be adjusted to point up or down the aorta, using a guide wire with a 6 mm J-tip. At the end of the procedure the needle or short catheter is removed and, because firm pressure at the aortic puncture site cannot be applied, significant bleeding into the periaortic retroperitoneal soft tissues is an inevitable consequence. The abdominal aorta can also be punctured or catheterized at the D12 level, a high puncture, with a skin puncture site above and medial to that already described and an angle of 30–45° to the aorta.

Arteriography of the lower limbs: lumbar aortography

The most common indication for lumbar aortography is the assessment of atherosclerotic peripheral vascular disease causing stenosis or occlusion in the lower-limb arteries. It is also used in the evaluation of peripheral aneurysmal disease, as well as embolism and trauma to the lower limbs, and in the investigation of arteriovenous malformations and bone or soft-tissue tumours in the legs.

Lumbar aortography via a femoral artery catheter is the preferred technique for arteriography of the lower limbs. If this is not possible, a translumbar, left transaxillary or brachial approach is used, unless a DVI facility is available. Femoral arteriography via a femoral artery catheterization is also suitable for arteriography of the calf and foot.

The aortogram should be performed using a 60 cm long 5F thin-walled pig-tail or straight catheter with an end-hole and multiple side-holes (Fig. 8.6). The tip of the catheter should be positioned in the lower abdominal or lumbar aorta, 5–10 cm above the aortic bifurcation at the L3/L4 level; 50–70 ml of non-ionic contrast medium, containing 370 mg iodine ml^{-1}, are injected at a rate of 8–12 ml s^{-1}. After a delay of 2 s, radiographs are exposed at a rate of 1 s^{-1} for 6 s and then one every other second for 12–24 s to cover the lower abdominal aorta, iliac, femoral, popliteal and tibial arteries and sometimes the feet in overlapping anteroposterior (AP) projections (Fig. 8.7). The contrast medium may take over 30 s to reach the ankles. In the assessment of stenoses in the iliac and femoral arteries, 30–45° posterior oblique views of the pelvis can be useful. Lateral views of the calf can be useful in the evaluation of the run-off vessels. Table 8.1 shows typical contrast medium volume and flow rates and film delay and programme sequences for the various types of angiography.

Arteriography of the thoracic aorta: arch aortography

The most common indication for arch aortography is the assessment of atherosclerotic vascular disease causing stenosis or occlusion in the carotid or vertebral arteries and in the innominate, subclavian or axillary arteries. It is also used in the evaluation

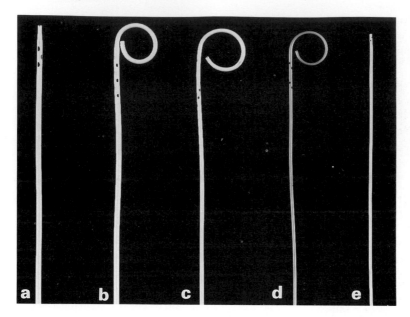

Fig. 8.6 Catheters used for aortography. (a) A 7F straight catheter for abdominal aortography in adult patients. (b) A 7F pig-tail catheter for arch aortography in adult patients. (c) A 5F pig-tail catheter for lumbar aortography in adult patients. (d) A 4F pig-tail catheter for lumbar aortography in adult patients. (e) A 4F straight catheter for abdominal aortography in paediatric patients.

of aneurysms and dissections of the thoracic aorta as well as aortitis, trauma to the chest and congenital anomalies of the great vessels. Arch aortography via a femoral artery catheter is the preferred technique for arteriography of the neck and upper limbs. A right transaxillary approach is suitable unless a DVI facility is available.

The aortogram should be performed using a 100 cm long 5F thin-walled pig-tail or curved catheter with an end-hole and multiple side-holes (see Fig. 8.6). The tip of the catheter should be positioned in the ascending aorta 5 cm proximal to the origin of the innominate artery. An anomalous origin of the left common carotid artery from the innominate artery occurs in 25% of patients. The patient is placed in a 45–60° right posterior oblique (RPO) position (Fig. 8.8), although subsequent 30–45° left posterior oblique (LPO) and AP projections can be useful in the evaluation of overlapping vessels. Non-ionic contrast medium (50 ml containing 370 mg iodine ml^{-1}) is injected at a rate of 20–25 ml s^{-1}. After a delay of 0.5 s, radiographs are exposed at a rate of 3 s^{-1} for 3 s and then 1 s^{-1} for 3 s to cover the thoracic aorta and the carotid and subclavian arteries.

Arteriography of the upper limbs

The most common indication for subclavian arteriography is the assessment of atherosclerotic vascular disease which is causing stenosis or occlusion in the upper-limb vessels. It is also used in the evaluation of the thoracic outlet syndrome, Raynaud's disease, emboli and trauma to the upper limb, and in the investigation of arteriovenous malformations as well as bone or soft-tissue tumours in the arms.

Selective arteriography via femoral artery catheterization is the preferred technique for arteriography of the upper limb, unless an i.v. DVI study is appropriate. Brachial artery catheterization is also suitable for arteriography of the forearm and hand.

The arteriogram should be performed using a 100 cm long 5F thin-walled Mani or headhunter catheter with an end-hole (Fig. 8.9). The tip of the catheter should be positioned 2–5 cm along the subclavian or innominate arteries, which originate from the arch of the thoracic aorta. The patient is placed in a 15–30° anterior oblique position. An AP projection with adduction and abduction of the shoulder can be useful in the assessment of extrinsic compression of the subclavian arteries in the thoracic outlet syndrome.

Non-ionic contrast medium (15–20 ml containing 300 mg iodine ml^{-1}) is injected at a rate of 6–8 ml s^{-1}. After a delay of 1 s, radiographs are exposed at a rate of 2 s^{-1} for 2 s and then 1 s^{-1} for 6–12 s to cover the subclavian, axillary, brachial, radial and ulnar

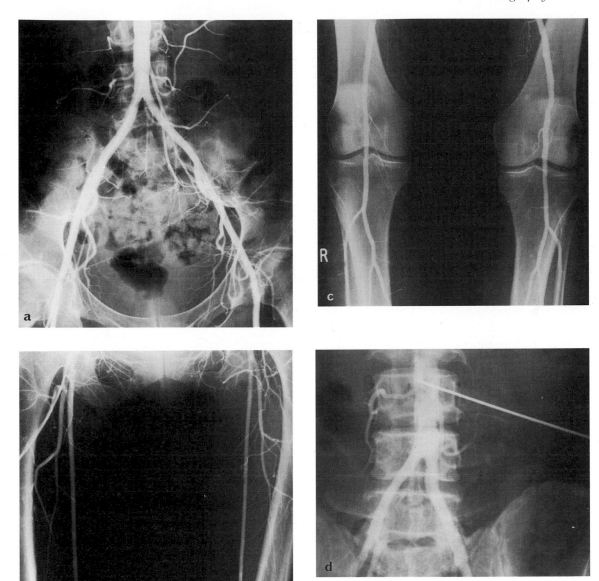

Fig. 8.7 Lumbar aortography via a right femoral artery catheter showing (a) the lower abdominal aorta and iliac arteries, (b) the femoral arteries, (c) the popliteal and tibial arteries, and (d) a translumbar aortogram with a needle.

arteries and sometimes the hand in overlapping AP projections (Fig. 8.10).

Neuroangiography

Indications for neuroangiography include cerebrovascular disease, subarachnoid haemorrhage and cerebral tumours. The types of neuroangiography are selective carotid and vertebral arteriography and spinal arteriography. Neuroangiography is considered in more detail in Chapter 19.

Carotid and cervical arteriography are also useful in the investigation of tumours and arteriovenous malformations in the head and neck as well as

Table 8.1 Aortography and selective arteriography

Type of examination	Contrast medium			Films	
	Conc.	Vol. (ml)	Rate	Delay	Programme
Lumbar aortography	370	50–70	8–12 ml s^{-1}	2 s	1 s^{-1} for 6 s 1 every other second for 12–24 s
Femoral arteriography	300–370	20–30	6–8 ml s^{-1}	1 s	1 s^{-1} for 4 s 1 every other second for 8–16 s
Popliteal arteriography	300	10–20	4–6 ml s^{-1}	1 s	1 s^{-1} for 4 s 1 every other second for 4–8 s
Thoracic aortography	370	50	20–25 ml s^{-1}	0.5 s	3 s^{-1} for 3 s 1 s^{-1} for 3 s
Subclavian arteriography	300	15–20	6–8 ml s^{-1}	1 s	2 s^{-1} for 2 s 1 s^{-1} for 4–8 s
Brachial arteriography	300	10–15	4–6 ml s^{-1}	1 s	1 s^{-1} for 4 s 1 every other second for 6 s
Common carotid arteriography	300	12–15	By hand	None	2 s^{-1} for 2 s 1 s^{-1} for 2–4 s
Internal carotid arteriography	300	8–10	By hand	None	2 s^{-1} for 2 1 s^{-1} for 4–8 s
External carotid arteriography	300	6–8	By hand	None	2 s^{-1} for 2 s 1 s^{-1} for 4–8 s
Vertebral arteriography	300	4–8	By hand	None	2 s^{-1} for 2 s 1 s^{-1} for 4–8 s
Left ventricular angiocardiography	370	35–50	10–12 ml s^{-1}	None	Cine
Left coronary arteriography	370	5–10	By hand	None	Cine
Right coronary arteriography	370	3–8	By hand	None	Cine
Pulmonary arteriography	370	40–50	20–25 ml s^{-1}	0.5 s	3 s^{-1} for 3 s 1 s^{-1} for 3 s
Abdominal aortography	370	50	15–20 ml s^{-1}	1 see	2 s^{-1} for 3 s 1 s^{-1} for 6 s
Coeliac arteriography	300–370	50–70	6–10 ml s^{-1}	0.5 s	2 s^{-1} for 3 s 1 s^{-1} for 3 s 1 every other second for 18–24 s
Superior mesenteric arteriography	300–370	50–70	6–10 ml s^{-1}	0.5 s	2 s^{-1} for 3 s 1 s^{-1} for 3 s 1 every other second for 18–24 s
Inferior mesenteric arteriography	300	15–25	3–5 ml s^{-1}	0.5 s	2 s^{-1} for 3 s 1 s^{-1} for 3 s 1 every other second for 12 s

Continued

Table 8.1 *Continued*

Type of examination	Contrast medium			Films	
	Conc.	Vol. (ml)	Rate	Delay	Programme
Splenic arteriography	300–370	50	6–8 ml s^{-1}	0.5 s	2 s^{-1} for 3 s 1 s^{-1} for 3 s 1 every other second for 18 s
Hepatic arteriography	300–370	50	6–8 ml s^{-1}	0.5 s	2 s^{-1} for 3 s 1 s^{-1} for 3 s 1 every other second for 12 s
Left gastric arteriography	300	10–15	3–5 ml s^{-1}	0.5 s	2 s^{-1} for 2 s 1 s^{-1} for 4 s 1 every other second for 6 s
Gastroduodenal arteriography	300	10–15	3–5 ml s^{-1}	0.5 s	2 s^{-1} for 2 s 1 s^{-1} for 4 s 1 every other second for 6 s
Renal arteriography	300	10–15	4–6 ml s^{-1}	0.5 s	2 s^{-1} for 3 s 1 s^{-1} for 3 s 1 every other second for 6 s
Adrenal arteriography	300	1–4	By hand	None	1 s^{-1} for 6–10 s
Internal iliac arteriography	300	10–15	4–6 ml s^{-1}	0.5 s	2 s^{-1} for 2 s 1 s^{-1} for 4 s 1 every other second for 4 s

epistaxis (Fig. 8.11). The technique of photographic subtraction is illustrated in Fig. 8.12.

Arteriography of the abdominal aorta

The most common indication for abdominal aortography is the evaluation of aneurysms of the abdominal aorta. It is also used in the assessment of atherosclerotic vascular disease causing stenosis or occlusion in the mesenteric and renal arteries, as well as being part of the assessment of the abdominal organs when selective catheterization of the arteries is not possible.

Abdominal aortography via a femoral artery catheterization is the preferred technique for arteriography of the abdomen. A left transaxillary approach is suitable unless a DVI facility is available.

The aortogram should be performed using a 60 cm long 5F thin-walled pig-tail or straight catheter with an end-hole and multiple side-holes (see Fig. 8.6). The tip of the catheter should be positioned in the lower thoracic and upper abdominal aorta, 5 cm above the origin of the coeliac axis at D12/L1 level.

Non-ionic contrast medium (50 ml containing 370 mg iodine ml^{-1}) is injected at a rate of 15–20 ml s^{-1}. After a delay of 1 s, radiographs are exposed at a rate of 2 s^{-1} for 3 s and then at 1 s^{-1} for 6 s to visualize the abdominal aorta and the mesenteric and renal arteries in an AP projection (Fig. 8.13). A lateral projection may be useful in the assessment of stenoses in the coeliac and mesenteric vessels. A 15–30° posterior oblique projection can be helpful in evaluating stenoses of the renal vessels.

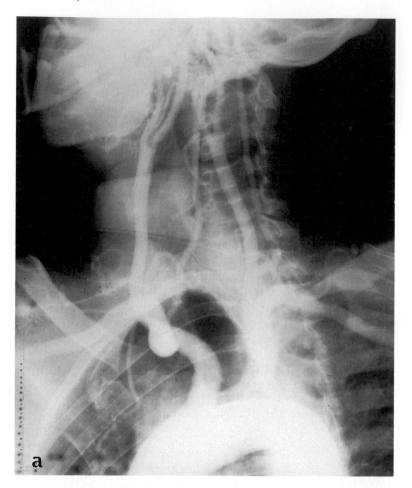

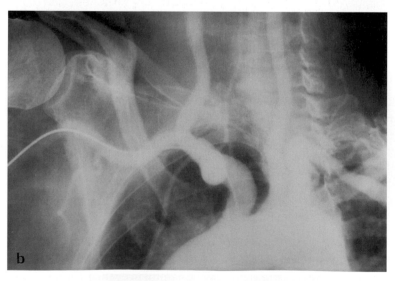

Fig. 8.8 (a) Arch aortography via a left femoral artery catheter showing thoracic aorta, carotid and subclavian arteries in a right posterior oblique (or left anterior oblique) position, and (b) a transaxillary arch aortogram with a catheter.

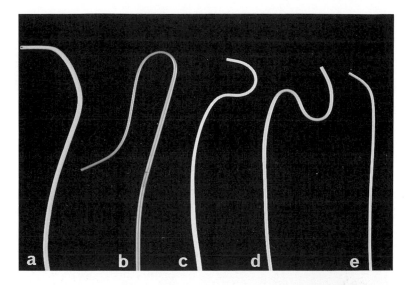

Fig. 8.9 Catheters used for selective arteriography of branches of the thoracic aorta. (a) A 7F headhunter catheter for easier manipulation in tortuous arteries. (b) A 6F Simmonds catheter for easier manipulation in tortuous arteries. (c) A 5F Kerber catheter for carotid arteriography in adult patients. (d) A 5F Mani catheter for carotid or subclavian arteriography in adult patients. (e) A 4F curved catheter for multipurpose use in paediatric patients.

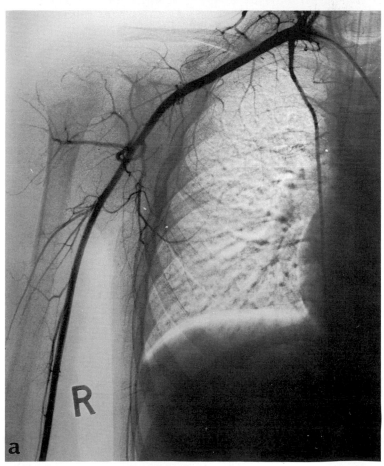

Fig. 8.10 (a) Selective right subclavian arteriography as a subtraction print using a 5F catheter.

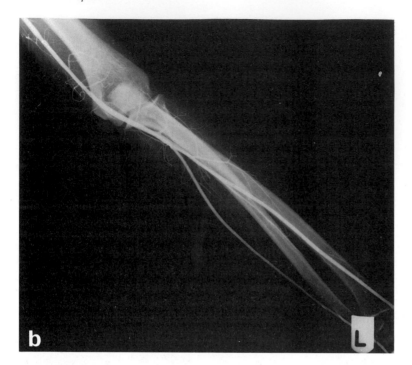

Fig. 8.10 *Continued.*
(b) Selective left brachial arteriography using a 5F catheter.

Mesenteric arteriography

The most common indications for mesenteric arteriography are the investigation of anaemia, haematemesis and melaena or rectal bleeding. Occasional indications include the investigation of a space-occupying lesion in the liver, spleen or gastrointestinal tract, portal hypertension, trauma to the liver, suspected endocrine or other tumour in the pancreas and the preoperative assessment of a primary hepatic tumour or hepatic metastases.

Selective arteriography via a femoral artery catheterization is the preferred technique, although a left transaxillary approach is possible. An i.v. DVI study is usually not appropriate.

Arteriography should be performed using a 50 cm long 5–7F cobra catheter or a 100 cm long 5–7F sidewinder catheter with an end-hole and two side-holes (see Fig. 8.3). The tip of the catheter should be positioned 2–5 cm along the coeliac axis or superior mesenteric artery and 1–2 cm along the inferior mesenteric artery. The coeliac axis originates anteriorly from the abdominal aorta at the D12/L1 level. The superior mesenteric artery also originates anteriorly from the abdominal aorta at the L1 level, while the inferior mesenteric artery originates anterolaterally on the left at the L3 level. An anomalous origin of the hepatic artery from the superior mesenteric artery occurs in 25% of patients.

Non-ionic contrast medium (50–70 ml containing 300 mg iodine ml^{-1}) is injected at a rate of 6–10 ml s^{-1} for coeliac axis or superior mesenteric arteriography. After a delay of half a second, radiographs are exposed at a rate of 2 s^{-1} for 3 s, 1 s^{-1} for 3 s and then one every alternate second for 18–24 s in the AP projection (Figs 8.14 & 8.15).

For inferior mesenteric arteriography, 15–25 ml of non-ionic contrast medium containing 300 mg iodine ml^{-1} is injected at a rate of 3–5 ml s^{-1}. After a delay of 0.5 s, radiographs are exposed at a rate of 2 s^{-1} for 3 s, 1 s^{-1} for 3 s and then one every alternate second for 12 s in the AP projection (Fig. 8.16). Oblique and lateral projections are occasionally useful.

Renal arteriography

The most common indications for renal arteriography are the investigation of suspected renovascular hypertension and renal haematuria. Occasional indications include the investigation of a space-occupying lesion in the kidney, a non-functioning kidney, trauma to the kidney, preoperative assess-

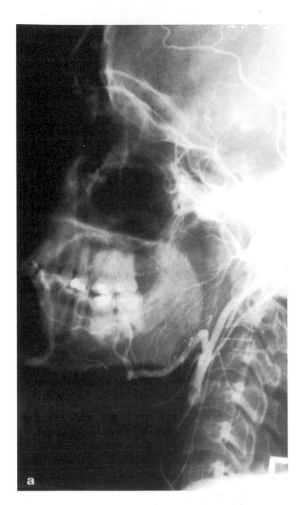 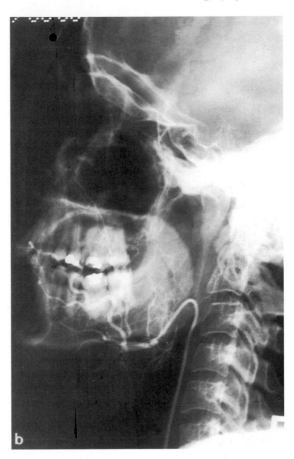

Fig. 8.11 (a) Selective left external carotid arteriography. (b) Superselective lingual arteriography using a 5F Mani catheter.

ment of a donor kidney and postoperative evaluation of a transplanted kidney.

Selective arteriography via a femoral artery catheterization is the preferred technique for renal arteriography, although a left transaxillary approach is possible. An i.v. DVI study is occasionally appropriate (see Chapter 12).

The arteriogram should be performed using a 50 cm long 5F cobra or a 100 cm long 5F sidewinder catheter with an end-hole and two side-holes (see Fig. 8.3). The tip of the catheter should be positioned 1–2 cm into the renal artery, which originates from the lateral aspect of the abdominal aorta, slightly posteriorly at the L1/L2 level. Accessory arteries to the lower or upper poles of the kidneys occur in 25% of patients.

Non-ionic contrast medium (10–15 ml containing 300 mg iodine ml^{-1}) is injected at a rate of 4–6 ml s^{-1}. After a delay of half of a second, radiographs are exposed at a rate of 2 s^{-1} for 3 s, 1 s^{-1} for 3 s and then one every alternate second for 6 s, visualizing the kidney in the AP projection (Fig. 8.17). Oblique projections are occasionally useful.

Adrenal angiography

Adrenal arteriography, adrenal venography and adrenal venous sampling are only very occasionally required in the radiological investigation of the adrenal glands, which are now largely assessed by CT, ultrasound and radionuclide imaging. Adrenal vein

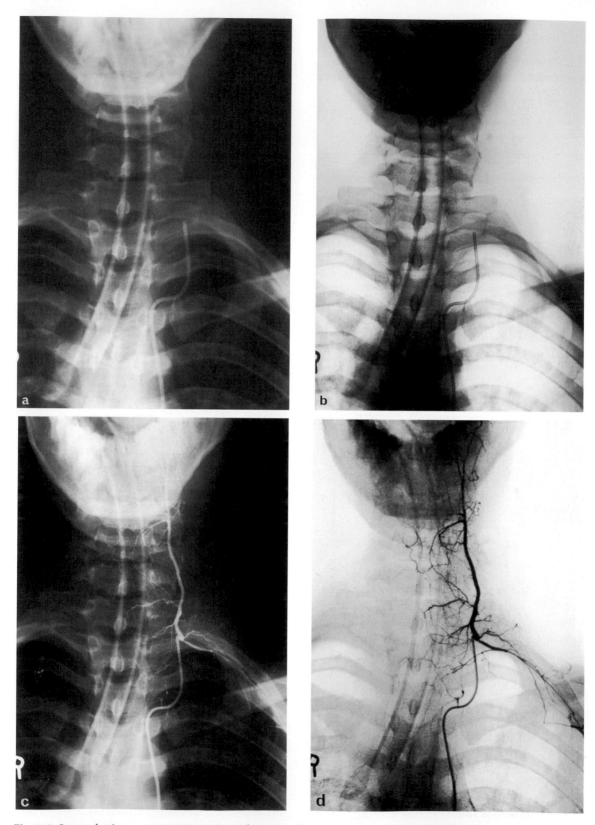

Fig. 8.12 Superselective costocervical arteriography using a 5F Mani catheter showing the radiographs required for the subtraction technique: (a) control radiograph, (b) mask radiograph, (c) angiogram radiograph, and (d) subtraction radiograph.

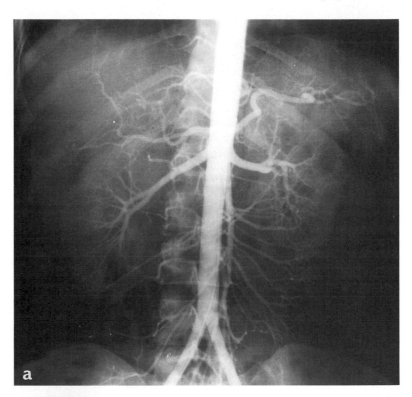

Fig. 8.13 Abdominal aortography via a right femoral artery catheter showing the abdominal aorta in (a) an anteroposterior and *(below)* (b) a lateral view.

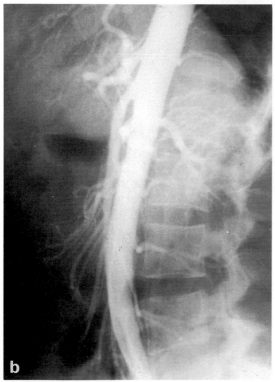

sampling for adrenal tumours and whole-body venous sampling for ectopic or extra-adrenal tumours, particularly phaeochromocytomas, is more accurate in the localization of adrenal tumours than aortography and selective arteriography. Arterial studies, however, can be useful in the assessment of phaeochromocytoma, neuroblastoma and adrenal carcinoma. Patients with a phaeochromocytoma should be controlled on α- and β-adrenergic blocking drugs to prevent a hypertensive crisis during the investigation.

The adrenal glands have a triple arterial blood supply: (i) the inferior adrenal artery arising from the renal artery; (ii) the middle adrenal artery from the aorta; and (iii) the superior adrenal artery from the inferior phrenic artery. The latter originates from the aorta or the coeliac axis. The right adrenal vein usually drains into the inferior vena cava and the left adrenal vein usually drains into the left renal vein and then into the inferior vena cava.

Renal arteriography via a femoral artery catheterization is the preferred technique for arteriography of the adrenal gland. The arteriogram

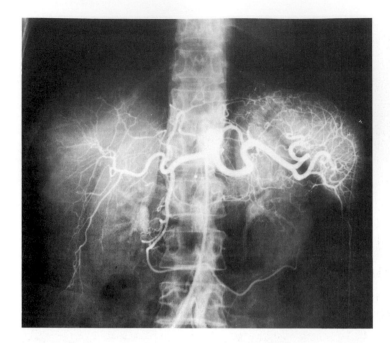

Fig. 8.14 Selective coeliac axis arteriography using a 6F catheter.

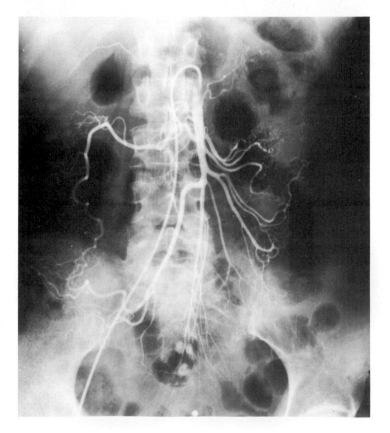

Fig. 8.15 Selective superior mesenteric arteriography using a 6F catheter.

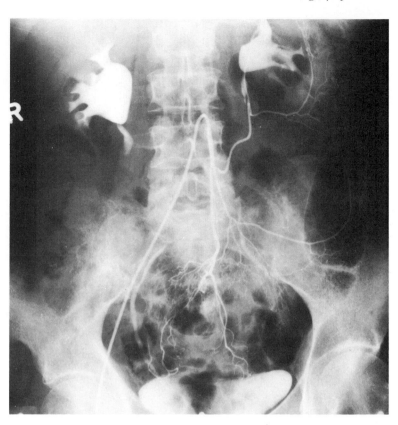

Fig. 8.16 Selective inferior mesenteric arteriography using a 6F catheter.

is performed as above for renal arteriography. Selective arteriography of one of the adrenal arteries via a femoral artery catheterization can also be performed for more detailed adrenal arteriography.

The arteriogram should be performed using a 50 cm long, 5F cobra or a 100 cm 5F sidewinder catheter with an end-hole (see Fig. 8.3). The tip of the catheter should be positioned at the origin of the artery and 1–4 ml of non-ionic contrast medium containing 300 mg iodine ml^{-1} are injected by hand after fluoroscopic assessment. Radiographs are exposed at a rate of 1 s^{-1} for 6–10 s in the AP projection (Fig. 8.18).

Pelvic arteriography

The most common indication for pelvic arteriography is as part of the assessment of atherosclerotic peripheral vascular disease causing stenosis or occlusion in the lower-limb arteries. It is also used in the evaluation of aneurysmal atherosclerotic peripheral vascular disease, as well as pelvic trauma, the investigation of haematuria from the bladder and arteriovenous malformations in the pelvis.

Lumbar aortography via a femoral artery catheterization is the preferred technique for arteriography of the pelvis. The aortogram is performed as described on p. 131 for lumbar aortography, except that only 30–40 ml of non-ionic contrast medium containing 370 mg iodine ml^{-1} are injected at a rate of 10–15 ml s^{-1}. After a delay of 1 s, radiographs are exposed at a rate of 2 s^{-1} for 2 s and then 1 s^{-1} for 4 s to demonstrate the pelvis in the AP projection.

Selective arteriography of the internal iliac artery, via an ipsilateral or contralateral femoral artery catheterization, can also be performed for more detailed pelvic arteriography. The arteriogram should be performed using a 50 cm long 5F cobra (or hook) catheter with an end-hole and two side-holes (see Fig. 8.3). The tip of the catheter should be positioned 1–2 cm into the internal iliac artery. Non-ionic con-

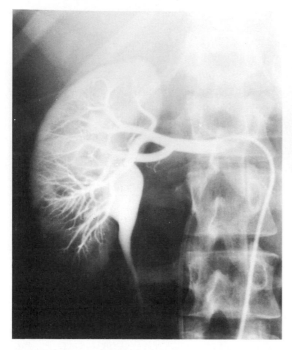

Fig. 8.17 Selective right renal arteriography using a 6F catheter.

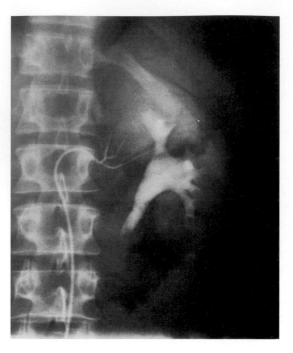

Fig. 8.18 Selective left middle adrenal arteriography using a 6F catheter.

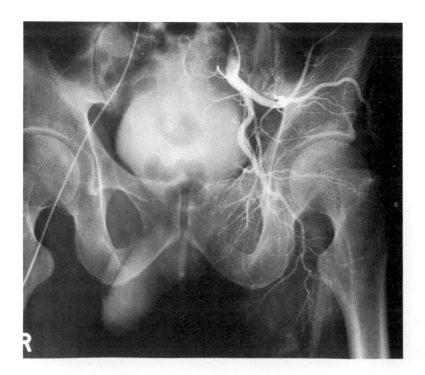

Fig. 8.19 Selective left internal iliac arteriography using a 5F cobra catheter from the right femoral artery across the aortic bifurcation.

trast medium (10–15 ml containing 300 mg iodine ml^{-1}) is injected at a rate of 4–6 ml s^{-1} . After a delay of half a second, radiographs are exposed at a rate of 2 s^{-1} for 2 s, 1 s^{-1} for 4 s and then one every alternate second for 4 s in the AP projection (Fig. 8.19). Oblique views are occasionally useful.

Complications

The complications of arteriography are usually due either to the arterial catheterization technique or to the contrast medium, but occasionally result from the drugs used in the premedication or the local, epidural or general anaesthetic used for the procedure. It is particularly important to remember that i.v. diazepam (Valium) in the elderly patient may produce respiratory arrest.

Reactions to contrast medium occur in about 3% of patients undergoing arteriography and venography (Shehadi, 1982). Major reactions occur in less than 0.15% and a fatal reaction in less than 0.005% of patients undergoing arteriography. Contrast media may cause either hypersensitivity or toxic reactions. The hypersensitivity reactions are not dose-related, being unpredictable. They are more common with the use of i.v. contrast medium, and in anxious or atopic patients. The toxic reactions are dose-related, not really predictable, and probably more common in dehydrated patients with generalized ischaemic disease. They are caused by the hyperosmolar effects of the contrast medium. Contrast medium reactions are undoubtedly reduced by the use of the new non-ionic intravascular contrast media such as iopamidol (Niopam), iohexol (Omnipaque), iopramide (Ultravist), ioversol (Optiray) and iodixanol (Visipaque). This reduction appears to be more marked when considering the toxic as opposed to the hypersensitivity reactions and is undoubtedly due to their low osmolarity (three to four times that of plasma) in comparison to the higher osmolarity (five to eight times that of plasma) of the ionic contrast media. The ionic contrast media should not be used for arteriography. The hypersensitivity or allergic type of reactions include urticaria, bronchospasm, angioneurotic/laryngeal oedema and acute anaphylaxis with cardiovascular collapse. The toxic type of reactions include a feeling of warmth, cardiac

arrhythmias, pulmonary oedema and cardiac arrest. Contrast media are considered in more detail in Chapter 30. Vasovagal reactions with bradycardia and hypotension can also occur during catheterization of the femoral artery.

The complications of arteriography can occur at the puncture site, in the arterial tree and within specific organs or systems.

Complications at the local arterial puncture site include haematoma, haemorrhage, arterial spasm, thrombosis, subintimal dissection, perivascular extravasation of contrast medium, false aneurysm, arteriovenous fistula, nerve trauma and local sepsis. These complications occur in about 5% of patients with 0.2% requiring surgery (Sigstedt & Lunderquist, 1978).

Haematoma formation and haemorrhage at the puncture site are undoubtedly the most common complications of arterial catheterization, but their incidence is reduced to a minimum by good angiographic technique. The large 7–8F diameter catheters, procedures exceeding 1 hour in length, multiple catheter changes and clumsy manipulations, clotting disorders, anticoagulation, systemic hypertension, aneurysmal arterial disease and inadequate compression of the artery at the puncture site all increase the risk of haematoma formation, haemorrhage and the rare false aneurysm formation. Arteriovenous fistula formation is very rare. Retroperitoneal haematoma is inevitable after a translumbar aortogram.

Arterial spasm at the puncture site is unusual but occurs with the use of large 7–8F diameter catheters, often in younger patients with normal arteries.

Thrombosis at the puncture site is one of the more common complications of arterial catheterization but, once again, its incidence can be reduced to a minimum by good technique. Arterial spasm, the large 7–8F diameter catheters, procedures exceeding 1 hour in length, multiple arterial punctures, multiple catheter changes and clumsy manipulations, polycythaemia, thrombocytosis, stenotic vascular disease and excessive compression of the

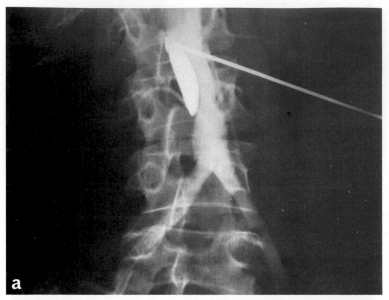

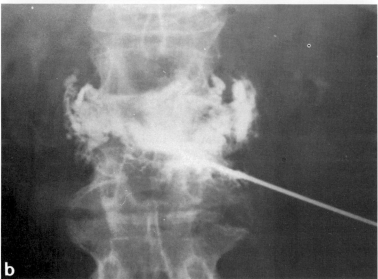

Fig. 8.20 Translumbar aortography using a needle and showing (a) subintimal dissection, and (b) perivascular extravasation of the contrast medium into the retroperitoneal soft tissues.

artery at the puncture site all increase the risk of thrombosis.

Subintimal dissection at the puncture site is also unusual, but occurs with the use of straight-tipped guide wires in older patients with atherosclerotic arteries.

Perivascular extravasation of the contrast medium is due to incorrect positioning of the needle tip and is most common in translumbar aortography (Fig. 8.20).

Nerve trauma is rare, being either due to primary nerve injury or secondary to extrinsic compression by haematoma, and is commonest in transaxillary catheterization.

The arterial complications distant to the puncture site include not only subintimal dissection, thrombosis and spasm, but also embolization, perforation, catheter knots and guide wire fracture as well as bacterial endocarditis and septicaemia.

These complications occur in about 0.5% of patients with 0.1% requiring surgery (Sigstedt & Lunderquist, 1978).

Subintimal dissection, one of the most common complications of arterial catheterization, occurs more frequently in the iliac artery during catheter positioning than in the common femoral artery during needle puncture. It is caused by the tip of the guide wire or catheter entering the wall of the artery, usually in relation to an atheromatous plaque, and stripping some of it off into the lumen. The use of soft 3 or 15 mm J-tipped guide wires, gentle catheter manipulations and small test injections of contrast medium under fluoroscopic control all decrease the risk of subintimal dissection. Perforation of the arterial wall is rare.

Arterial spasm is unusual in a selectively catheterized artery. The use of 5 or 6F diameter catheters, gentle catheter manipulations and withdrawal of the catheter tip all decrease the risk of spasm.

Thrombosis in an iliac or other selectively catheterized artery is rare and is usually due to subintimal dissection, particularly with an antegrade (as opposed to a retrograde) type of dissection, in which the direction of blood flowing in the artery tends to open the dissected flap.

Embolization into the arterial tree, one of the more common complications of arterial catheterization, occurs more frequently into the lower limb arteries than into the vascular bed of a selectively catheterized artery. It is caused by thrombus stripping off the guide wire or catheter during exchanges or by atheroma dislodging from the arterial wall during manipulations. The use of a soft 3 or 15 mm J-tipped Teflon-coated guide wire and 5 or 6F diameter catheters, short procedures, few catheter changes and gentle manipulation all decrease the risk of embolization. Heparin-bonded coatings for guide wires and catheters are also available. Cholesterol crystal embolization is due to trauma to an atheromatous plaque by the guide wire or catheter and can produce renal failure. Air embolization is due to accidental injection of air through the catheter and is more serious in the cerebral and coronary circulations than in the lower-limb vessels. Cotton fibre embolization also occurs.

Guide wire or catheter fracture is very rare. Catheter knotting is rare, but usually occurs when using a sidewinder catheter. The knot can be successfully untied with the use of a guide wire or a second catheter inserted through another puncture site (Thomas & Sievers, 1979).

Damage to specific organs or systems may be due to direct needle trauma to an organ, as in translumbar aortography, and/or catheter trauma or contrast medium toxicity to a system, as in catheter aortography or selective arteriography.

Retroperitoneal haematoma always occurs after translumbar aortography which increases the risk of myocardial or cerebral infarction in a patient with vascular disease. Other reported complications after translumbar aortography include acute pancreatitis, acute tubular necrosis, paraplegia, pneumothorax, cardiac tamponade, bowel perforation and damage to the cisterna chyli or thoracic duct. Most of these are very rare. Paraplegia and renal failure can also occur after catheter abdominal aortography. Hemiplegia and loss of vision can occur after thoracic (arch) aortography and carotid, subclavian or vertebral arteriography. Mesenteric, renal and adrenal infarction have occurred after selective catheter arteriography.

Interventional vascular radiology

Interventional vascular procedures have naturally developed from diagnostic angiographic techniques and therefore require the same angiographic apparatus, catheterization equipment and contrast media. These percutaneous endovascular procedures include transluminal angioplasty, embolization, selective intra-arterial drug treatment and the extraction and placement of intravascular foreign bodies.

Percutaneous transluminal angioplasty employs a balloon catheter to dilate an arterial stenosis or occlusion in order to increase perfusion to the ischaemic limb or organ. This is the most common vascular interventional procedure and has been performed not only in the iliac, femoral, popliteal, coronary and renal arteries, but also in the aorta and the tibial, sub-clavian, carotid and mesenteric arteries. The stenosis or occlusion is crossed with a guide wire and catheter combination and is then dilated with a suitable balloon. Rotating mechanical devices and lasers can be used to recanalize arterial occlusions. Metallic stents are available for complex vascular problems.

Percutaneous vascular embolization involves the introduction of occlusive material through a superselectively placed arterial catheter in the treatment of primary tumours, hepatic metastases, vascular malformations, the control of haemorrhage from any site and the ablation of function of the spleen, kidney and adrenal glands. The wide variety of both solid and liquid embolic agents for temporary or permanent occlusion includes gelfoam and polyvinyl alcohol fragments, metallic coils, detachable balloons, 50% dextrose, 100% ethyl alcohol and tissue adhesives.

Percutaneous intra-arterial drug treatment involves the perfusion or infusion of a drug through a selectively placed arterial catheter. This includes thrombolytic drugs for thrombotic or embolic occlusive vascular disease, cytotoxic drugs for malignant disease, vasoconstrictor drugs for haemorrhage, and vasodilator drugs for ischaemia.

Broken catheter fragments, thrombus and atheroma can be retrieved from the vascular system. Filters can be placed in the inferior vena cava. Catheters containing an ultrasound probe and angioscopes have also been developed for use in the vascular system.

Drugs in angiography

Both vasoconstrictor and vasodilator drugs are used in diagnostic pharmacoangiography. The vasoconstrictor adrenaline, in a dose of 5–10 μg, when injected into the renal artery is used to differentiate between normal and abnormal tumour blood vessels, as the latter do not have the usual vasoconstrictor response. Angiotensin, in a dose of 0.5–1 μg, when injected into the renal artery is used to produce a redistribution of blood flow to the adrenal gland if there is difficulty in selectively catheterizing the inferior adrenal artery, as renal vasoconstriction occurs. The vasodilator prostaglandin $F_{2\alpha}$, in a dose of 25–75 μg, when injected into the superior mesenteric artery enhances the venous phase of the arteriography.

Prostaglandin E, in a dose of 5–10 μg, when injected into the brachial artery accentuates the arterial phase in peripheral arteriography of the hand.

The vasoconstrictor vasopressin, in a dose of 0.2–0.4 U min^{-1} as an arterial infusion, can be used to stop active bleeding from the gastrointestinal tract. The vasodilators tolazoline (25 mg), papaverine (25 mg) and nitroglycerin (50–100 μg) as an intra-arterial bolus can be used to relieve spasm in popliteal or tibial arteries during angioplasty.

Thrombolytic agents, such as streptokinase, urokinase or recombinant tissue plasminogen activator as an arterial infusion, can be used to produce lysis of recent thrombus in any artery. Cytotoxic drugs, such as 5-fluorouracil or mitamycin C as an arterial infusion, can be used to treat hepatic metastases.

Comparison of uses of different types of arteriography and their relationship to other imaging modalities

DVI is described in Chapter 12. A DVI system is not available in all radiology departments performing angiography, but is part of all newly installed angiography equipment. The spatial resolution of a digital system is approaching that of film. High-definition arteriography such as coronary, cerebral and tumour/small-vessel angiography can now be performed by either technique. Intra-arterial DVI is particularly useful in interventional angiography, for instance embolization and angioplasty, paediatric angiography and patients in renal failure. Intravenous DVI is indicated in screening angiography, for instance in hypertension, for follow-up angiography after a surgical arterial graft and in patients with no suitable arterial puncture site.

The vascular system can also be investigated by other imaging techniques. These include ultrasound, CT, radionuclide imaging and magnetic resonance angiography (MRA).

Ultrasound is used in the management of aneurysms of the abdominal aorta for assessing their size, relationship to the renal arteries and rate of growth. Ultrasound can be used in the investigation of a pulsatile mass in the neck, groin or popliteal fossa. Duplex ultrasound, which is a combination of B-mode ultrasound imaging and pulsed Doppler, is used in the assessment of lower-limb arterial disease, surgical arterial graft surveillance, carotid artery stenosis and deep vein thrombosis in the lower limbs.

CT is the investigation of choice for confirming the diagnosis of a dissecting aortic aneurysm and showing its extent. CT is also used in the management of aneurysms of both the thoracic and the abdominal aorta for assessing their size and relationship to other arteries. CT can be used in the investigation of the complications of abdominal aneurysms before and after surgery.

Isotope studies using ^{99m}Tc sulphur colloid or ^{99m}Tc-labelled red cells can be used to locate the site of bleeding from the gastrointestinal tract. Isotope studies using ^{111}In-labelled white cells can be used to confirm the diagnosis of an infected surgical arterial graft.

MRA can be used to confirm the diagnosis of a dissecting aortic aneurysm and is particularly useful in imaging the thoracic aorta because of its multiplanar imaging facility. MRA can also be used in the assessment of carotid artery stenosis, renal artery stenosis, abdominal aortic aneurysms, lower limb arterial disease and thrombosis of the superior or inferior venae cavae.

References

Dyet, J.F., Hartley, W.C., Galloway, J.M.D., Wilkinson, A.R., Imrie, M.J. & Cook, A.M. (1990) Outpatient arteriography — a safe and practical proposition? *Clin. Radiol.*, **42**, 114–15.

Gaines, P.A. & Reidy, J.P. (1986) Percutaneous high brachial aortography: a safe alternative to the translumbar approach. *Clin. Radiol.*, **37**, 595–7.

Halpern, M. (1964) Percutaneous transfemoral arteriography: an analysis of the complications in 1000 consecutive cases. *Am. J. Roentgenol.*, **92**, 918–34.

Hawkins, I.F. (1982) Carbon dioxide digital subtraction angiography. *Am. J. Roentgenol.*, **139**, 19–24.

Hessel, S.J., Adams, D.F. & Abrams, H.L. (1981) Complications of angiography. *Radiology*, **138**, 273–81.

Levin, D.C. & Dunham, L. (1982) New equipment consideration for angiographic laboratories. *Am. J. Roentgenol.*, **139**, 775–80.

McIvor, J. & Rhymer, J.C. (1992) 245 transaxillary arteriograms in arteriopathic patients: success rate and complications. *Clin. Radiol.*, **45**, 390–4.

Rosch, J. & Grollman, J.H. (1969) Superselective arteriography in the diagnosis of abdominal pathology: technical considerations. *Radiology*, **92**, 1008–13.

Seldinger, S. (1953) Catheter replacement of needle in percutaneous arteriography: a new technique. *Acta Radiol.*, **39**, 368–76.

Shehadi, W.H. (1982) Contrast media adverse reactions: occurrence, recurrence and distribution patterns. *Radiology*, **143**, 11–17.

Sigstedt, B. & Lunderquist, A. (1978) Complications of angiographic examinations. *Am. J. Roentgenol.*, **130**, 455–60.

Stocks, L.O., Halpern, M. & Turner, A.F. (1969) Complete translumbar aortography: the teflon sleeve technique, *Am. J. Roentgenol.*, **107**, 835–9.

Thomas, H.A. & Sievers, R.E. (1979) Nonsurgical reduction of arterial catheter knots. *Am. J. Roentgenol.*, **132**, 1018–19.

Further reading

Belli, A.M. (ed.) (1994) *Interventional Radiology of the Peripheral Vascular System*. Edward Arnold, Sevenoaks.

Grainger, R.G. & Allison D.J. (eds) (1992) *Diagnostic Radiology*, chapter 102. Churchill Livingstone, Edinburgh.

Hillman, B.J. & Newell, J.D. (eds) (1985) *Digital Radiography. Radiological Clinics of North America 23, No. 2.*

Kadir, S. (1986) *Diagnostic Angiography*. WB Saunders, Philadelphia.

Koolpe, H.A. (ed.) (1986) *Vascular Imaging: Angiography and the New Modalities. Radiological Clinics of North America 24, No. 3.*

Reuter, S.R. & Redman, H.C. (1977) *Gastrointestinal Angiography*. WB Saunders, Philadelphia.

Ring, E.J. & McLean, G.K. (eds) (1981) *Interventional Radiology: Principles and Techniques*. Little, Brown & Co., Boston.

Sutton, D. (ed.) (1993) *A Textbook of Radiology and Imaging*, chapter 25. Churchill Livingstone, Edinburgh.

Veiga-Pires, J.A. & Grainger, R.G. (1982) *The Portuguese School of Angiography*. MTP Press, Lancaster.

Wilkins, R.A. & Viamonte, M. (eds) (1982) *Interventional Radiology*. Blackwell Scientific Publications, Oxford.

9 Venous System

H. L. WALTERS

Lower-limb phlebography

From the time when phlebography achieved a wide acceptance as a result of the work of Dos Santos (1938), the technique of ascending lower-limb phlebography has been developed and refined to such levels of accuracy and reproducibility that contrast phlebography is the standard by which other diagnostic techniques are assessed in the evaluation of venous diseases. It remains the only examination which provides direct evidence of the pathological process, its extent and its chronicity.

During phlebography, contrast medium is injected into one of the tributaries of the venous system. A variety of special techniques may be required to demonstrate veins in different regions. The main variations in technique are in the method of introducing the contrast medium and in the postural and other manoeuvres designed to obtain uniform or selective venous filling. No single method can encompass all the clinical indications and provide the required specific information in each case. The basic technique for lower-limb phlebography described below is, however, appropriate in the vast majority of cases. Variations of this technique, according to the clinical situation, are discussed on pp. 152–3.

Indications

The clinical situations where lower-limb phlebography may be of value can be summarized as follows:
1 The investigation of suspected deep-vein thrombosis: confirmation of the diagnosis and information regarding the site, extent and nature of the thrombus.
2 In establishing the source of pulmonary embolism and the demonstration of any residual thrombus.
3 The assessment of the deep venous system and demonstration of incompetent communicating veins prior to surgery of the superficial veins. The proce-

dure may also be of value following surgery in cases of recurrent varicosities.
4 The investigation of venous ulceration or oedema following deep-vein thrombosis — the post-thrombotic syndrome. Phlebography evaluates the patency of the deep veins, any damage to the venous valves and the localization of incompetent communicating veins.
5 The evaluation of the integrity of the venous system in patients with lower-limb oedema of unknown cause.
6 The investigation of venous dysplasia.

Contraindications

A known previous severe reaction to contrast medium requires a reappraisal of the need for examination. Possible alternative means of obtaining the desired information should be discussed with the referring clinician.

Although anticoagulant therapy is not a contraindication, special care must be taken to achieve haemostasis at the completion of the procedure.

Basic technique of ascending phlebography

Equipment

The basic requirement is a radiographic tilting table equipped for fluoroscopy and with a spot radiograph capability. This enables the flow of contrast medium to be monitored and exposures made only when there is optimal filling of the veins.

Patient preparation

1 The patient is fasted for 4–6 hours prior to the examination, thus anticipating any nausea or vomiting related to the use of contrast media.

2 In-patients with severe leg oedema should have the affected limb elevated to facilitate venepuncture.

Procedure

The patient is examined supine with a 20–40° foot-down table tilt. The provision of hand grips on the table enables patients to steady themselves and avoid any weight-bearing on the leg under examination (Fig. 9.1). This semi-upright position combined with the use of tourniquets gives maximal venous filling without flow artefacts, layering of the hyperbaric contrast medium occurring unless there is a uniform mixing with blood.

A tourniquet is applied above the ankle to distend the foot veins. The skin on the dorsum of the foot is cleaned. A 21 gauge butterfly needle is then inserted into a distal vein on the dorsum of the foot. If the needle is too proximal, the contrast medium may bypass the deep plantar veins and produce artefacts which give the false appearance of a deep venous occlusion. Whilst any of these distal veins is accept-

able, the most suitable vein is the medial digital vein of the great toe, which has the advantage of communicating directly with the plantar plexus through the first interosseous space. Thus, injected contrast medium flows preferentially into the deep veins. The butterfly needle is secured with adhesive strapping and is attached via a polyvinyl connection to a 10 ml syringe of saline, which allows the venepuncture to be checked by injecting saline under direct vision.

The presence of oedema may make venepuncture difficult, although a vein can usually be displayed if the area is locally massaged to disperse overlying oedema fluid. After an unsuccessful venepuncture, the needle should be left *in situ* and haemostasis achieved with firm local pressure. Possible leakage of contrast medium from the original failed venepuncture is thus reduced when there is a subsequent successful attempt at another site. Only rarely is it necessary to cut down on to a vein.

A second tourniquet is now applied above the knee in order to delay the flow of contrast medium from the calf veins, thus promoting adequate and more

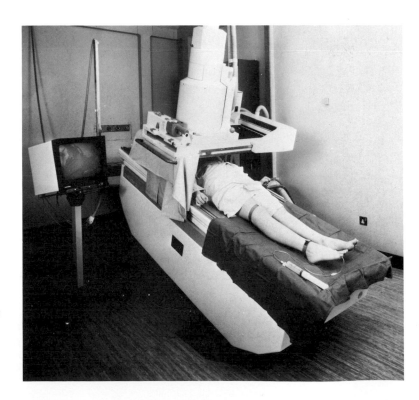

Fig. 9.1 The radiographic table has a 30° foot-down tilt. Hand grips provide support for this non-weight-bearing position. Tourniquets have been positioned just before starting the procedure.

uniform filling of all the deep distal veins. The alternative to the self-fastening Velcro tourniquet is a specially constructed pneumatic tourniquet consisting of two narrow cuffs connected by tubing to a manometer and an inflating hand bellows (Fig. 9.2). Separate control of each cuff by means of a stopcock permits independent alteration of pressure in the cuffs (Craig, 1972).

The saline syringe is replaced by syringe containing 60 ml of low-osmolar contrast medium. The concentration routinely employed is 250 mg iodine ml^{-1} and is obtained by diluting 50 ml of iohexol 300 or iopamidol 300 with 10 ml saline. The volume of contrast medium required varies between patients, reflecting the differing venous capacity of legs. Optimal venous opacification is determined by the appearances at fluoroscopy.

With the table tilted 20–40° in the foot-down position and the leg under examination internally rotated to separate the images of the tibia and fibula (Fig. 9.2), contrast medium is injected by hand under screen control. An injection flow rate of approximately 0.5–1 ml s^{-1} should be employed. The venepuncture site is checked to exclude extravasation. Progress of the contrast medium is observed to ensure that it passes into the tibial veins, the ankle tourniquet pressure perhaps requiring adjustment at this stage to ensure deep venous filling. The posterior tibial veins are normally the first to fill, followed by the fibular and anterior tibial veins. The muscular venous arcades draining the soleus and gastrocnemius often fill later than the main stem veins of the calf.

Films are exposed in the posteroanterior (PA)

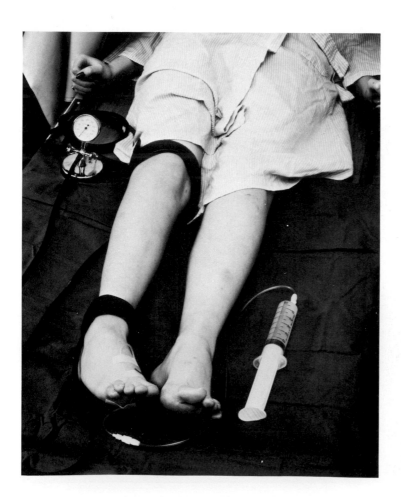

Fig. 9.2 Pneumatic tourniquets in position. The leg under examination is internally rotated to separate the images of the tibia and fibula.

position when there is uniform filling of the deep veins of the calf. Three exposures are made on a 35 × 35 cm radiograph, subdivided into three, to include the veins from the ankle to the knee (Fig. 9.3). Contrast filling of the popliteal venous segment is enhanced by employing gentle pressure on the deep calf veins just above the ankle. The leg is next externally rotated to obtain a lateral view of the deep calf veins, three similar exposures being made to include the veins from the foot to the knee (Fig. 9.4). These

lateral views are important in demonstrating the posterior tibial and soleal veins without superimposition of other veins. Whilst the majority of thrombi begin in these calf veins, some originate in the plantar veins and so a view of the foot should always be included in the lateral series (Lea Thomas & O'Dwyer, 1978). The leg is then repositioned to the front and the above-knee tourniquet is removed to allow contrast filling of the superficial and common femoral veins. Two exposures are made of the deep

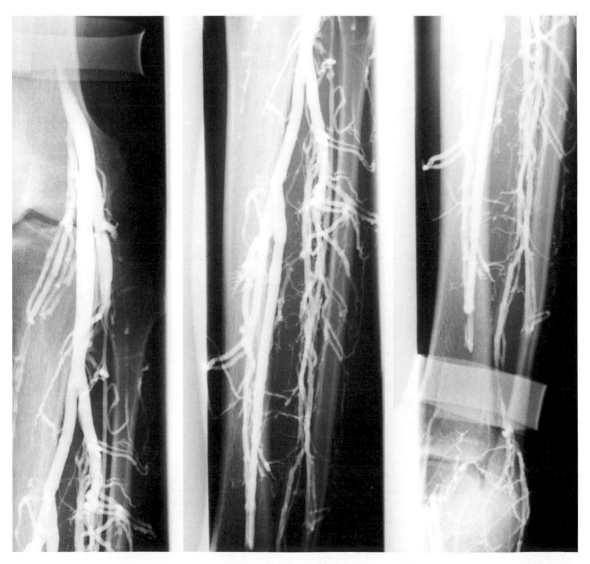

Fig. 9.3 Uniform filling of the deep calf veins exposed in the posteroanterior position on a divided 35 cm² film. The ankle tourniquet directs contrast into the deep veins; the above-knee tourniquet delays emptying of the calf veins.

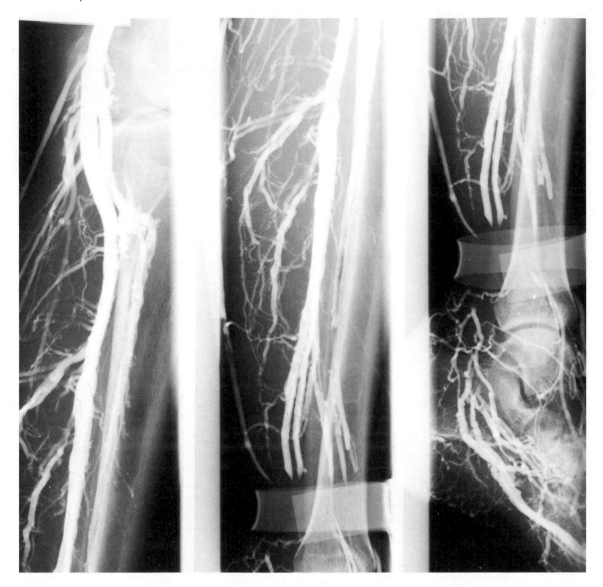

Fig. 9.4 Lateral exposures showing the main stem veins of the calf with good filling of the calf muscle veins. The plantar veins have been included on the first exposure.

veins in the thigh. The explorator is now positioned to include the area of the groin and pelvis. A third exposure is then made, following release of the ankle tourniquet and the application of firm pressure on the calf to propel contrast medium as a bolus, in order to demonstrate the iliac veins and the lower inferior vena cava (IVC) (Fig. 9.5). A Valsalva manoeuvre, performed when the common femoral and external iliac veins are filled with contrast medium, demonstrates the proximal segment of the deep femoral vein.

Following the procedure and while the radiographs are being processed, the veins are cleared of contrast medium by elevating the leg and injecting normal saline. Once the diagnostic adequacy of the radiograph is confirmed, early ambulation of the pa-

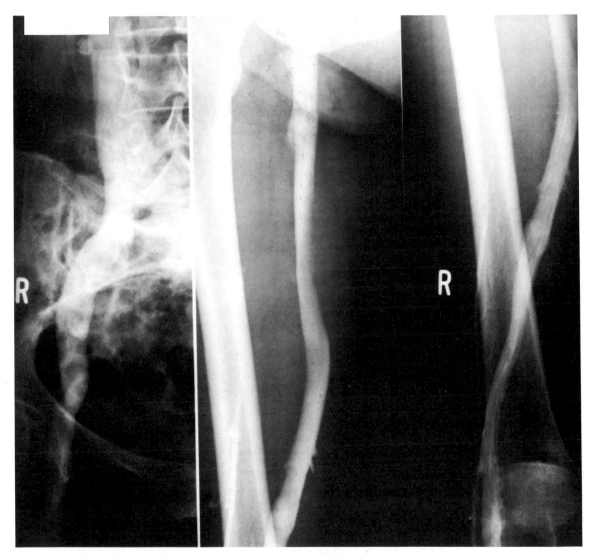

Fig. 9.5 Popliteal and superficial femoral veins demonstrated after tourniquet release. The final exposure to outline the iliac veins and lower inferior vena cava is made using the bolus technique following calf compression. The profunda femoris vein has not filled on this study.

tient is encouraged. Active leg movements should be performed when this is not possible. Possible thrombotic complications from stasis of the contrast medium are reduced in this way.

While this technique delineates the deep veins from the foot to the lower IVC, some segments of the venous system are difficult to fully demonstrate. The main difficulties arise in the following situations.

1 The anterior tibial vein may be occluded by the ankle tourniquet. A limited repeat examination after reducing the ankle tourniquet pressure, or dispensing with the tourniquet, demonstrates the patency or otherwise of the anterior tibial vein.
2 Even employing a non-weight-bearing technique, it is not possible to demonstrate the entire vast network of muscle veins in the calf (Cotton & Clark, 1965).

3 The deep femoral vein fills in only 50% of patients, either as a result of a loop connection with the superficial femoral vein or retrogradely during the Valsalva manoeuvre.

4 The internal iliac vein may fill during a Valsalva manoeuvre, but only as far as its valves will allow.

5 Occasionally the iliac veins and lower IVC are not adequately demonstrated by the technique of calf compression at the completion of the standard technique.

When it is necessary to show these venous segments in this situation, as in the delineation of the upper extent of a thrombus, a repeat examination with the following modification will demonstrate these veins in the majority of patients. An above-knee tourniquet is applied to each thigh, in order to delay calf emptying, and 50 ml of contrast medium are injected simultaneously into each leg. With the explorator centred over the pelvis and loaded with a 35 × 35 cm radiograph, an exposure is made immediately after the release of the tourniquet and the application of firm pressure to both calves. This bolus technique is a valuable method of demonstrating the iliocaval venous segment (Lea Thomas & Macdonald, 1977).

Variations of the basic technique

The objectives of ascending phlebography in defined clinical situations must be clearly understood. In many instances the basic technique will require little modification, merely particular attention directed to achieving those objectives. The aims of phlebography may be summarized in the following venous disorders.

Deep-vein thrombosis

Recent advances in treating venous thrombosis require more than simply the documentation of the presence of a thrombus. The phlebogram must aim to give an indication of the age of a thrombus, its extent and, as far as possible, its liability to embolize. The objectives are as follows.

1 To show that a filling defect in a vein is persistent and constant in shape on more than one radiograph excluding various artefacts (Lea Thomas & Carty, 1975).

2 To fill as many of the deep veins as possible, including established collateral vessels around occluded veins.

3 To demonstrate the upper extent of the thrombus or occluded vein.

Retrograde phlebography or intraosseous phlebography may be indicated when ascending phlebography, including the bolus technique, fails to demonstrate the iliocaval segment.

Varicose veins and incompetent communicating veins

Incompetent communicating veins allow the retrograde flow of blood from the deep to the superficial veins. Whilst most of these incompetent veins are recognized clinically and have a fairly constant position, some arise in an inconstant position. Phlebography shows their location and, further, confirms the integrity of the deep veins if there is doubt on clinical grounds prior to a radical stripping procedure.

An ankle tourniquet is applied sufficiently tightly to ensure that there is no superficial venous filling. The pneumatic cuffs, as described by Craig (1972) and referred to in the basic technique, are particularly useful in this context. The presence of ulceration around the ankle, or the suspicion of an incompetent communicating vein below the malleolus, may require the placement of a cuff around the forefoot.

The flow of the injected contrast medium is monitored and a radiograph is exposed when retrograde flow through the incompetent communicating vein is seen. These early radiographs are valuable since the varicosities may subsequently flood with contrast medium, making identification of the level of the incompetent vein difficult.

The precise level of these veins can be measured by means of a ruler with 1 cm radio-opaque markers. This allows for magnification and the level is determined by reference to the malleoli (Fig. 9.6).

The technique of varicography may be of value in patients with recurrent varicosities following surgery, or where the varicose vein follows an unusual course. The varix is directly punctured with a 21 gauge butterfly needle. Contrast injection

There is frequently involvement of the arterial, venous and lymphatic systems in these malformations (Kinmonth *et al.*, 1976). The investigation of each case must therefore be planned on an individual basis.

The demonstration of the presence or absence of a normal deep venous system is vital to the investigation of the mainly venous malformations. This information is essential when contemplating surgery. The phlebographic technique employed is similar to the modified approach in the investigation of incompetent communicating veins. It may occasionally be difficult to occlude the superficial venous system, especially if there are coexisting varicose veins, skin ulceration and soft-tissue hypertrophy. Intraosseous phlebography may be required to demonstrate the integrity of the deep venous system in these cases.

Having demonstrated the state of the deep veins and the presence of any incompetent communicating veins, the central connections of any superficial anomalous venous channel can best be evaluated by direct injection into the anomaly. Contrast medium then delineates the extent of the lesion and its central ramification.

Small localized venous anomalies are similarly dealt with by the direct injection of contrast medium into the dysplastic veins, using a 21 gauge butterfly needle (Fig. 9.7).

More extensive dysplasias which have arterial and venous components may best be demonstrated by arteriography. The film sequence is continued through into the venous phase following an arterial injection of contrast medium.

Pelvic phlebography

In those cases where the iliac veins and lower IVC have been inadequately demonstrated by the above technique, percutaneous perfemoral injections of contrast medium can demonstrate the iliocaval segments when the femoral vein is intact.

Indications

1 The demonstration of the upper extent of venous thrombosis.
2 To establish the source of pulmonary embolism.

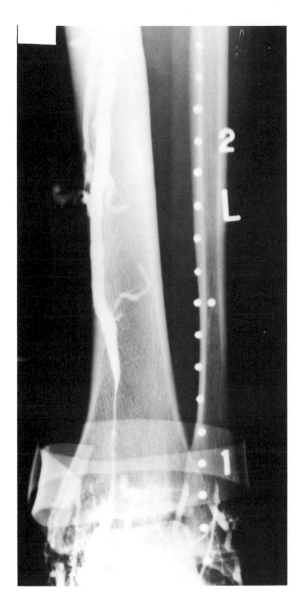

Fig. 9.6 An early exposure has been made to demonstrate this medial incompetent vein which, with the aid of the 1 cm marked ruler, is accurately measured as situated 11 cm above the tip of the medial malleolus.

will then identify the position of the incompetent communicating vein.

Venous dysplasias

The venous dysplasias form part of a wide clinical spectrum of congenital vascular malformations.

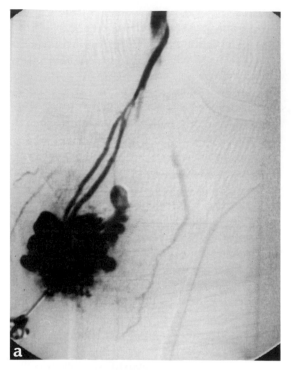

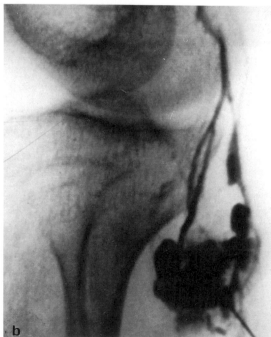

Fig. 9.7 Direct injection of venous angioma in upper calf demonstrating central connection with the popliteal vein. (a) Anteroposterior view. (b) Lateral view with landmark facility.

Iliac vein thrombosis carries a high risk of embolization.

3 The development of successful surgical procedures for the treatment of post-thrombotic states involving the iliac veins requires a precise anatomical demonstration of the pelvic veins and the venous collateral pathways.

Contraindications

As with ascending lower-limb phlebography, a previous severe contrast medium reaction is a contraindication and special care is required in patients receiving anticoagulant therapy.

Percutaneous perfemoral pelvic phlebography

The femoral vein, if patent, is the preferred approach to demonstrate the iliofemoral veins and lower IVC.

Technique

Equipment. A fluoroscopy unit with an overcouch tube and a rapid film changer is required.

Patient preparation. The patient is fasted for 4–6 hours prior to the procedure and both groins must be shaved.

The procedure. The patient is examined in the supine position. A control film of the pelvis, to include the area from the ischial tuberosities to the upper border of the 4th lumbar vertebra, checks the radiographic exposure and position.

The femoral vein lies medial to the femoral artery at the groin. Following aseptic skin preparation, local anaesthetic is infiltrated at a point 1 cm medial to the arterial pulsation and 2–3 cm below the inguinal ligament. Care is taken with the deeper subcutaneous infiltration to avoid intravascular injection by aspiration of the syringe before injecting local anaesthetic. A small 5 mm skin incision is made prior to femoral vein puncture.

A large-bore needle, such as a disposable Potts–Cournand needle*, is connected to a syringe con-

* Becton-Dickinson, Rutherford, New Jersey, USA.

taining saline via a polyvinyl connection. The needle is slowly withdrawn while, at the same time, applying gentle aspiration to the syringe. After a successful puncture, venous blood is aspirated and a small test injection of contrast medium is then made to confirm correct placement. The needle is then advanced a few centimetres over a flexible guide wire to ensure that it will not dislodge during the procedure. Venepuncture may be facilitated in difficult cases by asking the patient to perform a Valsalva manoeuvre, which distends the femoral vein. The same procedure is now performed on the other femoral vein.

The saline syringes are replaced by syringes which each contain 40 ml of contrast medium (iopamidol 300, iohexol 300 or ioxaglate 320). Simultaneous hand injections are then made by two operators. The injection must be forceful enough to deliver the volume in 4 s, in order to obtain a large bolus with uniform mixing with blood. The injection and filming sequence are started at the same time, eight

exposures being made at the rate of 1 s⁻¹ using the serial film changer (Fig. 9.8).

Whilst a single spot radiograph may be adequate for demonstrating an occlusion, a series of exposures gives a better display of any altered anatomy, shows the extent and direction of flow through venous collaterals and obviates the need for repeat examinations.

When the diagnostic adequacy of the radiographs has been confirmed, the needles are removed and firm pressure is applied to each venepuncture site until haemostasis is achieved.

Where the femoral vein is occluded, the proximal extent of the occlusion can be defined by one of three approaches:
1 Descending retrograde iliocavography.
2 Retrograde iliac phlebography, where the contralateral femoral vein is patent.
3 Pertrochanteric intraosseous phlebography (p. 157).

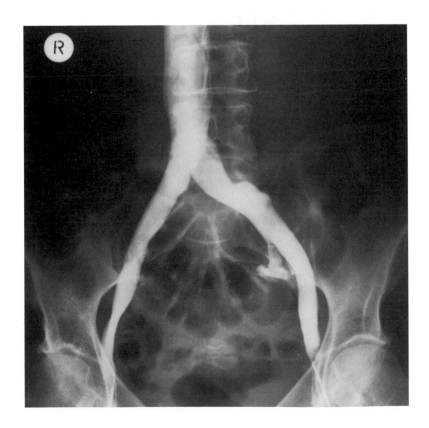

Fig. 9.8 Normal pelvic phlebogram showing external and common iliac veins and the lower inferior vena cava. There is slight filling of the left internal iliac vein and the left common iliac vein shows an indentation due to the right common iliac artery.

Descending retrograde iliocavography

This technique demonstrates the level of venous occlusion in the IVC or, more distally, down to the external iliac veins when the femoral approach is not possible or has provided insufficient anatomical detail. The technique also allows the internal iliac system to be examined and can be combined with pulmonary angiography (Dow, 1973).

The usual approach is via a catheter introduced into the median antecubital vein. Alternatively, a subclavian or jugular venous approach may be made. The jugular approach allows the subsequent insertion of a caval 'umbrella filter' as one of the management options in patients with, or at high risk of developing, pulmonary embolism in the presence of a loose venous thrombus.

The procedure involves the insertion of a 5F catheter with side-holes into the median antecubital vein at the elbow. The catheter is then advanced through the superior vena cava and, via the right atrium, into the IVC. As the catheter is slowly advanced down the inferior vena cava under screen control, test injections of contrast medium enable the catheter tip to be placed about 3 cm above the occlusion. The risk of dislodging any fresh thrombus or tumour is minimized in this way. The level of the occlusion is then recorded on a radiograph following the injection of contrast medium. A hand injection of contrast medium is sufficient when the caval flow is low as a result of the occlusion. Where flow is little impeded, a higher rate of injection is required.

Retrograde iliac phlebography

The upper extent of an iliofemoral occlusion can be demonstrated if the contralateral femoral and iliac veins have been shown to be patent on ascending phlebography of the lower limb.

The femoral vein is cannulated as described on p. 154 and a curved arterial catheter, for example a 5F renal catheter with side-holes, is introduced using the Seldinger technique (see Chapter 8). The catheter is then positioned in the contralateral common iliac vein. Care is taken, before placement of the catheter, to ensure that there is no thrombus projecting from the common iliac vein and that the catheter tip does not reach and dislodge any thrombus in this vein. The level and nature of the upper extent of the occlusion can thus be accurately defined. A hand injection of 20 ml contrast medium is sufficient to demonstrate an obstruction, because of the reduction in iliac venous flow.

Pertrochanteric intraosseous phlebography

This third approach, will demonstrate the pelvic veins and IVC but requires a general anaesthetic. The above techniques require only local anaesthesia.

Pelvic phlebography supplements ascending phlebography and enables the extent of the venous thrombosis to be assessed, particularly in the iliofemoral segment and IVC, by determining the upper extent of the disease, which is an important factor in case management.

Intraosseous phlebography

Intraosseous phlebography may be used when conventional phlebographic techniques are not possible because of venous occlusion or inaccessible veins. The technique is based on the observation that contrast medium injected into the bone marrow passes into the local venous drainage. This technique supplements conventional phlebography.

The application of the technique in various regions of the body has been widely studied by Schobinger (1960). The most frequent application of intraosseous phlebography has been to demonstrate the iliac veins and IVC in the presence of femoral vein occlusion. A combined approach may be made to examine the pelvic veins and IVC when lower-limb phlebography has revealed patency of the femoral vein on one side and occlusive disease on the contralateral side. The side of the patent femoral vein is examined by percutaneous perfemoral injection and the occluded side examined by pertrochanteric injection (Fig. 9.9). Intraosseous phlebography may occasionally be indicated to demonstrate the veins of the lower limb when i.v. access is not possible because of oedema.

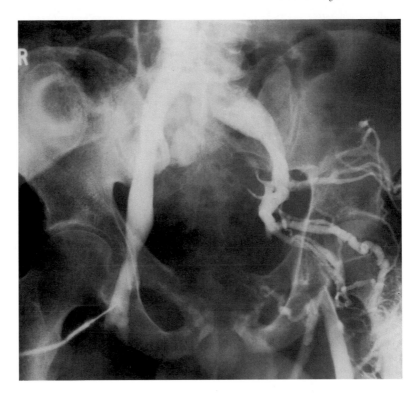

Fig. 9.9 Pelvic phlebography using a combined approach: a right perfemoral injection and left pertrochanteric intraosseous injection in a patient with an occluded left external iliac vein. The left femoral vein was punctured but the upper extent of the occlusion could not be defined (history of pelvic surgery followed by radiotherapy).

The procedure is painful and requires a general anaesthetic.

Indications

The only indication for intraosseous phlebography is failure of conventional intravenous phlebographic techniques, due to either venous occlusion or inaccessibility of veins. The technique has been largely supplanted with the advent of venous catheterization techniques but it remains a useful method in some situations.

Contraindications

1 The presence of local infection at the proposed puncture site is an absolute contraindication because of the attendant risk of osteomyelitis.
2 A known history of a bleeding diathesis, in particular haemophilia.

3 The technique is not undertaken in patients whose epiphyses are not fused because of the danger of impairing growth.
4 Previous severe contrast medium reaction.

Pertrochanteric intraosseous phlebography

Technique

Equipment. A fluoroscopy unit with an overcouch tube and rapid serial film changer is required.

Patient preparation. The patient is prepared for a general anaesthetic.

Procedure. A control film of the pelvis is used to check exposure and position, as described for pelvic phlebography.

The relatively slow clearance of contrast medium from the marrow cavity results in the hyperbaric contrast medium tending to gravitate to the most dependent veins. The internal iliac system is therefore preferentially demonstrated in the supine position, while the prone position better demonstrates the external and common iliac veins (Lea Thomas, 1970).

To demonstrate the iliofemoral segment, the patient is best examined in the prone position. A scrupulous aseptic technique is applied throughout the examination. Location of the greater trochanter is facilitated by an assistant who internally and externally rotates the leg while the bony prominence of the greater trochanter is located.

Puncture of the greater trochanter is undertaken with a 13 gauge Lea Thomas needle which has a drill tip to allow easy penetration of the outer cortex (Lea Thomas, 1970). Correct placement of the needle is confirmed by the aspiration of marrow blood and the free clearance of a small test injection of contrast medium from the marrow into the local draining veins. A second needle is inserted following an unsuccessful puncture, the first needle being left *in situ* to prevent extravasation of contrast medium along its track.

The needle is then connected to a pump injector and 40 ml of contrast medium (iohexol or iopamidol 300 or equivalent) are injected at the rate of 10 ml s^{-1}. Exposures are made at the rate of 1 s^{-1} for 10 s.

The needle is flushed with normal saline before its removal.

Intraosseous phlebography of the lower limb

Intraosseous phlebography demonstrates the deep veins when, as in the presence of gross oedema, it is not possible to locate a superficial vein. Although some workers carry out the procedure under local anaesthetic, the examination is painful and should be performed under general anaesthesia.

The most favourable access point in the lower limb is the medial malleolus. A 16 gauge bone-marrow needle is used and, with a strict aseptic technique, the upper part of the bony prominence of the medial malleolus is punctured with the needle tip angled cephalad to avoid entering the ankle joint. Correct placement of the needle is checked by the aspiration of marrow blood and by a small test injection of contrast medium which is screened to confirm free clearance into the local draining veins. Following an intraosseous injection, contrast medium passes preferentially into the deep venous system.

About 30–40 ml of contrast medium are usually adequate to demonstrate the deep venous system, the injection being made by hand. Exposures are made on a 35×35 cm radiograph, subdivided into three, as the contrast medium ascends the deep veins. These exposures are made when the veins are seen to be optimally filled.

Following the procedure, normal saline is infused to clear residual contrast medium. The needle is then removed.

Complications of intraosseous phlebography

Local complications

Incorrect needle position. The needle tip must be placed within the medullary cavity of the bone and its position checked by the aspiration of blood and the free clearance of a test injection of contrast medium from the medullary cavity into the local draining veins. This avoids extravasation into soft tissues and subperiosteal or intra-articular injections.

Osteomyelitis. Osteomyelitis is prevented by a scrupulous aseptic technique and avoiding injections at local sites of skin infection.

Bone infarction. Bone infarction has been described but appears to be a rare complication.

Distant complications

Fat embolism. Although rare, embolism represents the most serious complication and may be fatal. It has been suggested that the risk is increased when a pressure injection is made for intraosseous phlebography (Schobinger, 1960).

Inferior vena cavography

Indications

The main indications for inferior vena cavography are as follows:

1 IVC obstruction due to pathology arising within the vein, namely venous thrombosis, web obstruction, primary tumour or secondary tumour invasion. The examination must provide information on the extent of the obstruction and its upper limit.

2 Obstruction of the IVC due to pathology arising outside the vein, as with compression and displacement by tumour or retroperitoneal disease.

3 As a preliminary to confirm caval patency in suspected renal or hepatic vein thrombosis. Having excluded thrombus or tumour propagation into the IVC, selective examination of these veins can then be undertaken.

4 The complex embryological development of the IVC is reflected in the variety of congenital caval anomalies which may require investigation and interpretation by inferior vena cavography. The percutaneous bifemoral approach is the method of choice for their evaluation.

Technique

The approaches and techniques for inferior vena cavography are the same as those employed in pelvic phlebography. Cavography by a percutaneous bifemoral approach is the method of choice when both iliofemoral segments are patent.

Radiographs in both the anteroposterior (AP) and the lateral projections are required for a full evaluation of the IVC. The two projections can be obtained with the one injection if equipment providing biplane rapid serial radiography is available; otherwise two separate injections are required.

The control radiographs are centred on the region of interest. Suspected disease at the origin of the IVC requires a centring point at the level of the 5th lumbar vertebra, while disease near its termination must include the right atrium on the radiograph.

Simultaneous injections of 40 ml of contrast medium (iopamidol 370 or iohexol 350) are made on both sides, using a pump injector and a flow rate of 15 ml s^{-1}. The filming sequence is set for 2 s^{-1} for 3 s and then 1 s^{-1} for 4 s, the programme commencing half a second after the start of the injection. A delay may be incorporated for the last few radiographs if there is significant obstruction. In the absence of unilateral occlusive disease, such as an iliac vein block, a Y-connector joining both needles may be used and connected to a single injector.

Unilateral obstruction causes preferential flow through the unobstructed side.

When the patient has to be turned into a lateral position, in the absence of a biplane facility, it is safer to insert a 5F catheter with side-holes into each femoral vein using the Seldinger technique. The risk of displacing a cannula on turning the patient is thus avoided.

The IVC may alternatively be examined by introducing a catheter from the femoral vein by the Seldinger technique and advancing it to the required level in the IVC. This is the method of choice in examining the suprarenal segment of the IVC in cases of suspected obstruction. The catheter must have side-holes to allow uniform opacification of the IVC. With a catheter technique, 60 ml of contrast medium is injected with a flow rate of 20 ml s^{-1}. If digital subtraction angiography is available, smaller doses of contrast medium can be employed.

Upper-limb phlebography

The most common indication for investigation of the venous drainage of the arm is oedema associated with venous thrombosis. The site of obstruction is most commonly in either the axillary or the subclavian vein.

Technique

A fluoroscopy unit with a spot radiography capability is required. The patient is examined in the supine position on the fluoroscopy table. When the entire venous system of the arm is to be demonstrated, puncture of a peripheral vein on the dorsum of the hand is made with a 19 gauge butterfly needle, which is then secured. In the absence of the postural advantage of the semi-upright position used in lower-limb phlebography to retard venous return, a tourniquet is applied above the elbow to enable uniform mixing of the blood with the contrast medium and thus promote good venous opacification without artefacts. Exposures of the veins in the forearm are then made after injecting 30–40 ml of a low-osmolar contrast medium (iohexol 240).

Release of the tourniquet and firm compression of the forearm allows the contrast medium to delineate the upper-arm veins as a bolus, in particular the upper course of the basilic vein, which becomes the axillary vein and then the subclavian vein. This technique is of value when the median antecubital vein is not easily accessible for venepuncture.

The best approach to demonstrate the axillary and subclavian veins is via the median antecubital vein. In the presence of obstruction of the upper-arm veins the more peripheral veins are engorged and either a large-bore needle, such as a 16 gauge butterfly needle, or a 5F catheter with side-holes is introduced into the median antecubital vein. The catheter is then advanced to a point just distal to the occlusion with the aid of small test injections of contrast medium. Spot radiographs of the level and extent of the obstruction are then made during a hand injection of 30 ml of a low-osmolar constrast medium.

The cephalic vein is not used because contrast medium injected via this route bypasses the basilic vein and all but the termination of the axillary vein.

Following the procedure, firm pressure is applied to the venepuncture site until haemostasis is achieved.

Superior vena cavography

Superior vena cavography may be indicated in the following situations.
1 The evaluation of mediastinal disease, the vast majority of cases being related to neoplastic involvement of the superior vena cava.
2 The evaluation of venous thrombosis in the axillary, subclavian or innominate veins, with possible central extension into the superior vena cava.
3 The investigation of a congenital anomaly of the venous system.

Technique

Equipment

A fluoroscopy unit with spot radiography capability is used. As with the examination of the IVC, a biplane serial radiography unit is desirable to obtain AP and lateral projections with a single injection.

Patient preparation

If there is any oedema of the upper limb, the patient is encouraged to keep the arms elevated as much as possible before leaving the ward for the examination. This expedient may obviate the need for a modified cut-down procedure.

The patient is fasted for 4–6 hours prior to the examination.

Procedure

The examination is carried out with the patient lying in the supine position. Control radiographs are taken in the AP and lateral planes. The AP projection should be full field, extending from the root of the neck to the diaphragm and including the lateral chest walls. The lateral projection is coned to the mediastinum.

The arm veins are usually distended in the presence of superior vena caval obstruction. A tourniquet applied to the upper arm will further engorge the veins. Using an aseptic technique, the median antecubital vein at the elbow is identified and local anaesthesia infiltrated at the proposed venepuncture site. A small skin incision is made to facilitate catheterization. The venepuncture is made with an 18 gauge needle and, using the Seldinger technique, a 5F catheter with side-holes is advanced as close to the subclavian vein as the obstruction allows. Small test injections of contrast medium determine the level to which advancement is made.

Where the vein is not amenable to percutaneous

puncture, a modified cut-down is performed to expose the vein. The cephalic vein is best avoided because of its acute angle of entry near the termination of the axillary vein. The median antecubital vein has an obtuse angle of entry into the deep venous system, which facilitates catheter advancement.

The procedure is repeated for the other arm. Bilateral catheterization with simultaneous injections of contrast medium provides a full anatomical demonstration of the altered venous anatomy, avoiding the mixing artefacts due to the return of unopacified blood which occurs when examining only one arm.

The patient's arms are gently abducted to allow the lateral chest wall to be positioned as close as possible to the lateral film changer when a biplane facility is available. A separate injection is made into each catheter in preference to linking the catheters via a Y-connector. In the presence of obstruction, preferential flow occurs through the unobstructed or least obstructed side. A simultaneous injection of 30 ml contrast medium (iopamidol or iohexol 300 or equivalent) is made into each catheter and the radiographic sequence is started near the beginning of the injection. The radiographic sequence and rate of injection depend on the degree of obstruction. If test injections made during the positioning of the catheter suggest a complete obstruction, a hand injection is made and radiographs are exposed at the rate of 1 s^{-1} to demonstrate the level of obstruction, the collateral flow and whether or not there is any reconstitution of a main venous channel. The radiograph programme should be long enough to identify the venous anatomy beyond the obstruction, as well as the right atrium (Fig. 9.10). Where superior vena caval flow is less impeded, as with mediastinal deviation or compression, a more forceful injection is required, if necessary with a pump injector, to deliver contrast medium at a rate of 10 ml s^{-1}. The programme is then adjusted to take 2 radiographs s^{-1} for 4 s, followed by 1 s^{-1} for 10 s.

Where there is unequivocal clinical evidence of caval obstruction, for instance from involvement by a bronchial neoplasm, a large-bore needle, such as a 16 gauge butterfly needle, may be used instead of catheterization. A more rapid injection, which is possible with the catheter technique, is not required in these circumstances. Both arms are then examined as described in the technique above.

Having checked the diagnostic adequacy of the radiographs, the catheters are removed and firm pressure is applied to achieve haemostasis. Any sutures used when a cut-down has been necessary are firmly tied.

The technique of digital subtraction venography is of value in patients with limited venous access. Small peripheral veins may be successfully used to inject substantially smaller volumes of contrast medium (Andrews *et al.*, 1987).

Complications of phlebography

Complications which may arise during a phlebographic procedure may be due to the contrast medium or related to the technique.

Contrast media

Adverse reactions

These reactions are common to all situations where contrast media are injected into the vascular system and are not specific to phlebography. Adverse reactions, often of a minor nature, are more frequently seen after the i.v. injection of contrast medium than following an intra-arterial injection (Shehadi, 1975).

These adverse reactions may be classified as toxic, idiosyncratic and allergic. Toxic reactions are dose-related and it is probable that many of these reactions may be related to the hyperosmolar load imposed by conventionally used contrast media. The recent introduction of contrast media of low osmolality may significantly reduce these reactions.

Phlebography is contraindicated when there is a history of a previous severe reaction to contrast medium, unless there is an urgent need for information which the phlebogram can provide but which cannot be obtained by any other method. These high-risk patients may benefit from pretreatment with steroids (see Chapter 30). Emergency resuscitation equipment and drugs, a standard requirement in all radiology departments, should be immediately available.

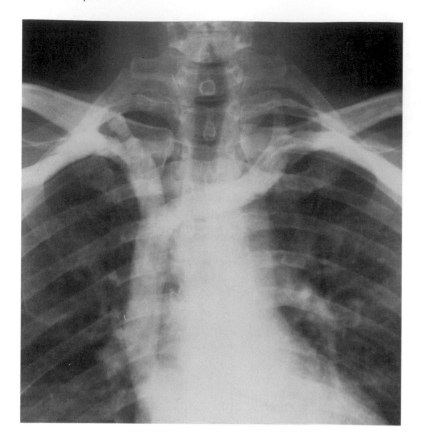

Fig. 9.10 Normal superior vena cavogram showing the subclavian and innominate viens and the superior vena cava down to the right atrium.

Local reactions

Pain. This is the most frequent complication of phlebography. It is not usually severe and is experienced locally in the foot and / or calf. The pain is related primarily to the hyperosmolality of the contrast medium but also to the sodium content of the medium. Dilution of the contrast medium (Betman & Paulin, 1977) and the use of sodium-free media reduces the incidence of pain and discomfort. There is, however, a limit to which any contrast medium can be diluted before the diagnostic adequacy of the phlebogram becomes adversely affected.

The advent of the low-osmolality contrast media has significantly improved patient acceptance of the examination. A comparative study, in which a conventional contrast medium (meglumine iothalamate 280) was injected into one leg and a low

osmolality medium (metrizamide 280) was used to examine the other leg, showed an incidence of leg pain of 68% with the conventional medium and only 15% with the non-ionic medium (Lea Thomas & Walters, 1979). Similar studies with the second-generation low-osmolar contrast media have consistently demonstrated significantly lower patient discomfort with these media.

Thrombosis. Thrombotic complications of phlebography, although well recognized, have been considered to be an uncommon or rare occurrence. This thrombogenic effect is due to the high osmolality of conventional contrast media. The incidence is minimized by clearing contrast medium from the veins at the completion of the examination by flushing with saline and encouraging early ambulation. Some workers routinely add heparin to the saline infusion. The aim in all cases is to allow contrast medium to remain in contact with veins for as short a time as possible.

Fibrinogen uptake tests show a significant incidence of thrombotic complications, but studies comparing conventional media with the low osmolality media have shown that the use of the latter virtually eliminates thrombotic complications (Walters *et al.*, 1980).

Technique

Local

Local extravasation. Although rare, serious complications may arise if contrast medium extravasates into the soft tissues during the injection. The extravasated contrast medium provokes a chemical cellulitis which may progress to a bullous eruption, skin ulceration and soft-tissue necrosis, gangrene having been described in extreme cases. Soft-tissue necrosis is more commonly seen in patients with peripheral ischaemia (Berge *et al.*, 1978).

Extreme care is therefore necessary with the venepuncture technique. The needle should be tested for its correct placement within the vein both by injecting saline under direct vision and by checking the flow of contrast medium on fluoroscopy as the injection is made. If the patient experiences severe local pain in the foot during the examination, extravasation may have occurred as a result of either needle dislodgement or bursting of the injected vein. The injection must then be stopped and the locally extravasated contrast medium diluted by injecting normal saline.

This complication, when it occurs in the groin during pelvic phlebography using a femoral vein puncture, does not appear to have such serious sequelae as in the foot. This is presumably because contrast medium is more readily dissipated and absorbed from the bulkier soft tissues of this region.

Haemorrhage and haematoma formation. Firm local pressure at the completion of the procedure avoids this complication. Special care is required in patients receiving anticoagulant therapy to ensure haemostasis.

Catheterization difficulties. Complications are rare, provided that the Seldinger technique is carefully undertaken and neither the guide wire nor the catheter is forced into the vein.

Distant

Pulmonary thromboembolism. The exact frequency of pulmonary embolism occurring in patients when phlebography has been performed in the presence of deep-vein thrombosis cannot be accurately defined because of the difficulties of diagnosing subclinical embolism. The complication has been described in a few cases but is a rare event.

Calf compression, employed in ascending lower-limb phlebography to demonstrate the iliofemoral venous segment, has been suggested as likely to provoke detachment of loose thrombus. This has not, however, been encountered in several large series.

Air embolism. This is prevented by ensuring that all connectors are tight and that syringes are air-free, always aspirating when a new syringe is connected, and by holding the syringe in a vertical position (plunger uppermost) when an injection is made.

Relationship to other imaging modalities and investigative techniques

Disorders of the venous system, in particular the immediate and delayed complications associated with deep-vein thrombosis, are the cause of a significant morbidity and mortality. Recent advances in treating venous thrombosis and in the surgical management of the post-thrombotic syndrome have stimulated the development of a number of new investigative procedures. The aims of these tests are the earliest diagnosis of thrombosis, when effective treatment may be instituted, and a functional assessment of the venous system to provide information of the underlying pathophysiology in the veins of patients with chronic venous insufficiency.

These techniques enable the venous system to be evaluated in a less invasive way than contrast phlebography. The accuracy of the contrast phlebogram, however, remains the baseline by which these newer techniques are assessed in terms of sensitivity and specificity. Kakkar (1980) has provided a detailed account of these techniques and a critical appraisal of their current status.

Doppler ultrasonic technique

The frequency of an ultrasound beam is altered when it is reflected by a moving object, the change in frequency being related to the velocity of the object due to the Doppler effect. The corpuscles in blood vessels act as the reflectors and ultrasound frequency therefore changes with the rate of blood flow. This frequency change can either be translated through an amplifier into an audible signal or be recorded on paper.

The normal venous flow signal in the legs of a patient lying supine varies with respiration, decreasing on inspiration and increasing with expiration. The velocity of flow in patent veins can briefly be increased by compression of the extremity to produce an augmented flow signal. There is thus a phasic flow signal which in the presence of venous obstruction, when the probe is placed distal to the obstruction, is replaced by a more or less continuous character signal. Augmented flow signals similarly become dampened. No signal is obtained when there is total occlusion.

The technique has a high degree of accuracy in detecting occlusions of the femoral, popliteal or iliac veins. Its main limitations arise from its failure to detect accurately non-occlusive thrombi in the proximal veins. Confusion and inaccuracy may also arise in the presence of an established collateral venous system which may simulate flow in a patent major vein. The major limitation is related to operator experience.

Radioisotope tests

Fibrinogen uptake test

Fibrinogen labelled with radioactive iodine follows the same pathways as endogenous fibrinogen and is converted to fibrin under the action of thrombin. A forming thrombus thus incorporates ^{125}I-labelled fibrinogen, which is then detected by external counting over the limb.

The levels of radioactivity are measured at marked positions on the legs. The criterion for the diagnosis of thrombosis is a count rate 15–20% greater than at adjacent points on the leg or the same point on the other leg, when compared with the reading at the same position on the previous day and provided this increase persists for more than 24 hours. Counting is repeated daily for up to 7–8 days.

The fibrinogen uptake test has found several clinical applications. Its most important contribution has been in the prospective surveillance of patients at high risk of developing venous thrombosis, for instance patients undergoing hip surgery. The technique also enables the natural history of venous thrombosis to be monitored, the rate of dissolution of the thrombus to be followed, and an assessment of the efficacy of prophylactic agents in preventing venous thrombosis to be made. A positive test is obtained in establishing venous thrombosis provided that a thrombus is still forming.

The important limitation of the fibrinogen test is its inability to detect iliac vein thrombosis and, to a lesser extent, thrombosis in the upper thigh because ^{125}I is a low-energy γ-ray emitter in a region where there is a high background activity in the bladder and adjacent vascular structures. There is also a delay of 24–48 hours between initiating the test and availability of results since the technique depends on the breakdown and deposition of the labelled fibrin. False positive results may be obtained in the presence of a haematoma, skin wound or inflammatory swelling.

Radionuclide phlebography

This technique is based on the principle that macroaggregates of albumin labelled with ^{99m}Tc, when injected into a superficial vein of the foot, may be trapped proximal to an occluding thrombus. Abnormal findings consistent with venous thrombosis are a cold area corresponding to decreased flow at the site of the thrombus, abnormal collateral flow, and stasis of radioactivity proximal to the thrombus. The transit of the isotope is recorded and the resulting γ-camera images resemble phlebograms, but have the major disadvantage of poor resolution in defining the exact anatomical site of the thrombus.

The technique produces a significant number of false positives and does not demonstrate the true extent of the disease. Its accuracy is, however, better for the thigh and pelvic region. The major advantage of this technique is that it can be incorporated with lung scanning procedures for the detection of pulmonary embolism.

Venous occlusion plethysmography

This technique is based on the principle of inflating a pressure cuff around the thigh to completely occlude the distal draining veins while not impeding the arterial supply to the leg distal to the cuff. The resulting increase in volume of the leg during venous occlusion can be determined by a plethysmograph. Sudden release of the cuff pressure causes a decrease in calf volume by venous emptying. Blood flow can be calculated, as a function of time, from the volume changes measured by the plethysmograph. The method thus provides functional information about venous flow. Several plethysmographic techniques have been used and include impedance, strain gauge and air cuff plethysmography. The most widely evaluated technique is impedance plethysmography, where venous outflow is measured by quantifying the changes in electrical impedance of a limb.

The presence of a deep-vein thrombosis reduces the maximum venous volume of the calf and, when the cuff is released, delays venous emptying. Thus thrombi which obstruct the venous outflow will be detected. The main limitation of the technique is in the detection of most calf vein thrombi since the main venous outflow tract is not obstructed. In the same way, small non-occlusive thrombi in the popliteal and femoral veins may be missed, as also may a venous occlusion which has a well established venous collateral system.

Thermography

This is, in the real sense, a non-invasive test which has recently been used to detect deep-vein thrombosis. Although the clinical diagnosis of deep venous thrombosis is inaccurate, the technique of thermography is based on one of the signs used in clinical diagnosis — the increased temperature or delayed cooling of a leg containing thrombosed veins. Whilst the temperature change may be subclinical and not apparent on palpation, a sensitive infrared camera accurately detects these abnormalities.

Exposure of the legs before recording any temperature change allows equilibration of the skin of the lower limbs at room temperature. The heat radiated from the legs is reflected by a mirror, so that the radiation strikes the lens of the infrared camera at right angles and thus prevents picture distortion.

Thermography has not been widely adopted, although studies have shown the technique to have a good accuracy when compared with phlebography and the ^{125}I fibrinogen uptake test. Its main limitation is its inability to detect thrombi in the pelvic veins and IVC. False positives are produced when there is a haematoma or in the presence of various inflammatory conditions.

The ideal non-invasive technique for detecting deep-vein thrombosis does not exist. The ^{125}I fibrinogen uptake test is the most sensitive method and detects calf vein thrombosis in its earliest stage. It is therefore the technique of choice for a prospective surveillance. Its main limitation is the incidence of false positives, so that a positive test may require verification. Techniques based on venous flow — venous occlusion plethysmography and Doppler ultrasound — are comparable in terms of their sensitivity and specificity in detecting major deep-vein thrombosis in the popliteal vein and above. Their limitation is in the failure to accurately detect thrombosis of the calf veins. Generally, the contrast phlebogram may be omitted when two (or occasionally one) of these non-invasive tests are unequivocally normal.

Ultrasound, computed tomography (CT) and magnetic resonance imaging (MRI)

In addition to the evaluation of the peripheral veins for venous thrombosis, ultrasound is employed in the visualization of the major veins — particularly the IVC and its tributaries. Its major role is in the detection of propagating tumour or thrombus in the IVC presenting as fixed echoes within the vessel. Whilst various abdominal tumours may extend into the IVC, the most common primary source is a renal cell carcinoma. The examination of the renal veins and IVC is thus an integral part of the complete ultrasound evaluation of a solid renal mass. Ultrasound is also useful in demonstrating mass effects upon the vena cava from adjacent nodal enlargement. Congenital anomalies of the IVC are rare, with an incidence of about 3%. Their importance lies in their possible misinterpretation, usually as nodal masses, if they are only imaged transversely. Longitudinal scans, supplemented where necessary with Doppler ultrasound, will clarify the venous origin of these structures.

CT will demonstrate both intrinsic and extrinsic lesions of the superior vena cava and IVC and their tributaries. Although not a primary indication for CT, venous thrombosis produces similar appearances to those seen with neoplastic invasion of the veins on contrast-enhanced scans. The technique elegantly displays caval displacement and compression by adjacent mass lesions or fibrotic processes. CT of the proximal course of the IVC is not limited by overlying bowel gas, the interposition of which may limit visualization by ultrasound. Most of the congenital venous anomalies of the mediastinum and of the IVC have been described using contrast enhancement combined with rapid sequential scanning.

Recent developments in vascular MRI have provided a non-invasive technique to evaluate the morphology and provide haemodynamic information on flow in the cardiovascular system. The signal void created by flowing blood enables vessel patency to be determined without the use of contrast media. However, slow-flowing blood in veins may produce an intraluminal signal which may closely simulate a thrombus. Differentiation between intraluminal thrombus and flow-related artefacts may be aided by phase image reconstruction (Erdman *et al.*, 1986) or by specific pulse sequences employing fast scan techniques (Spritzer *et al.*, 1988). When the techniques are fully developed and evaluated, MRI may well find an important application in the difficult area of the pelvis, where it has been used to detect deep-vein thrombosis (Erdman *et al.*, 1986).

References

Andrews, J.C., Williams, D.M. & Cho, K.J. (1987) Digital subtraction venography of the upper extremity. *Clin. Radiol.*, **38**, 423–4.

Berge, T., Bergqvist, D., Efsing, H.O. & Hallbook, T. (1978) Local complications of ascending phlebography. *Clin. Radiol.*, **29**, 691–6.

Bettman, M.A. & Paulin, S. (1977) Leg phlebography: the incidence, nature and modification of undesirable side effects. *Radiology*, **122**, 101–4.

Cotton, L.T. & Clark, C. (1965) Anatomical localization of venous thrombosis. *Ann. Roy. Coll. Surg. Engl.*, **36**, 214–24.

Craig, J.O. (1972) *In* Saxton, H.M. & Strickland, B. (eds) *Practical Procedures in Diagnostic Radiology*, 2nd edn, p. 250. H.K. Lewis, London.

Dos Santos, J.C. (1938) La phlébographie directe: conception, technique, premiers résultats. *J. Int. Chir.*, **3**, 625–32.

Dow, J.D. (1973) Retrograde phlebography in major pulmonary embolism. *Lancet*, **ii**, 407.

Erdman, A.E., Weinreb, J.C., Cohen, J.M. *et al.* (1986) Venous thrombosis: clinical and experimental MR imaging. *Radiology*, **161**, 233–8.

Kakkar, V.V. (1980) Diagnosis of deep vein thrombosis. *In* Verstraete, M. (ed.) *Methods of Angiography*, pp. 267–96. Martinus Nijhoff, The Hague.

Kinmonth, J.B., Young, A.E., O'Donnell, T.F. Jr *et al.* (1976) Mixed vascular deformities of the lower limbs. *Br. J. Surg.*, **63**, 899.

Lea Thomas, M. (1970) Pelvic phlebography. *In* McLaren, J.W. (ed.) *Modern Trends in Diagnostic Radiology*, pp. 201–9. Butterworths, London.

Lea Thomas, M. & Carty, H. (1975) The appearances of artefacts on lower limb phlebography. *Clin. Radiol.*, **26**, 537–3.

Lea Thomas, M. & Macdonald, L. (1977) The accuracy of bolus ascending phlebography in demonstrating the iliofemoral segment. *Clin. Radiol.*, **28**, 165–71.

Lea Thomas, M. & O'Dwyer, J.A. (1978) A phlebographic study of the incidence and significance of venous thrombosis of the foot. *AJR*, **130**, 751–4.

Lea Thomas, M. & Walters, H.L. (1979) Metrizamide in ascending venography of the legs. *Br. Med. J.*, **2**, 1036.

Schobinger, R.A. (1960) *Intraosseous Venography*. Grune & Stratton, New York.

Shehadi, W.H. (1975) Adverse reactions to intravascularly administered contrast media. *AJR*, **124**, 145–52.

Spritzer, C.E., Sussman, S.K., Blinder, R.A. *et al.* (1988) Deep venous thrombosis evaluation with limited flip-angle, gradient-refocused MR imaging. *Radiology*, **166**, 371–5.

Walters, H.L., Clemenson, J., Browse, N.L. & Lea Thomas, M. (1980) [125]I fibrinogen uptake following phlebography of the leg. *Radiology*, **135**, 619–21.

10 Heart and Pulmonary Circulation

C. ROOBOTTOM AND R. P. WILDE

The imaging of the heart and great vessels presents a unique series of challenges to the radiologist. There is a complex anatomical arrangement of chambers, valves and vessels; there is continuous movement and there is a wide range of imaging techniques available to examine these structures and their function. The heart and great vessels are supremely suited to the multimodal approach of system-based radiology. This chapter sets out the basis of the different modalities in common use. Table 10.1 shows some of the strengths and weaknesses of the different modalities in different diagnostic areas.

Echocardiography

Early work, following Edler's demonstration of mitral valve motion in 1954, led to simple 'M-mode' traces of cardiac valves and chambers being recorded as graphs of movement as the depth of structures changed with time. In the next two decades the deductive diagnosis, using M-mode traces and careful measurement of time and distance, became an important cardiological tool. In 1974 Griffith and Henry developed a real-time mechanical sector scanner and this stimulated the rapid development of real-time imaging of the moving heart structures.

Ultrasound Doppler techniques had been used in a variety of prototype applications since Satomura described frequency shifts in back-scattered ultrasound from cardiac structures in 1957. Pulsed Doppler techniques allowing sampling at specific depths was described by Wells and other in 1969. However, cardiac Doppler ultrasound had a long development period and it was only the development of the microchip that allowed the rapid processing that is necessary for real-time Doppler analysis.

Modern echocardiographic instruments form a complex integration of a variety of ultrasound imaging and Doppler modalities, usually incorporating M-mode (one-dimensional), two-dimensional imaging and pulsed, continous wave and colour flow Doppler options. The systems have inputs for electrocardiogram (ECG) signals, as well as dedicated software for the acquisition and processing of information. Recording of information is different from conventional ultrasound imagers and requires a videotape recorder and a continuous strip chart recorder as well as facilities for static image recording.

As well as mechanical and phased array sector probes for conventional transthoracic imaging, there are transoesophageal (single plane, biplane and multiplane) and high-frequency intravascular probes for specialist applications.

Echo studies have been adapted to many situations in adult and paediatric cardiology, including stress echocardiography, contrast echocardiography, fetal echocardiography, tissue characterization and intraoperative studies. Transoesophageal echocardiography has gained rapid acceptance in the clinical diagnosis of left atrial and mitral valve pathology, the study of prosthetic valves, the diagnosis of infective endocarditis, thoracic aortic disease and the clarification of some complex congenital abnormalities in the older child and adult.

Indications

Although very large or emphysematous patients can be difficult it is now possible in virtually all patients to assess and quantitate left ventricular function, the function of all four valves, structural abnormalities and pericardial disease. Quantitation may include assessment of stenoses by calculating pressure differences, measuring volume flow including cardiac output, and sometimes estimating intracardiac pressures. It is not possible to resolve fine detail of the

Table 10.1 Relative strengths and weaknesses of the various imaging techniques in cardiac radiology

Techniques	Major structures	Detailed structures	Coronary disease	LV function	Pulmonary arteries	Interventional guidance	Procedure costs	Radiation safety	Patient comfort	Haemo-dynamics
Chest radiograph	++	+	+	++	++	+	+++++	+++	+++++	+
Transthoracic echo	++++	+++	++	++++	+	+	++++	+++++	++++	+++
Transoesophageal echo	+++++	+++++	+++	++++	+	++	+++	+++++	++	+++
Nuclear medicine	++	–	++++	+++	–	–	+++	++	+++	+
Computed tomography	+++	–	+	++	++	+	+++	++	+++	+
Magnetic resonance imaging	+++++	++	++	++++	++++	+	++	+++++	+++	++
Cardiac angiography	+++++	+++++	+++++	+++++	+++++	+++++	+	+	++	+++++

LV, left ventricular.
The more plus symbols, the more advantages the technique has for the stated criteria. +++++ is essentially the gold standard, decreasing to + which is of minimal benefit and – which is of no perceived benefit.

coronary arteries, so only the secondary effects of coronary disease are seen. Echocardiography is a particularly valuable technique in infants and children where it has become a first-line diagnostic technique.

Indications for echocardiography are as follows.
1 Evaluation of the causes of heart murmurs, especially to exclude important valve lesions and to confirm 'innocent' murmurs.
2 Evaluation of the causes of heart failure, unexplained breathlessness or cyanosis.
3 Clarification of abnormal or unusual appearances on a chest radiograph.
4 Exclusion of a cardiac source of systemic embolus, especially in the case of young patients or recurrent symptoms.
5 Follow-up of known ventricular or valve pathology.
6 Assessment of cardiac function after cardiac surgery, especially after implantation of prosthetic valves.
7 Exclusion of structural cardiac pathology in the management of arrhythmias.
8 Assessment of pericardial fluid collections and guidance for their drainage.

Transoesophageal examination can be performed if more detailed information is required about the heart, either because of inadequate resolution or inadequate echocardiographic access to the structures of interest. The technique can easily be performed in the lightly sedated out-patient as well as in the intensive care unit and operating theatre. The technique is increasingly applied to the assessment of repairs in open heart surgery. The skills required must follow on from transthoracic echocardiography, descriptions of which are beyond the scope of this chapter.

Techniques

Two-dimensional imaging

Conventional echocardiography is based on a series of two-dimensional imaging planes which are defined by internal anatomical features of the heart. A high proportion of diagnoses can be achieved from these images alone but, in many cases, M-mode or Doppler measurements can add further important information.

The heart can only be imaged by gaining access through rib spaces or from below or above the sternum. The lungs prevent penetration of ultrasound. The patient is usually examined in a semi-recumbent position and half turned towards the left side. This ensures that the heart is exposed to the left of the sternum and the left lung is dependent and therefore less inflated than the right. The patient must be warm, comfortable and fully briefed about the details of the procedure.

There are three main windows from which the three scan planes are achieved: (i) the left parasternal window, in the second or third interspace; (ii) the apical window; and (iii) the subcostal or subxiphoid window. These are shown in Fig. 10.1. The three main scan planes are the long axis, the short axis and the four-chamber plane. In ideal circumstances two planes can be recorded from each window, thus allowing useful verification of findings in most situations (Fig. 10.2). The three planes are all orthogonal, or mutually at right angles, and thus allow a comprehensive evaluation of cardiac anatomy. In addition, each plane defined from a particular window can be adjusted to show a series of 'slices' in that plane.

The cardiac orientation, chamber sizes and chest configuration differ from patient to patient. The location of the optimal views must therefore be carefully sought in each patient. Figure 10.3 shows the main anatomical features of each plane.

M-mode examination

This technique is based on a single line or ultrasound beam that is passed through the heart at a rapidly repeated rate so that a trace of moving structures can be obtained at that point. The validity of M-mode measurements is highly dependent on the accurate placement of the beam in a standard or recognized position. Left ventricular function, one of the most important cardiac assessments, can only be accurately measured if the M-mode line is correctly placed across the ventricle without obliquity and without cutting the chamber tangentially. As the measurements are taken from only one position, the extrapolation to give figures for global left ventricular performance is only valid if there is no regional wall motion abnormality. Early instruments were

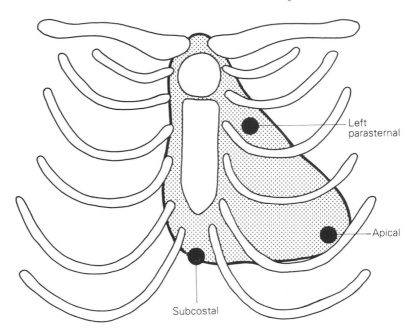

Fig. 10.1 The three main echocardiographic windows used to image the heart.

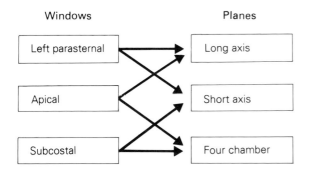

Fig. 10.2 The three main echocardiographic windows and the two imaging planes that can be obtained from each window.

based on M-mode examination alone, but virtually all modern systems use two-dimensional image guiding for accurately positioning the M-mode line.

M-mode studies can be used for assessing a variety of valvular chamber movements (Fig. 10.4), but the majority of assessments are now performed from two-dimensional images. M-mode studies are reserved for situations where accurate distance and time recordings are needed or where fast-moving structures need the high repetition rate of the technique.

Doppler studies

There are three main types of Doppler examination: pulsed, continuous wave and colour flow. All are commonly available on one instrument and all have different applications. While the fundamental Doppler principle is common to all, specific features are described below.

Pulsed Doppler. The pulsing allows specific range or depth 'gating'. This permits precise measurements of flow to be taken from specific anatomical sites, usually guided by the imaging system. Very clear traces of flow can be made, laminar and turbulent flow characteristics being clearly distinguished (Fig. 10.5). The major disadvantage of pulsed Doppler examination is that the pulsing is limited to a finite number of interrogations per second. This makes it difficult to record high-velocity signals without the artefact of aliasing. Most normal cardiac flow is less than 1.5 m s^{-1}, but pathological flow can be much faster and aliasing will considerably limit the study. In appropriate sites, pulsed Doppler recordings can be combined with cross-sectional area measurement at the same point to produce a calculated volume flow.

Continuous wave Doppler requires simultaneous emission and recording of a signal down the same line.

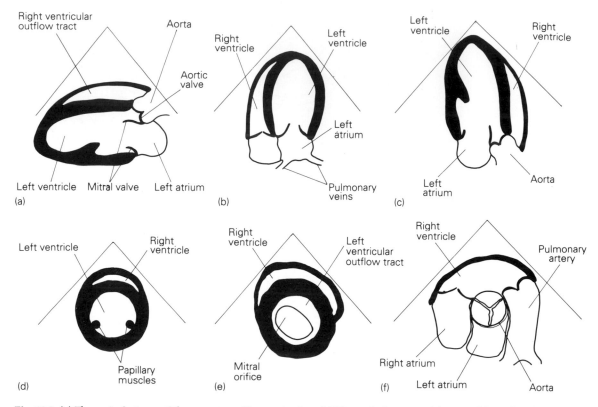

Fig. 10.3 (a) The main features of the parasternal long axis view. (b) The main features of the apical four-chamber view. (c) The main features of the apical long axis view. (d) The main features of the parasternal short axis view at ventricular level. (e) The main features of the parasternal short axis view at mitral valve level. (f) The main features of the parasternal short axis view at aortic valve level.

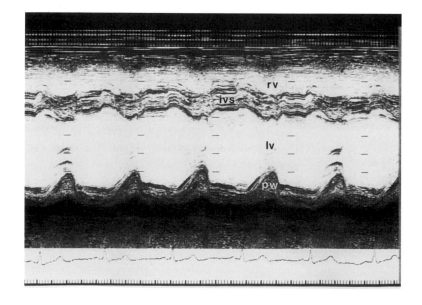

Fig. 10.4 Parasternal M-mode trace across the normal left ventricle. The right ventricular outflow tract (rv), interventricular septum (ivs), left ventricular cavity (lv) and left ventricular posterior wall (pw) are indicated.

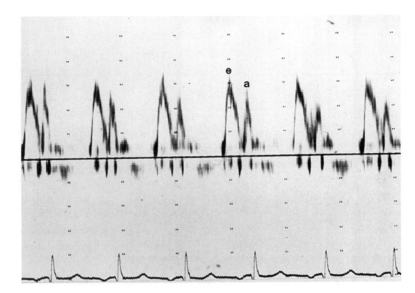

Fig. 10.5 Pulsed Doppler trace taken from the cardiac apex showing the normal inflow through the mitral valve. The trace shows well-organized flow in two diastolic phases, an initial passive flow phase (e) followed by the atrial contraction phase (a).

The technique can be used to record the highest velocities but it has no depth resolution, recording all flow along the beam. This technique is particularly important in cardiac pathology as the velocity of jets in stenotic valves can be used to determine the pressure drop across the obstruction, or 'gradient', by the application of the simplified Bernoulli equation $p = 4v^2$, where p is pressure drop in mmHg and v is the velocity in m s^{-1}. Other applications include assessment of regurgitant valves and the use of pressure differentials to estimate absolute pressures in some cardiac chambers. An example of this is the use of the tricuspid regurgitant jet to determine right ventricular pressure and hence pulmonary artery pressure.

Colour flow Doppler. Although giving a dramatic appearance, this is merely an extension of the principle of pulsed Doppler examination. Doppler shifts are calculated across the image by multiple Doppler lines being added to the imaging lines in the sector. Frequency shifts and hence flows are plotted as colours, blue away from the transducer and red towards. Normal flows are clearly seen (see Plate 10.1, facing p. 310) but abnormalities are much more quickly identified using this technique. Regurgitant jets or abnormal communications are instantly identified and may need more careful assessment using other modalities. The major

limitation of colour flow Doppler studies is the reduction in frame rate inherent in the technique. Additional lines of Doppler interrogation account for this and so the colour area is usually kept to a minimum within the overall image.

Complications

There are no significant complications of the technique, but it is very operator-dependent and mistakes and misinterpretations are easily made by inexperienced or untrained operators.

Transoesophageal echocardiography

This technique requires a specially designed probe (single plane, biplane or multiplane) mounted on a flexible endoscope. Intubation requires proper training but is similar to that used in gastrointestinal endoscopy. A variety of transverse and longitudinal planes are achievable as well as transgastric views and views of the thoracic aorta. Providing proper precautions are taken, including monitoring of the sedated patient and exclusion of contraindications such has oesophageal pathology, the technique has a very low complication rate. However, there have been occasional reports of oesophageal damage and informed consent must be obtained.

A variety of imaging and Doppler modalities can

be used in conjunction with the technique. Plate 10.1 and Fig. 10.6 show some examples of transoesophageal examinations.

Stress echocardiography

The examination of the heart under conditions of stress, either exercise or pharmacological, can offer important insights into cardiac function, especially ischaemic heart disease. Dobutamine stress echo studies are now increasingly used to evaluate left ventricular function. The principles underlying stress studies are more fully covered on pp. 175–6.

Relation to other techniques

Cardiac ultrasound is undoubtedly the most important 'non-invasive' diagnostic technique in cardiology after the chest radiograph and ECG. Nevertheless, it has important limitations. Structures as small as coronary arteries cannot be routinely imaged and angiography remains the main technique for the diagnosis of coronary artery pathology. Hilar and pulmonary structures cannot be imaged by ultrasound due to the surrounding air and angiography, computed tomography (CT) or magnetic resonance imaging (MRI) may be necessary for their assessment. Detailed intracardiac haemodynamic calculations often need full cardiac catheterization but this is partly superseded by some Doppler measurements. MRI perhaps has the potential to replace many of the characteristics of echocardiography. Nuclear medicine studies still have a place, particularly in the functional evaluation of the heart. Thallium perfusion scanning still offers something not achieved easily by ultrasound. Nuclear angiography (multiple gated acquisitions, MUGA scans) is complementary, being particularly useful in subjects with difficult ultrasound imaging characteristics.

Nuclear medicine techniques

Cardiac imaging was one of the first disciplines to

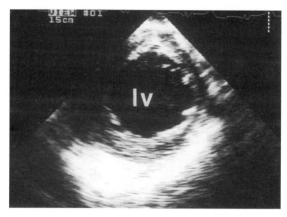

(a)

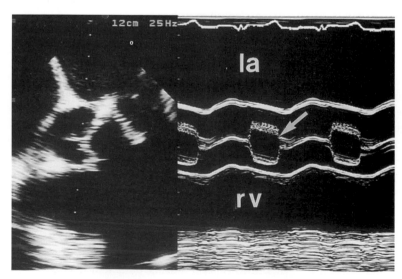

(b)

Fig. 10.6 (a) Transoesophageal examination with the probe advanced to the gastric fundus from where it is possible to achieve a short axis view of the left ventricular cavity (lv). This can be useful in monitoring left ventricular function during surgery. (b) Transoesophageal examination of the aortic valve with the accompanying M-mode study of the aortic leaflet movements. The position of the M-mode trace is shown on the two-dimensional image as a dotted line. The left atrium (la), aortic valve leaflets (arrow) and right ventricle (rv) are labelled.

which radionuclide tracer technology was applied. In 1943 Blumgart used the injection of tracer into a peripheral vein to measure circulation times. It has gained in application since the mid-1970s and has since undergone steady growth. Its primary functions are the assessment of myocardial perfusion and angiocardiography utilizing MUGA scanning.

Stress testing

Stress protocols are primarily used in perfusion imaging. In patients with coronary disease, infarcted areas show as defects on myocardial perfusion scintigraphy but areas supplied by vessels with significant stenoses are usually normal at rest. As the ability of stenotic vessels to dilate with increased oxygen demand is small, uptake post-exercise or on pharmacological stress is reduced relative to the areas supplied by normal vessels. Stress, therefore, significantly increases the sensitivity of myocardial perfusion scintigraphy. Stress testing is sometimes used during angiocardiography to assess myocardial reserve. Contraindications for stress testing include unstable angina, severe cardiac failure or valvular disease and uncontrolled hypertension.

The most frequently used method is a physical stress test. Patients should ideally stop all cardiac medication prior to stress testing, especially β-blockers which reduce exercise capacity and maximum heart rate. Testing requires appropriate exercise equipment, a treadmill being the most physiological means. ECG monitoring (there is a small but significant risk of arrhythmia) and regular measurement of blood pressure are maintained during and after stress. Stress testing requires supervision by an experienced physician. A number of protocols are available, the Bruce protocol being the most widely used. If adequate stress is not achieved, reversible ischaemia may be missed. A significant degree of stress is achieved when the heart rate is above 85% of predicted maximum. At this stage the radiopharmaceutical is injected and exercise continued for 2 min to ensure maximum myocardial uptake of the tracer. End-points for discontinuing exercise are chest pain, dyspnoea, a fall in blood pressure of more than 10 mmHg below the resting value, ventricular tachycardia or a run of three premature ventricular beats.

Pharmacological testing can be used in patients who are unable to undergo conventional exercise testing. Specificity of pharmacological testing is superior to exercise testing. The sensitivity of pharmacological testing is comparable to that achieved by maximum exercise, but is superior to suboptimal exercise. Side effects are more frequent with pharmacological stress testing, although ST changes are less marked.

The most frequent indication for pharmacological stress testing is an inability to undergo physical stress. A number of pharmacological agents can be used to highlight heterogeneities in myocardial perfusion. Dobutamine primarily acts through stimulation of β_1-receptors within the myocardium and, like physical exercise, results in increased oxygen demand. A perfusion abnormality on exercise or dobutamine infusion therefore represents true ischaemia. Dipyridamole and adenosine are both vasodilators. Regional variations during their infusion are not accompanied by increased myocardial oxygen demand and therefore do not represent true ischaemia.

Selection of the agent used depends upon personal experience and preference. Consideration must, however, be given to the following groups of patients.
1 Patients with asthma and chronic airways disease — dobutamine should be used. Both adenosine and dipyridamole induce bronchospasm.
2 Patients with heart block — avoid adenosine as it increases atrioventricular block.
3 Patients with known aneurysms — theoretical risk of rupture due to hypertension induced by dobutamine.

Patient preparation involves cessation of dipyridamole, theophylline and caffeine products for adenosine and dipyridamole and calcium channel blockers and β-blockers for dobutamine. With all agents, blood pressure and ECG should be monitored regularly.

Dobutamine is administered by infusion initially at 10 μg kg^{-1} min^{-1} and increasing by 10 μg kg^{-1} increments to a maximum of 40 μg kg^{-1} min^{-1} if tolerated. End-points are achievement of maximum dose or 85% of predicted maximum heart rate, severe angina, hypertension, ST depression of more than 2 mm, syncope, dyspnoea, or systolic blood pressure of less than 90 mmHg. Adenosine is also administered via infusion, initially at 50 µg kg^{-1} min^{-1} and increasing to a maximum of 140 µg kg^{-1} min^{-1}. End-points of adenosine are a high degree of atrio-ventricular block, systolic blood pressure of less than 80 mmHg, ST depression, intolerable shortness of breath, flushing, headache or chest pain. With both agents, the tracer is injected towards the end of the infusion. Dipyridamole is injected slowly by hand with injection of the tracer 3 min afterwards. Suboptimal exercise is also used by some workers at this stage. There are no specific end-points with dipyridamole as side effects are seen after the infusion is complete.

Complications

Cardiac death, non-fatal infarction and serious arrhythmia (ventricular fibrillation and sustained ventricular tachycardia) are rare and occur with the same frequency for both treadmill and pharmaco-logical stress testing.

Regarding pharmacological stress testing, minor side effects occur in 30–80% of patients and are probably most common with adenosine. They include the following:
1 Chest pain — frequent with adenosine and dipyrid-amole. Can occur without coronary artery disease.
2 Shortness of breath — bronchospasm with adenos-ine and dipyridamole. Stimulation of carotid chemo-receptors induces hyperventilation.
3 Hypotension— induced by systemic vasodilation or arrhythmia
4 Atrioventricular block — rare with dobutamine and dipyridamole. Most common with adenosine.
5 Myocardial ischaemia — due to increased demand with dobutamine and coronary artery steal, and re-duced distal pressure with adenosine and dipyridamole.

Radionuclide myocardial perfusion imaging

Indications

While regional wall abnormalities can be assessed by echocardiography, MRI and nuclear ventri-culography, these modalities do not differentiate between ischaemic myocardium, with reduced con-tractility, and irreversibly damaged myocardium. At present nuclear medicine techniques represent the only widely available method of doing so. This can be performed with 'conventional' radiopharma-ceuticals and positron emission tomography (PET; see below). Indications include the following:
1 Diagnosis and assessment of extent and degree of reversibility of coronary artery disease.
2 Evalution of interventional procedures.
3 Demonstration of old myocardial infarction.
The technique is particularly useful where clinical suspicion of myocardial ischemia is high but the ex-ercise ECG is equivocal, impossible to perform or difficult to interpret, for instance in patients with conduction abnormalities, previous infarcts or digi-talis effect. Compared to the exercise ECG, myocar-dial perfusion imaging has a higher sensitivity and specificity (approximately 85%).

Radiopharmaceuticals

Myocardial perfusion imaging can be performed by using ^{99m}Tc-based radiopharmaceuticals and ^{201}Tl chloride.

^{201}Tl chloride

Myocardial uptake of thallium is an active process via the membrane-based sodium–potassium pump. It is initially rapidly taken up by cardiac and other tissues with uptake directly proportional to myocar-dial metabolism and subsequent coronary blood flow. After the initial rapid uptake there is a redistri-bution, with thallium being washed out of cells from various tissues. This is available for uptake by the myocardium and forms the basis of the exercise redistribution technique.

Exercise and resting images can be obtained from one injection using the exercise redistribution tech-nique. Following either physical or pharmacologi-cal stress, 80 MBq of thallium chloride is injected. Stress phase images are begun within 5 min of injec-tion. Both ischaemic and infarcted areas show as photon-deficient areas. Differentiation of the two can be made by rescanning the patient at 3 hours. At this stage there is redistribution of thallium. Ischaemic but viable myocardium will show increased uptake while infarcts remain photon-deficient (see Plate 10.2, facing p. 310). If a photon-deficient area is seen at this stage, particularly in a patient with no history of infarct, delayed images (at 18–24 hours), preferably following a second smaller dose of ^{201}Tl (40 MBq) are recommended because approximately 30% of fixed defects in this group will show reversibility.

False positive results can occur with cardiomyopathies, aortic stenosis, infiltrative cardiac disease (amyloidosis and sarcoidosis), any cause of reduced cardiac perfusion other than infarction (coronary artery spasm, myocardial contusion or fibrosis) and left bundle branch block. False positive results may also be secondary to attenuation from overlying tissues, cardiac pacemakers, breast implants or metallic objects in shirt pockets, or simulated by normal variants such as apical ventricular thinning.

False negative images can be obtained in balanced ischaemia with symmetrical three vessel disease; inadequate stress; or by anti-angina medication, particularly β-blockers which should ideally be stopped prior to the examination.

^{99m}Tc-based compounds

Technetium-based myocardial perfusion agents have been introduced recently. Compounds such as teboroxime and sestamibi localize either within the mitochondria or the cytosol of myocardial cells with uptake being proportional to blood flow. Sestamibi shows long retention within the myocardium with no redistribution. Imaging of resting and stress images therefore requires two separate injections. Two-day protocols are optimal but it is usually more convenient to utilize a one-day protocol. This is most effective when the resting study is performed first. A typical protocol would involve an initial injection of 250 MBq of sestamibi with resting images 60 min afterwards. Two hours after the initial injection, exercise or pharmacological stress protocols are applied and 750 mBq of radiopharmaceutical is injected at peak exercise. Rescanning takes place after a further 60 min. As excretion of sestamibi is via the biliary system, gallbladder activitiy should be reduced by ingestion of a milk drink prior to imaging on both occasions.

^{99m}Tc-based compounds have a number of advantages over thallium, including the following:
1 No redistribution and long retention in the myo-

cardium allows greater time for imaging, permitting the utilization of both single photon emission CT (SPECT) imaging and ECG gating.
2 Improved dosimetry due to shorter half-life allows greater dosages to be used with less patient radiation.
3 Greater photon flux allows faster imaging; ECG gating and SPECT are therefore more easily applied.
4 The ^{99m}Tc tracer doses are adequate for first-pass angiocardiography, thereby affording a functional evaluation of both ventricles as well as perfusion data.
5 Higher photon energy results in less attenuation artefact (see above) and less scatter.
For these reasons there is a gradual shift from thallium to ^{99m}Tc-based agents. At the time of writing the balance is about equal within the UK.

Image acquisition

If ^{99m}Tc-based agents are injected in a tight bolus, angiocardiographic images can be obtained to assess myocardial contractility and ejection fraction. This is not possible with thallium. Digital and analogue data acquisition should occur simultaneously, the former improving diagnostic accuracy. A 128×128 matrix is optimal. Post-processing using subtraction techniques as well as circumferential profiles, improves image interpretation. The following projections are routinely used: (i) supine anterior; (ii) supine left anterior oblique (LAO) 45°; and (iii) LAO 70°, supine unless the left hemidiaphragm results in attenuation of inferior wall activity when a right decubitus view is used. ECG gating can be used but increases acquisition time with little improvement in diagnostic accuracy.

SPECT imaging is now frequently used, although requiring a longer acquisition time (less so with ^{99m}Tc-based agents due to increased photon flux). SPECT improves diagnostic accuracy by increasing contrast between normal and photon-deficient areas and permitting image reconstruction, both in long and short axis as well as the two-dimensional 'bull's eye' views (see Plate 10.3, between p. 310 and p. 311). Three-dimensional displays are possible. Tomographic images with a single-headed camera are through an arc of either 360 or 180°, from 45° right anterior oblique (RAO), to 45° left posterior oblique (LPO), spending the acquisition time where maximum cardiac activity is detectable. The total imaging time is approximately 30 min. ECG gating improves specificity at the expense of increased scanning times. With such long scanning times, movement artefact may result in severe image degradation.

Radionuclide angiocardiography

Indications

Radionuclide angiocardiography can be performed using either a first-pass technique or following uniform mixing of the radiopharmaceutical in the body blood pool. The most commonly used radiophar-maceutical is ^{99m}Tc-labelled red blood cells because of the good heart to lung ratio. These are routinely labelled *in vivo*, although *in vitro* labelling is a valid alternative. To label red blood cells, an injection of 'cold' stannous pyrophosphate is given 20 min before an injection of ^{99m}Tc (800 MBq maximum dose).

First-pass technique

This records the initial passage of the tightly administered bolus of radiopharmaceutical through the heart and lungs (see Plate 10.4, between p. 310 and p. 311). Acquisition at a minimum of 20 frames s^{-1}, while the bolus travels through the cardiac chambers, will show the sequence of cardiac chamber filling and permit measurement of ejection fractions of the right and left ventricles. The latter is, however, better assessed by gated blood pool images. The RAO 30° projection gives best visualization of the right atrium and ventricle, the LAO 45° optimally separates the ventricles.

Indications for first-pass radionuclide angiography are as follows.
1 Demonstration of superior vena caval obstruction.
2 Assessment of right ventricular function and ejection fraction.
3 Assessment of right ventricular infarction.
4 Detection and quantification of cardiac shunts, using a time activity curve from the pulmonary region. The technique only requires 15 s of patient co-operation and subsequent repeated studies are possible (using diethylenetriame penta-acetic acid (DTPA)).

Multiple gated acquisition scanning

Gated blood pool imaging is usually performed after a first-pass study or in isolation. Imaging begins after the radiopharmaceutical has reached equilibrium in the blood, about 1 min post-injection, in the supine position. Gated images demonstrate abnormalities of contractility and provide a reproducible accurate measurement of ventricular function, in particular left ventricular ejection fraction. Indications include the following.
1 The demonstration of regional wall abnormalities, including demonstration of left ventricular aneurysms.
2 Evaluation of left ventricular ejection fraction, in ischaemic heart disease and in the follow-up of oncology patients receiving cardiotoxic drugs such as doxorubicin.
3 Assessment of left ventricular functional reserve, utilizing cardiac stress usually in the form of a bed-mounted bicycle.
4 Evaluation of valvular regurgitation.

Technique

Images are acquired during selected portions of the cardiac cycle gated by the R-wave of the ECG. Each image is composed of more than 200 000 counts obtained over several hundred cycles. It is important to obtain images from several different projections, in order to demonstrate the complete anatomy of the ventricles with separation of both ventricles on at least one view. An LAO projection with 15–30° caudal tilt (to separate the ventricles) and LPO (to separate atria and ventricles) are usually performed.

Arrhythmias are a relative contraindication and cause significant degradation of image quality. Mild arrhythmias can be overcome by software rejection.

Qualitative information about the left ventricle is obtained by viewing the images in a cine mode format, showing the contractile motion of both ventricles in a number of projections. Assessment is made of myocardial contractility and chamber size. Static images in systole and diastole are usually performed and are complementary to cine images.

The most important quantitative measurement is left ventricular ejection fraction. The count obtained from a ventricle is directly proportional to the volume of blood in the chamber and is not dependent on geometric assumptions, making it relatively accurate particularly in the presence of regional wall abnormalities or abnormal ventricular shape. A time–activity curve is generated from a region of interest drawn around the left ventricle, the end diastolic and systolic frames are identified and the left ventricular ejection fraction calculated from:

$$\text{ejection fraction} = \frac{\text{end diastolic counts} - \text{end systolic counts}}{\text{end diastolic counts}}.$$

The information in the gated blood pool images can be expressed in the form of a parametric image. The two most commonly used are amplitude images, which demonstrate count changes in each pixel, and phase images which reflect the timing in changes of activity (see Plate 10.5, between p. 310 and p. 311). The former gives an appreciation of wall motion while the phase images give appreciation of abnormal contraction that occurs in aneurysms or conduction abnormalities.

Miscellaneous techniques

Infarct avid imaging

It is possible to demonstrate myocardial damage using technetium-labelled phosphates and phosphonates, probably secondary to local temporary elevation of calcium levels, and indium-labelled antibodies which accumulate on intracardiac myosin exposed by damaged cell membranes. Avascular areas do not show significant uptake.

These proceedures have a limited use — for right ventricular infarction, when enzyme patterns are equivocal or not possible to obtain, or the ECG is difficult to interpret (bundle branch block, digitalis effects or left ventricular hypertrophy) and occasionally in the diagnosis of myocarditis. There is a time lag of up to 18 hours post-infarction until significant uptake is seen. Maximal uptake occurs between 24 and 72 hours with return to normal at 10–14 days.

Sensitivity is a reflection of the site and thickness of myocardium involved. Full thickness infarcts, particularly on the anterior wall, are shown very well whilst the sensitivity for non-transmural and inferior infarcts is below 50%. False positive scans occur in approximately 10% of cases and can be due to any cause of myocardial damage (contusion, myocarditis, cardioversion, radiation and cardiotoxic drugs), uptake in calcified valves or uptake in extracardiac structures: costal cartilage, rib lesions, uptake in breast tumours or inflammation, paddle burns from cardioversion and lung tumour uptake.

Positron emission tomography scanning

PET scanning is an alternative method for assessing myocardial viability on the basis of residual perfusion and metabolic activity in ischaemic but viable areas. PET emitting tracers can be incorporated into a variety of organic compounds without altering their biological properties. Assessment can be made of metabolism (18-labelled fluorodeoxyglucose), blood flow (N13-labelled ammonia) and innervation (C11-labelled hydroxyephedrine). It has the advantage of high spatial resolution due to electrical collimation and high count density but is expensive, has limited application and is not widely available. It therefore remains primarily a research tool.

Imaging of myocardial sympathetic innervation with metabenzylguanidine (MIBG)

The heart is supplied with a high density of sympathetic innervation. Heterogeneity of this innervation or autonomic imbalance have been suggested as a major mechanism of sudden cardiac death. Iodine-labelled MIBG is taken up by sympathetic cells within the myocardium and distribution maps can be generated. Its clinical application is, as yet, to be realized.

Magnetic resonance imaging

Of the techniques available for assessment of cardiovascular disease, MRI is the most recent and the one with the most potential for producing both anatomical and physiological information. Its multiplanar capability allows imaging of the heart and great vessels in different perspectives. This makes it useful in delineating complex cardiac anomalies as well as cardiac and pericardial tumours. MRI also allows imaging of the ventricles, valves, outflow tracts and great vessels in both long and short axes, with no limitation of acoustic windows as is experienced with echocardiography. Rapid imaging sequences permit images to be obtained in various phases of the cardiac cycle, allowing functional assessments of cardiac volumes, cardiac muscle mass and ejection fractions. These sequences can be placed in a cine-loop format, thereby giving an appreciation of cardiac movement.

MRI also confers angiographic information. Gradient echo sequences produce high signals in flowing blood and hence the 'cine MRI angiogram' similar in appearance to conventional angiograms. This facility permits assessment of valvular function as well as flow in the systemic and pulmonary vasculature.

The MR signal contains information regarding the phase of spins. It is possible to derive flow information because the phase acquired by spins can be made proportional to their velocity. This may be valuable in the quantification of cardiac output, assessment of the degree of valvular stenoses, regurgitant volumes and shunt quantification.

Indications

Despite its relative infancy, MRI has an established role in many myocardial disorders (Table 10.2).

Contraindications

Because of the high magnetic field strengths, consideration should always be given to the presence of ferromagnetic objects either in or on the patient. Absolute contraindications include the presence of cardiac pacemakers or defibrillators, which may malfunction in the field. Implanted infusion pumps may also malfunction. Cardiac valves are safe within the scanner, with the exception of pre-6000 series Starr–Edwards valves. Intravascular coils, stents and filters, being firmly fixed in the vessel and unlikely to be displaced, are also safe.

Care should also be taken to ensure there are no metallic lines within or on the patient, such as ECG pulse oximeter or Swan–Ganz thermodilution catheters. Localized heating of the wires may cause burns.

Technique

Cardiac imaging is possible on the majority of MRI

scanners over a wide range of field strengths. Higher field strengths produce a higher signal to noise ratio, improved resolution and are generally best for MRI angiography. They do, however, result in longer repetition times as well as increased chemical shift and movement artefact.

Gating techniques

Movement artefact is a particular problem with cardiac MRI. MR images require the sampling of data over a relatively long time, longer than a single cardiac cycle. Cardiac morphology is therefore blurred because of cardiac motion. Cardiac gating, using ECG triggering of the imaging sequence at comparable times in the cardiac cycle, freezes cardiac motion and thereby improves resolution. Respiratory motion also results in a degree of image degradation but the effect is less marked, gating is more difficult and respiratory gating significantly lengthens scanning times. It is therefore not routinely used.

Spin-echo sequences

The classic spin-echo sequence uses a 90° radio frequency (RF) pulse which is ECG gated followed by a 180° RF pulse and subsequent signal sampling. Each separate slice is constructed from a number of samples. An individual slice can only be sampled once per cardiac cycle. However, multiple separate slices can be sampled per cycle. The limitation of this technique is that the number of slices obtainable is determined by patient heart rate and each slice of the multislice acquisition is imaged during a different portion of the cardiac cycle. The signal intensity returned from tissues is dependent upon the proton density, the relaxation parameters of the tissue T_1 and T_2 and the imaging sequence used. Blood flowing rapidly through the imaging plane does not have time to experience all of the necessary imaging pulse sequences and therefore appears as a signal void (black blood). The primary role for spin-echo sequences in cardiac imaging is determination of cardiac morphology (Fig. 10.7).

Gradient-echo sequences

In this sequence, the sampled echo is generated by

Table 10.2 Role of magnetic resonance imaging (MRI) in myocardial disorders

Disorder	MRI information	Relation to other techniques
Congenital heart disease	Three-dimensional structure and connections of great vessels; shunt identification; identification of valvular insufficiency	Echocardiography and angiography remain the primary investigative tools; MRI useful in complicated anomalies
Cardiac masses	Site and extent, appreciation of vascular involvement	Superior to other techniques; shows greater intracardiac detail than CT
Pericardial disease	Thickening, masses, adhesions; effusion volume and functional consequence	Method of choice; CT and echocardiography may give similar information and are more widely available
Ischaemic heart disease	Site and extent of infarction; identification of aneurysms and thrombus; quantification of chamber size, valvular insufficiency, regional ventricular motility, global function and indices	Thallium and isonitrile perfusion studies preferred method of detecting ischaemia; echocardiography and nuclear medical techniques are simpler and more widely available; angiography only method of visualizing coronary arteries
Cardiomyopathies	Site and extent of hypertrophy; ventricular mass, volume, function and indices; associated valvular insufficiency	Echocardiography remains primary diagnostic tool; consider in patients with poor acoustic windows
Valvular heart disease	Chamber volumes; regurgitant jets, fractions and volumes; valve areas	Echocardiography remains primary diagnostic tool
Aorta	Identification of major branches, their patency and distribution; aortic dimensions; thrombus identification; site of dissection/intimal flap	Investigation of choice; CT, echocardiography (including transoesophageal) and angiography may give similar information

CT, computed tomography.

Fig. 10.7 Spin-echo magnetic resonance images. The secions are all in a transverse plane, starting superiorly and moving inferiorly through the heart and great vessels. (a) At the level of the aortic arch (r). Both arteries and veins (s, superior vena cava) show low signal, as does the air-containing trachea (t).

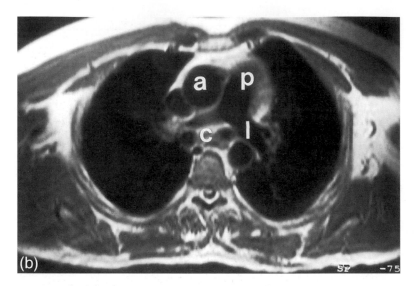

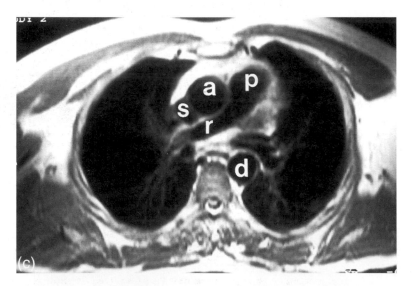

Fig. 10.7 *Continued.* (b) At the level of the carina (c) the main pulmonary artery (p) can be seen bifurcating. The left pulmonary artery (l) is well seen at this level. a, ascending aorta. (c) At the next level down the right pulmonary artery can be seen going between the ascending (a) and descending (d) aorta. The left pulmonary artery is not seen at this level.

the rapid reversal of gradient coil polarity rather than the application of an additional RF pulse as in spin-echo imaging. Sampling times are shorter, improving temporal resolution and allowing multiple samples to be obtained in one cardiac cycle. The mechanism of image contrast in gradient-echo imaging is different. Rapid sampling rates lead to partial saturation of static tissues, thereby producing less than maximal image intensity from these structures. The most intense signal is seen from spins that have not been exposed to repeated sampling

volume, that is flowing blood. Flowing blood therefore shows high signal, except in areas of disturbed flow as in regurgitant and stenotic valvular jets, probably secondary to intravoxel dephasing of spins with cancellation of the net signal. These rapidly acquired images can be viewed in a cine-loop format which gives an appreciation of cardiac movement and therefore areas of impaired contractility. Combination of the images in various stages of the cardiac cycle with mathematical formulation allows assessment of cardiac volumes and ejection

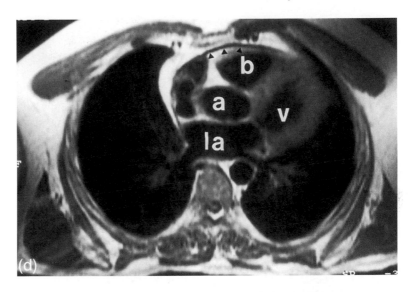

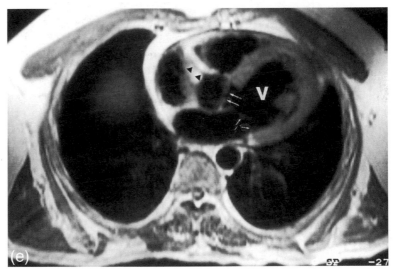

Fig. 10.7. *Continued.* (d) The left atrium (la) with pulmonary veins entering posteriorly can be seen. The right (b) and left ventricles (v) are just visible. The pericardium (arrowheads) is seen as low signal intensity within the high-signal pericardial fat. a, ascending aorta. (e) The aortic root is seen at this level with the right coronary artery being seen (arrowheads). The mitral and aortic valves (arrowed) can be seen at the base of the left ventricle (v).

fractions. The most widely used application in cardiac MRI is the assessment of flow.

Imaging planes

The multiplanar capability of MRI allows imaging of cardiac structures in any plane. It is usual to perform axial and sagittal images initially and from these the subsequent imaging planes can be chosen to assess the primary structure of interest. As in all radiological techniques it is preferable to image the area of interest in two planes, usually in the long and short axes.

Computed tomography

Non-enhanced CT scans give no appreciation of internal cardiac architecture as myocardium and blood have similar attenuation. Assessment of internal cardiac structure therefore requires the use of i.v. contrast medium. As with MRI cardiac motion is a problem and brings about image degradation. The

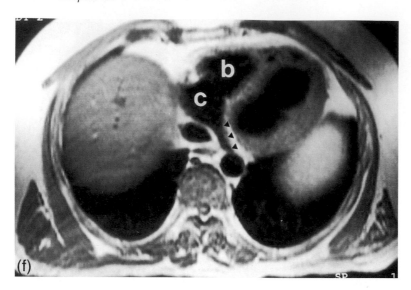

Fig. 10.7 *Continued.* (f) The coronary sinus (arrowheads) can be seen to enter the right atrium (c). b, right ventricle.

use of prospective or retrospective ECG gating is possible but not widely used with conventional CT. In order to improve temporal resolution, efforts have been made to reduce scanning times and have resulted in the development of ultrafast CT scanners. The first of these was developed at the Mayo clinic and employed numerous X-ray tubes around the patient, fired in rapid sequence. Subsequent commercial units employ a powerful electron beam generated by an electron gun (cathode). This is passed through an electromagnetic coil which focuses and steers the beam to impact on a circular anode. The generated X-rays are collimated and pass through the subject to detectors, as in conventional CT. This information is digitized and stored for later image reconstruction.

Indications

CT is useful in the assessment of mediastinal, pericardiac and paracardiac pathology. In patients with contraindications to MRI, for example cardiac pacemakers, ultrafast CT can give both anatomical and functional information similar to MRI. Its ability to detect calcium allows detection of coronary artery calcification, an indicator of high-risk coronary disease. Coronary graft patency detection is another important potential application, particularly in the early postoperative period, CT being at present superior to MRI. Radiation burden is similar to con-

ventional CT, therefore its frequent use should be avoided when echocardiography or MRI can give similar information.

Technique

Both conventional and ultrafast CT require i.v. contrast medium to depict internal cardiac anatomy. It is important when giving contrast medium to use an adequate amount, approximately 100 ml of 60% iodine being usually sufficient. The contrast medium is injected into a large peripheral vein via a large-bore needle, for instance 18 gauge, with rapid administration to achieve a good bolus. Timing and image sequencing are modified to address the clinical problem. The area of interest should be imaged during the phase of maximum contrast enhancement — the right-sided structures are reached at approximately 5 s and the left at 10 s with normal cardiac output.

Both conventional and ultrafast CT usually give adequate anatomical information. Ultrafast CT, with its reduced scanning times, has improved spatial resolution. Machines are also equipped with larger scanning apertures and mobile tables to allow flexible although limited imaging planes in oblique and short axes.

Images with ultrafast CT can be obtained in cine, flow and volume modes. The cine mode is triggered by the ECG. Images are obtained at 50 ms intervals with 8 ms pauses throughout the cardiac cycle. With a normal heart rate. up to eight levels of cardiac anatomy can be depicted during one imaging sequence. These can be viewed as a cine loop in order to show sectional cardiac anatomy. This mode is useful for the evaluation of global and regional ventricular function. As in MRI static end systolic and diastolic images can be used for assessment of cardiac mass, volumes and output.

The flow mode acquires 50 ms images in relationship to ECG. Each image can be obtained at any point in the cardiac cycle. This allows acquisition of images as contrast medium traverses the left ventricle and aorta and subsequently enters the myocardium. Using the indicator dilution theory and image analysis software, it is possible to determine regional myocardial perfusion from the changes of density that occur with the passage of contrast medium through the heart. The technique also allows quantification of cardiac output and cardiac shunts.

The volume mode acquires up to 40 scans in a single imaging sequence at 50 or 100 ms intervals. The volume mode is usually employed to define cardiac anatomy and, because of short scanning times, has excellent temporal resolution with no requirement for respiratory gating.

Cardiac angiography

Although Forssman first passed a venous catheter to the heart in 1928, angiography was a relatively slow technique to develop. This was mainly because of the technical difficulties in achieving the short exposure times necessary to 'freeze' cardiac motion. The most rapid advances in cardiac angiography took place in the 1960s and were related to the new and more convenient cine recording technique, the development of safe and reliable contrast media and the introduction of purpose-designed catheters. The simultaneous rapid development of cardiac surgery, especially coronary artery surgery and paediatric surgery, was a powerful stimulus for the refinement of these angiographic techniques.

Modern cardiac angiographic systems are based on a variation of the C- or U-arm suspension of the X-ray tube and image intensifier which rotate round a radiolucent carbon fibre table. There must be a very wide range of movement around the patient, with a full range of obliques being possible as well as facilities for caudocranial ('cranial') and craniocaudal ('caudal') angulation of at least 30°. This axial angulation is essential in achieving satisfactory profiles of anatomical features whose major orientation lies in the transverse plane of the patient. The movement around the patient is usually based on the heart lying at the 'isocentre' or point of rotation of the equipment, which allows easy changing of views. Some systems have a biplane arrangement where two independent suspensions can move around the patient to allow rapid alternate screening in different projections and simultaneous cine acquisition in two views. This biplane facility is useful in complex situations such as paediatric studies or cardiac interventional techniques.

The generator and X-ray tube are capable of producing high current pulses of very short duration, typically 2–5 ms, at rates of between 12.5 and 75 frames s^{-1}; 25 frame s^{-1} are most commonly used in adults. High currents are required for these short pulses in order to avoid the 'quantum mottle' effect of too low a dose of radiation per frame. A voltage of around 70 kV is optimal for cardiac studies. It is usual to record on an image intensifier-based medium, for instance cine or digital, rather than on to X-ray film. Cine film recording still offers the highest spatial resolution but the slightly better contrast resolution of digital recording makes the two methods broadly similar in terms of image quality at today's level of technology. Digital systems have the advantages of speed, potential for radiation reduction and image data manipulation. It is likely that digital systems will become the dominant recording method in the next few years.

Contrast media with an iodine content of not less than 320 mg ml^{-1} are required for cardiac angiography, most centres using 340–370 mg ml^{-1}. Traditional ionic media formulated for cardiac use can still be safely used in the majority of situations but, if financial pressures allow, most centres prefer to use non-ionic media. Not only does this reduce contrast reactions, but the fluid load to the patient is considerably reduced, which is important in infants, ill or unstable patients. Patient comfort is undoubtedly better with non-ionic media.

Indications

Coronary arteriography

This is the most common type of cardiac angiogram. Over 100 000 of these procedures are performed in the UK annually and the figure for the USA probably exceeds 1 million studies per year. The procedure usually involves left ventriculography and multiple views of the coronary arteries. There is currently no alternative technique for examining the coronary arteries. Indications for coronary arteriography are as follows.

1 Assessment of patients with known or suspected coronary artery disease prior to coronary revascularization by surgery or angioplasty. These patients include those with stable angina of effort, unstable angina and a minority of cases with recent myocardial infarction.

2 Diagnosis of patients with chest pain of unknown or equivocal type. These patients may have atypical symptoms with a negative or equivocal stress test. The exclusion of coronary disease is an important prognostic feature.

3 Examination of the coronary arteries in patients without symptoms of ischaemic heart disease who are to have cardiac surgery for valve disease or other cardiac disease, in whom the status of the coronary arteries needs to be known for surgical planning.

4 Follow-up of patients who have had previous revascularization by angioplasty or surgery but in whom there is evidence of recurrent disease.

Other types of angiography in adults

Aortography is indicated in the examination of pathology of the aortic valve, particularly regurgitation, but also in cases of aortic root aneurysm, dilatation or dissection. Right ventricular angiography is very rarely required but pulmonary angiography is often important in the diagnosis and treatment of pulmonary embolism, the catheter being used to administer thrombolytics as well as to inject the contrast medium. Right or left atrial angiography is rarely indicated in adults.

Structural abnormalities are increasingly diagnosed by other means, such as echocardiography (including transoesophageal), CT scanning or MRI.

Paediatric cardiac angiography

As with adults, but perhaps even more so, the use of non-invasive imaging techniques has considerably modified the use of cardiac angiography. A high proportion of patients can have a full presurgical diagnosis without angiography. Indications for paediatric cardiac angiography are as follows:

1 Patients in whom there is persisting doubt about structural abnormalities after echocardiography.

2 Cases where imaging of small structures such as coronary arteries is critical to future management.

3 Imaging of structures in or near the lungs where satisfactory ultrasound imaging cannot be performed, particularly the assessment of pulmonary artery anatomy.

4 Situations where the imaging data need to be accompanied by catheter-derived haemodynamic data such as intracardiac pressures and oxygen saturations. Although some haemodynamic data can be derived from Doppler studies, sophisticated calculations such as that of pulmonary and systemic vascular resistance can only be obtained by invasive means.

5 In association with interventional cardiac techniques.

Techniques

Catheterization room

As well as the X-ray equipment described above, the room must have facilities for continuous monitoring of ECG and blood pressure, at least two channels for each, and must be fully equipped for dealing with ill patients and those needing resuscitation. A full range of emergency cardiovascular drugs and a defibrillator must be in the room itself. All staff must be fully conversant with all available equipment. Although serious complications are rare in the catheter room, it should be possible to treat the majority of them successfully.

Approach to the heart. The most common route to the left-sided cardiac structures is the percutaneous (Seldinger) approach to the femoral artery, usually on the right. The next most common route is the right brachial artery, using either a cut-down or a percutaneous approach. Venous access to the right-sided cardiac structures can be achieved by percutaneous femoral vein puncture, femoral vein cut-down or via a brachial vein. The jugular route is occasionally used in children. In small infants a cut-down to artery or vein is commonly required due to the small size of the vessels and the difficulty of percutaneous puncture.

General principles of angiography in the heart

Percutaneous or cut-down? The trend is moving substantially to percutaneous techniques, even for difficult cases. Those operators who favour the cut-down to the brachial artery can perform very quick and safe procedures but only if they are very experienced. There is a high complication rate, usually ischaemia, associated with cut-down to the brachial artery by inexperienced operators. Care with haemostasis is important. Pressure on the correct site should not be excessive and a distal pulse should be palpable during the period of pressure. The operator should always have felt the distal pulses before the procedure.

Heparin. With modern catheters and a percutaneous route, heparin is not usually used if the angiogram proceeds quickly and no unusual manipulations are required. If the procedure is prolonged, the patient should receive systemic heparin, usually 50–100 IU kg^{-1} and repeated if necessary. A single dose of heparin 30 min or more before the procedure is completed should not significantly impair haemostasis.

Catheter size. Slightly larger catheters are generally required for cardiac angiography because (i) the manipulations are usually round the bend of the aortic arch, and (ii) larger doses of contrast medium are often given at high flow rates. In adults 6 French (F) or 7F arterial catheters are usually used, with 4 and 5F catheters being common in children.

Catheter selection. The first choice is whether to use an end-hole or a multihole catheter. The former is used in selective angiography, for example preshaped coronary catheters such as Judkins left and right or Amplatz, or for careful pressure measurements made at precise sites. The latter are used for large volume angiography, the pig-tail catheter being commonly used in the left ventricle. The NIH catheter, which is commonly used in children, has no end-hole but multiple side-holes and must be used through a sheath. The Gensini catheter, which has end and side-holes, also has a variety of applications.

Large volume angiography. This is for injections into cardiac chambers or the great vessels. A pump injection is required and the following are guidelines for dose and flow rate, assuming a 70 kg adult.

A typical ventricular injection for assessment of contractility is 35–40 ml at 12 ml s^{-1}, over three to four cardiac cycles to minimize ectopic beats and to give a 'functional' assessment. For the anatomical demonstration of a large cardiac chamber or great vessel, 40 ml at 20 ml s^{-1} will give a dense bolus over two cycles. Volumes and rates should take into account chamber size, any volume overload, catheter position and risk of recoil. If in doubt, a preliminary injection of 20% volume is given to check the catheter position.

Suggested projections are as follows.
1 Left ventricle. 30° RAO and 60° LAO with 30° cranial tilt to demonstrate better the length of the main part of the septum.
2 Aortic root. 30° RAO and 60° LAO.

Pulmonary angiography is best performed with two injections, each of 35 ml, selectively to left and right. For the left pulmonary artery posteroanterior (PA) with 30° cranial tilt and 60° LAO; and right pulmonary artery, PA with 30° cranial tilt and 60° RAO. The cranial tilt is not used if a good view of venous return is required.

Coronary arteriography. A typical technique for a patient with stable angina (70 kg adult) is for the left ventricular angiogram, 35 ml of non-ionic contrast medium, 370 mg iodine ml^{-1} at 12 ml s^{-1}. A pig-tail catheter is placed in the ventricle between the papillary muscles, so as not to cause ectopics or be caught in the mitral valve. The ejection fraction can be calculated by a variety of tested algorithms that are based on geometric models of the left ventricular cavity. The modern digital systems can calculate this quickly and automatically with a high degree of reliability (Fig. 10.8). Left ventricular end diastolic pressure is measured before and after the angiogram. A withdrawal trace as the catheter is pulled out of the ventricle after the angiogram will exclude aortic stenosis. A single plane 30° RAO projection is commonly used but an LAO is added if there is a biplane facility.

Coronary injections. Depend on the size of the vessel and the flow down the vessel. The catheter must lie free in the coronary ostium with no tendency to obstruct flow and with the tip away from the vessel wall. A small (0.5 ml) test injection should wash away freely and the pressure trace from the catheter tip should show no obstruction. Typical doses are 5–8 ml for the left coronary and 2–3 ml for the right coronary artery. The rate of the hand injection should be fast enough to reflux to the ostium but not to flood the sinus of Valsalva. The right coronary artery may be small and the catheter tip may then wedge.

Projections depend on the anatomy and pathology. The coronary anatomy varies considerably in branch size and orientation, so that the study must be carefully interpreted as it proceeds in order that the proximal parts of all major vessels and branches are fully demonstrated. Typical projections are as follows.

1 Left coronary: LAO 60°; left lateral; LAO 30° with 30° cranial tilt (Fig. 10.9a); 25° RAO; 40° RAO with 15° caudal tilt.

2 Right coronary: LAO 60° (Fig. 10.9b), LAO 30° with 30° cranial tilt; RAO 30°.

Paediatric angiography

In general contrast doses of 1 ml kg^{-1} in infants, falling to 0.6 ml kg^{-1} in larger children, are used for ventriculography. Doses are increased or decreased according to chamber size and flow in the chamber to a maximum of 2 ml kg^{-1} in infants. An injection rate which allows the contrast to be injected in 1.5 to two cardiac cycles is selected. In some cases where a small infant has a high flow lesion, such as a large ventricular septal defect, a flow rate might not be achievable if too small a catheter size has been selected. When using non-ionic media, a total procedure dose of 4 ml kg^{-1} is a very safe level. This may be extended to 6 ml kg^{-1} but only if the patient is

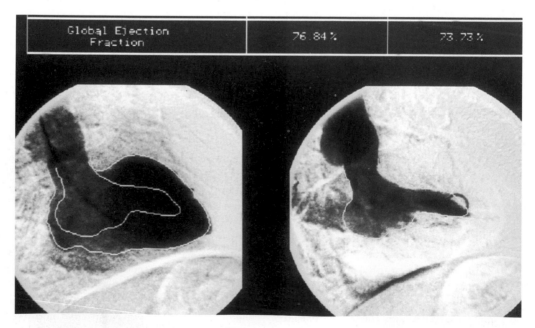

| Global Ejection Fraction | 76.84 % | 73.73 % |

Fig. 10.8 Left ventricular angiogram performed on a digital imaging unit which has facilitated the calculation of the left ventricular ejection fraction.

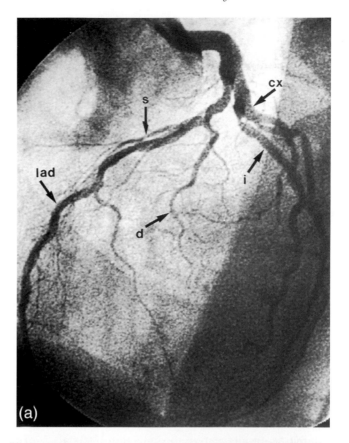

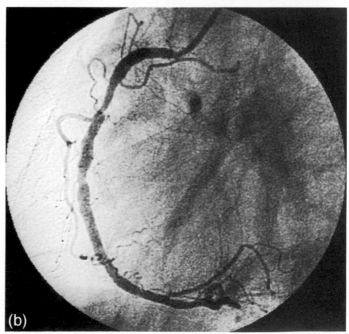

Fig. 10.9 (a) Selective left coronary arteriogram recorded as a digital image in the left anterior oblique projection with caudocranial angulation. The left anterior descending (lad), diagonal (d), septal (s), intermediate (i) and circumflex (cx) branches are shown. (b) Left anterior oblique view of a selective right coronary arteriogram.

well hydrated and there are no grounds for concern over the condition of the infant.

Complications

In spite of the complications outlined below, the technique of coronary arteriography, and cardiac catheterization in general, has become very safe. In well-conducted centres the mortality rate is around 0.1%.

Puncture site

1 Haematoma. The most common complication can be avoided with careful technique and local pressure afterwards. Haemostasis may take longer if the patient has been on aspirin. Moderate and large haematomas must be treated carefully and investigated by ultrasound if necessary.
2 Dissection is avoided by not pushing against resistance. If in doubt, a small careful angiogram should be obtained through the needle, dilator or catheter.
3 Haemorrhage is rarely a major problem unless it is concealed. Retroperitoneal bleeding must be considered in a patient with signs of haemodynamic collapse.
4 Thrombus is rare nowadays but should be considered as an alternative to dissection if distal ischaemia develops.

General

1 Contrast reaction (see Chapter 30).
2 Embolus. Meticulous technique should be observed in connecting catheters, flushing and using guide wires. If a guide wire is used for any length of time the catheter and wire should periodically be brought to the descending aorta, the wire withdrawn and cleaned, and the catheter flushed. The usual coronary injection system should be carefully set up in the descending aorta to avoid the risk of air or thrombotic embolus to the coronary or carotid vessels.

Cardiac

1 Arrhythmias are common and usually benign, being related to stimulation of myocardial tissue by the catheter. The operator must be able to distinguish those caused by catheter manipulation from those due to more serious causes. In the latter case, common treatments for the arrhythmias must be available, including emergency pacing and defibrillation.
2 Cardiac trauma. Aggressive pushing of stiff catheters can damage cardiac tissue and, especially in the right ventricle, can penetrate the wall and cause tamponade. Means of diagnosing and treating this uncommon occurrence should be available.

Coronary artery trauma is particularly dangerous and, if the catheter tip dissects the proximal left coronary artery, can be rapidly fatal. Fortunately this is a rare occurrence and is avoided by meticulous care with catheter tip positioning.
3 Hypotension. Transient hypotension is not uncommon but care must be taken to treat any significant drop in pressure. In patients with severe coronary artery disease, especially those with critical stenosis of the left main coronary artery, sustained hypotension can be dangerous and occasionally fatal. If the severity of the left main stenosis is clear from the first one or two views, it is prudent to reduce the number of injections to the potentially large ischaemic territory.
4 Radiation protection should be of a high quality for the patient and also for the staff. The throughput of many cardiac catheter rooms is now very high and staff and operators, if not properly protected, can be subjected to considerable cumulative amounts of radiation.

Diagnostic quality

One of the greatest hazards to the patient is to subject them to the risks outlined above without producing an angiogram of optimal diagnostic quality.

Cardiac intervention

One of the earliest transcatheter treatments of cardiac disease was the Rashkind atrial balloon septostomy. This method rapidly gained acceptance in the 1960s and is still the primary palliation for cyanotic infants with transposition of the great arteries. In 1977, Gruntzig reported a successful coronary artery dilatation. Hundreds of thousands of percutaneous transluminal coronary angioplasties (PTCA) are now performed worldwide every year.

A great variety of techniques offer valuable alternatives to conventional surgical methods.

The principle of balloon dilatation is the most widely used, with pulmonary valve stenosis being the most commonly treated valve lesion. Selected cases of mitral stenosis can be dilated as well as lesser numbers of aortic and tricuspid valves. Aortic coarctation, recoarctation, peripheral pulmonary stenosis and stenotic surgical conduits have all proved amenable to balloon dilatation. Occlusion of abnormal communications is now common, a special 'umbrella' closure device being used for closure of patent ductus arteriosus and a variety of coils and detachable balloons to close abnormal fistulae. Radiofrequency ablation catheters are now used to perforate some atretic valves and to ablate some abnormal conduction pathways. Devices are available for retrieving fragments of foreign material from the heart and circulation. Some catheters also incorporate a blade for enlarging the atrial septal communication in some cases of congenital heart disease.

Percutaneous transluminal coronary angioplasty

Indications

The mortality rates for both PTCA and coronary artery bypass graft (CABG) are similar at about 1%. The indications for both procedures are clinically similar, namely symptomatic ischaemic heart disease that is not fully responsive to medical therapy or that affects the future prognosis of the patient. PTCA patients tend to have more localized disease, commonly confined to one or two main sites and generally without chronically occluded vessels. CABG is not restricted in this way and multiple occluded vessels can be treated. However, the situation is a rapidly changing with PTCA indications widening.

An uncomplicated PTCA is associated with a short hospital stay, as little as 1–2 days, and low morbidity with a rapid return to normal activity. CABG usually involves 12–24 hours' postoperative intensive care, 7–10 days in hospital and a minimum of 2–3 months' convalescence. The major problem with PTCA is the recurrence rate. Early vessel closure, in less than 24 hours, occurs in about 5% of cases and requires either repeat PTCA or CABG. Cardiac surgery facilities should always be available where PTCA is carried out. Restenosis of the vessel occurs in 20–40% of cases within the first 6 months and is a major drawback of PTCA. Repeat PTCA, however, is not a difficult procedure and will solve the problem in many patients. An increasing number of patients with recurrent symptoms after surgery can be helped by angioplasty to the grafts or to native vessels.

Technique

Patient preparation involves proper explanation and a 4-hour fast. It is preferable for the patient to be on aspirin for its antiplatelet action. The procedure is generally performed from the femoral artery using an 8F guiding catheter. Once optimal angiographic views of the lesion are obtained, the patient is fully heparinized with a clotting time above 300 s. Intracoronary nitrates or calcium antagonist drugs are sometimes administered. Initial crossing of the lesion is usually achieved with a 'steerable' guide wire of 0.014 in. with a soft tip. A low-profile PTCA balloon is advanced to the lesion and inflated, generally to 6–8 atm pressure for at least 60 s. Balloon size is judged from the angiogram but is commonly 2.5–3.5 mm in expanded diameter. Most patients tolerate inflations well but continuous careful monitoring of the patient's symptoms, blood pressure and ECG is required. In a few cases there is inadequate distal perfusion and a special perfusion balloon must be used. This allows a small amount of flow to pass through the inflated balloon. Figure 10.10 shows stages in a typical successful PTCA of a severe left anterior descending artery stenosis.

After the procedure, sheaths are left in the femoral artery and vein, the latter for urgent venous and pacing access if required. Sheaths are generally removed 6 hours after the procedure.

Complications

The most common complication is a dissection of the artery which causes partial or complete occlusion of the lumen. This can often be repaired using repeated inflation or an intracoronary stent, but in some cases (2–5%) the patient must be referred for immediate CABG to avoid prolonged ischaemia. Other complications of PTCA include thrombosis and spasm at

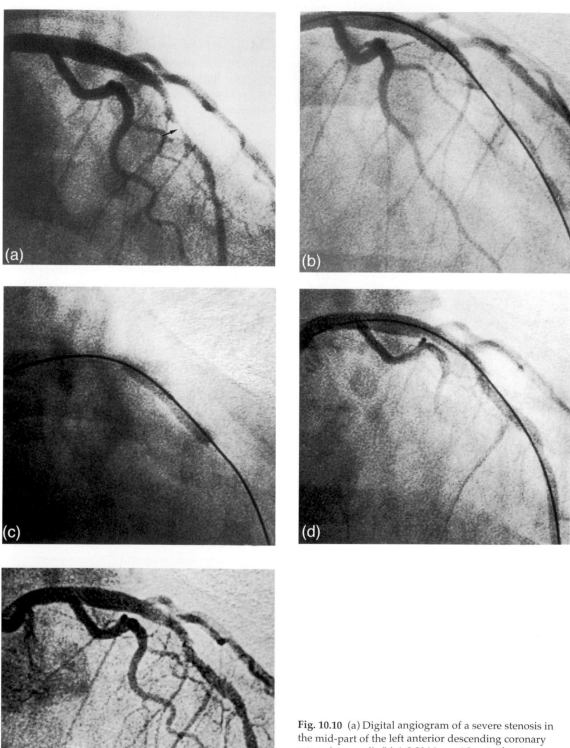

Fig. 10.10 (a) Digital angiogram of a severe stenosis in the mid-part of the left anterior descending coronary artery (arrowed). (b) A 0.014 in. guide wire has been passed across the lesion, almost obstructing the flow. (c) A 3 mm balloon inflated in the stenosis. (d) Post-dilatation: the guide wire is still in position. (e) The final result after the guide wire has been withdrawn. There is almost complete resolution of the stenosis.

the site of dilatation, but these can generally be managed or prevented by appropriate drug therapy.

Relationship to other techniques

New devices are constantly being introduced. For example, atherectomy techniques involve the use of a catheter-mounted cutter in a small chamber to remove rather than rupture or displace the atheromatous deposits.

Trials are being conducted on the use of intravascular ultrasound catheters in the assessment of disease and for monitoring the effects of angioplasty and stent placement.

The problem of restenosis after PTCA is not yet solved, but one line of current research involves techniques for local drug delivery on impregnated stents.

Acknowledgements

We would like to thank Dr G. Vivian, Derriford Hospital, Plymouth for her advice on the nuclear medicine section.

Further reading

Blackwell, G.G., Cranney, G.B. & Pohost, G.M. (1992) *MRI: Cardiovascular System*. Gower Medical, London.

Edler, I. & Hertz, C.H. (1954) The use of the ultrasonic reflectoscope for the continuous recording of the movements of heart walls. *K. Fysiogr. Sallsk. Lund. Forh.* **24**, 40–58.

Elliot, L.P. (1991) *Cardiac Imaging in Infants, Children and Adults*. JB Lippincott.

Griffith, J.M. & Henry, W.L. (1974) A sector scanner for real time two dimensional echocardiography. *Circulation* **49**, 1147–52.

Marcus, M., Schelbert, H.R., Skorton D.J., & Wolf, G.L. (1991) *Cardiac Imaging*. WB Saunders, Philadelphia.

Miere, H., Cosgrove, D., Dewbury, K. & Wilde, P. (1993) *Clinical Ultrasound*, Vol. IV *Cardiac Ultrasound*. Churchill Livingstone, Edinburgh.

Pohost, G.M. & O'Rourke, R.A. (1991) *Principles and Practice of Cardiovascular Imaging*. Little, Brown, Boston.

Satomura, S. (1957) Ultrasonic Doppler method for the inspection of cardiac function. *J. Acoust. Soc. Am.* **29**, 1181–5.

Sutton, D. (1993) *A Textbook of Radiology and Imaging*. Churchill Livingstone, Edinburgh.

Sutton, D. & Young, J. (1990) *A Short Textbook of Clinical Imaging*. Springer-Verlag, New York.

Wells, P.N.T. (1969) A range-gated ultrasonic Doppler system. *Med. Biol. Eng.* **7**, 641–52.

11   Portal and Hepatic Venous System

R. DICK

The variety of methods for introducing contrast medium into the portal system is matched only by their degree of ingenuity. A direct portogram via the splenic parenchyma was first described over 40 years ago (Abeatici & Campi, 1951). It was followed by the transhepatic approach (Lunderquist & Vang, 1974), both techniques being performed under local anaesthesia in the vascular suite. Other access routes include haemorrhoidal or jejunal vein injection, reopening the umbilical vein, and catheterization of the internal jugular vein with subsequent entry to a hepatic vein. All but the last of these direct venous entries requires surgery in an operating theatre and more straightforward methods are therefore desirable.

Kreel and Williams described the use of indirect portography in 1964 and this technique has stood the test of time. It results when contrast medium, delivered during coeliac or superior mesenteric angiography, is collected in the capillary beds of gut end organs and returned to the liver by the portal venous system.

Percutaneous splenoportography (PSP)

PSP is no longer a common procedure in Europe, but it retains its popularity elsewhere. Many would be unhappy to undertake PSP on an out-patient basis, yet Dilawari *et al.* (1987) claim this is safe. The risk of bleeding from the entry site is negligible if the tract is embolized during withdrawal.

Indications

Portal hypertension

Direct PSP delineates portal venous anatomy well and allows measurement of portal pressure (elevated if more than 11 mmHg). A normal PSP demonstrates only the splenic and portal veins and their radicles (Fig. 11.1), reversed flow into gastro-oesophageal collaterals being accepted as evidence of portal hypertension (Fig. 11.2). Sometimes the splenic or portal veins may be displaced or invaded by inflammatory or neoplastic disease of the pancreas, bile-ducts or liver.

Contraindications

1 Coagulopathy with persistently high INR.
2 Platelet count less than $75\,000/mm^3$.
3 Gross ascites.

Technique

In adults, PSP can be performed under local anaesthesia following explanation. However, children require general anaesthesia. After estimating splenic size by palpation and fluoroscopy, a skin site is identified in the mid-axillary line at least 3 cm below the left costophrenic angle and towards the middle of the spleen. After skin and subcutaneous infiltration with 5 ml 1% lignocaine, a 9 cm long 6 French (F) gauge needle–cannula* is inserted for 4–6 cm in a steady movement and during absolute apnoea. After needle withdrawal, blood from the splenic pulp will exude from the cannula. A pressure recording is taken (Fig. 11.3) followed by a contrast study (40 ml of non-ionic contrast medium, 300 mg iodine ml^{-1}, at 8 ml s^{-1}). Twelve images are acquired at the rate of 1 s^{-1}. Ivalon (150–300 U) is injected into the pulp during cannula withdrawal and the patient is returned to the ward for 12 hours' pulse and blood pressure monitoring during bed rest, initially lying on their left side to compress the spleen.

* Vygon Intranule, Ecouen, France.

194

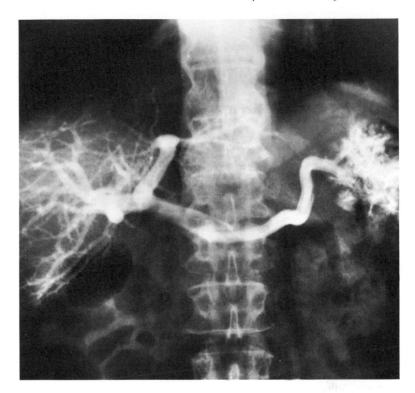

Fig. 11.1 Normal splenic portogram. Note dilution in main portal vein by superior mesenteric venous flow. Pulp pressure 10 mmHg. Portal hypertension excluded.

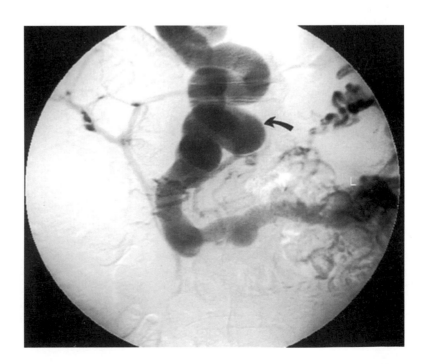

Fig. 11.2 Digital subtraction angiography percutaneous splenoportogram. Note thinned portal vein due to 'steal' by huge left gastric vein (arrowed). Earlier ultrasound and coeliac and superior mesenteric arteriography had been equivocal in regard to portal vein status.

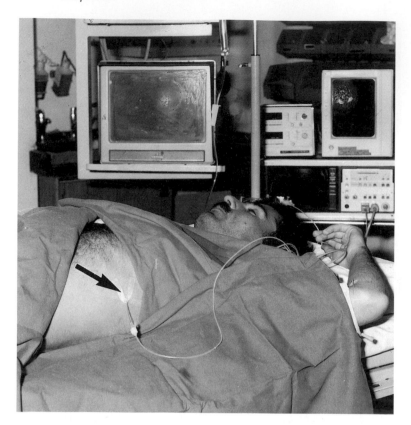

Fig. 11.3 Patient having transsplenic portogram. Cannula entering splenic pulp through intercostal space just behind mid-axillary line (arrow). A pressure line connects to the transducer in the background.

Variations

Using digital subtraction angiography (DSA), PSP can be performed quickly and safely using a 20 or 21 gauge spinal needle, 20 ml of non-ionic contrast medium injected at 5 ml s^{-1} being sufficient to give a diagnostic study. In patients with splenomegaly of unknown cause, possible infection or lymphoma, splenic aspirates may be obtained under ultrasound or computed tomographic (CT) control. Focal defects can be identified for fine-needle aspiration biopsy (FNAB) or culture.

Complications

Severe complications are rare, the incidence being 0.7% following many thousands of studies. Surgery has confirmed the efficacy of needle tract plugging to control bleeding and the safety of PSP has been proven in a retrospective review by Brazzini *et al.* (1987).

Relationship to other techniques

Despite its simplicity and its ability to diagnose portal hypertension definitively, PSP has severe limitations.

1 Altered blood flow patterns may cause a false impression of portal vein occlusion and need clarification by later coeliac and superior mesenteric arteriography (CSMAP) or PSP.
2 Arteriography is necessary if a vascular liver lesion or an arterial gut bleeder is to be identified.
3 Additional hepatic vein pressure measurements would be needed in many patients to localize correctly the site and type of obstruction causing the high pressure found in the splenic pulp.
4 It is not possible to proceed to embolize varices via the spleen, whereas this may be performed following transhepatic or transjugular portography.
5 Dynamic enhanced CT and magnetic resonance angiography (MRA) will in future provide most of the information yielded by PSP.

Coeliac and superior mesenteric arterioportography

Contrast medium delivered into the territory supplied by these arteries will, in the venous phase, fill the splenic/portal vein and the superior mesenteric/portal vein, respectively (Figs 11.4 & 11.5).

Indications

1 To show arterial and capillary abnormalities in the liver, spleen, pancreas and viscera of patients with chronic liver disease, suspected neoplasms, aneurysms of major arteries and haemangiomas.
2 In portal hypertension — to demonstrate fully anatomy and abnormal flow.
3 To indicate the state of major arteries and mesenteric/portal veins prior to a shunt procedure or in the work-up for liver transplant.
4 To search for an active non-variceal bleeding point in the stomach or bowel, for example erosion, ulceration or angiodysplasia.
5 For demonstration of previously performed surgical portosystemic shunts where Doppler ultrasound has been difficult or requires supplementary information (Fig. 11.6).
6 Occasionally to treat variceal bleeding by intra-arterial vasopressin.

Contraindications

These are as for femoral artery catheterization (see Chapter 8).

Technique

Preparation is as for arteriography. If bleeding is active, an inflated Sengstaken balloon catheter is inserted before transport to the hospital and angiogram suite. Blood is transfused and the patient sedated

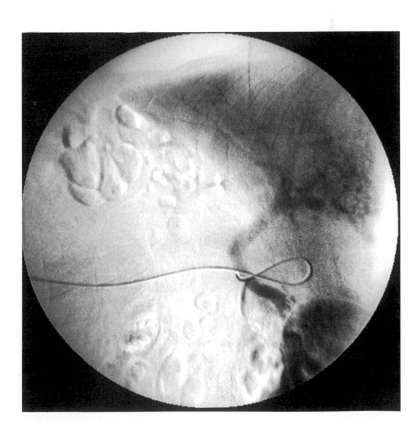

Fig. 11.4 Digital subtraction angiography: venous phase coeliac arteriogram. Normal splenic/portal veins, and dense regular portogram extending to periphery of liver, which has a smooth outline.

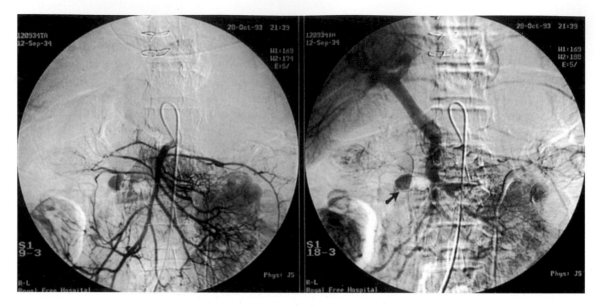

Fig. 11.5 Digital subtraction angiography: superior mesenteric arteriogram — normal study. Good delineation of SMV and PV, with no variceal filling (subtraction artefact indicated by arrow).

with 5 mg Diazemuls or midazolam. A 5F sidewinder type 1 or 2 catheter is suitable in patients with coagulopathy, side-holes being important to stabilize catheter position during injection.

It is best to perform coeliac axis angiography first, since the finding of malignancy, other liver pathology or fistulae may alter the management of a patient with portal hypertension. Using DSA, 35 ml of non-ionic contrast medium (300 mg iodine ml^{-1}) are injected at a rate of 7 ml s^{-1}. Bowel paralysis and at least 25 s absolute apnoea are required for clear arterial and venous delineation unimpeded by subtraction artefact. The catheter may subsequently be placed deeply into the splenic artery and a further run acquired. The use of gas distension of the stomach and intra-arterial vasodilators prior to contrast injection used to be recommended but is now only occasionally employed should DSA facilities be unavailable. Due to reversed or variable flow patterns, suspected varices may not fill from the above studies; the coeliac study should always be followed by superior mesenteric arterioportography. Contrast medium (40 ml) is injected at 8 ml s^{-1}, with an image acquisition rate of 1 s^{-1}. It is vital to extend the

run to at least 30 s, as the timing of intrahepatic portal vein filling is variable and may be very late. Pharmacoangiography is occasionally employed (Fig. 11.7).

Variations

Two catheters have been advocated to improve the contrast density of CSMAP, the splenic and superior mesenteric arteries being injected simultaneously, along with vasodilators, resulting in rich venous filling (Zannini *et al.*, 1979). DSA, if available, renders this unnecessary. Occasionally, selective left gastric arteriography, using a sidewinder type 1, or 'femorovisceral' type 1 catheter, will highlight oesophageal varices or a gastric bleeder.

Finally, should complex surgical liver resection be planned for tumours, cysts and so on, a catheter is placed deeply into the superior mesenteric artery and the patient transported to the CT department for CT portography. Dynamic scanning commences simultaneously with the start of an injection of 130 ml of contrast medium at a rate of 2 ml s^{-1}. Provided some well-described flow

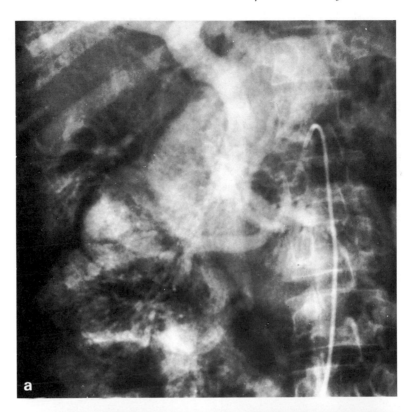

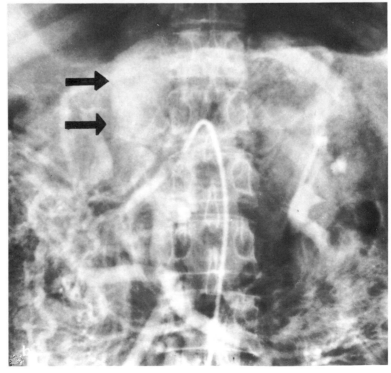

Fig. 11.6 (a) Superior mesenteric arteriogram. Venous phase in patient with portal hypertension. Superior mesenteric and portal veins fill. (b) Same patient with repeat study 9 months after successful mesocaval shunt. Contrast medium enters inferior vena cava (arrowed) through the patent shunt.

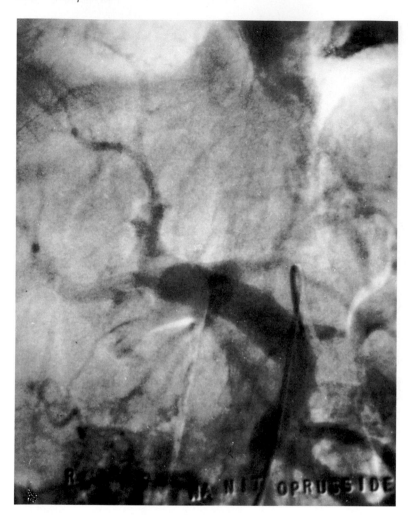

Fig. 11.7 Photographic subtraction of venous phase from a superior mesenteric arteriogram after intra-arterial nitroprusside to highlight veins. Initial angiogram gave poor venous information.

artefacts are recognized, this technique will provide highly accurate preoperative differentiation between normal and abnormal tissue (Fig. 11.8). It is usually followed by intraoperative ultrasound (Dick & Gibson, 1993).

Relationship to other techniques

CSMAP is timed according to the clinical setting. It is used if more information is required about the arterial or portal system than has been provided by non-invasive means, or if the patient is to proceed to an interventional procedure such as arterial or venous embolization, or to transjugular intrahepatic portosystemic stent shunt (TIPSS).

A further advantage is that, should an abnormal focal area be seen within the liver, an accurate biopsy may be considered at the time with the arterial catheter *in situ*. Many of these patients are at risk, and the tract is plugged with a spongiostan (Gelfoam) or polyvinyl alcohol (Ivalon) embolus before checking for haemostasis by a repeat arterial injection. In the unlikely event of a haemoperitoneum, the arterial catheter should be advanced to embolize the liver close to the site of biopsy.

Finally, both magnetic resonance imaging (MRI) and CT may give both arterial and venous information in portal hypertension (Fig. 11.9).

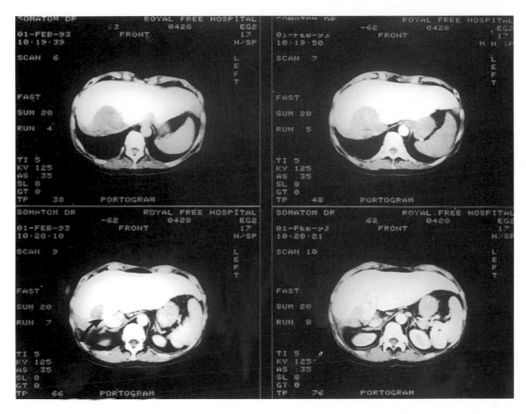

Fig. 11.8 Computed tomographic (CT) portogram. Previous partial right hepatectomy for fibrolamellar carcinoma. Non-opacified tissue on CT is the recurrent tumour which has engulfed portal vein (arrowed) and vena cava. The study indicated that further study was not possible.

Transhepatic portography (THP)

Prior to the development of the TIPSS procedure, THP was an important technique for treating patients with acutely bleeding varices (Smith-Laing *et al.*, 1981).

Indications

Portal hypertension

THP is superior to both PSP and CSMAP in demonstrating the portal system, particularly the left lobe of the liver. Causes of failure of these other studies to show the portal vein include portal vein thrombosis, 'stealing' collaterals preventing portal vein opacification, and hepatofugal blood flow in the

* William Cook Europe, Bjaeverskov, Denmark.

portal vein. By employing a tip deflecting handle and wire*, the catheter may be manoeuvred from the portal and splenic vein into the left and short gastric veins (Fig. 11.10), followed by injection and embolization of varices (Fig. 11.11). Variceal bleeding is arrested in 80% of patients but the rebleeding rate is up to 50%. THP is therefore used in patients with recent acute variceal bleeding rather than in those with chronic bleeds.

Venous sampling

Selective catheterization allows access to all the veins which drain the portal system. The main application is searching for endocrine tumours in the pancreas or surrounding territory (Fig. 11.12). As an alternative to the tip deflecting catheter, a catheter with a short preformed curve at its tip may be exchanged over a guide wire.

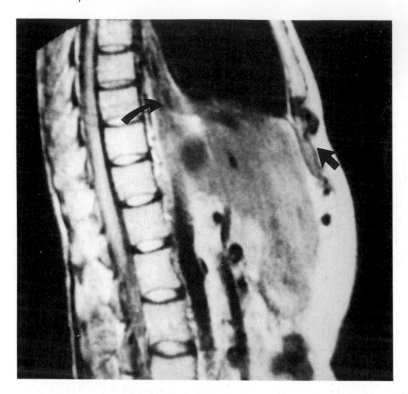

Fig. 11.9 Magnetic resonance image in a patient with cirrhosis and portal hypertension. Straight arrow on anterior abdominal wall indicates enlarged umbilical vein. Curved arrow over the spine shows varices in the oesophagus. Courtesy of Dr A. Leung.

Contraindications

Defective clotting should be corrected and gross ascites reduced as much as possible. Embolization is often performed during bleeding, the patient being ventilated and resuscitated *pari passu* with the procedure.

Lack of available expertise is a major contraindication. Failure to enter the portal vein occurs with experience in only 6%. Nevertheless, THP is both technically difficult and time-consuming, taking longer than 1.5 hours.

Technique

The portal vein is located by ultrasound or earlier CSMAP. Under local anaesthesia of the skin and subcutaneous tissue, the liver is approached with a 40 cm long needle sheathed in a matching length 5F polyethylene catheter*. This is advanced during suspended respiration towards the anticipated site

of a large portal vein radicle above the liver hilum. After needle removal, aspiration is performed during slow catheter withdrawal until venous blood is obtained. The delineation of the main trunk of the portal vein by injected contrast medium confirms correct entry into the portal vein. If initial passes are unsuccessful, the catheter must be embolized with particulate fragments prior to its final withdrawal in order to prevent liver haemorrhage. Up to five attempts may be required to enter the portal system.

Using a series of guide wires of varying flexibility and rigidity, the catheter is advanced deeply into the extrahepatic portal system. Full portography is obtained, injecting 30 ml of contrast medium at 10 ml s⁻¹. The procedure thereafter is determined by the particular indications. During final catheter withdrawal from the liver, the extravascular hepatic tract must be sealed with Gelfoam (spongiostan).

Variations

Kimura-Tsuchiya *et al.* (1981) carried out THP after puncturing, and thus localizing, a major portal vein

---

* William Cook Europe, Bjaeverskov, Denmark.

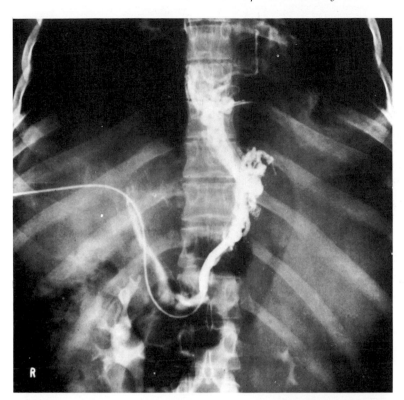

Fig. 11.10 Transhepatic portogram. Selective catheterization of left gastric vein demonstrating gastric and oesophageal collaterals. Gross splenomegaly.

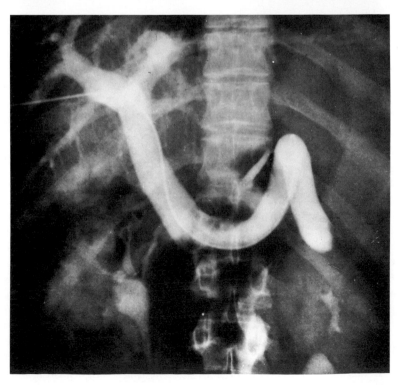

Fig. 11.11 Same patient as Fig. 11.10. Free portogram after transoesophageal obliteration of varices. Note contrast medium trapped in a short segment of left gastric vein from previous study.

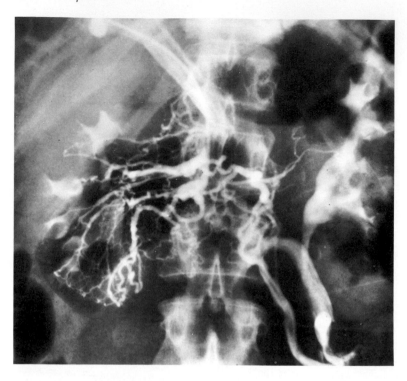

Fig. 11.12 Transhepatic portogram with selective catheterization of posterosuperior pancreaticoduodenal veins for sampling in patient with suspected insulinoma.

branch with a fine Chiba needle (15 cm long, 0.7 mm outer diameter). By exchanging through the Chiba needle and introducing a larger catheter, THP succeeded in all 67 patients with no complications.

Complications

Transient fever is common. Subcapsular and subcutaneous haematoma occur, particularly in those with a bleeding tendency. Major complications are rare. Two deaths have so far been reported worldwide, both resulting from haemoperitoneum before the sealing of exit liver tracts became routine practice. Thrombosis of the portal vein is an important sequel if varices are not injected with scrupulous care to prevent reflux into the main vascular trunks. Endophlebitis and wall thickening of the portal vein are of serious concern to the surgeon if liver transplantation is considered in the future.

Relationship to other techniques

THP has superior accuracy to PSP in showing true flow patterns in the portal vein and its tributaries (Burcharth & Aagaard, 1988). It has, nevertheless, recently lost popularity because of the advances in endoscopic variceal injection for the treatment of bleeding oesophageal varices and the development of the TIPSS procedure for creating a non-surgical portosystemic shunt.

Hepatic venography (HV)

A technique for hepatic vein catheterization was first described by Warren and Brannon in 1944. Many methods have been tried to demonstrate the hepatic veins, some of these being crude and lacking practicality. They included the use of single- and double-balloon catheters in the inferior vena cava, forced retrograde filling of hepatic veins after raising intrabronchial pressure, the i.v. injection of carbon dioxide and the direct percutaneous introduction of contrast medium into the liver.

The aims of HV are (i) to record pressures within the hepatic venous tree, inferior vena cava and right atrium; and (ii) to obtain an angiogram following occlusion of the hepatic vein which has been entered.

Ideally, HV should be simple, cause the minimum hazard and discomfort, and give maximum morphological and haemodynamic information. It should be reproducible.

Technique

The examination is not painful and is performed under local anaesthesia with premedication. The patient is fasting and is reassured that the study is neither unpleasant nor lengthy. The hepatic vein may be approached from above the diaphragm via an antecubital or jugular vein. Depending upon patient anatomy, the first site may require a time-consuming venous cut-down. Both methods need cardiac monitoring because the catheter traverses the heart. The recommended method is from the common femoral vein by the Seldinger technique, and is straightforward unless there is gross oedema or a previous thrombosis.

Catheters should have no side-holes because of the manometry. The types of catheter used are the disposable Cournand catheter* 7F, 100 cm and the 7F, 65 cm Meditech occlusion balloon catheter †, straight yet formable at 80–90°C. These are the most satisfactory for HV. Straight and movable core J wires at 145 cm (0.038 in.) are employed to guide catheters up the inferior vena cava and into a selected vein, the balloon being protected during femoral vein entry by passing the catheter through a Cordis 7 and 8F introducer sheath. Up to three hepatic veins are usually studied, namely a major and middle right hepatic vein and the single left hepatic vein. Pressures may be averaged from three sets of readings, although contrast studies are usually only performed in one vein.

To engage the right hepatic vein, both catheter and guide wire are advanced to the high inferior vena cava. After withdrawal of the wire into the body of the catheter, the latter is rotated to face the right side just below the right hemidiaphragm. Gentle manipulations and variations in respiration cause the catheter to engage the hepatic vein orifice and, with guide

* Cordis.
† Keymed.

wire help, it is advanced into the main trunk of the vein.

After a free hepatic venous pressure measurement is obtained, the balloon on the catheter is inflated until it completely occludes the vein, as shown by a small injection of contrast medium through the catheter channel. The occlusion pressure is read, corresponding to the peripheral wedge pressure if a Cournand catheter had been used. Occlusion hepatic venography (Fig. 11.13) is now performed by filling the hepatic venous tree beyond the catheter, 20 ml of contrast medium being injected at 5 ml s^{-1} and 10 images being acquired at a rate of 1 s^{-1}. The balloon is then decompressed and the catheter inserted distally or into another vein with further pressure recordings. Finally, pressures are taken in the right atrium and at the high, middle and low levels of the inferior vena cava.

Occlusion balloon catheters have greatly improved the safety of earlier wedge studies where contrast medium flooding the sinusoids caused liver cell damage (Fig. 11.14). With a balloon catheter facility, contrast medium is injected into the lumen of a hepatic vein and both free and occlusion (wedge) pressures can be obtained with ease (Novak *et al.*, 1977).

Indications

Cirrhosis of the liver with suspected portal hypertension

The normal wedge pressure lies between 8 and 12 mmHg (Ruzicka *et al.*, 1972). If the figure does not exceed this range in a patient being investigated for suspected portal hypertension, the diagnosis is refuted and the study terminated. When there is elevation of the wedge pressure, it is necessary to obtain a corrected pressure by subtracting the wedge pressure reading from the free hepatic venous pressure. This is because there are many factors which may raise the wedge pressure, including (i) heart failure; (ii) compression of the hepatic portion of the inferior vena cava; and (iii) any cause of raised intra-abdominal pressure such as ascites. The normal gradient between wedged and free hepatic vein pressure is 3–5 mmHg. Higher values indicate the degree of elevated intrasinusoidal pres-

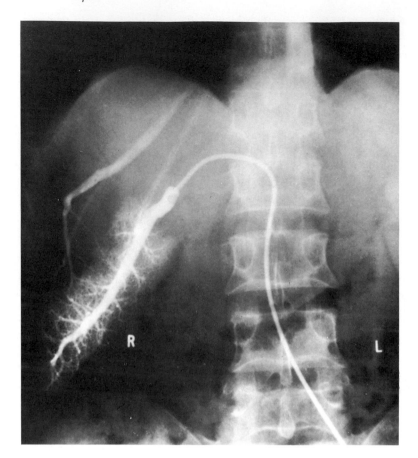

Fig. 11.13 Occlusion balloon catheter hepatic venography. Normal study. Note filling of hepatic vein radicles (5th and 6th divisions) in a subsegment of the right lobe and free flow to other patent hepatic veins.

sure due to disease, for instance cirrhosis, affecting the sinusoidal or postsinusoidal territories. Such patients have similar elevation of their splenic pulp pressures, in contradistinction to the group of patients with either presinusoidal portal blocks or extrahepatic portal venous obstruction who will have normal corrected venous hepatic pressures yet raised splenic pulp pressure. Thus pressure readings taken on both sides of the liver indicate the causative level of portal hypertension.

A corrected wedge pressure of 5–10 mmHg is considered slightly elevated, 10–15 mmHg being moderately raised, while greater than 15 mmHg represents marked elevation (Cavaluzzi *et al.*, 1977). The appearance of a hepatic venogram with a balloon inflated in the main trunk of a vein may provide a useful assessment in cirrhosis, the extent of pruning and irregularity correlating closely with the severity of the liver disease (Van Leeuwen *et al.*, 1989).

Portal hypertension patients before or after shunt surgery

Should only a small pressure difference exist between the corrected hepatic pressure in an inferior vena cava compressed by an irregular liver, it can be predicted that a portosystemic shunt will not function well. In patients with established surgical shunts, the hepatic venous study permits pressure measurements and shows altered haemodynamics, including newly developed portosplanchnic collaterals.

Suspected Budd–Chiari syndrome (BCS)

Hepatic vein obstruction is often due to thrombosis affecting either large or multiple small veins. Thrombosis may result from hypercoagulability states, venous invasion by neoplasms, or some unknown

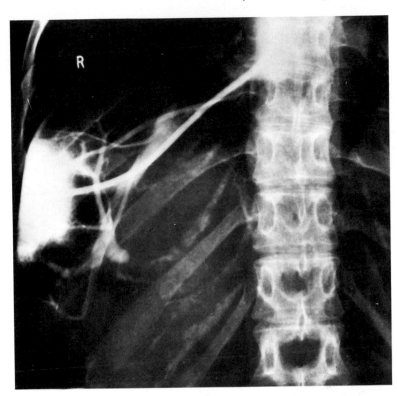

Fig. 11.14 Wedge hepatic venogram. Normal study. The catheter has been introduced from an antecubital vein and has wedged peripherally in the liver. Contrast medium demonstrates normal sinusoidogram and flow to portal vein branches as well as other hepatic veins. Direct injection of contrast medium following this type of wedge catheter is undesirable.

cause. Occasionally, obstruction is due to a congenital venous web, dilatable by a balloon catheter using the technique described above. In BCS it is necessary to take pressure measurements in the inferior vena cava and hepatic veins. The wedge pressure will be elevated, a corrected reading being important since most patients have ascites. Thrombus in a hepatic vein allows only partial entry of a catheter. When the catheter is impeded, 20 ml of injected contrast medium demonstrates a 'spider's web' and no sinusoidogram. The web probably represents multiple small tortuous collateral veins (Sherlock & Dooley, 1993) (Fig. 11.15). Thrombi can cause intraluminal filling defects, or extend into the cava. In complete thrombosis, it may be impossible to catheterize any hepatic vein, although there may be sparing of multiple small veins draining the caudate lobe.

Inferior venacavography must be undertaken in both anteroposterior (AP) and lateral projections, the first showing side-to-side narrowing due to hepatomegaly and the latter demonstrating a prominent anterior shelf indenting the high hepatic portion of the inferior vena cava as a result of liver swelling and caudate lobe hypertrophy. Thrombus may also be seen in the inferior vena cava.

Contraindications

There are no absolute contraindications to the safe technique of hepatic venography.

Complications

None should occur providing balloon catheters are used. Contrast medium injected through simple wedged catheters may cause pain, local necrosis and seepage of contrast medium under the capsule. A push-through effect of contrast medium from any injection at a peripheral site in a hepatic vein may cause a degree of retrograde filling of the portal venous system. Although this may occur in normal subjects, gross retrograde flow

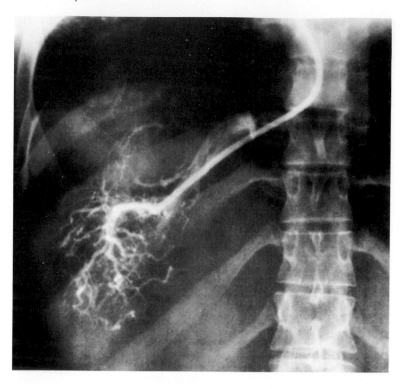

Fig. 11.15 Wedge hepatic venogram in Budd–Chiari syndrome. The catheter is unable to pass any further along the hepatic vein and injection of contrast medium demonstrates a spider's web pattern of numerous collateral hepatoportal and hepatocapsular veins.

into the extrahepatic portal vein indicates hepatofugal flow within it.

Relationship to other techniques

Ultrasound and CT regularly show hepatic veins, Duplex doppler studies giving even fuller information. The precise anatomy or pathology of the entire tree is best shown by catheter hepatic venography. Accurate pressure studies are generally of more clinical value than the venous angiogram, although there is a general agreement that cirrhosis causes several alterations in the unsupported hepatic veins before affecting the portal vein.

If it is impossible to enter hepatic veins in suspected BCS, Ruzicka *et al.* (1972) recommend transhepatic intraparenchymal angiography (hepatography). Here a percutaneously introduced catheter forces the liver parenchyma to handle 20 ml contrast medium delivered over 6 s. Contrast medium leaves the liver either by the portal vein, from reversed or hepatofugal flow, or by a network of multiple intercommunicating collaterals which are probably of both portal and hepatic origin and enter

capsular veins. In this way a suspected diagnosis of complete hepatic vein outflow obstruction is confirmed. Earlier in the patient's course, an isotope scan may have shown pronounced uptake in the caudate lobe, while hepatic arteriography demonstrated 'pseudometastases' within the liver as a result of sinusoidal stasis.

Transvenous liver biopsy

In patients with severe coagulopathy, liver biopsy may be performed from either the transjugular or the transfemoral route. If necessary, transjugular liver biopsy using the long Ross or Brockenburg needle may be combined with hepatic venography at the same session. The procedure is safe, with low morbidity and mortality, any bleeding subsequent to biopsy being into the patient's own circulation.

More recently, Teare *et al.* (1994) described a transfemoral technique. Transfemoral access is familiar to most radiologists and the technique uses long curved biopsy forceps which are passed through an 11F sheath placed in the femoral vein. Inside this sheath is an inner 9F sheath with a 5 cm diameter distal curve and this end is guided into the proximal right hepatic vein. Specimens are small and multiple passes are undertaken. The procedure is safe provided a postbiopsy venogram is done to demonstrate the biopsy tract and ensure no perforation has occurred. Should a leak be demonstrated, it must be sealed with a wire coil.

Image-guided percutaneous liver biopsy should be in the armamentarium of any general radiologist. There are a variety of automatic spring-loaded biopsy devices available, some being disposable. It is advisable in any patient with a bleeding tendency to embolize the tract, either by introducing the biopsy needle through a sheath or removing the central core of the needle which contains the specimen, immediately after the biopsy and so allowing embolization through the outer cannula of the apparatus.

A comparison of transjugular and plugged percutaneous liver biopsy shows that the latter is quicker to perform and provides large specimens but does carry a minimal but real haemorrhagic risk (Sawyer *et al.*, 1993).

Transjugular intrahepatic portosystemic stent shunts

Rosch *et al.* (1987) were the first to describe in animals the use of an expanding metal stent to link the portal and hepatic venous systems. This followed much earlier experimental work. Shunts in humans had been described 4 years earlier, but their patency was limited as the tract was merely dilated with a balloon. Current clinical enthusiasm for TIPSS follows the development of metallic expandable stents in humans in 1990 by Richter *et al*.

Indications

1 Treatment of acute haemorrhage in patients with portal hypertension, oesophageal/gastric varices or ectopic varices such as occur at an ileostomy.
2 Control of recurrent haemorrhage following failed endoscopic sclerotherapy.
3 As a prelude to liver transplant in patients with chronic liver disease and portal hypertension.
4 Control of intractable ascites.

Technique

It is helpful if the patient has had Doppler ultrasonography and/or superior mesenteric angiography to access the patency and flow in the portal vein. An approach via the right internal jugular vein under local anaesthesia is recommended. A 9F introducer set and sheath* is inserted into the jugular vein and used to cannulate the right or middle hepatic vein under fluoroscopy control. A simple cardiac transseptal sheathed needle may be used, although several assemblies are available commercially (Fig. 11.16). The Ritcher set may prove to be the least traumatic since, after removal of the mandrel, a blunt-ended cannula remains in the hepatic vein.

The stages of the procedure are shown in Fig. 11.17. The most difficult parts of TIPSS are finding the portal vein, then the formation of a tract between the right hepatic vein and the selected right portal vein branch. For this a floppy-tipped heavy duty 0.035 in. guide wire (Amplatz extra-stiff†) is recommended. The blunt end of the wire is initially introduced into the cannula and thence directed anteriorly through the liver parenchyma towards the portal vein radicle, the latter being identified by an experienced ultrasonographer working via a right intercostal space.

With optimum factors, the confidence and orientation of the ultrasonographer in the team being vital, the echogenic wire is clearly seen. If necessary the direction of the needle is altered, so that the wire is seen to indent and enter the portal vein. The cannula is now advanced over the wire into the vein and the wire removed. Aspiration during fractional withdrawal of the cannula will yield free flow of portal venous blood, checking with contrast medium to indicate the length of the tract to be bridged, following which the floppy end of the guide wire may be introduced and passed deeply into the superior mesenteric vein. After a short contrast study, a pressure measurement is taken in the portal system and compared with that in the right atrium, this latter pressure being taken via the side-arm of an introducer sheath.

* William Cook (UK) Ltd, Letchworth, Hertfordshire, UK.
† Boston Scientific Co., UK.

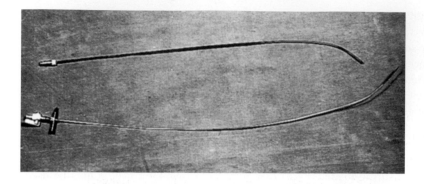

Fig. 11.16 Standard 16 gauge transjugular biopsy needle and sheath. The needle tip is available with standard or reversed bevel (William Cook Europe).

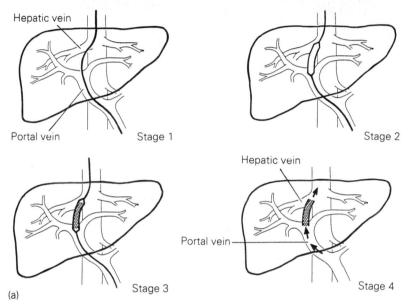

(a)

Fig. 11.17 (a) Four stages of transjugular intrahepatic portosystemic stent shunt (TIPSS).

An extra-stiff exchange wire is now introduced, the added length being required since many metal stents are carried on a long catheter. Next a 5F low-profile balloon dilating catheter (8 mm diameter balloon) is passed over the wire and through the liver tract, the tract then being fully dilated. This part of the procedure is painful and the patient may require 25–50 mg i.v. pethidine. It is especially important to dilate the portal and hepatic venous ends of the tract.

A metallic prosthesis of suitable length and diameter for the tract is selected. Both Wallstent* and Memorex† stents are satisfactory, the latter being

especially radio-opaque, available in a choice of diameters up to 12 mm and undergoing minimal shortening during its expansion. Prior to stent release, the sheath in the neck must be withdrawn several centimetres so that its lower end is well above the hepatic vein/right atrial junction, otherwise the proximal part of the stent will not open. With the stent open, a repeat portogram is obtained to show shunt patency (Fig. 11.18) and further pressures are taken in the portal vein and right atrium. Portal pressure should drop significantly, so that the post-TIPSS gradient between portal and systemic venous systems should be 10 mmHg or less. The sheath assembly is removed from the neck and the patient returned to intensive care or the ward. A follow-up Doppler is important in the next 48 hours and is

* Surgimed, UK.
† Angiomed, UK.

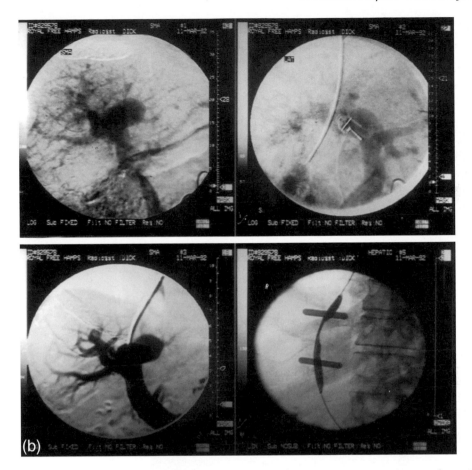

Fig. 11.17 *Continued.* (b) TIPSS study. Top images (from left): venous phase superior mesenteric artery (sometimes performed immediately prior to TIPSS); needle pass towards portal vein, needle too distal and readjusted. Lower images (from left): portal vein entered with needle and wire, then balloon dilatation of tract.

repeated after 3 months, when repeated TIPSS portography from the jugular or femoral route may be undertaken (Fig. 11.19) and, if necessary, lavage of the shunt performed.

Many series show TIPSS to succeed in over 90% of patients and, once the steep learning curve is mastered, the procedure takes less than 2 hours (McCormick *et al.*, 1993). Embolization of gastro-oesophageal collaterals may also be undertaken at the time of TIPSS.

Complications

1 Haemoperitoneum. This is the most feared com-plication, but will occur only if the portal vein has been punctured extrahepatically. It could also result from a tear in the liver capsule during earlier at-tempts at TIPSS when using a percutaneous transhepatic approach.

2 Accelerated liver failure in Childs–Pugh B or C pa-tients. Any deviation of blood supply from the liver via a shunt can sometimes precipitate early liver fail-ure and death.

3 Septicaemia. Antibiotic cover is necessary in all cases and a rigorous aseptic technique must be observed, as many series report deaths from sepsis.

4 Encephalopathy. As with surgical shunts, this is an expected complication of TIPSS. It is usually

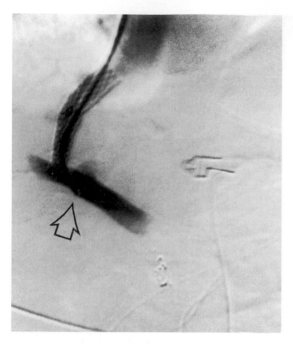

Fig. 11.18 Good functioning transjugular intrahepatic portosystemic stent shunt. Note some preserved blood flow to liver. Arrow, portal vein.

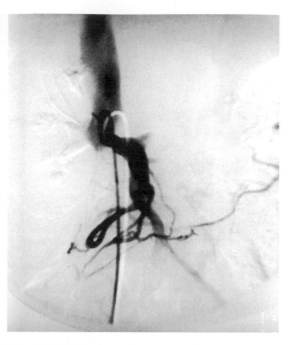

Fig. 11.20 Digital subtraction angiography: patent surgical portocaval shunt. A sidewinder Z-shaped catheter has passed from inferior vena cava into portal vein.

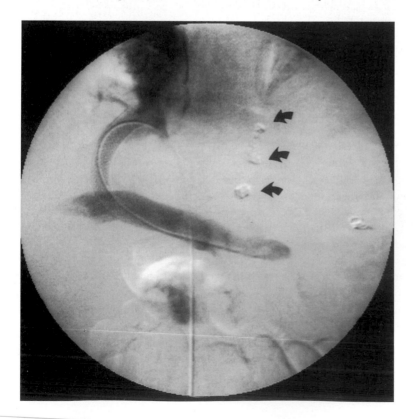

Fig. 11.19 Follow-up study of transjugular intrahepatic portosystemic stent shunt via femoral vein confirms patency at 3 months. Arrows indicate coils in the left gastric vein which was embolized via the stent during initial procedure.

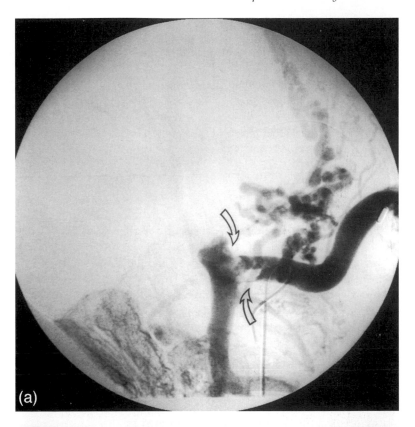

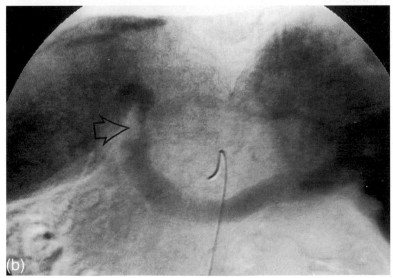

Fig. 11.21 (a) Superior mesenteric artery — venous phase; 24 hours after liver transplantation the portal vein has acutely occluded with thrombus which extends to splenic vein (arrows). Note reversed flow into collaterals. Treatment: surgery. (b) Coeliac arteriogram — venous phase. A portal vein stenosis has developed 1 year after transplantation (arrow).

satisfactorily treated clinically and only on rare occasions will it be necessary to narrow an existing shunt by placing a further stent inside the initial one.

5 Intimal hyperplasia. With time, all metal stents will develop some intimal overgrowth. If excessive, this can be treated by balloon angioplasty or restenting. There is no evidence that chemical thrombolysis is of benefit. Atherectomy devices have not yet been employed.

Relationship to other techniques

TIPSS is performed as either an emergency or an elective procedure.

In the former, resuscitation with blood products and clotting factors is the first line of patient management. TIPSS patients are often gravely ill, being on life support with a Sengstaken tube *in situ*.

An arteriogram and serum α-protein are important in the work-up. These will exclude underlying tumour. The angiogram will confirm the presence of a patent portal vein immediately before the TIPSS commences. Surgical cover is also required for TIPSS although the recorded mortality rate (5%) is considerably less than for surgical shunts performed in acute variceal bleeding.

Surgical portosystemic shunts

Should malfunction or occlusion be suspected, Doppler studies are the first investigation. If thought to be non-definitive or abnormal, the shunt may be entered from the inferior vena cava and its state and patency shown together with the pressure gradient (Fig. 11.20). Percutaneous angioplasty may be successful in treating an occluding shunt (Sherlock & Dooley, 1993).

Hepatic transplantation

Portal and hepatic vein status is clarified by the methods described above (Fig. 11.21). An acute portal vein thrombosis is an emergency, whereas stenosis of hepatic or portal veins may be considered for elective angioplasty.

References

Abeatici, S. & Campi, L. (1951) La visualizzazione radiologica della porta via splenica. *Minerva Med.*, **42**, 593–605.

Brazzini, A., Hunter, D.W., Darcy, M.D. *et al.* (1987) Safe splenoportography. *Radiology*, **162**, 607–9.

Burcharth, F. & Aagaard, J. (1988) Total hepatofugal portal blood flow in cirrhosis demonstrated by transhepatic portography. *Fortschr. Rontgenstr.*, **148**, 47–9

Calaluzzi, J.A., Sheff, R., Harrington, D.P. *et al.* (1977) Hepatic venography and wedge hepatic vein pressure measurements in diffuse liver disease. *AJR*, **129**, 441–6.

Dick, R. & Gibson, M. (1993) Imaging for planned hepatic resection. *Ann. Chir. Gynaecol.*, **82**, 109–16.

Dilawari, J.B., Chawla, Y.K., Raju, G.S. *et al.* (1987) Safety of splenoportovenography as an outpatient procedure. *Lancet*, **i**, 101.

Kimura-Tsuchiqa, Y., Ohto, M., Ono, T. *et al.* (1981) Single puncture method for percutaneous transhepatic portography using a thin needle. *Radiology*, **139**, 748–9.

Kreel, L. & Williams, R. (1964) Arteriovenography of the protal system. *Br. Med. J.*, **2**, 1500–3.

Lunderquist, A. & Vang, J. (1974) Transhepatic catheterization and obliteration of the coronary vein in patients with portal hypertension and oesophageal varices. *N. Engl. J. Med.*, **290**, 646–9.

McCormick, P.A., Dick, R., Chin, J. *et al.* (1993). Transjugular intrahepatic portosystemic stent shunt. *Br. J. Hosp. Med.*, **49**, 791–7.

Novak, D., Butzow, G.H. & Becker, K. (1977) Hepatic occlusion venography with a balloon catheter in portal hypertension. *Radiology*, **122**, 623–8.

Richter, G.M., Noeldge, G. & Palmaz, J.C. (1990) The transjugular intrahepatic portosystemic shunt (TIPSS); results of a pilot study. *J. Cardiovasc. Intervent. Radiol.* **3**, 200.

Rosch, J., Uchida, B.T., Putnam, J.S. *et al.* (1987) Experimental intrahepatic portocaval anastomosis: use of expandable Gianturco stents. *Radiology,* **162**, 481–5.

Ruzicka, F.F. Jr, Carilo, F.J., d'Alesandro, D. & Rossi, P. (1972) The hepatic wedge pressure and venogram vs. the hepatic intraparenchmal liver pressure and venogram. *Radiology*, **102**, 252–8.

Sawyer, A.M., McCormick, P.A., Dick, R. *et al.* (1993) A comparison of transjugular and plugged percutaneous liver biopsy techniques in patients with impaired coagulation. *J. Hepatol.*, **17**, 81–5.

Sherlock, S. & Dooley, J.S. (1993) The hepatic artery and veins. *In* Sherlock, S. & Dooley, J.S. (eds) *Diseases of the Liver and Biliary System*. Blackwell Scientific Publications, London.

Smith-Laing, G., Scott, J., Long, R.G. *et al.* (1981) Role of percutaneous transhepatic obliteration of varices in the management of haemorrhage from gastro-oesophageal varices. *Gastroenterology*, **80**, 1031–6.

Teare, J.P. Watkinson, A.F., Erb, S.G. *et al.* (1994) Transfemoral liver biopsy — a review of 104 consecutive procedures. *J. Cardiovasc. Intervent. Radiology* (in press).

Van Leeuwen, D.R. Sherlock, S., Scheuer, P.J. & Dick, R. (1989) Wedged hepatic venous pressure recording and venography for the assessment of precirr-

hotic and cirrhotic liver disease. *Scand. J. Gastroent.*, **24**, 65–73.

Warren, J.V. & Brannon, E.S. (1944) A method for obtaining blood samples directly from the hepatic vein in man. *Proc. Soc. Exp. Biol. Med.*, **55**, 144–6.

Zannini, G., Masciariello, S., Sangiulo, P. *et al.* (1979) Splenoportographie: une technique toujours actuelle. Nouvelles perspective. *J. Chir.*, **116**, 577–82.

12 Digital Subtraction Angiography

J. F. COCKBURN AND A. P. HEMINGWAY

Digital subtraction angiography (DSA) has been shown to be as useful as conventional angiography in many vascular territories (Goldberg *et al.*, 1986; Lee *et al.*, 1986; Roeren *et al.*, 1986; Kim *et al.*, 1991; Smith *et al.*, 1992). It is now the standard, not only because its efficacy rivals the conventional technique despite its lesser spatial resolution, but also because of its excellent contrast resolution, ease of use and relative cost-effectiveness. There are still circumstances where the spatial resolution of conventional angiography may be desirable, for instance in the investigation of an occult bleeding lesion in the gastrointestinal tract. However, it is rare for rapid sequence analogue films to disclose a lesion in the presence of a perfectly normal and technically ideal digital subtraction angiogram.

DSA is a *sine qua non* for many vascular interventional procedures, particularly embolization, because it allows instantaneous imaging of the vascular occlusion as it happens. The recent advances in embolization and other transcatheter therapies, including improvements in coaxial catheter, guide wire and balloon technology, have been prompted by the ability of DSA to allow monitoring of therapy with unprecedented accuracy.

In the 12 years since the first edition of this book (Whitehouse & Worthington, 1983) the importance of angiography as a diagnostic tool has reduced considerably. Colour Doppler ultrasound has made significant inroads into areas which were the exclusive preserve of angiography, for instance the diagnosis of extracranial carotid disease, although the angiogram remains the gold standard in this area. Ultrasound serves as an excellent, cheap screening tool in this particular situation but cannot be relied upon as the sole preoperative test. Peripheral angioplasty performed solely under ultrasound control is being investigated in several centres. The introduction of ultrasound contrast media is likely to lead to an even greater role for this modality in the assessment of vessels and vascularity.

Spiral contrast-enhanced computed tomography (CT) with three-dimensional reconstruction allows the exquisite depiction of vascular anatomy without the need for central vascular access. Abdominal aortic aneurysms and their relationship to the renal arteries are particularly well demonstrated using this technique, and surgery can be adequately planned without the need for angiography in most cases.

Magnetic resonance angiography (MRA) is making progressively greater inroads into the assessment of vasculature, in particular of the cerebral circulation (Furuya *et al.*, 1992; Chiesa *et al.*, 1993). Although it is likely to become the initial technique of choice for the identification of intracerebral aneurysms in the future (Gouliamos *et al.*, 1992), the mainstay of preoperative planning in patients with subarachnoid haemorrhage remains the 'four-vessel angiogram' (Schuierer *et al.*, 1992).

It is clear, therefore, that DSA is being challenged on several fronts. In order to understand why it will continue to be a valuable diagnostic modality, providing information unavailable by other techniques, it is necessary to understand what is being imaged and the mode of image production.

Physical principles (Fig. 12.1)

An ideal subtraction image shows only those blood vessels which contain radiographic contrast medium, the bones, bowel gas and soft tissues having been subtracted. Prior to the advent of DSA, subtraction was performed photographically after completion of an examination. It was not possible to enhance or manipulate the information contained in these images, nor was it possible to correct for patient movement. In DSA, a computer-based technology,

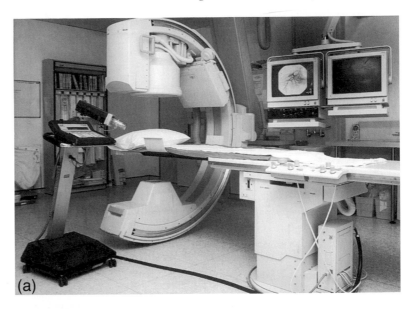

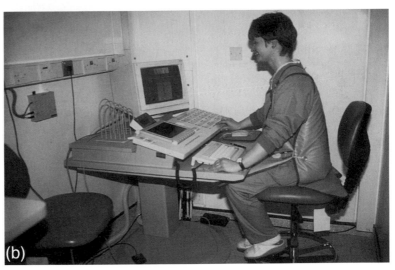

Fig. 12.1 (a) State-of-the-art digital subtraction angiography equipment — a Philips Integris V3000. (b) The operating console.

virtually instantaneous subtracted images are displayed provided that at least one 'mask' is obtained at the start of an angiographic sequence or 'run'. The mask is no more than a simple digital radiograph of the area to be examined, acquired via the image intensifier–television chain prior to the arrival of the contrast medium. An example is shown in Fig. 12.2a. Assuming that this mask is the first image to have been acquired in the sequence, the digital informa-

tion contained within this radiograph is logarithmically subtracted from every subsequent image taken during the injection of the contrast medium. In theory even the smallest change in contrast between the mask and subsequent images can be displayed. In practice this is not possible because of the noise inherent in the images. Successful subtraction requires that the density of contrast medium exceeds the background noise level. Satisfactory images can be achieved with concentrations of contrast medium far lower than required for conventional angiography. Figures 12.2b and 12.2c show what happens when the mask image in Fig. 12.2a is subtracted from images taken during and after the injection of contrast medium. The computer has removed bone and soft tissue from the images. The advantages in terms of increasing the conspicuity of pathological lesions are obvious. Movement caused by breathing, bowel peristalsis or patient movement creates artefacts which are not present on the mask. During the process of electronic subtraction, the computer renders these changes opaque. Such opaque artefacts corrupt the images and may lead to errors in diagnosis. A summary of techniques to minimize artefacts is presented later in this chapter.

Unlike conventional angiography, which relies on film processing to produce hard-copy images for diagnostic purposes, digitally subtracted images appear virtually instantaneously on the VDU screen. The angiographer can see immediately if the examination is satisfactory and, of equal importance, can terminate an examination if all is not well. This is particularly important during embolization and other interventional procedures when the timing of the cessation of the procedure is crucial to its safety and success.

The data can be reviewed immediately at the end of a sequence and a variety of postprocessing algorithms can be applied to improve the image and allow qualitative and quantitative analysis. The available processes differ widely between various machines and manufacturers.

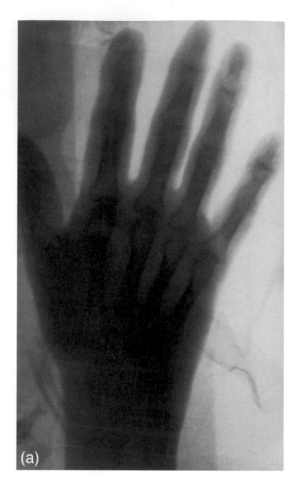

(a)

Fig. 12.2 (a) 'Mask' image for a 'digitally subtracted' digital angiogram.

Qualitative processing techniques

1 Magnification/zoom. The basic image is made up of pixels in either a 512×512 or a 1024×1024 matrix. In simple $\times 2$ magnification or zoom, each pixel is increased to four pixels, each containing the same data. In another technique, known as interpolation, the pixels in the area of interest are expanded to fill the entire 512×512 matrix and those pixels in between are electronically calculated.

2 Pixel-shifting/reregistration. This process allows the mask to be shifted relative to a subsequent contrast-containing image in order to correct for artefacts

created by patient movement. Newer machines such as that illustrated in Figure. 12.1 allow the mask to be shifted using a computer mouse controller. Pixel shift often allows the retrieval of diagnostic information from what would otherwise be an unsatisfactory image.

3 Vascular tracing/picture integration allows data from, for example, an early arterial phase to be added to those from a later image in the study so that the final image shows contrast in all areas of the vascular tree.

4 Contour enhancement/crisping allows a sharper image to be produced, improves the visibility of smaller vessels and allows see-through when two vessels cross each other.

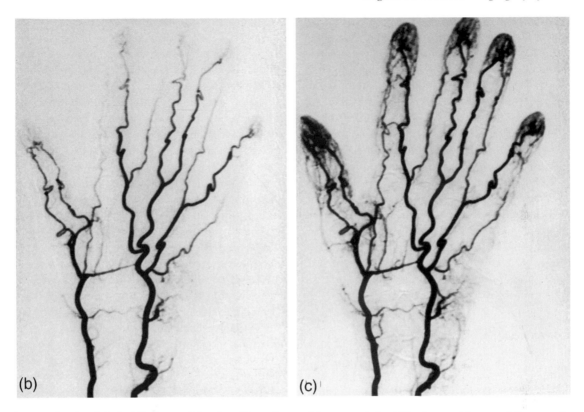

(b)

(c)

Fig. 12.2 *Continued.* (b & c) Early arterial and capillary phases of the same study. All background bone, soft tissue and so on, have been subtracted.

Quantitative processing techniques

1 Length of measurement allows structures in the image to be measured by reference to an object of known length, for instance a catheter with centimetre markers. It is important to remember that the reference object may be in a different geometric plane from the structure being measured.

2 Vessel analysis is an attempt at quantification of stenoses within vessels. Different manufacturers employ different algorithms for this type of analysis. The vessel diameter at the site of the stenosis is determined in relation to a non-stenotic area and is expressed as a percentage patency. The analysis is usually based on contrast density and many, but not all, computer programs assume that the vessel's lumen is circular at the point of measurement, which is rarely true in atheromatous stenoses.

Image storing/archiving

Initially data are stored on a hard disk from which transfer to floppy, compact or optical disc can be made. Where picture archiving and communications systems (PACS) are in operation, the data on optical disc can be stored in a jukebox for future rapid retrieval. The data are usually sent to a laser imager for the production of hard copy.

Digital subtraction angiography in practice

Contrast medium may be introduced into the vascular tree either i.v. or intra-arterially. The principal differences between the two techniques are the quality of the angiographic result (superior with i.a. injections) and the invasiveness of the procedure (less with the i.v. technique). The initial enthusiasm for i.v. DSA has not been sustained, not only because of the considerably superior images obtainable using arterial DSA, but also because the smaller catheters now available have made the arterial route safer and less invasive than before. Furthermore, arterial studies permit transcatheter therapy, for instance balloon dilation of a stenosis or thrombolysis at the time of the examination. Many departments now perform out-patient arterial studies, although there is an increased risk of complications at the puncture site caused by early ambulation. Intravenous DSA may be performed safely on out-patients but, as Dawson (1988) has argued, many of the patients referred specifically for i.v. DSA are unsuitable for this examination either because poor image quality is to be expected and/or because the large load of contrast medium inherent in this type of examination is undesirable.

Intravenous DSA

Indications

The indications for i.v. DSA are difficult to summarize dogmatically as the decision to perform this investigation depends on the equipment and degree of expertise available in any given department. The authors have observed that those departments with state-of-the-art equipment which can produce excellent i.v. DSA tend to use that equipment to produce the best arterial images. Some of the indications for i.v. DSA that have been described in the literature are shown in Table 12.1.

Table 12.1 Indications for i.v. digital subtraction angiography

Extracranial carotid arterial disease (Fig. 12.3)
Subclavian artery disease (Fig. 12.4)
Aortic arch anomalies
Pulmonary embolic disease
Pulmonary vascular anomalies (Fig. 12.5)
Abdominal aortic anomalies (Figs 12.6 & 12.7)
Renal vascular disease
Visceral artery stenosis
Peripheral vascular disease
Postoperative graft follow-up (Fig. 12.8)

The least controversial indication for i.v. DSA is the assessment of proximal disease in large arteries. Good examples are the evaluation of suspected aortic disease (see Figs 12.6 & 12.7), and preoperative renal artery assessment in young transplant donors. Problems with the i.v. technique begin when smaller calibre vessels need to be assessed. Such problems occur when trying to define its role in the diagnosis of renal artery stenosis. Intravenous DSA is good at detecting proximal stenoses due to atheroma (Wilms et al., 1986; Dunnick et al., 1989) but some authors have found it disappointing when the pathology lies more distally (Illescas et al., 1988). Intravenous DSA is generally not used for the assessment of transplant kidney arterial supply, as the volume of contrast medium required in these patients should be kept to a minimum. A typical i.v. study in this situation might require 100 ml of contrast medium whereas arterial injections can demonstrate the arterial supply in greater detail using a fraction of this amount (Roeren et al., 1986).

Follow-up DSA studies of peripheral arterial grafts lend themselves to i.v. injection of contrast medium as the entire graft, including both the proximal and distal anastomoses, can be satisfactorily demonstrated without puncturing them (Ameli et al., 1991) (Fig. 12.8). Some vascular surgeons insist on operating on 'virgin' femoral arteries and, in this situation, i.v. DSA can successfully demonstrate proximal atheromatous disease.

The assessment of extracranial carotid disease (see Fig. 12.3) using i.v. DSA is contentious (Cebul & Paulus, 1986; Crocker et al., 1986; Borgstein et al., 1991). As already mentioned, this technique is at its best when proximal disease is present. Distal carotid or intracerebral disease is less likely to be picked up by the i.v. technique. However, selective i.a. DSA of the carotid arteries has a permanent neurological deficit rate of 0.3–1% (Waugh & Sacharias, 1992; Warnock et al., 1993). This is felt by some to be a strong argument in favour of i.v. DSA (Stevens et al., 1989), particularly when this technique is accompanied by Doppler ultrasound examination.

Complete cessation of cerebral blood flow is the single best sign of brain death and some believe it should be demonstrated before brain death is declared (Nau et al., 1992). Intravenous DSA is reliable in diagnosing this state (Vatne et al., 1985).

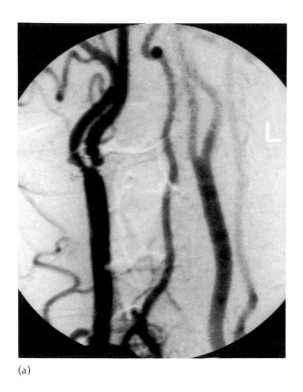

(a)

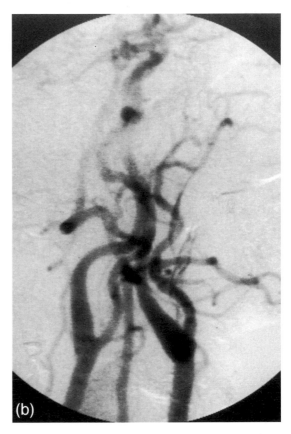

(b)

Fig. 12.3 Intravenous digital subtraction angiography (DSA) of extracranial carotid vessels in the left anterior oblique projection. The left bifurcation is normal. Severe atheromatous narrowing of the right bifurcation involving the internal and external carotid vessels is clearly seen. (b) Intravenous DSA study of the extracranial carotid vessels.

Relative contraindications to i.v. DSA are a history of severe allergy or previous contrast medium reaction, the presence of congestive cardiac failure or other low-output states, renal failure (because of the effects of large volumes of contrast medium) and conditions requiring detail which cannot be achieved with the technique, such as small intracranial vascular pathology, or the demonstration of extremity arcades.

Technique

Most i.v. DSA examinations are performed on an out-patient basis. Contrast medium is delivered, under sterile conditions, as a bolus into the venous system and images of the arterial tree in the area of interest are obtained during the first pass of con-

trast medium. It is possible to deliver an adequate volume (35–40 ml) of contrast medium at a fast enough rate (20–25 ml s^{-1}) into a vein in the antecubital fossa via a short wide-bore cannula, for instance the Venflon (Meaney, 1982; Ludwig, 1986), but there is a greater risk of venous rupture with this technique compared with central delivery of contrast medium. If this route is chosen, non-ionic contrast media must be employed to minimize potential complications.

In order to deliver the contrast medium centrally a 4 or 5 French (F) high-flow catheter, either pig-tail or straight with open end and multiple side-holes (Table 12.2) is introduced under local anaesthetic into the superior vena cava or right atrium. Venous access is invariably obtained in one or other antecubital fossa. Ideally, the operator should choose the basilic

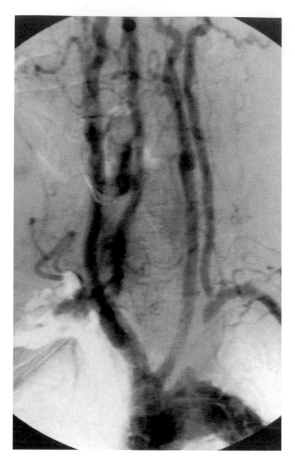

Fig. 12.4 Intravenous digital subtraction angiography in a patient suspected clinically of having a subclavian steal syndrome. The occluded portion of the left subclavian artery is clearly visible.

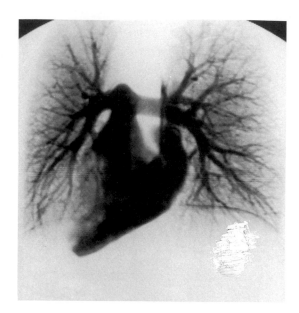

Fig. 12.5 Intravenous digital subtraction angiography in a child with suspected pulmonary vascular anomalies. Contrast medium was injected via a 5F central catheter. Further projections were performed and were all normal, thus excluding pulmonary artery branch vessel stenosis.

vein as this poses very few problems for negotiation of the axillary and subclavian veins.

The patient lies with the right arm lying on an arm rest at 45° to the table. A loose tourniquet is positioned high above the elbow and the upper and lower arm are swabbed with antiseptic solution. After drapes are applied, leaving only the antecubital fossa exposed, the tourniquet is inflated and an 18 gauge cannula is inserted into the basilic vein using a single wall puncture technique. Either an 0.035 J-shaped or Newton cerebral 15 cm floppy tip wire is introduced into the cannula and guided up the arm under continuous screening. If even slight resistance is met (this usually happens first at the junction of axillary and subclavian vein) no further advancement

is attempted; the wire is withdrawn slightly, and the cannula removed while applying pressure over the venous entry site. The vessel is dilated to the appropriate size and the catheter delivered over the wire. The properties of the catheter, usually a 65 cm 5F pig-tail catheter, can be employed to negotiate the area of non-advancement. If this is inserted over the wire until only a couple of centimetres of wire remains exposed, taking care to screen continuously during catheter advancement to ensure that the wire does not advance against the area of resistance, it assumes an angled shape which allows the direction of the tip of the wire to be changed when gentle torque is applied to the catheter. It is unusual for this method to fail and one rarely needs to resort to removing the wire and injecting contrast medium to identify the route ahead. In particularly difficult situations, raising the straightened arm to the level of the shoulder or beyond may be useful. If it has proved necessary to puncture a cephalic vein, there is a significant chance that difficulty will be encountered in negotiating the vessel in the region of the claviopectoral fascia. The wide-angled or 15 mm J-tip

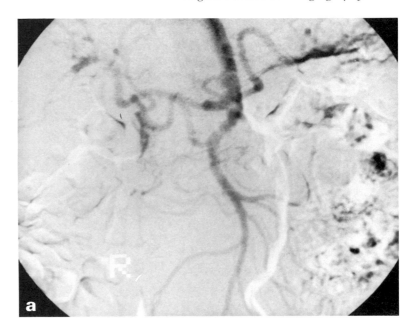

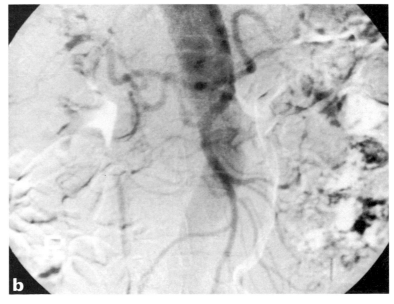

Fig. 12.6 Intravenous digital subtraction angiography in a patient suffering from hypertension and abdominal pain. The early phase study (a) shows filling of the superior mesenteric artery and renal vessels; it is not until a later phase (b) that the aortic lumen is visualized. This confirmed the diagnosis of aortic dissection.

wire or movable-core 3 mm wire is very useful in this situation. Once the subclavian vein is entered, the wire generally passes easily into the superior vena cava. The catheter is then advanced over the wire, which is then withdrawn. The tip of the catheter is left in either the lower superior vena cava or the right atrium. Once positioned, the catheter is kept well flushed with heparinized saline. The injection

pump is loaded with undiluted low-osmolar non-ionic contrast medium and connected to the catheter. Typical injection parameters are 40 ml at 20 ml s^{-1}. A delay is programmed into the computer so that sufficient time elapses between injection of the contrast medium and arterial opacification: 5 s for the aortic arch and 10 s for the aortic bifurcation are acceptable initial delay times. The timing of the second run

Table 12.2 Characteristics of catheters used in digital subtraction angiography

Vessel	Catheter	Contrast delivery volume (ml/ml s^{-1})	Contrast strength (relative to Omnipaque 350 or Urografin 370)	Filming rate frames s^{-1}	Other
Non-selective					
Aortic arch	Pig-tail	45/25	1:3	3	
Abdominal aorta (including renals)	Pig-tail	45/15	1:3	2–3	Buscopan
Peripheral angiography (first two positions)	Pig-tail	35/12	1:3	2	Buscopan
Peripheral angiography (second three positions)	Pig-tail	40/12	1:2	1	
Selective					
Subclavian, carotids	Headhunter or Sidewinder	10 (hand injection)	1:3	3	
Coeliac axis	Sidewinder	36/6	1:2	2	Buscopan
Splenic artery (and indirect splenoportogram)	Sidewinder	36/6	1:2–3:4	1	Buscopan
Superior mesenteric artery	Sidewinder	42/7	1:2	2	Buscopan
Inferior mesenteric artery	Sidewinder	10 (hand injection)	1:3	2	Buscopan
Renal artery	Cobra or Sidewinder	18/6	1:3	2	Buscopan

can be accurately determined by noting when contrast medium first appears on the screen. Bowel relaxation can be achieved with 10–20 mg of hyoscine butylbromide (Buscopan) and great emphasis must be placed on breath-holding. Rapid image acquisition and multiple masks maximize the post-processing capabilities. Each examination is tailored to suit individual problems.

Femoral vein punctures are made with an 18 gauge two-part needle, introduced medial to the common femoral arterial pulse at an angle of 45° to the skin. It is useful to ask the patient to perform a Valsalva manoeuvre during vessel puncture. After inserting the needle as far as its hub, the stylet is removed and suction is applied to the needle with a 5 ml syringe, containing 2 ml of saline, as the needle is slowly withdrawn. This procedure is best performed with the hub of the needle displaced dorsally so that it just touches the skin surface. This causes the needle to

'pop' into the centre of the vessel lumen when it has cleared the posterior wall of the vein. As soon as good flow of venous blood into the syringe is detectable, the syringe is removed and a wire of a size compatible with the catheter is gently introduced under fluoroscopic guidance. The needle is withdrawn, maintaining firm pressure on the puncture site, and a catheter with end-holes and multiple side-holes is introduced over the wire into the upper inferior vena cava or right atrium.

Intra-arterial DSA

Indications

This technique is the 'gold standard' of vascular imaging in many circumstances. Arteriography remains the mainstay for the investigation of peripheral and coronary arterial disease. Many surgeons are un-

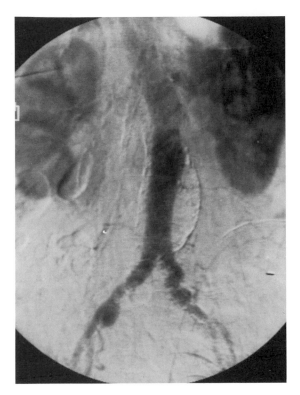

Fig. 12.7 Intravenous digital subtraction angiography in a patient with an aortic aneurysm. Deliberate slight misregistration in the patient clearly shows the aortic lumen and the surrounding unopacified thrombus with calcium in the wall of the aneurysm.

willing to proceed with operations on extracranial carotid disease without i.a. DSA, despite the apparent values of duplex ultrasound, i.v. DSA and MRA (Crocker *et al.*, 1986; Colquhoun *et al.*, 1992; Chiesa *et al.*, 1993) (Fig. 12.9). It is also possible, using i.a. DSA, to study at the same examination the carotid and peripheral vascular territories in a patient with widespread vascular disease. Similarly, i.a. angiography persists in major neurosurgical centres as the definitive procedure for the detection of intracerebral aneurysms. It also allows the demonstration of normal and variant vascular anatomy in advance of abdominal operations, particularly those involving the hepatic arterial and portal venous systems (Figs 12.10 & 12.11). Intra-arterial DSA has a major role in the diagnosis of pancreatic neuroendocrine tumours, as well as other functioning endocrine tumours, by facilitating venous sampling. DSA in the

assessment of the trauma patient is of major importance but is becoming progressively underrated with the advent of contrast-enhanced CT. This is regrettable as even major arterial injury may be missed using the latter technique.

Excellent studies of abdominal vessels can be obtained, provided meticulous attention is paid to reducing motion artefact (Figs 12.12 & 12.13).

Despite their limitations, contrast and non-contrast enhanced Doppler ultrasound, spiral CT and MRA are likely to progressively encroach on the territory of diagnostic i.a. DSA, particularly as they are able to demonstrate anatomy and pathology outside the vessel lumen. Technological advances in these areas are forging ahead while recent improvements in DSA are limited in comparison. The introduction of carbon dioxide as a contrast medium is one of the more exciting developments in DSA, promising a cheap and safe alternative to iodinated media (Weaver *et al.*, 1990, 1991). It remains to be seen how widespread a role this will have in practice.

Good quality diagnostic angiography always precedes transcatheter therapy. This area is one which will not be replaced by new imaging techniques, at least in the foreseeable future. DSA is extremely important in the treatment of acutely bleeding lesions (after surgery, obstetrical delivery or penetrating trauma), arteriovenous fistulas and malformations, and intracranial aneurysms. DSA has facilitated the recent rapid advances in interventional radiological technology and techniques. Vascular stents, caval filters, coaxial catheter embolization systems, coronary and peripheral angioplasty balloon catheters, atherectomy devices and percutaneous devices for treating cardiac septal defects owe their continued existence and development to the ease and speed with which interventional procedures may be performed using DSA compared to conventional angiographic monitoring. The ability of DSA to provide virtually real-time images on the VDU, available for immediate review, is central to its success in interventional procedures. Furthermore, the feature known as road-mapping, which allows the projection of fluoroscopic guide wire manipulation superimposed on an angiographic run, facilitates the catheterization of difficult vessels.

Another very significant advantage of real-time imaging is that the operator has control over the

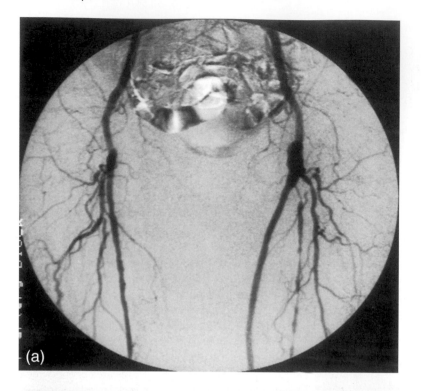

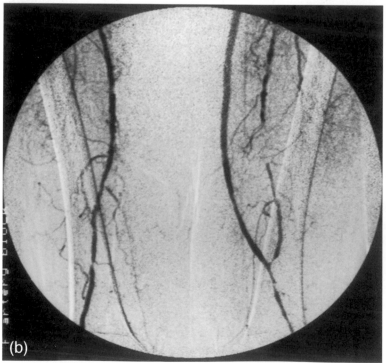

Fig. 12.8 (a) Intravenous digital subtraction angiography showing the upper anastomosis of a left femoropopliteal bypass graft. (b) The lower anastomosis. Severe native vessel disease noted above and below the anastomosis. Some early narrowing of the lower segment of the graft is also noted. There is a tight stenosis of the distal right superficial femoral artery.

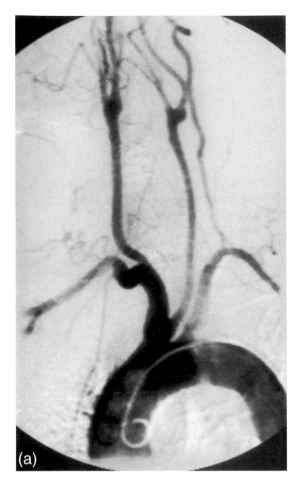

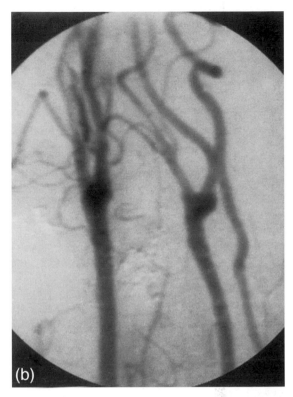

Fig. 12.9 Intra-arterial digital subtraction angiography of extracranial carotid vessels and leg vessels in a patient with severe peripheral vascular disease and transient ischaemic attacks. (a) Left superior oblique arch and great vessels. (b) Magnified view of carotid bifurcations in left anterior oblique projection.

length of each period of data acquisition. An example of this is in peripheral angiography when there is extensive disease and differential flow in the leg vessels. In conventional filming in this situation the flow on one side can frequently be missed, necessitating a repeated injection. In DSA the acquisition continues until all the necessary data are obtained on both sides (Fig. 12.14).

Indirect venography using arterial DSA renders direct splenic puncture unnecessary for demonstrating the portal vein, and allows abdominal venography to be performed (for instance, portal vein, renal vein, superior mesenteric vein) by extending imaging time beyond the arterial phase into the capillary and venous phases. However duplex Doppler ultrasound is increasingly relied upon to demonstrate venous patency in the abdomen. Spiral contrast-enhanced CT can provide much of the same information if the injection of contrast medium is optimally timed.

The indications and contraindications for i.a. DSA are identical to conventional arteriography.

Technique

The principles of arterial puncture and vessel catheterization are exactly the same as for conventional studies (see Chapter 8).

In peripheral studies, the legs are positioned ap-

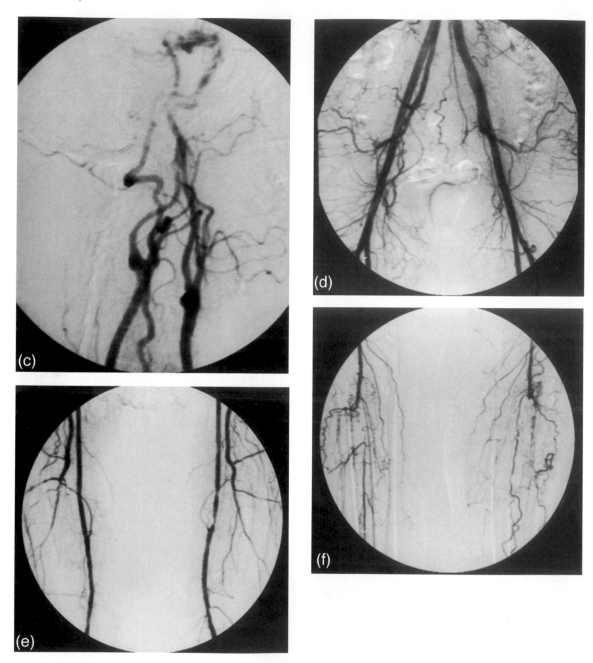

Fig. 12.9 (*Continued*). (c) Right anterior oblique view of carotid bifurcations. (d) Pelvic vessels showing some atheroma of the internal iliac vessels. (e) Superficial femoral arteries (SFAs) and distal profundas. Diffuse atheroma most marked in left SFA. (f) Bilateral severe trifurcation disease. Entire study completed (nine runs plus test shots) with a total of 160 ml Omnipaque 350.

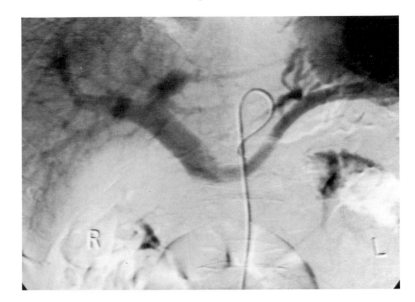

Fig. 12.10 Indirect splenoportogram. Contrast medium (20 ml with approximately 260 mg iodine ml^{-1}) was injected into the splenic artery. Venous phase clearly shows the splenic vein, main portal vein and its right and left intrahepatic branches.

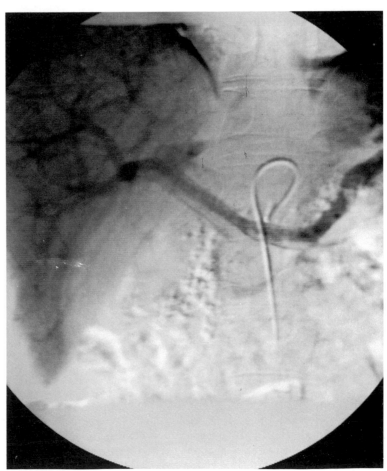

Fig. 12.11 Indirect splenoportogram. This example clearly shows the streaming effect of unopacified blood entering the portal vein from the superior mesenteric vein. Good intrahepatic portal vein detail is also present.

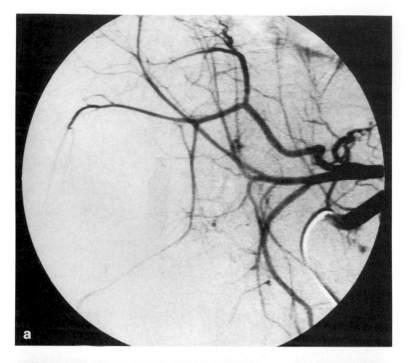

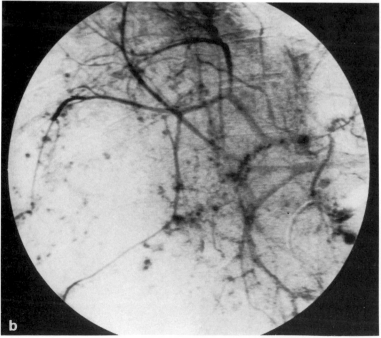

Fig. 12.12 Arterial (a) and capillary (b) phase of a selective hepatic arteriogram in a patient with a large hepatic mass. The vessels are stretched and in the later phase pooling of contrast medium in vascular lakes characteristic of the presence of a benign haemangioma is noted.

propriately prior to the start of the procedure and immobilized by binding them together and securing them to the table top. Pelvic and abdominal studies require attention to breath-holding techniques (Hemingway *et al.*, 1985). Examinations in these territories are conducted in mid-inspiration or mid-

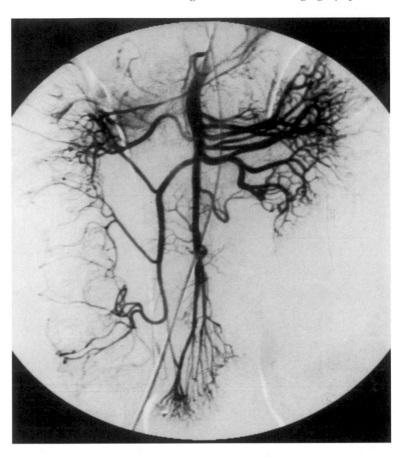

Fig. 12.13 Intra-arterial digital subtraction angiography of the superior mesenteric arteriogram showing clarity of vascular detail that can be obtained by obliterating movement artefacts of all types.

expiration. Extremes of the respiratory cycle are avoided as they induce movement artefact because the patient tends to tense the abdomen. The patient is required to learn the correct breathing technique at the start of the procedure and this can be checked with fluoroscopy when the patient is instructed to stop breathing and moving. Some patients have difficulty with this and compression applied to the nose by an assistant at the time of each injection can improve compliance. Occasionally, no useful breath-holding can be achieved by the patient. Cardiorespiratory failure is often responsible for this. The only way to get satisfactory images in this situation is to take masks at 2 s^{-1} through a whole respiratory cycle before injecting contrast medium. Eight or more masks may be needed to make allowance for variations in breathing, but the results often justify the extra radiation, retrieving an otherwise substandard angiogram.

In thoracic studies, breath-holding is clearly important, but several masks are always needed to allow for normal cardiac motion. In the neck the added movement which occurs when the patient swallows needs to be discouraged. The chances of swallowing during a run are minimized by asking the patient to swallow immediately before starting the angiographic run. Breath-holding is also important in the neck as respiratory movement in the chest is invariably accompanied by changes in the position of the neck. Even intracerebral studies may benefit from breath-holding as the instruction to suspend respiration helps to concentrate the patient's attention on remaining motionless.

The radiologist may be responsible for introducing 'patient movement' by leaning on the examination table during the injection. It is surprising how common this elementary error is even among experienced personnel.

Bowel peristalsis can be difficult to eradicate, and

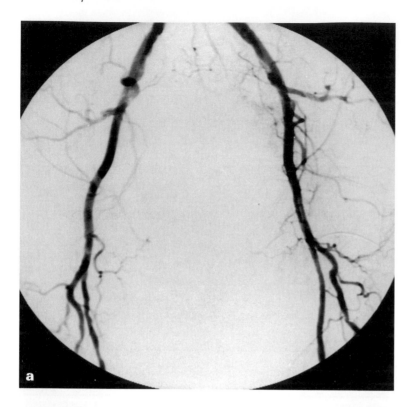

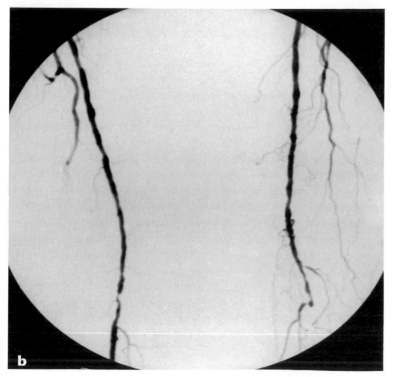

Fig. 12.14 Intra-arterial digital subtraction angiography femoral aortogram. The aortic segment was normal. No significant disease detected in the iliac or common femoral segments (a). Diffuse atheromatous disease noted in both superficial femoral arteries, with complete occlusion noted just above the knee on the left (b).

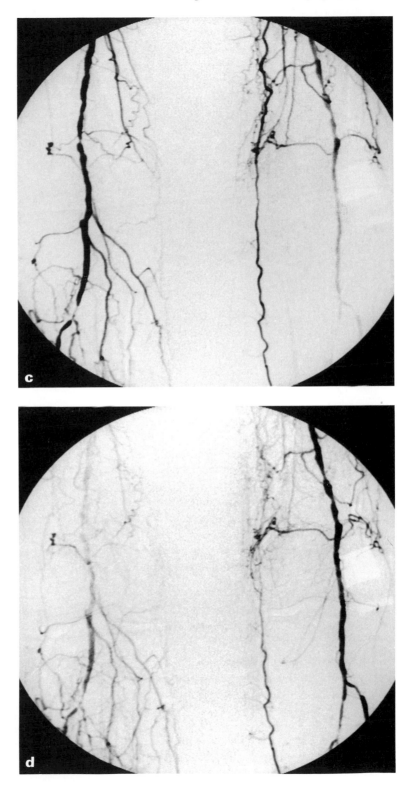

Fig. 12.14 *Continued.* (c) The earlier phase shows that the right popliteal and calf vessels fill first but are severely diseased. Contrast medium has almost disappeared from the right by the time the left popliteal is adequately demonstrated (d).

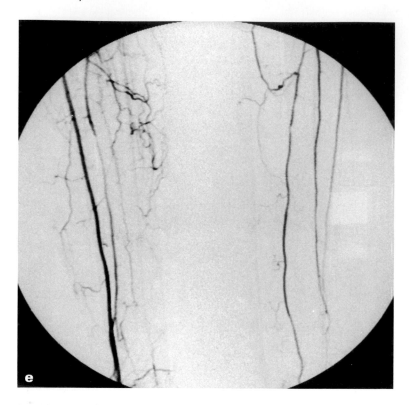

Fig. 12.14 *Continued.* (e) Calf vessel detail seen here.

appears to be a particular problem among anxious young adult males. Some authorities favour abdominal compression, others rely on hyoscine-2-butylbromide (Buscopan) in incremental doses of 20 mg to an arbitrary maximum of 60 mg i.a. per case to achieve bowel paralysis, bearing in mind its contraindications. If this fails, glucagon 0.5 mg i.a. can be administered and repeated once only. More than 1 mg of glucagon is reliably emetic. Refractory bowel peristalsis can make repeated angiographic runs necessary for a diagnostic study to be performed and should not be underestimated.

Conclusion (Zeitler, 1992)

DSA has virtually replaced conventional angiography. Although in its early years it was justified on the grounds of reduced cost per procedure, the total amount of contrast medium used by a department may be the same or increased after the installation of a DSA system. This reflects the ease and speed with which multiple runs in several projections may be obtained, and also the change in refer-

ral patterns (particularly in relation to peripheral angioplasty) which DSA brings with it.

Constantly challenged as a diagnostic medium by CT, Doppler ultrasound and MRI, the role of DSA as a linchpin of transcatheter therapy seems secure. The success of the technique relies on sufficient emphasis being put on the reduction of patient movement. Time taken to learn how to maintain a constant background for subtraction will be repaid by dramatic improvements in the angiographic results.

References

Ameli, F., Rooney, M., St Louis, E., Stein, M., Grosman, H. & Gray R. (1991) Intravenous digital subtraction arteriography in the evaluation of vascular grafts. *Ann. Vasc. Surg.*, **5**(3), 223–8.

Borgstein, R., Brown, M., Waterston, J. *et al.* (1991) Digital subtraction angiography of the extracranial cerebral vessels: a direct comparison between intravenous and intra-arterial DSA. *Clin. Radiol.*, **44**(6), 402–5.

Cebul, R. & Paulus, R. (1986) The failure of intravenous digital subtraction angiography in replacing carotid arteriography. *Ann. Intern. Med.*, **104**(4), 572–4.

Chiesa, R., Melissano, G., Castellano, R. *et al.* (1993) Three dimensional time of flight magnetic resonance angiography in carotid artery surgery: a comparison with digital subtraction angiography. *Eur. J. Vasc. Surg.*, **7**(2), 171–6.

Colquhoun, I., Oates, C., Martin, K., Hull, K. & Whittingham, T. (1992) The assessment of carotid and vertebral arteries: a comparison of CFM duplex ultrasound with intravenous digital subtraction angiography. *Br. J. Radiol.*, **65**(780), 1069–74.

Crocker, E.J., Tutton, R. & Bowen, J. (1986) The role of intravenous digital subtraction angiography in the evaluation of extracranial carotid artery disease. Can the decision for carotid artery surgery be made solely on the basis of its findings? *J. Vasc. Surg.*, **4**(2), 157–63.

Dawson, P. (1988) Digital subtraction angiography — a critical analysis. *Clin. Radiol.*, **39**(5), 474–7.

Dunnick, N., Svetkey, L., Cohan, R. *et al.* (1989) Intravenous digital subtraction angiography: use in screening for renovascular hypertension. *Radiology*, **17**(1), 219–22.

Furuya, Y., Isoda, H., Hasegawa, S., Takahashi, M., Kaneko, M. & Uemura, K. (1992) Magnetic resonance angiography of extracranial carotid and vertebral arteries including their origins: comparison with digital subtraction angiography. *Neuroradiology*, **35**(1), 42–5.

Goldberg, H., Moses, J., Fisher, J., Tamari, I. & Borer, J. (1986) Diagnostic accuracy of coronary angiography utilising computer-based digital subtraction methods. Comparison with conventional cineangiography. *Chest*, **90**(6), 793–7.

Gouliamos, A., Gotsis, E., Vlahos, L. *et al.* (1992) Magnetic resonance angiography compared to intra-arterial digital subtraction angiography in patients with subarachnoid haemorrhage. *Neuroradiology*, **35**(1), 46–9.

Hemingway, A.P., Virjee, N. & Allison, D. (1985) DSA in gastrointestinal disease. *Med. Mundi.*, **31**, 91–5.

Illescas, F., Braun, S., Cohan, R., Sussman, S., Saeed, M. & Dunnick, N. (1988) Fibromuscular dysplasia of renal arteries: comparison of intravenous digital subtraction angiography with conventional angiography. *Can. Assoc. Radiol. J.*, **39**(3), 167–71.

Kim, D., Porter, D., Brown, R., Crivello, M., Silva, P. & Lemming, B. (1991) Renal artery imaging: a prospective comparison of intraarterial digital subtraction angiography with conventional angiography. *Angiology*, **42**(5), 345–57.

Lee, K., Cox, G., Price, H., Johnson, J. & Neff, J. (1986) Intraarterial digital subtraction arteriographic evaluation of extremity tumours: comparison with conventional arteriography. *Radiology*, **158**(1), 255–8.

Ludwig, J.W. (ed.) (1986) *Digital Subtraction Angiography in Clinical Practice*. Best, the Netherlands.

Meaney, T.F. (1982) DSA in the thorax. *Ann. Radiol.*, **25**, 470–2.

Nau, R., Prange, H., Klingelhofer, J. *et al.* (1992) Results of four technical investigations in 50 clinically brain dead patients. *Intens. Care Med.*, **18**(2), 82–8.

Roeren, T., Hauenstein, K., Dinkel, E. & Kirste, G. (1986) Intraarterial digital subtraction angiography of renal transplants. *Urol. Radiol.*, **8**(2), 77–80.

Schuierer, G., Huk, W. & Laub, G. (1992) Magnetic resonance angiography of intracranial aneurysms: comparison with intra-arterial digital subtraction angiography. *Neuroradiology*, **35**(1), 50–4.

Smith, T., Cragg, A., Berbaum, K. & Nakagawa, N. (1992) Comparison of the efficacy of digital subtraction angiography of the lower limb: prospective study in 50 patients. *Am. J. Roentgenol.*, **158**(2), 431–6.

Stevens, J., Barter, S., Kerslake, R., Schneidau, A., Barber, C. & Thomas, D. (1989) Relative safety of intravenous digital subtraction angiography over other methods of carotid angiography and impact on clinical management of cerebrovascular disease. *Br. J. Radiol.*, **62**, 813–16.

Vatne, K., Nakstad, P. & Lundar, T. (1985) Digital subtraction angiography in the evaluation of brain death. A comparison of conventional cerebral angiography with intravenous and intraarterial DSA. *Neuroradiology*, **27**(2), 155–7.

Warnock, N., Gandhi, M., Bergvall, U. & Powell, T. (1993) Complications of intraarterial digital subtraction angiography in patients investigated for cerebral vascular disease. *Br. J. Radiol.*, **66**, 855–8.

Waugh, J. & Sacharias, N. (1992) Arteriographic complications in the DSA era. *Radiology*, **182**(1), 243–6.

Weaver, F., Pentecost, M. & Yellin, A. (1990) Carbon dioxide digital subtraction arteriography: a pilot study. *Ann. Vasc. Surg.*, **4**(5), 437–41.

Weaver, F., Pentecost, M., Yellin, A., Davis, S., Finck, E. & Teitelbaum, G. (1991) Clinical applications of carbon dioxide/digital subtraction arteriography. *J. Vasc. Surg.*, **13**(2), 272–3.

Whitehouse, G.M. & Worthington, B.S. (eds) (1983) *Techniques in Diagnostic Imaging*, 1st edn. Blackwell Scientific Publications, Oxford.

Wilms, G., Baert, A., Staessen, J. & Amery, A. (1986) Renal artery stenosis: evaluation with intravenous digital subtraction angiography. *Radiology*, **160**(3), 713–15.

Zeitler, E. (1992) Digital subtraction angiography (DSA). Myth or reality? *Eur. Radiol.*, **2**, 279–81.

13   Lymphatic System

G. R. CHERRYMAN

The structure and function of the lymphatic system were for many years evaluated by direct visualization of the lymphatic channels and nodes with contrast media. This technique is known as either lymphangiography or lymphography. Today there are few indications for direct lymphangiography. The lymphatic system is best studied through a combination of X-ray, cross-sectional and radionuclide investigations. In the future, there is likely to be a greater emphasis on functional lymphatic vessel imaging using magnetic resonance imaging (MRI) and ultrasound in combination with radionuclide studies.

In the normal adult, approximately 3 litres of excess interstitial fluid drains into lymphatic capillaries each day. The lymphatic capillaries converge to form larger lymphatic vessels that finally drain into the systemic circulation through the right and left thoracic ducts. The lymphatic system consists of this fluid, known as lymph, the lymphatic capillaries and vessels and the lymph nodes through which the lymph drains.

Lymph nodes are scattered throughout the body in groups. Each node has a fibrous capsule, an outer cortex containing densely packed lymphocytes and an inner medulla. Lymph drains in sinuses from cortex to medulla before leaving the node in one or two efferent lymphatic vessels, which lead to another node in the same group or a node in a proximal group. A normal node is bean shaped and between 1 and 25 mm in length. The efferent vessels usually leave through the hilum. Blood vessels enter and leave the node through the hilum. The nodes function as filters of the lymph. Macrophages destroy filtered foreign substances. In addition, the node can produce plasma cells and T lymphocytes which can leave the node and circulate in the blood.

In addition to nodes, there are discrete aggregations of lymphoid tissue within the body. Many of these are tiny, but the spleen, thymus, tonsils and adenoids are much larger and clinically important lymphoid structures.

The lymphatic system has a key role in the control of infection and immunity. Knowledge of the location of lymph nodes and the direction of lymphatic flow is important to radiologists. Lymphatic vessels contain valves. Lymph is moved by a combination of skeletal muscle movement, respiratory movement and the one-way action of the valves.

Inflamed or malignant nodes will increase in size. At present, no radiological test can determine the cause of lymph node enlargement and reliably differentiate benign from malignant enlargement. However, in the right clinical context, the demonstration of enlarged nodes will help determine the correct management of patients with malignant disease.

Radiology of lymph node enlargement

Lymph node enlargement may be recognized on plain radiographs, especially in the pulmonary hila and mediastinum. Elsewhere, grossly enlarged or calcified nodes may be seen. Ultrasound may be helpful in detecting enlarged cervical, pelvic and abdominal nodes. The imaging method of choice for nodal staging of cancer is computed tomography (CT). CT will detect normal lymph nodes in soft tissues if the nodes are surrounded by fat. Enlarged nodes may be confidently demonstrated, even when not surrounded by fat. As a node increases in size the probability of it containing tumour increases, thus the larger the node in a patient with cancer the more confident the radiologist can be that the node contains metastatic disease. In many areas of the body, size criteria indicate the probability of an enlarged node representing metastatic disease in appropriate circumstances and are sufficient to base a management decision on the observation (Table

13.1). Filling defects are often seen within the node on CT after bolus contrast enhancement, especially in the pelvis. These filling defects are often due to fibrofatty change and should not be regarded as malignant foci. This is a particular problem in older people, especially in the groin and pelvic regions. The exception to this is the patient with squamous carcinoma of the neck in whom a focal non-enhancing centre to an appropriate neck node should be regarded as malignant, even if the node remains within normal size.

MRI is of similar value to CT in the local staging of many cancers. It is no better than CT for staging distant nodal involvement as size remains the only confident sign of involvement.

The use of lymphangiography in patients with malignant disease to demonstrate the location, size and internal architecture of the lymph node is currently only of historical interest. The technique had been widely used to demonstrate pelvic and abdominal nodes after the bipedal injection of an oily lymphangiographic contrast material. Patients found the procedure uncomfortable. It was time-consuming and complicated for the operator. There were slight risks to the patient associated with the procedure, especially following the injection of oily contrast media, and not all patients were suitable. The technique was most helpful in planning the management of patients with lymphoma and testicular tumours. Its use in the pelvis has always been limited by its failure to opacify internal iliac and deep pelvic nodes, as well as an unacceptable number of false positives arising from benign enlargement of pelvic nodes and the high frequency of fibrofatty node replacement. Important lymph node groups in the abdomen fail to opacify, including mesenteric nodes and many of the upper abdominal, periportal and peripancreatic nodes.

It is often said that CT has replaced lymphangiography. This is not strictly true. The treatment of both lymphoma and teratoma has changed, mainly towards an increased reliance on chemotherapy. The information currently necessary to stage, treat and monitor patients can be obtained from CT. This may alter again in the future and some form of direct lymph node imaging may once again become mandatory. The possibility of endolymphatic therapy is a further reason why the technique of lymphatic cannulation remains worthwhile.

Radiology of the lymphatics

Lymphatic imaging may be required for the investigation of both lymphoedema and lymphatic leakage. Lymphoedema is a consequence of reduced lymphatic function leading to the accumulation of interstitial fluid in the tissues. It is secondary to surgery, radiotherapy, inflammation such as rheumatoid arthritis, infection including filariasis and leprosy, or neoplasia. Primary lymphoedema is less common and falls into one of three clinical scenarios: (i) simple congenital lymphoedema; (ii) familial lymphoedema or Milroy's disease, which is also present from birth, involves the lower limbs, and is a result of too few and poorly functioning lymphatics; and (iii) lymphoedema praecox which is seen in teenage women with progressive oedema of lower limbs and trunk. Direct visualization of the lymphatics is still occasionally required to make the diagnosis, but this can often be done on clinical grounds and by excluding other causes of leg swelling, such as venous obstruction. Lymphoscintigraphy may also be helpful in establishing the diagnosis of lymphoedema. In the future much greater use is likely to be made of Doppler ultrasound examination of the lymphatic flow and MRI examination of swollen soft tissues.

Lymphatic leakage is typically postoperative or post-traumatic in origin. Direct opacification of the lymph vessels may still be required to confirm the presence of a leak. This will often require injection of oily contrast medium. Intraoperative lymphangiography with sulphan blue has also been used as a guide to the surgeon.

Radiological techniques

The use of X-ray, CT, MRI and ultrasound is covered elsewhere (Chapters 26, 28 and 29). This chapter will

Table 13.1 Size criteria for normal lymph nodes

Neck	< 1 cm
Thorax	< 1.5 cm
Retrocrural region	< 0.7 cm
Abdomen	< 1.5 cm
Pelvis	< 1.5 cm

outline the techniques of direct lymphatic cannulation with contrast media injection and indirect injection of radionuclide to perform lymphoscintigraphy. Further radionuclide studies of lymphatic function, for instance indium-labelled white cells and ^{67}Ga scanning, are described in Chapter 27.

Lymphatic cannulation

Lymphatic cannulation requires a cut-down into the subcutaneous tissue under local anaesthesia, followed by the identification and cannulation of an appropriate lymphatic. The technique is considerably easier if the lymphatics are opacified with a blue dye prior to cut-down.

Method

The patient lies supine on an X-ray table. Fluoroscopic screening is helpful, otherwise one or more plain radiographs of the calf will be required.

If the leg is swollen, its elevation in a hospital bed for 48 hours prior to the procedure may be helpful. The patient should be normally hydrated.

The skin over the dorsum of the patient's feet and the web spaces between the toes are cleaned with chlorhexidine.

The patient gives informed consent and is checked for allergies, especially to iodine and sulphan blue. Further precautions are required if the injection of an oily contrast medium is contemplated (see below).

Sulphan blue (1 ml of 2.5%)* is injected into each of the first two web spaces on both feet, a total of 4 ml of sulphan blue being used. Local anaesthetic may be mixed with the sulphan blue prior to injection.

The lymphatics will take up the sulphan blue within a few minutes and fine blue lines should be visible under the skin of the dorsum of the foot. A strong light is often helpful. In difficult cases it may be helpful to ask the patient to walk around for 30 min. Dermal backflow may be seen in patients with lymphoedema. The diagnosis of lymphoedema can then be made and the procedure terminated.

If a suitable lymphatic vessel is visualized cannulation may proceed. Under local anaesthesia (1%

* Patent Blue V, Laboratoire Guerbet, Paris, France.

lignocaine without adrenalin), an opacified lymphatic vessel (typically just lateral to the tendon of extensor hallucis longus) is located following cut-down (Fig. 13.1), gently dissected free of fatty tissue and snared with a loop of 3/0 silk thread. Two loops may be used to pull the lymphatic vessel taut (Fig. 13.2)

A 30 standard wire gauge attached to a giving set, for example Macarthy's Surgical St Thomas' Hospital pattern, is used. The lymphangiogram needle is gently but firmly inserted into the opacified lymphatic channel (Fig. 13.3). Magnification (×2) is helpful. The needle is best held with the hand resting on the patient's foot for stability. The tip of the needle is then firmly tied with the silk thread (Fig. 13.4). The thread and cannula are then taped to the patient's foot. Finally a small dose of water-soluble contrast is slowly injected, while watching the needle tip for leakage. Opacification of the lymphatics is confirmed by fluoroscopy and/or radiograph of the calf immediately following injection. The opacified lymphatic vessel will be seen as a thin steady line of contrast medium in the calf (Fig. 13.5). Venous in-

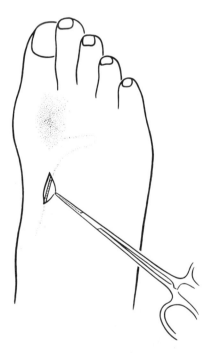

Fig. 13.1 A 1 cm longitudinal incision is made on the dorsum of the foot to expose the blue-coloured lymphatic vessel.

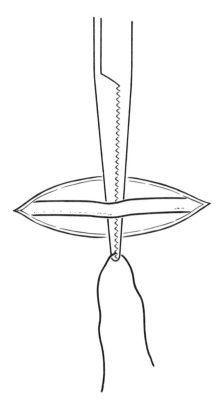

Fig. 13.2 Silk ties are passed below the lymphatic vessel. Many operators use two ties, one proximal and the other distal, to steady the lymphatic vessel at the time of cannulation.

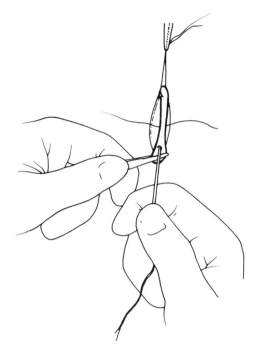

Fig. 13.3 While the lymphatic vessel is held taut, the needle is inserted into it and threaded about 0.5 cm along the vessel before being firmly tied.

jection or venous cross-flow will be seen as fragmentation of the contrast column and a more rapid transit of the contrast medium up the calf.

If the injection is unsuccessful, further attempts can be made either in other lymphatics through the same incision or by repeating the cut-down procedure proximally. The needle is removed after the procedure. The wound is then cleaned and sutured. The patient is advised to elevate the foot as much as possible for the next few days and to avoid wearing shoes. The patient is also advised that the blue stain in the foot may persist for several weeks. The patient may also notice a blue colour to a urine for a few days. Sutures are removed after 10 days.

Injection with oily contrast medium is occasionally required in patients with lymphatic leakage. An iodized oil such as Lipiodal Ultrafluid* is used.

* Laboratoire Guerbet, Paris, France.

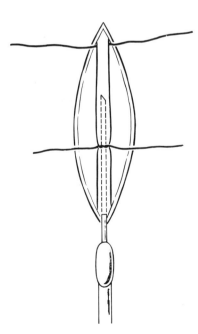

Fig. 13.4 This shows the needle in position immediately prior to injection.

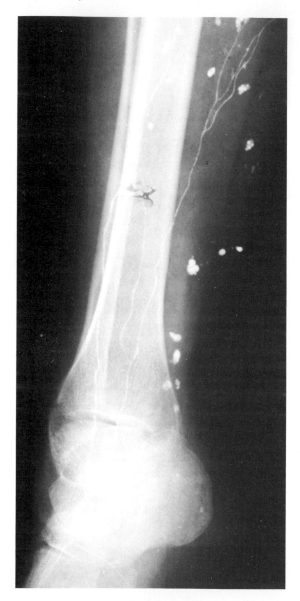

Fig. 13.5 The thin continuous line of contrast medium is seen to outline a lymphatic vessel in the calf. Fragmentation of the contrast medium column is the hallmark of venous injection.

Additional precautions must be taken prior to its use as the oily contrast medium will pass into the systemic and pulmonary circulation. This will result in pulmonary embolism and reduced respiratory function. Patients with poor respiratory function, including the elderly and those with chronic obstructive

airway disease or pulmonary fibrosis, should be excluded. Situations where a large dose of oil could reach the lung within a short space of time should be avoided. These include recent radiotherapy, immunosuppressives and steroids, which all cause lymph node atrophy and consequent hurry of the injected oily contrast medium through the lymphatics and lymphaticovenous communications, as well as trauma and surgery or as malignant disease. In all cases the injected dose of oily contrast medium should be limited to a maximum of 7 ml per limb (14 ml overall), with a reduced dose if there is any concern over respiratory embarassment. Finally, the rate of injection should be limited to 4 ml hour^{-1} through a lymphangiogram injector and the progress of the oily contrast medium carefully monitored with fluoroscopy and/or radiographs. As soon as the cisterna chyli is seen, contrast medium injection must stop. Lymphatic leakage is seen as a collection of oily contrast medium in the soft tissues and/or abdominal cavity. The early radiographs are often the most helpful in locating the leak. In traditional lymphangiography, the immediate abdominal and pelvic radiographs were followed by serial radiographs at 24 and 48 hours to examine the uptake of the oily contrast medium into the lymph nodes. Oblique radiographs were helpful in interpretation.

Direct lymphangiography

In patients with lymphoedema, non-ionic water-soluble contrast medium (240 mg iodine ml^{-1}) should be used. A slow injection of contrast medium should opacify any lymphatics, distinguish hypoplasia from hyperplasia and show any lymphaticovenous communications. This procedure should be directly monitored and discontinued when the necessary diagnostic information has been obtained.

Indirect lymphangiography

Sulphan blue injection into the subdermal tissues may be helpful to surgeons seeking to repair lymphatic leakage. This is usually performed in theatre by the surgeon. An indirect injection taken up by the lymphatics forms the basis of lymphoscintigraphy, which is a study of lymphatic function. In the future similar information may be available from MRI following injection of paramagnetic materials into either the circulation or the subdermal tissues.

Lymphoscintigraphy is performed at a greater range of sites than traditional direct lymphangiography, including subcostal injection for the internal mammary and axillary nodes in patients with breast cancer. Following skin anaesthesia a small volume (less than 1 ml) of ^{99m}Tc-labelled microcolloid (18–38 MBq) is injected intradermally and scintigraphic images obtained 2–3 hours later. Lymphoedema is shown by obstruction of normal ascent, node uptake in unusual sites and absence of liver and spleen uptake following bipedal injection.

Further reading

Clouse, M.E. & Wallace, S. (1985) *Lymphatic Imaging. Lymphography, Computed Tomography and Scintigraphy.* Williams & Wilkins, Baltimore.

Fogelman, I., Maisey, M.N. & Clarke, S.E.M. (1994) *An Atlas of Clinical Nuclear Medicine*, pp. 707–11. Martin Dunitz, London.

Kinmouth, J.B. (1982) *The Lymphatics. Surgery, Lymphography and Diseases of the Chyle and Lymph Systems.* Edward Arnold, London.

Macdonald, J.S. (1987) Lymphography. In Ansell, G. & Wilkins, R.A. (eds) *Complications in Diagnostic Imaging*, 2nd edn, pp. 300–9. Blackwell Scientific Publications, Oxford.

Section 3
Respiratory Tract

14   Larynx

G. A. S. LLOYD

Conventional techniques

Plain radiography, high kilovoltage techniques and linear tomography have a limited place in the investigation of the larynx. Essentially, they only show the mucosal surfaces and these are better assessed endoscopically. However, these methods can usefully demonstrate subglottic extension of tumour and, in some patients, cord fixation.

Plain radiographic examination

The larynx is best examined in the lateral position since the cervical spine largely obliterates the outlines of the air-containing structures of the larynx in the anteroposterior (AP) projection. The lateral radiograph is obtained by centring the incident ray at a point just behind the prominence of the thyroid cartilage. The film is placed against the shoulder and the anode film distance increased to 1.8 m in order to minimize geometric distortion.

High kilovoltage technique

This may be used in both the AP and lateral projections. The advantage of lateral high kilovoltage radiographs over the standard soft-tissue lateral radiograph is that any obscuring calcification in the thyroid cartilage is obliterated, thus allowing better visualization of structures at glottic level (Fig. 14.1).

AP radiographs of the larynx using a voltage of 145 kV or more and 3 mm of brass filtration give obliteration of the superimposed cervical vertebrae, allowing almost bone-free studies of the larynx. High kilovoltage studies are used to show cord mobility, radiographs being obtained in quiet inspiration and during phonation (Fig. 14.2). This may demonstrate cord fixation (Fig. 14.3), which is important in the preoperative staging of laryngeal carcinoma since it immediately classifies the tumour as T3 or T4 by the Union International Contre le Cancer (UICC) classification.

Tomography

This technique is easy to perform and free from discomfort to the patient. It allows the outline of the laryngeal soft tissues to be seen clearly without the overlap of the bony density of the cervical spine, in addition to showing the lower limits of tumour extension into the subglottic space — an area difficult to examine by endoscopy.

A linear or elliptical tomographic movement of the tube in a direction longitudinal to the patient is recommended for studies of the larynx. The incomplete blurring of structures lying in the direction of tube swing, which is a feature of linear tomography, tends to enhance the definition of laryngeal structures against the contrast of the air, generally giving better results than circular or hypocycloidal movements (Fig. 14.4).

Tomographic sections are made to 0.5 cm intervals with the patient lying supine and phonating 'ee'. This causes approximation of the vocal cords, their outlines being more clearly shown in relation to the surrounding air. Tomograms are obtained with both expiratory and inspiratory phonation, the latter usually producing better air distension of the ventricles and allowing compression of the ventricle to be distinguished from infiltration.

Computed tomography (CT) of the larynx

CT imaging of the larynx is a significant improvement on conventional techniques. It demonstrates the larynx in axial section, providing a view of the laryngeal structures in the horizontal plane, with the

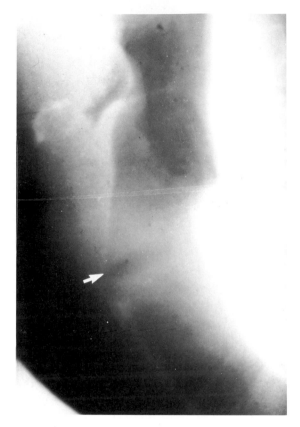

Fig. 14.1 Lateral high kilovoltage radiograph of a normal larynx showing ventricles (arrow), with true and false cords below and above.

possibility of showing cartilage invasion in addition to the soft-tissue extent of tumour.

Technique and normal anatomy

The patient lies supine with the head slightly extended. Contiguous sections of 5 mm are obtained from the base of the tongue to the thoracic inlet. Scans are normally made in quiet respiration but the new fast scanners enable patients to hold their breath during the scan and this may permit images to be obtained with the cords in abduction and adduction (Phelps, 1992).

As sequential scans are made from above downwards, the level is easily identified from the characteristic features of the oropharynx and larynx. The epiglottis and valleculae are seen at the level of the hyoid (Fig. 14.5), while the thyroid laminae become

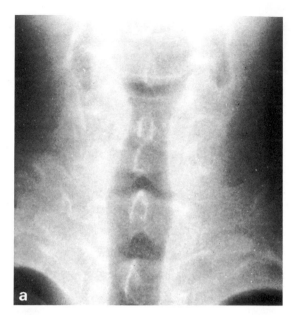

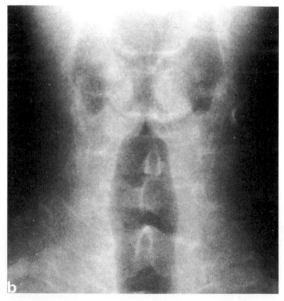

Fig. 14.2 Anteroposterior views taken by high kilovoltage technique. (a) Film taken in inspiration with abduction of the cords. (b) Film taken in phonation showing true and false cords, ventricles and pyriform fossae distended with air.

apparent below this level. The shape of the thyroid cartilage changes in a very characteristic way on scans at a lower level. Above the cords the laminae do not meet in the mid-line where the thyroid notch

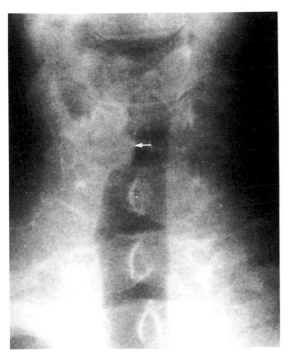

Fig. 14.3 High kilovoltage anteroposterior radiograph taken in inspiration showing fixation of vocal cord (arrow) due to carcinoma.

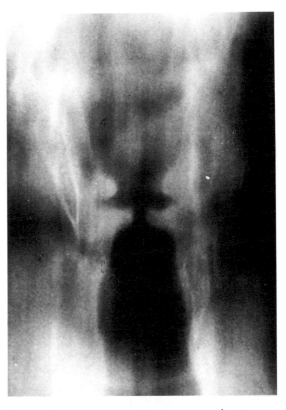

Fig. 14.4 Normal anteroposterior tomogram showing true and false cords, ventricles and subglottic space.

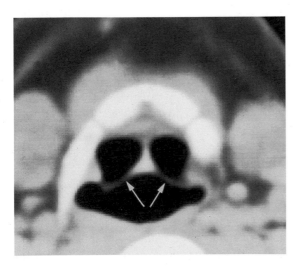

Fig. 14.5 Computed tomography scan at the level of the hyoid. The crescentic epiglottis is shown within the air translucency (arrows) with the valleculae anterior to it.

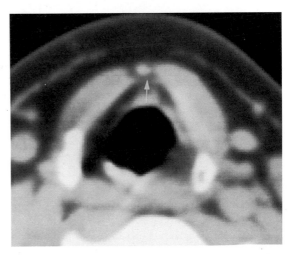

Fig. 14.6 Computed tomography scan at the level of the thyroid notch, which is shown as a gap between the thyroid laminae anteriorly (arrow).

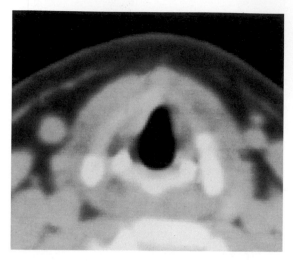

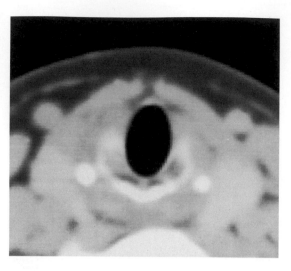

Fig. 14.7 Computed tomography scan made at glottic level. The arch formed by the thyroid laminae is shown with the boat-shaped air gap between the cords. Note that normally there is virtually no soft-tissue gap between the air space and the junction of the thyroid laminae.

Fig. 14.8 Computed tomography scan showing the shape of the subglottic air space with the cricoid cartilage posteriorly and the inferior cornua of the thyroid cartilage on either side.

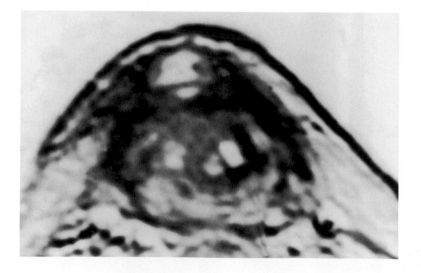

Fig. 14.9 Gadolinium-enhanced magnetic resonance subtraction print showing a stage T_4 laryngeal carcinoma with massive spread to the local soft tissues.

is present and are arranged at approximately 80° to one another (Fig. 14.6). The two thyroid laminae fuse just above the vocal cord level and assume the shape of an arch (Fig. 14.7), which becomes more rounded at a lower level and forms the anterior portion of an oval which is completed posteriorly by the cricoid. The shape of the airway also alters on sequential scans. The airway is bisected by the crescentic epiglottis at the level of the hyoid (see Fig. 14.5). Below this level the airway assumes a triangular shape and the two pyriform sinuses are seen as two lateral appendages separated by the aryepiglottic folds. The shape changes at the level of the cords to the characteristic glottic chink or boat shape, with the sharp anterior commissure extending right up to the thyroid cartilage in the mid-line (see Fig. 14.6). In the subglottic area there is an even, symmetrical oval shape (Fig. 14.8) which changes at the level of the first tracheal ring to an oval flattened posteriorly, similar in shape to a horseshoe.

Magnetic resonance imaging (MRI)

The role of MRI in the imaging of the larynx is similar to CT in that it is used to define the deep extension of disease. However, the multiplanar facility and superior soft-tissue definition of MRI mean that it is now replacing CT as the imaging investigation of choice for this purpose. An anterior or wrap-around surface coil is necessary to obtain high signal-to-noise images of the larynx.

A standard spin-echo technique with short TR is used in the axial plane and coronal sections are obtained if craniocaudal extension of tumour needs to be assessed. Gadolinium-enhanced T_1 sequences can be used instead of T_2 weighted images to give better spatial resolution and shorter scan time. The latter is especially useful in the larynx, where respiratory movement and swallowing are liable to degrade the image. Fast gradient echo images can also be applied after gadolinium (Phelps, 1992). Subtraction studies in the larynx are difficult to apply because of cord movement but in large tumours with cord fixation the full extent of tumour invasion is optimally demonstrated by this technique (Fig. 14.9).

Reference

Phelps, P.D. (1992) Carcinoma of the larynx — the role of imaging in staging and pre-treatment assessments. *Clin. Radiol.*, **46**, 77–83.

Bronchial Tree, Lungs and Pleura

S. P. G. PADLEY AND C. D. R. FLOWER

Lung needle biopsy

Both localized and diffuse pulmonary disease may produce a diagnostic problem which is not resolved by clinical and radiographic means. Although the clinical history and examination of the sputum for organisms and malignant cells reduces the number of patients in this problem group, a significant number require some form of biopsy to establish the correct diagnosis. An open lung biopsy performed via a thoracotomy provides a large piece of tissue for histological examination. Less invasively, percutaneous needle biopsy may be performed for focal lung masses and bronchoscopically guided transbronchial biopsy for diffuse lung disease. Both are safe procedures with a very low morbidity and mortality in experienced hands.

Percutaneous lung biopsy

Although percutaneous needle biopsy has been used in the investigation of diffuse lung disease (McKenna *et al.*, 1986; Gunther, 1992), it is not generally regarded as a suitable alternative to transbronchial or open biopsy and all further discussion relates to the biopsy of focal pulmonary masses.

The type of needle used to obtain tissue from a pulmonary mass varies quite widely (Fig. 15.1). In most circumstances cytological samples are obtained from fine-gauge needles (20–22 gauge) of the aspirating or screw variety. Occasionally, these needles will yield tiny tissue fragments which are suitable for histology. Immunocytochemical and immunohistochemical staining techniques have helped to improve the accuracy of diagnosis. Larger tissue samples consistently suitable for histological examination can be obtained from cutting needles of a slightly larger calibre, usually 16–18 gauge. There is a greater risk of significant pneumothorax and

pulmonary haemorrhage with these needles (Sinner, 1976; Berquist *et al.*, 1980). This, coupled with the accuracy of cytopathology for most lung tumours, means that cutting needle biopsy can usually be reserved for focal masses in the periphery of the lung which are regarded from computed tomography (CT) findings as likely to represent a benign condition with a complicated histological pattern, such as cryptogenic organizing pneumonia.

Indications

The major indication for percutaneous needle biopsy is the diagnosis of localized intrapulmonary disease (Fig. 15.2). In the majority of patients this means differentiating between a benign or a malignant process. Accuracy in the diagnosis of malignant lesions is around 90% in experienced hands. False positive results for malignancy are very low but a false negative rate of around 10% is the major weakness of the technique. The false negative rate is related to a variety of causes, including inaccurate targeting, inadequate sampling, sampling of adjacent pneumonia or infarction, tumour necrosis, poor sample preparation and inadequate cytopathology. Whilst high diagnostic rates for benign lesions have been reported, most series state a specific diagnostic rate for benign masses of 6–44% (Calhour *et al.*, 1986). This is because it is virtually impossible to make a specific diagnosis on cytology for granulomatous lesions and focal masses due to chronic pneumonia or infarction.

In a patient with a solitary intrapulmonary mass, a percutaneous biopsy should only be undertaken if the result is likely to affect patient management and obviate the need for a diagnostic thoracotomy. If the radiographic appearances are characteristic of a bronchial carcinoma, a 'negative' biopsy will probably not prevent a thoracotomy (Charig *et al.*, 1991).

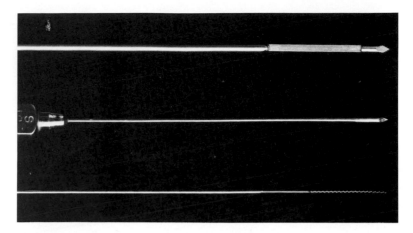

Fig. 15.1 Biopsy needles (cutting, aspiration and screw types).

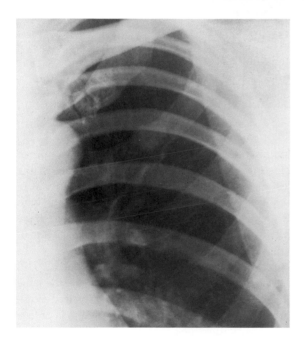

Fig. 15.2 A 1 cm mass as an isolated finding on the chest radiograph. Metastasis from a renal carcinoma.

Nevertheless, confirmation of the diagnosis and establishment of cell type can be of considerable help in patient management, whilst occasionally one is surprised by a diagnosis of a solitary metastasis or some benign condition such as tuberculosis, for both of which a thoracotomy would be inappropriate. In patients with a presumed bronchial carcinoma, but in whom a thoracotomy is contraindicated, biopsy gives confirmation of the diagnosis and allows cell typing prior to radiotherapy or chemotherapy. It also has a role in establishing the nature of a solitary intrapulmonary mass in a patient with a known extrathoracic primary malignancy, as well as distinguishing between metastases and benign disease in some patients with multiple intrapulmonary masses and no known primary malignancy. Needle aspiration is an excellent method for obtaining organisms from a presumed lung abscess. In this regard it is the method of choice for establishing the cause of focal lung opacities in immunosuppressed patients and for confirming the diagnosis of tuberculosis when sputum culture is negative in patients with an abscess (Fig. 15.3). It is obviously imperative that the smears are appropriately stained and that the correct cultures are set up.

Mediastinal masses can also be biopsied using fine or cutting needles (Herman *et al.*, 1991). This is of most use for confirming a suspected recurrence of lymphoma or in presumed mediastinal metastatic spread. Inconclusive results may be obtained from biopsy of tumours arising in and adjacent to the thymus even when histological samples are obtained.

Contraindications

Biopsy should not be performed if the pulmonary mass is likely to represent an echinococcal cyst or an arteriovenous malformation because of the respective risks of anaphylactoid reaction and haemorrhage. Anticoagulant therapy or a bleeding diathesis are relative contraindications, although anticoagulant levels can be adjusted to provide a satisfactory prothrombin index and platelet deple-

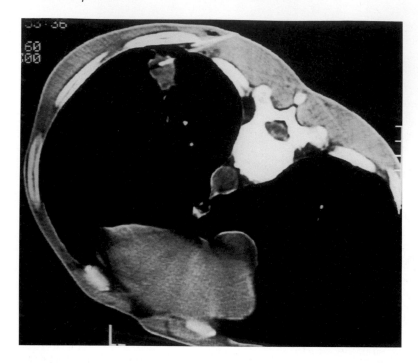

Fig. 15.3 Computed tomography-guided needle aspiration biopsy of a solitary pulmonary nodule. Tubercle bacilli identified on smear from the needle biopsy. The aspiration biopsy needle tip is in the centre of the lesion. The local anaesthetic needle is still in place.

tion can be partially overcome by platelet transfusion. The likelihood of pneumothorax is increased in patients with emphysema, in whom such an occurrence is particularly liable to cause respiratory embarassment. Similarly, patients who have had a pneumonectomy are unlikely to be able to withstand a pneumothorax. Haemorrhage following biopsy is a potentially life-threatening complication in patients with pulmonary hypertension.

Technique

The lesion must be accurately localized prior to biopsy. This requires well centred and adequately exposed posteroanterior (PA) and lateral radiographs. CT will also be required in a significant number of cases. Premedication is best avoided in order that the patient can cooperate. The procedure is performed under fluoroscopic or CT guidance, depending on the site of the lesion and operator preference. For fluoroscopic biopsy, single-plane intensification is acceptable for large or peripherally placed lesions but is inadequate for small or central masses which require biplane intensification or a C-arm. The patient is placed under the image intensifier in a prone or supine position, depending on the site of the lesion. A mark is then made on the skin under fluoroscopic control, in a position directly in line with the lesion. Local anaesthetic is injected down to the pleura. By moving the position of the arms, it is usually possible to project the lesion between the ribs and thereby obtain an unimpeded approach.

Prior to insertion, the needle is marked at the same distance from its tip as the lesion is measured radiographically to lie from the skin surface. It is preferable to introduce the needle over, rather than under, a rib in order to avoid damage to intercostal vessels and nerves. After making a small incision in the skin, the needle is introduced vertically under fluoroscopic control in line with the lesion and central X-ray beam. The needle tip is then advanced smoothly during quiet respiration and under fluoroscopic guidance directly to the lesion, which it is often felt to enter. Satisfactory positioning of the needle is suggested when the lesion is seen to move with the tip of the needle and can be confirmed with fluoroscopy at right angles. For aspiration biopsies, the central stylet is removed and suction applied with a 20 ml syringe whilst the needle tip is rotated and moved backwards and forwards within the lesion. A potential hazard is the introduction of air after removal of the stylet and before application of the syringe. This is avoided by instructing the patient not to breathe and placing a finger over the aspirating needle during the change-over. The performance of screw and cutting needle biopsies follows the same approach, the needle tip being advanced to the proximal margin of the lesion prior to biopsy. CT guidance is required for lesions which are not visible at fluoroscopy, either because of their size or, more commonly, because of their position. It is preferable to use CT guidance for lesions which arise within or lie adjacent to mediastinal structures, or if it is important to traverse the minimum amount of lung in patients who are at increased risk of pneumothorax. Accurate localization of the biopsy needle tip is aided by the use of a spiral scanning sequence.

The biopsy specimen is smeared on slides and is air dried or rapidly fixed in a suitable agent such as 74% alcohol. Histological material may also be placed in formalin. Material for culture is placed in sterile saline or broth. Following biopsy, the patient should remain recumbent, lying on the site from which the biopsy has been taken, for 3–4 hours, at which time a chest radiograph is obtained to check for a pneumothorax. In selected cases and when a 4-hour post-biopsy radiograph reveals no evidence of complications, the patient may be discharged with clear instructions on what to do if symptoms suggestive of a pneumothorax occur. In the majority of cases it is usually more appropriate to keep the patient in hospital overnight with a second chest radiograph obtained prior to discharge.

Complications

Pneumothorax is the commonest complication and occurs in 10–25% of patients, but is usually small and clinically insignificant (Weisbrod, 1990). Approximately one in every 10–15 patients who develop a pneumothorax requires intercostal tube drainage because of respiratory embarassment. The risk of a significant pneumothorax is increased in patients with emphysema and in patients who have difficulty in cooperating. The size of biopsy needle, number of

passes through the pleura, duration when the needle is *in situ*, size of the lesion and expertise of the operator are all factors which influence the likelihood of a pneumothorax. Radiologists performing lung biopsy should be able to deal with this complication, if necessary on an emergency basis, by inserting a trocar catheter to which can be attached a unidirectional airflow valve (Heimlich valve).

Haemoptysis is an infrequent complication, occurring in approximately 5–10% of patients (Weisbrod, 1990). Although it is usually small, haemoptysis invariably frightens the patient. A large haemorrhage is more likely to occur when using needles greater than 19 gauge. Haemoptysis may be extremely difficult to control and is the major cause of death. Treatment includes turning the patient onto the side that has been biopsied followed by immediate bronchoscopy with suction and, if necessary, by occlusion of the appropriate bronchus with a balloon catheter. It follows that lung biopsy should only be undertaken where these facilities are available.

Air embolism should be prevented by meticulous technique and by always performing the biopsy with the patient in the horizontal position. The implantation of tumour cells along the needle track has been rarely described and is more likely to occur following the use of larger gauge cutting needles. Mesotheliomas are particularly likely to seed to the skin (Sinner & Zajicek, 1976).

Transbronchial biopsy

The advent of fibreoptic bronchoscopy in the 1960s heralded a major advance in pulmonary medicine. Bidirectional tip flexion combined with a wide angle of vision permits precise guidance within the bronchial tree. A central 2 mm channel provides the opportunity for suction, the passage of a large variety of biopsy forceps and brushes as well as the instillation of local anaesthetic and contrast media. The instrument is best introduced transnasally under local anaesthesia after some form of premedication. The procedure is well tolerated, remarkably safe and may be performed on an out-patient basis. The small size of the instrument, coupled with its flexibility, allows visualization of the bronchial tree down to subsegmental level, which is a great advantage over the rigid bronchoscope. Whilst there are increasingly wide applications of the fibrescope, only its role in the diagnosis of localized and diffuse pulmonary disease is discussed here.

Localized disease

Lesions in the trachea and the lobar and segmental bronchi are biopsied under direct vision. Centrally situated pulmonary masses may directly involve the adjacent bronchial mucosa but frequently distort the bronchi and lie outside the mucosa, in which case transbronchial needle aspiration is required. Circumscribed peripheral opacities which are beyond the direct visual range of the fibrescope may be biopsied by advancing biopsy forceps, firstly into the appropriate segmental bronchus under direct vision, and secondly into the lesion under fluoroscopic control (Fig. 15.4). Nylon brushes, used in a similar fashion, enable specimens to be obtained for histological and cytological examination and for culture. The procedure is more time-consuming than percutaneous needle biopsy and is less successful at providing diagnostic material from a peripheral pulmonary mass. However, a complete examination of the bronchial tree can be performed by this technique. Other advantages are the very low incidence of pneumothorax and the much better control of pulmonary haemorrhage. The choice of technique frequently depends upon the referring clinician's preference and experience. The ideal is to have operators available who are experienced in both techniques, which can then be used in a complementary fashion. As a general rule, circumscribed lesions under 5 cm in diameter in the outer half of the lung are best approached by the percutaneous method. More central and ill-defined or cavitating lesions are often best approached via the fibrescope (Fig. 15.4).

Diffuse disease

The ability to obtain representative, albeit small, histological samples in a high percentage of patients has been a major advance in the differential diagnosis of diffuse disease. Transbronchial biopsy is particularly valuable in the diagnosis of sarcoidosis, carci-nomatosis, tuberculosis, extrinsic allergic alveolitis and opportunistic infections (Fig. 15.5). It is less useful in fibrosing alveolitis and drug-induced disease, where the distribution of histological change varies throughout the lung and the small samples obtained may be unrepresentative of the disease. If biopsy is necessary in these patients, it is often preferable to perform an open biopsy via a limited thoracotomy or thoracoscope.

Bronchography

Bronchography, first described by Sicard and Forestier (1922), was until recently the imaging investigation of choice in the diagnosis of bronchiectasis. High-resolution CT (HRCT) is an extremely accurate technique for examining the lungs and has almost completely superseded bronchography, such that in many centres in the UK and North America it is no longer practised at all. Should bronchography be undertaken it should be performed via the fibreoptic bronchoscope (see Whitehouse & Worthington, 1990 for a description of bronchography).

Pleural intervention

Contraindications to pleural intervention relate to poor patient cooperation and abnormal clotting. Pleural intervention may still be undertaken after correction of any clotting abnormality. Indications for pleural interventions are given in Table 15.1.

Pneumothorax drainage

A pneumothorax is usually treated by drainage, when it is large or causing respiratory embarassment or other significant symptoms. Drain inser-

Table 15.1 Indications for pleural intervention

Pneumothorax drainage
Pleural fluid aspiration
Empyema drainage
Pleural sclerotherapy
Pleural biopsy

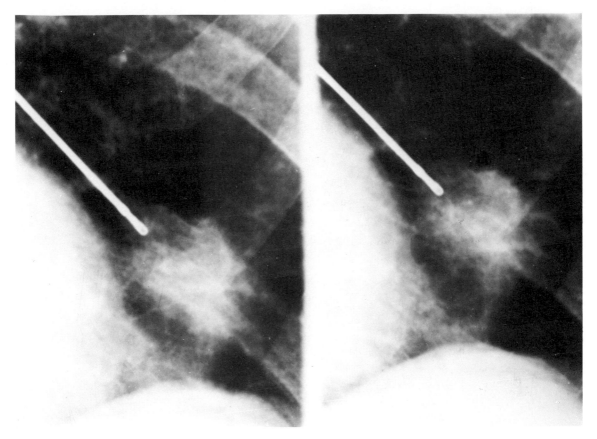

Fig. 15.4 Irregular mass (carcinoma) adjacent to heart. Unsuitable for percutaneous biopsy. Spot radiographs obtained during bronchoscopic biopsy.

tion is usually performed at the bedside by clinicians using relatively large-bore 22–28 French (F) tubes, although many pneumothoraces may be equally well treated with a smaller bore catheter (Perlmutt *et al.*, 1986). Radiologists are occasionally required to drain a pneumothorax when it is loculated or when it is difficult or impossible to identify on the chest radiograph because of its site or the patient's position. Fluoroscopy and CT are the imaging techniques usually employed. Radiologists should also be prepared to drain pneumothoraces resulting from percutaneous biopsy, when the decision to insert a chest drain depends on the development of respiratory compromise or increase in size of pneumothorax between the immediate post-biopsy radiograph and the 4-hour post-biopsy film to greater than 50% estimated lung volume. In the

emergency situation, a small-bore tube (7–9F) can be inserted through either the second intercostal space anteriorly or into the 5th or 6th intercostal space in the mid-axillary line. In cases of loculated pneumothorax, best delineated by CT, alternative sites of insertion may be more desirable. Depending on the degree of urgency, prior skin preparation and instillation of local anaesthetic is performed at the selected site and a small skin incision is made. Either a trocar method or the Seldinger technique may be used to insert the drain. The former is more appropriate in patients with little chest wall musculature and the latter in those patients with substantial intervening soft tissues. As with all pleural interventions, care should be taken to avoid the neurovascular bundle. When trocar catheter insertion is employed, the trocar is ad-

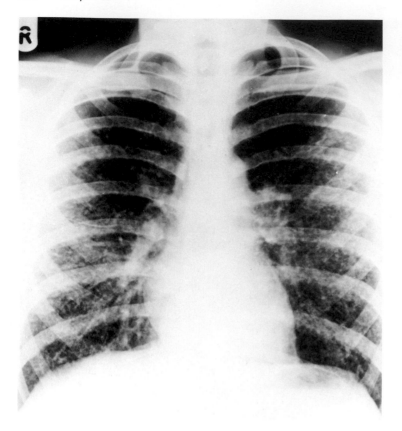

Fig. 15.5 Sarcoidosis producing diffuse fine nodular shadowing. Diagnosis established by transbronchial biopsy.

vanced over the top of the underlying rib. If the operator is right handed the left hand is used to control the degree of trocar insertion while the right hand provides a twisting motion and forward pressure. Usually a sudden give indicates entry into the pleural space. When a Seldinger technique for drain insertion is employed, the method is the same as that described for therapeutic pleural fluid aspiration.

Following insertion, free aspiration of air confirms placement in the pleural space and the catheter is advanced over the trocar which is held in place. The trocar is subsequently removed and a two-way tap attached, followed by evacuation of air by a large-volume syringe until mild resistance is encountered. Alternatively, an underwater drain system or one-way flutter valve may be attached to the cannula, which should be firmly secured to the skin. Wall suction should be limited to –20 cm of water. Immediate confirmation of adequate catheter placement with both PA and lateral chest radiographs should be un-

dertaken, with subsequent radiographic confirmation of lung re-expansion. The presence of a bronchopleural fistula should be suspected from a continuing air leak which, when persistent, may require further pleural or bronchoscopic intervention. Drains should not be removed until drainage of air has ceased.

Complications of a small-bore chest tube insertion are unusual but include laceration of underlying structures, particularly the intercostal artery or vein, and may result in the development of a haemothorax.

Pleural fluid aspiration

Pleural intervention as a bedside procedure without the benefit of radiological guidance has a relatively higher complication and failure rate than when performed with the benefit of radiological guidance (Westcott, 1985). In most instances ultrasound is the most appropriate imaging modality.

With the exception of large free pleural effusions, attempts at pleural aspiration should be conducted at the time of, or immediately following, radiological confirmation of the extent and site of pleural fluid.

Sonography is the ideal imaging technique to guide interventional procedures when pleural fluid is present and is easily employed at the bedside. Diagnostic aspiration is most commonly performed to determine whether an effusion is due to infection or related to malignancy. Therapeutic thoracentesis presupposes that the nature of the underlying pleural fluid has already been established and is most frequently employed in patients with large incapacitating malignant or parapneumonic effusions, or when effusions of any kind are causing respiratory difficulty or significant discomfort.

Diagnostic aspiration

Ultrasound-guided pleural fluid aspiration may be undertaken in the radiology department or at the bedside. CT should be reserved for complicated fluid collections. Sonographic confirmation of the presence and site of fluid should include an assessment for the presence of debris and loculation. Aspiration is performed in ambulant patients in a comfortable sitting position with support for the forearms, while bed-ridden patients are normally managed in the supine or supine oblique position. The skin is marked under ultrasound guidance, cleaned and draped. Local anaesthetic (1% lignocaine) is then instilled down to the pleural surface. Frequently aspiration of pleural fluid into the local anaesthetic syringe will occur. If this is the case, 20–50 ml of fluid is aspirated, having exchanged the local anaesthetic needle for one of suitable length as judged sonographically. When the pleural fluid is an exudate rather than a free-flowing transudate, a relatively large-bore needle (up to 14 gauge) may be required to obtain a diagnostic sample. When there is difficulty in aspirating what appears to be a pleural fluid collection, care should be taken not to advance the needle too far, traverse the pleural collection and enter the underlying lung. Insertion of the needle under direct ultrasound control, in order to confirm tip position, should avoid this problem. While fluid collections are accurately identified on ultrasound in most cases, a pleural or pulmonary tumour will occasionally appear completely transonic and mimic pleural fluid. If pleural aspiration is unsuccessful and a tumour is suspected, the patient should proceed to a CT examination. Other circumstances in which aspirations may prove difficult are the presence of very thick exudate or poor patient positioning.

Therapeutic aspiration

Following skin preparation and draping, local anaesthetic is instilled down to the pleural surface and a small scalpel incision is made. A 14 or 16 gauge Teflon sheath needle cannula, attached to a 20 ml syringe, is inserted across the chest wall above the adjacent rib, applying gentle aspiration until fluid is obtained. The sheath is then advanced a further 1–2 cm, depending on the size of the effusion, and the needle removed. Care should be taken to occlude any cannula or needle entering the pleural space. Although an angiographic guide wire may be employed, a shorter (60 cm) guide wire is more appropriate and easier for a single operator to manage. Passage of serial dilators followed by the chest drain minimizes resistance from the chest wall. The drain is then temporarily occluded and firmly secured to the chest wall, preferably with a purpose-designed self-adhesive hub, following which it is attached to low-pressure (–20 cm of water) suction via an underwater seal or closed tube and bag drainage.

While it is appropriate to remove a large volume of the fluid at the time of drain insertion, too rapid drainage of very large and long-standing effusions should be avoided in order to prevent the rare but well-recognized complication of re-expansion pulmonary oedema. This is effected by clamping the drainage system for 1–2 hours after the initial drainage of 1 litre of fluid.

Should the catheter cease to drain, particularly when there is evidence of debris within the drainage system, the catheter should be flushed with 20–50 ml of sterile saline 4–6 hourly. The inclusion of a two- or three-way tap within the drainage system is useful for this purpose. Catheter flushing may be safely undertaken at the bedside by appropriately trained nursing staff.

Empyema drainage

Once the diagnosis of an empyema has been established, usually by diagnostic aspiration, successful treatment depends upon prompt and adequate drainage together with appropriate antibiotic therapy. Although some patients will eventually proceed to surgical decortication, the management of empyema with radiologically guided catheters has a success rate of over 80% (Hunnam & Flower, 1988). As with unguided diagnostic and therapeutic thoracocentesis, unguided empyema drainage, traditionally with large-bore surgically placed drains, has a higher complication rate (trauma to lung, oesophagus, liver and spleen) and a lower success rate (35–50%) than imaging-guided empyema drainage (van Sonnenberg *et al.*, 1984). Imaging with CT or ultrasound permits accurate tube placement and confirmation of tube position at the time of the procedure. Loculated empyema collections may fail to drain adequately from a single chest tube insertion and multiple drains are sometimes required. Due to the viscid nature of empyema fluid and the frequent presence of debris, larger bore radiological drains (12–14F) are employed than for simple pleural fluid aspiration.

The method for tube insertion is similar to therapeutic thoracentesis, with a Seldinger technique and use of serial dilators prior to insertion of the pig-tail drain. While complicated or multiloculated empyemas are best assessed and drained under CT guidance, a combination of ultrasound and fluoroscopy is otherwise used. Following drain insertion, PA and lateral chest radiographs should be obtained to document tube position. When catheter insertion is performed with CT guidance, correct drain position may be confirmed by subsequent CT scans (Fig. 15.6).

Following tube placement, as much empyema fluid as possible should be aspirated at the bedside until gentle resistance is encountered. The catheter should subsequently be connected to an underwater seal and low-pressure (–20 cm water) suction applied. Regular (4–6 hourly) catheter irrigation with 50 ml sterile saline should be performed via a three-way tap to ensure continuing catheter patency and to prevent blockage by debris. As with therapeutic thoracentesis, the catheter should be firmly secured to the chest wall to prevent tube kinking at the exit site.

Successful treatment is best confirmed by a combination of clinical improvement and either chest radiography or repeat ultrasound scanning. A residual pleural rind is often evident, but if there is clinical improvement and irrigation confirms catheter patency, with either a minimal or absent fluid residue, the empyema can be considered adequately drained and the drain removed.

Several studies have documented the utility of instilling fibrinolytic agents such as streptokinase or urokinase into loculated pleural collections, with a resultant increase in fluid drainage (Moulton *et al.*, 1989; Lee *et al.*, 1991). Subsequent empyema resolution varies from 44 to 100% in reported series. Typically, 100 000 U of urokinase in 50 ml of normal saline is instilled through the tube drain and the catheter clamped for 1 hour. Suction drainage is then re-established, with intermittent catheter irrigation as before. Instillation of urokinase may be repeated on a daily basis. There is no firm limit on the duration of this form of treatment, but a maximum of 500 000–600 000 U is probably appropriate. Significantly increased drainage is normally encountered after the first instillation. It is seldom necessary to use the maximum dose of fibrinolytic agent. This technique has not been associated with an increase in bleeding or other complications and there has been no evidence of significant systemic absorption of the fibrinolytic agent (Moulton *et al.*, 1989).

Complications of empyema drainage are rare and include haemothorax, pneumothorax and bacteraemia. Failure to drain adequately under radiological guidance should be followed by further appropriate imaging (usually CT) and either image-guided tube insertion or referral for decortication.

Pleural sclerosis (sclerotherapy)

Pleural sclerosis is usually reserved for patients with malignant pleural effusions that reaccumulate rapidly following therapeutic thoracentesis. Systemic chemotherapy is often inappropriate and, for many patients with recurrent effusions, obliteration of the pleural space offers the best form of palliation. Surg-

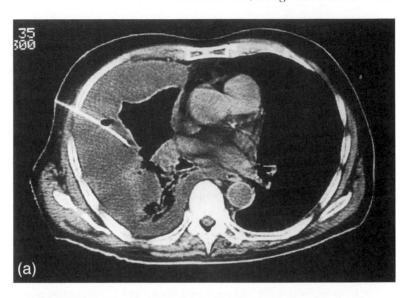

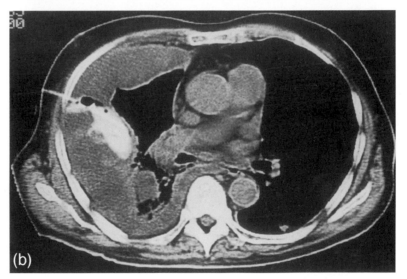

Fig. 15.6 (a) Computed tomography-guided drainage of parapneumonic empyema. (b) The heavily loculated nature of the collection is evident following insertion of 30 ml of normal saline containing 2 ml of non-ionic contrast medium.

ical pleurectomy has a high success rate but carries a high morbidity and mortality.

Chemical pleurodesis may be performed with a variety of agents, including talc, bleomycin, tetracycline, mepacrine and *Corynebacterium parvum*, but there are few controlled trials (Morrison *et al.*, 1992). As a result, the choice of sclerosing agent frequently reflects local practice. Currently, tetracycline is the most widely used pleural sclerosant in the UK, al-

though it may shortly become unavailable in the USA. *Corynebacterium parvum* is no longer available. High success rates have recently been reported with iodized talc (Webb *et al.*, 1992). Unlike tetracycline, which frequently produces considerable pain requiring instillation of intrapleural local anaesthetic and systemic narcotic analgesia, talc appears to be well tolerated without significant side effects in the majority of patients. Adult respiratory distress syndrome and acute pneumonitis are recognized complications following instillation of intrapleural talc.

Success rates depend upon the agent used, varying between 50 and 100%. Successful pleural sclerosis depends primarily on initial successful thoracentesis allowing complete lung re-expansion, thus re-establishing contact between the visceral and parietal pleura. Initial complete drainage of the pleural space, prior to sclerosant instillation with subsequent drainage of less than 100 ml of fluid per day, is therefore required. Failure to achieve this state makes successful pleurodesis unlikely (Reid & Rudd, 1993).

Tetracycline (2–3 g in 20–50 ml of normal saline) or talc (5 g of talc and 3 g of thymol iodide as a slurry) is instilled through the tube drain which is then clamped. The patient is rotated to ensure even distribution through the pleural cavity. Suction drainage is re-established for 24 hours and then subsequently removed.

Pleural and chest wall biopsy

Fine-needle aspiration cytology or cutting needle biopsy of chest wall masses arising from or involving the pleura may be performed under CT, ultrasound or fluoroscopic guidance (Fig. 15.7). The choice of imaging depends on operator preference, patient cooperation and lesion accessibility. Most focal masses are best targeted with ultrasound or CT, diffuse pleural thickening with CT and rib lesions with either fluoroscopy or ultrasound. Complications are rare but include haemothorax, pneumothorax and local haematoma formation. When a cutting needle is used, a suitably angled approach ensures the throw of the cutting needle chamber does not traverse the visceral pleura and lung (Gleeson *et al.*, 1990).

Mediastinal abscess drainage

Mediastinal abscesses are usually secondary to thoracic trauma, particularly penetrating trauma, and oesophageal perforation (either spontaneous rupture or secondary to carcinoma) or oesophageal intervention such as dilatation manoeuvres. The prognosis is grave and prompt drainage is required. This is often most appropriately performed by open surgery, but occasionally a percutaneous approach is prefer-

able and the results from a limited number of studies are encouraging (Gunther, 1992). CT guidance is always required (Fig. 15.8). Anterior collections are drained via a parasternal approach, taking care to avoid the internal mammary vessels. Abscesses in the middle and posterior mediastinal compartments are drained by a paravertebral and extrapleural approach and it is often necessary to place catheters on both sides of the spine.

Pericardial fluid aspiration

Pericardial effusions are readily diagnosed by sonography and CT. It is therefore not uncommon for radiologists to perform pericardial aspirations, particularly when dedicated imaging guidance is required. Most collections are evacuated using a subcostal or subxiphoid approach. The distal puncture is performed with an 18 gauge needle or a small gauge (5F) Teflon sheath needle. A 5F pig-tail catheter is inserted if continuous aspiration is required.

Lung abscess drainage

There is a limited need for percutaneous catheter drainage of lung abscesses, since the majority are adequately dealt with by antibiotic therapy and generally drain spontaneously into the bronchial tree. The technique is reserved for those patients in whom there is a persistent abscess despite appropriate antibiotic therapy. Such lesions occur particularly in debilitated patients for whom limited surgical resection was performed in the past. The technique should only be used when the abscess lies in the periphery of the lung with part of its circumference in contact with the pleura. Such conditions, which exist in the majority of cases, greatly reduce the likelihood of a secondary empyema. CT is required to delineate precisely the abscess and adjacent anatomy prior to catheter insertion, and is also usually used for the procedure itself (van Sonnenberg *et al.*, 1991). As with abscess cavities elsewhere, relatively large calibre catheters (12–14F) are often required to drain tenacious abscess contents. They are introduced in the same way as for empyema drainage, using a line of approach which ensures that aerated lung is not traversed. Complications include pulmonary haem-

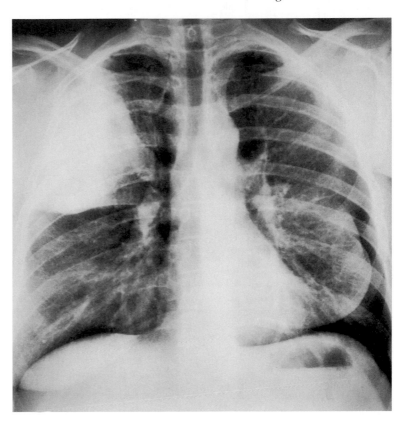

Fig. 15.7 Chest wall mass associated with a rib fracture following minor trauma. There has been previous surgery and radiotherapy to the left breast, which is reduced in size. Ultrasound-guided biopsy using an 18 gauge cutting needle confirmed metastatic adenocarcinoma of the breast.

orrhage, bronchopleural fistula and empyema formation.

In patients with *Aspergillus* colonization of lung cavities who are systemically unwell, direct instillation of amphotericin may be desirable. CT usually provides the most appropriate imaging guidance. Amphotericin prepared as a gel may be injected on separate occasions or via an indwelling catheter.

Tracheobronchial stent insertion

Narrowing of the trachea and major bronchi produces marked airflow reduction and significant symptomatic relief can be provided by the insertion of expandable or self-expanding metallic stents.

The most common indication for stent insertion is unresectable malignant disease causing narrowing of the airway, either prior to palliative radiotherapy or chemotherapy or at the time of recurrence, particularly if the tumour is largely extrinsic to the air-

way. Despite the relatively short life expectancy of these patients quality of life and respiratory distress can be dramatically improved by stent insertion. Since they are not removable, tracheobronchial stents are usually reserved for patients with incurable disease. However, they are occasionally used in patients with benign inoperable stenoses due to sarcoidosis, relapsing polychondritis and amyloid and also for strictures secondary to bronchial or tracheal anastomotic ischaemia following lung transplantation (Egan *et al.*, 1994).

The most commonly inserted devices are the Wallstent* and Gianturco stent†. The Wallstent has been extensively used in the biliary tree and is composed of a cylinder of braided steel monofilaments which can be elongated and mounted on a catheter to produce a small diameter delivery system of 7–

* Schneider (UK), Staines, Middlesex, UK.
† William Cook (UK), Letchworth, Hertfordshire, UK.

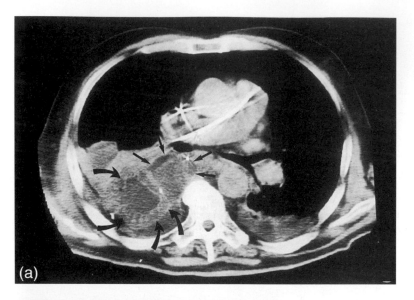

(a)

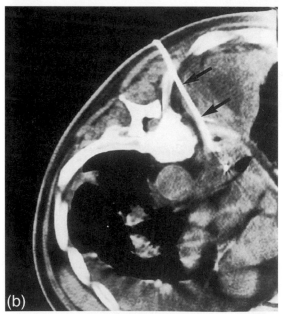

(b)

Fig. 15.8 (a) Posterior mediastinal collection (straight arrows) complicating breakdown of anastomosis following oesophagectomy and gastric conduit formation (curved arrows). (b) Narrow-bore drain insertion (arrows) under computed tomography guidance with the patient in a semi-prone position.

9F. The stent is contained within a constricting covering which is removed once positioned across the area of narrowing. The Gianturco stent is composed of stainless spring steel monofilaments fashioned into a double zigzag and introduced on a 12F delivery system, fixation hooks engage the side-wall of the airway. Both varieties are introduced bronchoscopically and the range of diameters permits a stent of appropriate gauge to be inserted. It is usual to select a stent diameter slightly larger than the normal lumen of the airway in question, so that radial stress forces are maintained once the stent has re-expanded. If necessary, multiple stents may be inserted to cover the area of airway abnormality adequately (Fig. 15.9).

Prior to stent insertion, the severity of airway narrowing is documented with conventional tomography or CT and pulmonary function tests, including measurement of the flow–volume loop. Fibreoptic bronchoscopy is undertaken immediately prior to stent insertion and correlated with the imaging findings. Stenting is usually best carried out under general anaesthesia. Following bronchoscopic assessment, a guide wire is placed via the bronchoscopy channel across the stenotic segment. The bronchoscope is removed and the delivery system railroaded into position under fluoroscopic guidance, following which the stent is released and allowed to expand across the stenosis.

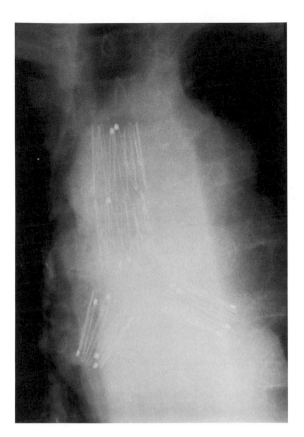

Fig. 15.9 Metallic stents (Gianturco) in the trachea and major bronchi in a patient with stidor due to a central carcinoma.

Stent migration or malpositioning is uncommon and there is usually rapid relief of respiratory symptoms and improvement in the flow–volume loop. In patients with malignant disease, restenosis by ingrowth of tumour through the stent may occur and require surgical curettage. Incorporation of a plastic or silicone membrane into the stent is a possible solution to this. Spontaneous stent fracture has been reported with the Gianturco stents, although this problem now appears to have been rectified.

Computed tomography

Whilst the chest radiograph remains the first-line imaging investigation of thoracic disease, it is frequently necessary to elucidate more fully the nature of detected or suspected abnormalities of the lung, pleura and mediastinum by means of CT.

The scanning technique and protocol depend upon a variety of factors, including the clinical requirements, the nature of the pathological process being studied and the technical facilities of the scanner being used. Generally no specific prior preparation is required for CT of the chest. Scans are normally obtained at full inspiration with most patients being able to reliably reproduce the same level of inspiratory effort for contiguous scans. However, elderly and dyspnoeic patients may require careful instruction and several practice inspirations immediately prior to the start of scanning. When lack of cooperation or the degree of dyspnoea preclude scanning during suspended inspiration, adequate images may still be obtained during gentle continuous respiration.

When contrast-enhanced scans are required, these should be acquired in spiral or dynamic mode. Between 50 and 150 ml of i.v. contrast medium (300–350 mg ml^{-1} of iodine) is administered, ideally with a power injector. Contrast volumes, rates of infusion and relative timing of scanning depend greatly on the capability of the scanner and the clinico-radiological requirements. Modern scanners with continuous image acquisition and spiral capability provide the opportunity for significantly improved data acquisition and high-quality images, often with a relatively small volume of contrast medium.

Images are displayed at soft-tissue and lung window settings. Typically soft tissues are best diplayed with a window level of 35 Hounsfield units (HU) and a width of 300 HU, and lung window settings with a level of –600 HU with a width of 1600 HU.

Lung cancer

Contiguous 10 mm scans are obtained from the lung apex into the upper abdomen to include the liver and adrenals. Enhanced scans are obtained from just above the aortic arch to the inferior pulmonary veins, to assist in the assessment of direct tumour invasion and spread to regional lymph nodes. Contiguous 5 mm thick sections are sometimes useful for assessing the major airways and hila. In some institutions, particularly when a histological diagnosis of small cell carcinoma has been established, a head scan is also performed.

Mediastinal tumours

Unenhanced continguous 10 mm scans from the lung apex to include the entire ling volume are followed by i.v. contrast-enhanced scans from a level above to a level below the tumour.

Lung metastases

Unenhanced contiguous 10 mm scans are obtained from the apex of the lung to include the entire lung volume. Scans are imaged on mediastinal and lung window settings. Limited high-resolution CT slices through a representative nodule may occasionally be of value.

Solitary pulmonary nodule

It is sometimes appropriate to perform CT to confirm the presence of the lesion, determine its exact position and assess its contour and contents. Thin slices (1–2 mm) are best obtained using a spiral sequence. A high spatial frequency algorithm permits identification of calcium and fat within the lesion. Three-dimensional images, following a spiral sequence with 5 mm thick slices, are valuable for the demonstration of pulmonary arteriovenous malformation.

Empyema

Scanning should always be performed following suitable i.v. contrast enhancement with 10 mm thick slices at 10–15 mm increments. Unenhanced scans are seldom required.

Oesophageal carcinoma

The patient should fast for 8 hours and oral contrast medium should be given as for standard abdominal scanning. Contiguous 10 mm scans are obtained from the lung apices to the apex of the diaphragm, followed by contrast-enhanced scanning to the level of the aortic bifurcation. This protocol provides optimal assessment of direct tumour spread and nodal metastases of oesophageal carcinoma arising in the lower third of the oesophagus.

Diffuse lung disease

HRCT is used in the assessment of patients with diffuse chronic infiltrative lung disease, bronchiectasis, emphysema and selected cases of diffuse acute lung disease (Padley *et al.*, 1993).

A recent chest radiograph should be scrutinized prior to the scan and the investigation appropriately tailored to the clinical and radiological probabilities. Contrast enhancement is not required. Scans are obtained from the lung apices to the diaphragm, using a slice width between 1 and 2 mm and reconstructing with a high spatial frequency algorithm to optimize resolution. Table increments of 10 mm are appropriate for most conditions, but large increments (15–20 mm) are acceptable if the disease is likely to be profuse and detailed assessment of extent is not required. In the assessment of bronchiectasis, 5 mm increments and a $-20°$ gantry angle may be used to scan along the plane of the middle lobe and lingular bronchi.

Prone scans are occasionally required in patients suspected of having asbestosis or early cryptogenic fibrosing alveolitis, as well as for the occasional patient in whom there is difficulty in differentiating dependent increased attenuation from true structural abnormalities. Expiratory scans at selected levels are used to identify air trapping in patients with suspected obliterative bronchiolitis and in the assessment of bullae.

Thoracic outlet syndrome

CT scanning can provide useful diagnostic information in selected patients with suspected thoracic outlet syndrome. CT identifies osseous abnormalities other than cervical ribs, such as abnormally long and drooping C7 transverse processes, and allows assessment of the relationship between the C7 transverse process and the scalene triangle and scalene muscles (Bilbey *et al.*, 1989).

Scans are obtained from the middle of the C6 pedicles to the bottom of the T2 vertebral body. Contiguous 2.5 mm thick slices are obtained without i.v. contrast medium. Images are displayed on mediastinal window settings.

Pulmonary embolism

There is now evidence that CT is an accurate method for detecting emboli in vessels up to and including segmental level (Remy-Jardin *et al.*, 1992). A spiral sequence from a level just above the aortic arch to the level of the inferior pulmonary veins is required with a 5 mm table feed and reconstruction at 3–5 mm intervals. Strict attention should be paid to the i.v. contrast medium enhancement in order to provide correct opacification of the pulmonary vessels. Contrast medium (100–150 ml) of a concentration of 150 mg ml^{-1} is delivered at a rate of 5 ml s^{-1} and scanning commenced after a delay of 5–10 s.

Aortic dissection

A preliminary scanogram permits the selection of the appropriate levels for continuous scanning without table movement during the passage of a bolus of contrast medium. It is usual to scan at the level of the aortic arch, just the above the aortic valve and at a level midway between these two points. Alternative protocols are a spiral sequence with a table feed of 5 mm s^{-1} and reconstruction at 5 mm intervals or a dynamic sequence with sequential scans at 10 mm intervals.

References

Berquist, T.H., Bailey, P.B., Cortese, D.A. *et al.* (1980) Transthoracic needle biopsy. Accuracy and complications in relation to location and type of lesion. *Mayo Clin. Proc.*, **55**, 475–81.

Bilbey, J.H., Muller, N.L., Connell, D.G., Luoma, A.A. & Nelems, B. (1989) Thoracic outlet syndrome: evaluation with CT. *Radiology*, **171**(2), 381–7.

Calhoun, P., Feldman, P.S., Armstrong, P. *et al.* (1986) The clinical outcome of needle aspirations of the lung when cancer is not diagnosed. *Ann. Thorac. Surg.*, **41**, 592–6.

Charig, M.J., Stutley, J.E., Padley, S. & Hansell, D.M. (1991) The value of negative needle biopsy in suspected lung cancer. *Clin. Radiol.*, **44**, 147–9.

Egan, A.M., Dennis, C. & Flower, C.D. (1994) Expandable metal stents for tracheobronchial obstruction. *Clin. Radiol.*, **49**(3), 162–5.

Gleeson, F., Lomas, D.J., Flower, C.D. & Stewart, S. (1990) Powered cutting needle biopsy of the pleura and chest wall. *Clin. Radiol.*, **41**(3), 199–200.

Gunther, R.W. (1992) Percutaneous interventions in the thorax. *J. Vasc. Intervent. Radiol.*, **3**, 379–90.

Herman, J.H., Holub, R.V., Weisbrod, G.L. & Chamberlain, D.W. (1991) Anterior mediastinal masses: utility of transthoracic needle biopsy. *Radiology*, **180**, 167–70.

Hunnam, G.R. & Flower, C.D. (1988) Radiologically guided percutaneous catheter drainage of empyemas. *Clin. Radiol.*, **39**(2), 121–6.

Lee, K.S., Im, J.-G., Kim, Y.H., Hwang, S.H., Won, K.B. & Lee, B.H. (1991) Treatment of thoracic multiloculated empyemas with intracavitary urokinase: a prospective study. *Radiology*, **179**, 771–5.

McKenna, R.J., Campbell, A., McMurtrey, M. & Mountain, C.F. (1986) Diagnosis for interstitial lung disease in patients with acquired immunodeficiency syndrome: a prospective comparison of bronchial washing, alveolar lavage, transbronchial lung biopsy, and open lung biopsy. *Ann. Thorac. Surg.*, **41**, 318–21.

Morrison, M.C., Mueller, P.E., Lee, M.J. *et al.* (1992) Sclerotherapy of malignant pleural effusions through sonographically placed small bore catheters. *AJR*, **158**, 41.

Moulton, J.S., Moor, P.T. & Mencini, R.A. (1989) Treatment of loculated pleural effusions with transcatheter intracavitary urokinase. *Am. J. Roentgenol.*, **153**, 941–5.

Padley, S., Adler, B. & Müller, N.L. (1993) HRCT of the chest: current indications. *J. Thorac. Imaging*, **8**, 189–99.

Perlmutt, L.M., Braun, S.D., Newman, G.E. *et al.* (1986) Transthoracic needle aspiration: use of a small chest tube to treat pneumothorax. *AJR*, **148**, 849–51.

Reid, P.T. & Rudd, R.M. (1993) Management of malignant pleural effusion. *Thorax*, **48**, 779–80.

Remy-Jardin, M. Remy, J, Wattine, L & Giraud, F. (1992) Central pulmonary thromboembolism: diagnosis with spiral volumetric CT with the single breath hold technique — comparison with pulmonary angiography. *Radiology*, **185**(2); 381–7.

Sicard, J.A. & Forrestier, J. (1922) Méthode générale d'exploration radiologique par l'huile iodée. *Bull. Soc. Med. Hop. Paris*, **38**, 463–7.

Sinner, W.N. (1976) Complications of percutaneous transthoracic needle aspiration biopsy. *Acta Radiol. Diagn.*, **17**, 813–28.

Sinner, W.M. & Zajicek, J. (1976) Implantation of metastases after percutaneous transthoracic needle aspiration biopsy. *Acta. Radiol. Diagn.*, **17**, 473–80.

vanSonnenberg, E., Nakamato, S.K., Mueller, P.R. *et al.* (1984) CT and ultrasound guided catheter drainage of empyemas after chest tube failure. *Radiology*, **151**, 349–53.

vanSonnenberg, E., D'Agostino, H.B., Casola, G., Halasz, N.A., Sanchez, R.B. & Goodacre, B.W. (1991) Percutaneous abscess drainage: current concepts. *Radiology*, **181**(3), 617–26.

Webb, W.R., Ozmen, V., Moultier, P.V., Shabahang, B. & Breux, J. (1992) Iodized talc pleurodesis for the treatment of pleural effusions. *J. Thorac. Cardiovasc. Surg.*, **103**(5), 881–5.

Weisbrod, G.L. (1990) Transthoracic percutaneous lung biopsy. *Radiol. Clin. N. Am.*, **23**(3), 647–55.

Westcott, J.L. (1985) Percutaneous catheter drainage of pleural effusion and empyema. *Am. J. Roentgenol.*, **144**, 1189–93.

Whitehouse, G.H. & Worthington, B.S. (eds) (1990) *Techniques in Diagnostic Imaging*, 2nd edn. Blackwell Scientific Publications, Oxford.

Section 4
Genitourinary Tract

16 Urinary Tract

C. EVANS, S. McGEE AND G. H. WHITEHOUSE

Intravenous urography (IVU)

Once the dominant examination in the radiological diagnosis of urinary tract disease, IVU is now performed far less frequently. This has arisen out of concerns about radiation dose and the extra costs incurred with the use of expensive low-osmolar contrast media (LOCM). In addition, the past two decades have seen the development of alternative, less invasive imaging techniques, particularly ultrasound. These factors have forced a reappraisal of the place of IVU in urological diagnosis and the total number of examinations performed has fallen by upwards of 50%. In selected patients, however, IVU remains as a first-line investigation.

Indications

1 Haematuria.
2 Renal colic.
3 Renal trauma.
4 Persistent pyuria.
5 Prior to percutaneous urological procedures to define renal anatomy.
6 Prior to surgery involving risk of significant ureteric injury, for example gynaecological or colorectal malignancy.
7 As part of the work-up of a live donor in renal transplantation.
8 After surgery, for example ureteric surgery.
9 When other investigations are equivocal or puzzling.

Poorly localizing symptoms such as haematuria or persistent pyuria are best investigated by IVU as it provides an overview of the whole urinary tract from the kidneys to the bladder. Haematuria, particularly when overt and not associated with urinary tract infection, warrants prompt urography and cystoscopy, preferably in one hospital visit at a haematuria clinic. The advantage of IVU over ultrasound in this clinical setting is the exquisite calyceal detail it provides, enabling the diagnosis of early transitional cell tumours, small calculi and renal papillary necrosis.

Limited IVU is of considerable value in renal colic, particularly when performed during an attack of pain. The study will confirm a plain radiographic opacity as the cause of urinary tract obstruction and occasionally demonstrates the underlying aetiology for stone formation, for example medullary sponge kidney. It has been suggested that the combination of a plain abdominal radiograph and a renal ultrasound scan are as accurate as IVU in the assessment of patients with acute renal colic (Haddad et al., 1992). This study showed sensitivity and specificity of more than 90% for this combination in the diagnosis of acute urinary tract obstruction. However, ultrasound cannot differentiate mild pelvicalyceal dilatation in acute obstruction from normal distension of the collecting system in a well-hydrated individual and is unreliable in the diagnosis of non-dilated obstruction. For these reasons IVU remains the investigation of choice in renal colic. In renal trauma the value of IVU is twofold: (i) evaluation of the form and function of the injured kidney; and (ii) confirmation of a functioning contralateral kidney.

The IVU is no longer routinely indicated in the investigation of hypertension, renal failure, urinary tract infection in children and adult females, or complications following renal transplantation. Should the findings from other imaging modalities be equivocal or non-diagnostic, IVU remains available in reserve.

The use of IVU as a screening examination in men with prostatism cannot be justified. A plain abdominal radiograph to exclude calculi, together with an ultrasound examination of the kidneys and bladder in association with a urinary flow rate measurement, yields adequate information in virtually all cases.

Contraindications

1 Previous serious reaction to injected contrast medium.
2 Pregnancy and in women who indicate the possibility of pregnancy.
3 Diabetes mellitus with renal insufficiency.

While not an absolute contraindication to IVU, caution is needed in patients who have previously experienced adverse reactions to contrast media. It is wise to obtain a detailed clinical history and discuss the problems with the referring clinician before proceeding with the study. In most cases the IVU may be performed safely using a different contrast medium and following premedication with oral corticosteroids (dexamethasone 6 mg orally 12 and 2 hours prior to injection of contrast medium). The evidence for the protective effects of steroid premedication is not yet conclusive (Dawson & Sidhu, 1993) but this approach constitutes reasonable medical practice, given the available evidence at this time.

It is clearly preferable to avoid irradiating a woman who is or may be pregnant, particularly in the first weeks of pregnancy when the developing fetus is especially susceptible to the effects of ionizing radiation. IVU may precipitate acute renal failure in patients with diabetic nephropathy and so should be avoided whenever possible.

In infants and patients with myeloma, sickle cell disease and asthma one should question whether the information could be obtained by other means, for example isotope studies, before proceeding with IVU.

Technique

All IVUs should ideally be supervised by a radiologist so that the maximum amount of diagnostic information can be obtained in the shortest time using the fewest number of radiographs and with minimum radiation dose to the patient. The exact conduct of the investigation varies from department to department but should be tailored to answer the clinical questions.

Patient preparation

Patients undergoing IVU should be instructed to avoid the meal immediately prior to the examination. No other special preparation is necessary. This protocol avoids overhydration and limits abdominal gas, both of which may adversely affect the quality of the urogram, as well as reducing the chances of contrast-induced vomiting.

There is no evidence that routine bowel preparation is advantageous (George *et al.*, 1993). Dehydration has no significant effect on image quality and should be avoided, particularly in the very young, the elderly and in patients with diabetes mellitus, multiple myeloma and sickle cell anaemia where dehydration may be positively harmful. The patient should micturate immediately prior to the study in order to avoid dilution of contrast medium in the bladder.

Radiographic procedure

It is important that the patient is as relaxed as possible and to this end a calm, quiet atmosphere in the IVU room is helpful, as is a courteous attitude from radiographer and radiologist. An anxious patient is prone to fidget and may swallow significant amounts of air, resulting in image degradation from motion unsharpness and overlying gas. There is, moreover, some evidence to indicate that anxiety is associated with an increased risk of adverse reactions to contrast medium.

Preliminary radiographs

These radiographs are a fundamental component of the IVU and most diagnostic errors are due to mistakes in their interpretation. In a male patient of average build the following radiographs will usually be obtained.
1 35×43 cm of the abdomen in arrested inspiration to include the symphysis pubis.
2 24×30 cm (30×40 cm in a large patient) collimated to the renal areas in arrested expiration.
A single 35×40 cm radiograph may suffice in children and small adults.

The 'control' radiographs are obtained at a relatively low kilovoltage (65–75 kV) to optimize soft-tissue detail and are taken for the following reasons.
1 To demonstrate opacities that may lie within the urinary tract.
2 To check positioning and radiographic exposure factors.

3 To determine if there is any other abnormality within the abdomen which may account for the patient's symptoms, for example bowel obstruction, aortic aneurysm, and so on.

Further radiographs (renal area in inspiration, oblique, lateral) may be required to determine whether an opacity lies within the urinary tract.

Linear tomography is occasionally necessary prior to the injection of contrast medium, particularly when the kidneys are obscured by bowel gas or faeces. The tomographic mid-point of the kidneys has been estimated to lie one-third of the way along a line from the table top to the anterior abdominal wall at the inferior costal margin, usually 7–11 cm above the table top. Nephrotomography employs a wide angle of swing (25–40°), producing relatively thin slices in sharp focus. An alternative technique, zonography, uses smaller angles of swing, typically 8–10°, and slices are correspondingly thicker.

Nephrotomography is probably superior to zonography in demonstrating subtle calyceal deformity but departments vary in their preference in this respect.

Contrast medium

The most commonly used contrast media in IVU are shown in Table 16.1. Iohexol and iopamidol are examples of second generation non-ionic LOCM, while iothalamate and diatrizoate salts are conventional ionic substituted tri-iodobenzoic acid derivatives with significantly higher osmolality.

All these agents are excreted virtually exclusively by glomerular filtration. Most of the water in the glomerular filtrate is then reabsorbed in the proximal convoluted tubules (PCT). PCT reabsorption is independent of the state of hydration but is influenced by the osmolality of the contrast medium and, in the case of ionic agents, by whether sodium or meglumine is the dominant cation in the contrast medium used. High-osmolar contrast media (HOCM) produce a larger osmotic diuresis than LOCM and this is greater for meglumine than for sodium salts. Final adjustment of the water content of the filtrate is regulated by antidiuretic hormone (ADH) at the distal convoluted and collecting tubules. Dehydration may influence events at this stage by its effects on circulating levels of ADH. The nephrogram phase of the IVU is essentially due to filtered contrast medium in the PCT. The maximum density of the nephrogram is determined by the peak plasma level of contrast medium, the glomerular filtration rate (GFR) and PCT reabsorption of sodium and water. The peak plasma level of contrast is dependent on the total administered dose, the rate of injection and patient weight.

The quality of the pyelogram phase of IVU depends on the urinary iodine concentration, which in turn depends on the administered dose of iodine together with the total amount of tubular water reabsorption, i.e. the renal concentrating ability. The degree of calyceal distension is also a factor. There are differences in the renal handling of HOCM and LOCM. The peak nephrogram is slightly delayed with LOCM. Distension of the pelvicalyceal system is less with LOCM than with HOCM, because of the

Table 16.1 Low- and high-osmolar contrast media (LOCM and HOCM)

	Generic name	Proprietary name
Conventional ionic media (1.5 ratio HOCM) sodium and meglumine salts of:	Diatrizoate	Hypaque/Urografin
	Iothalamate	Conray
	Iodamide	Uromiro
	Metrizoate	Triosil/Isopaque
Ionic dimer (3 ratio LOCM):	Ioxaglate	Hexabrix
Non-ionic (3 ratio LOCM):	Iopamidol	Niopam
	Iohexol	Omnipaque
	Iopromide	Ultravist
	Ioversol	Optiray

smaller osmotic diuresis, suggesting that abdominal compression may be more important when a non-ionic agent is used. Urinary iodine concentrations are theoretically higher with LOCM due to greater tubular reabsorption of water but clinically this does not result in a denser pyelogram. Indeed, the available evidence suggests that there is no significant difference between conventional HOCM and non-ionic LOCM in the quality of IVU obtained (Gavant *et al.*, 1992). For the contrast media in Table 16.1 a minimum dose in an adult of average build and normal renal function is 50 ml. Higher doses, for instance 75 ml, are frequently given in elderly patients, to compensate for the decline in glomerular filtration rate with age, and in obese patients. The standard dose may be doubled in renal failure but IVU is rarely indicated in these patients. For infants and small children the dose depends on body weight but is relatively higher because of the relatively poor concentrating ability of the immature nephron. Thus doses of 1.5 ml kg^{-1} may be given in small children and 4 ml kg^{-1} in neonates. Contrast medium should be administered by rapid injection over 30–60 s in adults, but more slowly (up to 3 min) in small children, the elderly and any patient at risk of cardiac arrhythmia. There is no advantage in the use of a drip infusion technique, as has been advocated in the USA.

In recent years there has been a significant change in the use of contrast media in IVU as well as in angiography and computed tomography (CT) with a marked shift away from HOCM and much greater use of LOCM. There is very strong evidence of the greater safety and better patient tolerance of LOCM (Bagg *et al.*, 1986) and their use is associated with a significant reduction in the incidence of all grades of adverse reaction attributed to contrast media (Palmer, 1988), although not in the number of deaths (Caro *et al.*, 1991). There is some evidence (Lasser *et al.*, 1987) that premedication with oral corticosteroids offers a degree of protection against adverse reactions to HOCM, but the benefit is significantly less than that obtained by using an LOCM alone.

At present the only argument against wholesale conversion to LOCM as the agents of choice for IVU is economy. Grainger and Dawson (1990) have produced guidelines for the use of i.v. contrast media on behalf of the Royal College of Radiologists. They acknowledge the evidence from large-scale Australian (Palmer, 1988) and Japanese (Katayama *et al.*, 1990) studies of the greater safety of LOCM and state that the ultimate objective should be to replace HOCM with LOCM as soon as the necessary funding is available. Until then they recommend priority use of LOCM.

Applying these guidelines to IVU, LOCM are indicated in the following groups of patients.
1 Those at higher risk of anaphylactoid reaction:
   (a) previous reactors,
   (b) asthmatics,
   (c) atopic individuals,
   (d) those allergic to other drugs or agents.
2 Those unable to tolerate a high osmotic load:
   (a) poor cardiac reserve,
   (b) oliguric or anuric renal failure (IVU rarely indicated).
3 Infants and babies.
4 Elderly patients.
5 Sickle cell disease or trait.
6 Patients with pre-existing renal impairment to minimize the risk of contrast-induced nephrotoxicity. These guidelines are followed by many departments in the UK and patients outside the high-risk categories continue to receive conventional HOCM. It is likely that in the next few years LOCM will completely replace HOCM as i.v. contrast media. Although the case for pretreatment with corticosteroids is not proven, current practice is to give oral steroid 'cover' to any patient who has previously experienced an adverse reaction to i.v. contrast medium, asthmatics who have required oral steroid therapy or previous hospital admission, and atopic individuals.

Radiographic sequence

The radiographic sequence following injection of contrast medium depends on the clinical problem but the following is suggested as an appropriate routine for a patient's first IVU (Fig. 16.1).
1 A 1-min post-injection radiograph of the renal areas in arrested inspiration to demonstrate the nephrogram phase. In practice, this radiograph is often omitted as the renal outlines are usually adequately visualized on the 5-min radiograph, especially as the nephrogram phase occurs later with LOCM.

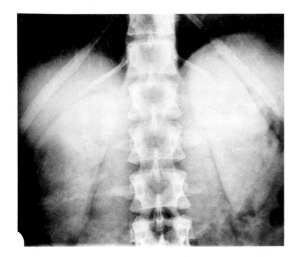

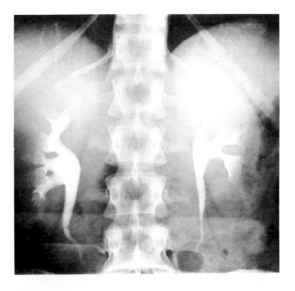

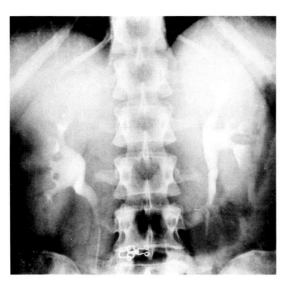

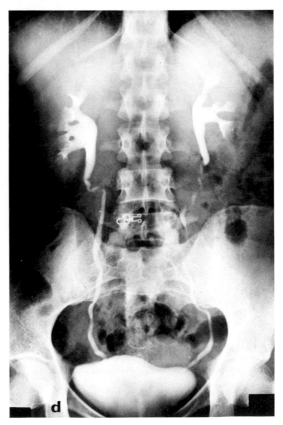

2 A 5-min post-injection radiograph of the renal areas in arrested inspiration to demonstrate contrast in the pelvicalyceal systems. Abdominal compression is now applied, if not contraindicated. This effectively produces partial ureteric obstruction, resulting in more complete distension of the collecting systems, improved calyceal detail and more reliable ureteric opacification upon release of compression (Mawhinney & Gregson, 1987). This is achieved using an inflatable balloon placed on a rigid wooden or plastic board. The whole apparatus is strapped to the patient using a belt (Fig. 16.2) with the balloon placed between the anteriosuperior iliac

Fig. 16.1 Phases of the standard intravenous urogram. (a) Nephrogram. (b) A 5-min radiograph. (c) A 15-min radiograph with abdominal compression. (d) Full length radiograph at 20 min, with release of compression.

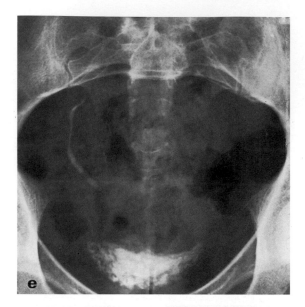

Fig. 16.1 *Continued.* (e) Post-micturition radiograph of the bladder.

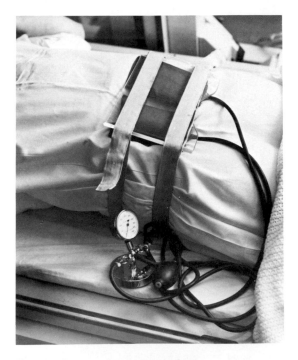

Fig. 16.2 Compression device used in intravenous urography. Two inflatable balloons lie on a plastic board and are maintained in position by two belts.

spines and inflated using a sphygmomanometer immediately after the 5-min post-injection radiograph. Effective compression invariably results in some discomfort for the patient, but this is usually tolerable for the short time during which it is applied. Compression is contraindicated in (i) urinary tract obstruction; (ii) ureteric colic; (iii) patients with an abdominal mass or aortic aneurysm; (iv) following trauma or recent abdominal surgery; (v) in any patient with abdominal pain or tenderness, stoma and IVC filter; (vi) renal failure; and (vii) myeloma. Compression should be released immediately if the patient becomes unwell.

3 A 10-min post-injection film of the renal areas in arrested inspiration to demonstrate distended collecting systems and proximal ureters.

4 A 15-min 'release' full length abdominal radiograph — a 35 × 43 cm radiograph of the abdomen is exposed immediately following release of compression to demonstrate the entire urinary tract, but particularly the lower ureters.

5 Post-micturition radiograph of the bladder area — immediately after the patient has completely emptied the bladder a 18 × 14 cm radiograph is exposed with the X-ray tube angle 15° caudad and centred 2.5 cm below the anterosuperior iliac spines.

Additional radiographs

Further images are occasionally required.

1 Linear nephrotomography. This is indicated to improve visualization of the renal outlines and/or improve visualization of the collecting systems. The need for tomography can often be predicted from the control radiographs and an appropriate tomographic level established before injection of contrast medium. The renal outlines are optimally demonstrated on a 5-min tomograph of the renal areas with calyceal detail usually well shown by a 10-min tomograph during abdominal compression.

2 Oblique radiographs. Oblique views 15 min post-injection with abdominal compression are occasionally useful in clarifying subtle calyceal abnormalities.

3 Full length prone abdominal radiograph. This view may demonstrate contrast medium in the lower ureters when these have not been adequately seen on the 'release' radiograph.

4 Full length post-micturition radiograph. This view

is of value in evaluating a suspected calculus at the vesicoureteric junction when the IVU has shown a 'standing column' of contrast medium in the ureter in question.

5 Fluoroscopy. This is underutilized but is very useful in distinguishing a pelvic phlebolith from a non-obstructing lower ureteric calculus, when the radiographs are indeterminate.

Modifications of basic technique

Urinary tract obstruction

The aims of IVU in urinary tract obstruction are to confirm the presence of obstruction, demonstrate the level of obstruction and, if possible, establish its cause.

In acute obstruction presenting as renal or ureteric colic, a control radiograph together with a full length radiograph at 15-min post-injection are obtained. Delayed films may be required up to 24 hours to confirm suspected ureteric obstruction, particularly if caused by a radiolucent calculus. Abdominal compression is contraindicated and care is taken to avoid large doses of contrast medium. Both these factors increase the risk of spontaneous ipsilateral rupture of the renal pelvis, which may proceed to a perirenal collection.

In chronic obstruction with significant hydronephrosis, larger doses of contrast medium are often required and delayed radiographs are frequently necessary to establish the level of obstruction. The study is invariably difficult if there is marked impairment of excretion. While tomography and prone full length radiographs can be useful, provided there is sufficient contrast medium in the collecting system, this situation is most often an indication for an alternative imaging modality.

Pelviureteric junction (PUJ) obstruction presents a particular challenge as the symptoms and radiographic signs are frequently intermittent. The patient may give a history of episodic loin pain, typically after drinking large volumes of fluid, but IVU may only demonstrate an extrarenal pelvis. In these circumstances it is occasionally possible to demonstrate significant obstruction by giving frusemide 40 mg i.v. after the release radiograph and exposing a further full length abdominal radiograph 15 min later.

The contrast will wash away if there is no obstruction, whilst the renal pelvis distends in the presence of obstruction. Increasingly, however, the diagnosis and follow-up of these patients is made by isotope renography.

Pregnancy

IVU is occasionally required in pregnancy, for example in suspected ureteric colic in late pregnancy when ultrasound is unable to differentiate pathological from physiological dilatation of the urinary tract. In these circumstances a limited study is performed. A preliminary radiograph is followed by a full length erect abdominal radiograph 20 min after the injection of contrast medium. Abdominal compression is contraindicated. The relative delay in obtaining the post-contrast radiograph ensures adequate opacification of the pelvicalyceal systems, while the erect position minimizes physiological distension.

'One-shot' IVU

A preliminary radiograph followed by a full length abdominal radiograph 15 min after the injection of contrast medium will suffice to demonstrate ureteric anatomy, particularly unsuspected duplex systems, prior to surgery where there may be risk of ureteric injury. Typically, this is in patients awaiting resection of extensive neoplasms of the sigmoid colon or gynaecological malignancies.

Such a study is also of value as a check following urological surgery, as an emergency examination in suspected colic and following blunt abdominal trauma.

High-dose urography

The urogram in renal failure has been largely superseded by ultrasound and plain radiographs (Evans, 1987). These are able to answer the following questions: (i) What is the renal size? (Small kidneys denote chronic disease.) (ii) Is there hydronephrosis to indicate postrenal obstruction as the cause of dysfunction?

Very occasionally in the presence of mild renal failure, high-dose urography may provide valuable diagnostic information, for instance, in demonstrating renal scarring or papillary necrosis. In such cases, there must be no dehydration, a double dose (600 mg iodine kg⁻¹) of non-ionic contrast medium should be given following preliminary tomograms of the renal areas, and the tomograms repeated post-injection at 1, 15 and 30 min. Delayed radiographs may be necessary in questionable obstruction, but nowadays this diagnosis is excluded by other means, for example ultrasound and antegrade or retrograde pyelography.

Complications

Adverse reactions to contrast medium

Adverse reactions and their treatment are discussed in full in Chapter 30. Most reactions commence within 15 min of administration of contrast medium and patients should not be left unattended during this period. Full resuscitation equipment, including defibrillator, should be available in or close to the IVU room. The needle should be kept in the arm vein throughout the examination.

Spontaneous rupture of the collecting system

This may occur in acute calculus obstruction as discussed earlier. For this reason, large volumes of contrast medium are avoided and abdominal compression is contraindicated. The diuretic effect of the contrast medium may cause increased pain during the examination.

Contrast medium-induced nephropathy

Acute renal failure can be the direct result of contrast medium administration, and is said to be the third most common cause of in-hospital renal failure after hypotension and surgery. The risk in patients with normal renal function is very low. Pre-existing renal failure in association with diabetes mellitus is a strong risk factor (Parfrey *et al.*, 1989). Other risk factors include old age, myeloma, dehydration, cardiovascular disease and the use of diuretics. The effect may range from a transient rise in creatinine without oliguria to severe oliguria requiring dialysis. LOCM are probably less nephrotoxic than HOCM,

although the data are incomplete. Patients with risk factors, for example diabetic nephropathy, should not be dehydrated, have large volumes of contrast medium nor have repeated contrast examinations within short periods of time.

The nephrogram in contrast medium-induced nephropathy is dense and persistent in most cases, with poor or no visualization of the collecting system. The kidneys may be enlarged and smooth. Thankfully, most cases are transient and do not lead to long-term renal failure.

Relationship to other techniques

The situations where urography is a first-line investigation have declined in number in recent years, as new competitive imaging modalities have become available. However, IVU remains an extremely valuable back-up examination in many different clinical situations.

Retrograde pyelography

Retrograde pyelography is the radiological examination of the pelvicalyceal systems and ureters by direct retrograde injection of contrast medium into the ureter.

Indications

1 Absent or unsatisfactory visualization of the pelvicalyceal systems and ureters at IVU.
2 To evaluate filling defects, obstructive lesions and fistulae in the urinary tract seen on IVU; and to enable collection of appropriate specimens for laboratory examination.
3 Distension of the renal collecting system prior to percutaneous interventional procedures, for example percutaneous nephrolithotomy or balloon dilatation of PUJ obstruction.

Contraindications

1 Hypersensitivity to contrast medium. This is a relative contraindication as, in practice, systemic absorption is minimal provided pyelorenal extravasation due to overdistension of the collecting system is

avoided and care is taken to prevent prolonged stasis of contrast medium in the renal pelvis.

2 Urinary diversion. Retrograde catheterization of ureters is not possible in these patients.

Technique

The procedure involves catheterization of the ureter and positioning of the catheter in the renal pelvis. This is followed by the injection of contrast medium (Fig. 16.3). Pre-existing urinary tract infection should be treated prior to the examination and prophylactic antibiotics given in cases of ureteric obstruction.

Ureteric catheterization takes place in theatre under general anaesthetic at the time of cystoscopy. A 4 or 5 French (F) gauge radio-opaque catheter is passed through the relevant ureteric orifice and advanced under fluoroscopic guidance until the tip lies in the renal pelvis. The catheter has a blunt end in order to minimize ureteric trauma and is passed very gently along the ureter to prevent spasm and avoid perforation. Urinary samples may be collected via the ureteric catheter at this stage and sent for laboratory analysis.

The patient is then transferred to the imaging department for the injection of contrast medium. The external component of the catheter is taped securely to the patient's thigh in theatre to prevent the catheter slipping out while the patient is being moved.

The investigation is performed under sterile conditions. The catheter position is checked and contrast medium injected under fluoroscopic control. The contrast medium is warmed to body temperature and injected from a syringe, care being taken to remove any bubbles from the system. The contrast media used are fairly dilute, for example Urografin 150, so that small filling defects such as non-opaque calculi are not obscured.

The injection should be slow with as little applied pressure as possible. At least 10 ml of contrast medium are required to delineate the pelvicalyceal system and radiographs are exposed in the anteroposterior (AP) and both oblique projections. After inspection of these radiographs, more contrast medium is gently injected as the catheter is slowly withdrawn down the ureter until the entire ureter is delineated and the catheter tip lies in the distal ureter just proximal to the vesicoureteric junc-

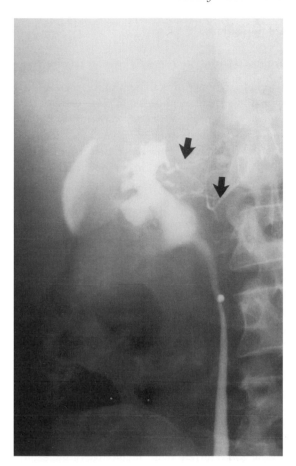

Fig. 16.3 Retrograde pyelogram. Subcapsular extravasation of contrast medium. There is also pyelolymphatic backflow (arrows).

tion. Spot radiographs are exposed during the injection and a 35 × 35 cm radiograph split into three is usually most convenient. If ureteric detail is inconsistent, better images may often be obtained by turning the patient into the prone position. The catheter is left *in situ* until the findings have been discussed with the referring urologist as selective urine collection for cytology may be required, for instance in the case of a transitional cell carcinoma.

Modifications of basic technique

Increasingly, operating theatres are now equipped with portable image intensifiers so that some urologists are content to rely on fluoroscopy only, without a hard copy record of the examination.

Complications

Traumatic injury to the ureter and/or renal pelvis

Urothelial damage or even perforation is more likely with difficult catheter insertions, poor operator technique or when the retrograde catheter used is too rigid. Soft catheters are preferable as they are more likely to coil up on themselves rather than perforate the ureteric wall. Perforation may result in retroperitoneal infection and prophylactic antibiotics are indicated if perforation is known to have occurred.

Urinary tract infection

This can be a problem in cases of uretric obstruction and a hydronephrosis may be converted into a pyonephrosis, especially if aspiration is not performed before withdrawal of the catheter.

Extravasation

Overdistension of the collecting system with contrast medium may cause rupture of the calyceal fornices and extravasation of contrast into the renal sinus, lymphatics and veins (see Fig. 16.3). This is not usually important but may increase the risk of sepsis and interfere with the quality of the examination.

Relationship to other imaging modalities

The technique remains important prior to interventional uroradiological procedures, but antegrade pyelography is frequently the preferred method for investigating ureteric obstruction demonstrated by IVU or ultrasound. The number of retrograde studies is greater when urograms are of poor quality or badly supervised.

Urinary diversion

Urinary diversions are surgical procedures to redirect urine flow and are performed most frequently for the relief of urinary tract obstruction or incontinence secondary to congenital, traumatic or neoplastic disease of the bladder.

The classification of urinary diversions is a complex subject which is beyond the scope of this text. This section discusses the radiological management of the most commonly encountered forms of urinary diversion, the ileal conduit (cutaneous ureteroileostomy) and the various continent urinary diversions. The ileal conduit consists of a surgically isolated loop of distal small bowel, 15–25 cm in length, into which the ureters are implanted. The distal end of the loop forms a stoma in the right iliac fossa and the patient wears an appliance.

There are many forms of continent urinary diversion. The basic principle is to create a pouch, using loops of bowel, to take the place of the bladder. The pouch may be anastomosed to the skin (cutaneous pouch) and be emptied by intermittent self-catheterization. Alternatively, the pouch is anastomosed to the urethral stump (orthotopic pouch) and the patient voids in the normal way.

Radiology

Imaging has an important role in both the immediate postoperative period and in the long-term follow-up of these patients.

Postoperative studies

Imaging is routinely performed between 7 and 14 days postoperatively in continent urinary diversion to assess pouch integrity, the ureteric anastomoses and ureteric patency (Fig. 16.4).

Stent studies

Stents are placed in the renal pelves at operation and the distal ends are externalized through the stoma or urethra. Contrast medium, for example Urografin 150, is dripped under gravity into each of the stents in turn until the collecting system and ureter are opacified. Spot radiographs are taken to demonstrate the collecting system, the position of the stent and the integrity and patency of the ureteropouch anastamosis.

Pouchography

This is performed via an indwelling catheter placed

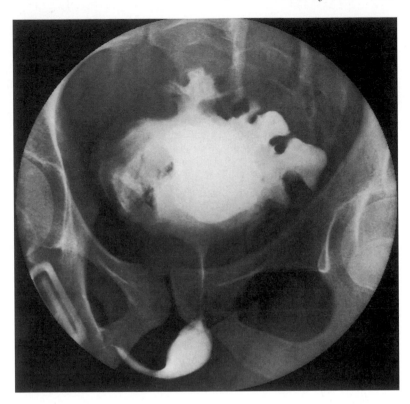

Fig. 16.4 Postoperative cystogram to exclude leakage following bladder reconstruction. The bladder is constructed of large bowel and peristalsis is visible on fluoroscopy.

at the time of surgery. Up to 250 ml of contrast medium may be infused into the pouch. The drip technique is again used to maintain low pressure and avoid stressing the suture lines. Spot radiographs are taken (oblique and lateral) to examine all sides of the pouch. A post-drainage radiograph may be useful if extravasation is suspected but unconfirmed.

Follow-up

Annual plain abdominal radiography and urinary tract ultrasound are indicated routinely in these patients, so that disease recurrence, in cases of urinary tract malignancy, and long-term complications of urinary diversion may be detected at an early stage. Other indications for imaging studies in long-term management include the following.
1 Persistent urinary tract infection.
2 Symptoms of urinary tract obstruction.
3 Evidence of renal dysfunction.
4 Abnormal ultrasound findings.

Loopography (conduitography)

This technique is used to image the ileal loop and to exclude obstruction (Fig. 16.5). A medium-sized Foley catheter is passed retrogradely through the stoma and the balloon is inflated. Gentle traction on the catheter occludes the stoma. Urografin 150 is slowly infused until the whole loop is filled and bilateral ureteric reflux is observed. Spot radiographs are obtained, including drainage views to demonstrate that emptying of the kidneys, ureters and loop is adequate. If reflux from an ileal conduit into both ureters does not occur, then ureteric obstruction is a serious consideration. Poor drainage from the stoma at the end of the procedure may indicate stomal stenosis.

Pouchography imaging in the late postoperative period is performed to document the capacity of the pouch, to assess the degree of urinary stasis, to detect pouch–ureteric reflux and to exclude distal obstruction.

Cystography and micturating cystourethrography (MCU)

These studies involve the introduction of contrast medium directly into the bladder. The bladder is demonstrated when filled with contrast medium and the urethra is shown when the patient voids.

Indications

Children

1 *Recurrent urinary tract infection* in infants and small children. MCU is performed to detect vesico–ureteric reflux.
2 *Suspected anatomical abnormalities of the bladder neck and urethra.* The examination may demonstrate posterior urethral valves as a cause of lower urinary tract obstruction in boys. Urethral strictures may be shown or, in the female, urethral diverticula.

Adults

1 *Functional disorders of the bladder and urethra.* A complete urodynamic assessment is indicated. This involves pressure–flow studies (see later) together with cystography.
2 *Suspected vesicovaginal or vesicocolic fistula.*
3 *Suspected bladder trauma.* Cystography will confirm bladder rupture. It may also be useful postoperatively in evaluating a suspected bladder leak.

Contraindications

1 *Urinary tract infection.* Appropriate antibiotics are prescribed to clear any infection before cystography is performed via a bladder catheter.
2 *Hypersensitivity to contrast medium.* A relative contraindication as there is some systemic absorption of contrast medium from the bladder.

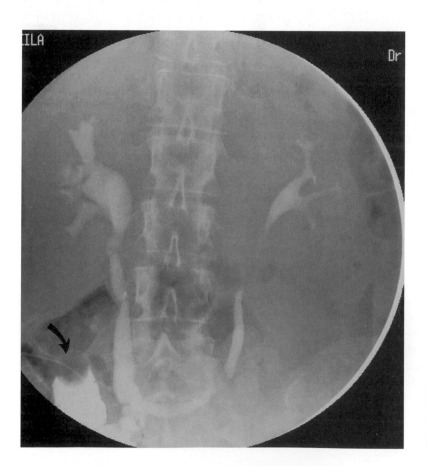

Fig. 16.5 Conduitogram. Balloon catheter in the ileal loop with reflux into both kidneys demonstrating normal collecting systems and no obstruction.

Technique and radiographic sequence

Infants and small children (Fig. 16.6)

Close cooperative between the referring paed-
iatrician and the radiologist is essential to ensure that
this invasive technique is carried out with minimal
distress to the child and parents. The procedure is
explained to the parents and informed written consent is obtained. The examination is most commonly
performed via a bladder catheter with the child sedated. Sedation and catheterization of the bladder
are preferably carried out by the paediatric team. Prophylactic antibiotics, for example trimethoprim
4 mg kg^{-1}, are also given at this time. The bladder is
catheterized with a fine-bore feeding tube (6 or 8F).
A catheter specimen of urine is collected and sent
for microscopy and culture. The catheter is taped
securely to the thigh and the patient is then brought
to the examination room. Residual urine is drained
from the bladder.

Any excess tape should be removed prior to the
introduction of contrast medium so that the
catheter may be removed quickly once voiding has
begun.

A conventional ionic tri-iodinated contrast medium, for example Urografin 150 or Hypaque 25%,
is appropriate for MCU. The bladder is steadily
filled with contrast medium. For children over 2
months of age the contrast medium is delivered
from a 250 ml bottle elevated 1 m above the examination table. Hand injection of contrast medium
from a syringe is usually adequate in younger children as much smaller volumes are required. Intermittent fluoroscopy is performed to assess bladder
filling and to check for vesico–ureteric reflux. A spot
radiograph is obtained during early bladder filling
as this is the optimal time to demonstrate a
ureterocoele. Spot radiographs are taken of any
vesico–ureteric reflux. The bladder is filled until the
patient is seen to start voiding. The catheter is withdrawn and further spot radiographs are taken as
the child micturates onto absorbent paper on the
table. Images should include oblique views of the
bladder, ureters and urethra during voiding together with a post-voiding view to include the kidneys. Satisfactory images are acquired using a 100
mm camera.

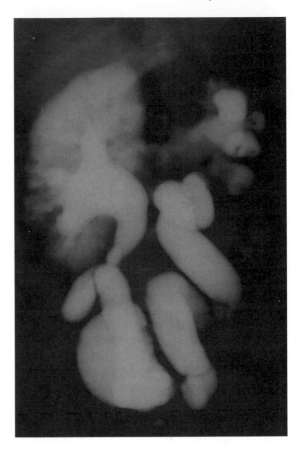

Fig. 16.6 Micturating cystogram showing gross bilateral
ureteric reflux with intrarenal reflux on the right side.

The timing of catheter withdrawal is important to
satisfactory imaging of the voiding phase. Children
frequently become extremely restless as the bladder
is distended to maximum capacity and it is easy to
remove the catheter prematurely before voiding has
commenced.

If the child does not void immediately, a long wait
may follow. Bladder emptying may be incomplete
due to the effects of sedation, because of dysuria following catheterization, in cases of neurogenic bladder, or because of refilling from above where there is
significant vesico–ureteric reflux. Occasionally, it is
necessary to complete bladder emptying by manual
expression of contrast medium.

Adults

The examination is performed under sterile conditions, usually via a bladder catheter. The patient is requested to empty the bladder prior to the procedure and then lies supine on the examination table. The external urethral meatus is cleaned with a mild antiseptic solution and local anaesthetic gel is applied. A medium-sized Harris or Foley catheter is passed into the bladder and any residual urine is drained. The balloon of a Foley catheter need not be inflated and will avoid overdistension of the bladder.

Urografin 150, or a similar conventional contrast medium, is warmed to body temperature and infused through the catheter from a bottle suspended 1 m above the fluoroscopy table. Spot radiographs are obtained in posteroanterior (PA) and oblique projections to demonstrate the bladder and any associated abnormalities. Lateral views are required in cases of vesicocolic or vesicovaginal fistula. It is important to fill the bladder until there is an uncomfortable urge to micturate, particularly when a voiding study is required, as a well-distended bladder is most likely to be associated with successful micturition. The patient micturates in the upright position either into a bottle or a gourd-shaped urinal placed between the thighs. Further oblique radiographs are obtained during micturition to demonstrate any vesico–ureteric reflux and to show the bladder neck and urethra.

Stress incontinence is no longer evaluated by cystography alone. Previously, erect lateral views of the full bladder were obtained during cystography with the urethral catheter in position. The relationship of the bladder to the bony pelvis could then be evaluated, with and without straining. The angle between the urethra and the bladder base could also be determined. This technique is now invariably combined with pressure studies (urodynamics) (Fig. 16.7).

Alternative techniques

1 *Suprapubic bladder puncture.* In infants this approach may be used in some cases of lower urinary tract obstruction, for example posterior urethral valves. In adults pelvic trauma is the most common indication for a suprapubic approach. In many of these cases it has been impossible to pass a catheter per urethram or an elective decision has been made to insert a suprapubic catheter because injury to the bladder and/or urethra is suspected.

2 *Urethrocystography.* Contrast medium may be introduced into the bladder during ascending urethrography using a Foley catheter or Knutsson clamp. Indeed, this may be necessary for adequate visualization of the posterior urethra.

3 *Following IVU.* This technique is no longer widely employed but imaging of micturition after the bladder has become uncomfortably full at the end of an IVU allows some basic questions to be addressed, such as the presence or absence of lower urinary tract obstruction.

Complications

1 *Urinary tract infection.* The incidence of urinary tract infection following cystography in adults and children has been estimated at 30%. The most severe complications of urinary infection — septicaemia and death — are fortunately rare, but are more likely in patients with urinary retention, gross hydronephrosis and vesico–ureteric reflux. Children are routinely given antibiotic cover for this procedure and there is a case for extending this policy to all patients, irrespective of age.

2 *Complications of catheterization* include (i) urethral trauma; (ii) bladder trauma; and (iii) insertion of a suprapubic catheter into the peritoneal cavity or extravesical space. Trauma can cause transient haematuria, dysuria, urinary frequency and urinary retention. Urethral oedema may convert a previous partial obstruction into a complete obstruction. When catheterization is difficult there is a risk of creating a false urethral passage. The risk of bladder rupture is negligible if use of a balloon catheter is avoided and if the patient is not under general anaesthesia or heavy sedation.

3 *Complications of contrast media* include (i) adverse reactions due to absorbed contrast medium; and (ii) contrast-induced cystitis. The risk of adverse reactions from contrast medium absorbed via the urothelium is much smaller than the risk from an IVU.

Relationship to other imaging modalities

There is unquestionably still a place for MCU in the

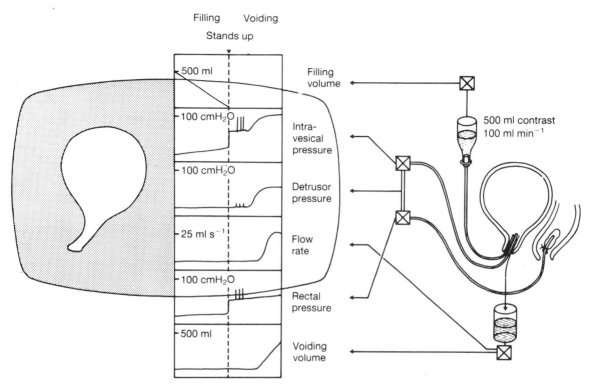

Fig. 16.7 Videocystourethrography. Simultaneous recording of bladder and rectal pressure changes during supine cystometry, combined with a display of bladder filling volume, is shown on the left-hand side of the polygraph trace. The bladder and rectal pressures during voiding, with the voiding rate and volume, are recorded on the right side of the trace. A television camera selects three parameters (intravesical pressure, detrusor pressure and voiding rate) which are added to the radiographic image of the bladder and recorded with sound commentary on videotape. Courtesy of S.L. Stanton and Harper & Row.

investigation of infants and small children with urinary tract infection, say under the age of 2 years. In older children with urinary tract infection cystography is now rarely performed, as it does not affect clinical management. If reflux needs to be excluded in an older cooperative child, this may be done by indirect isotope cystography.

Antegrade pyelography

This is the direct percutaneous injection of contrast medium into the pelvicalyceal system.

Indications

1 Urinary tract obstruction when information from IVU is inadequate and retrograde pyelography has failed or is contraindicated because of the greater risk of introducing infection, or the risks of general anaesthesia.

2 Prior to the insertion of a nephrostomy drainage tube.

3 Prior to interventional urinary tract procedures; for example percutaneous removal of a calculus, ureteric stent insertion or ureteric stricture dilatation.

4 Following ureteric reimplantation. Retrograde pyelography is impossible when the ureters have been reimplanted into a loop of ileum or sigmoid colon. Antegrade pyelography is of value when loopography or urography are inconclusive in defining an upper tract abnormality.

5 To define a ureteric fistula following radical cystectomy, ureterosigmoidostomy or hysterectomy.

6 In renal transplantation where ureteric obstruction or leakage is suspected.

7 To carry out urodynamic studies in cases of doubtful urinary tract obstruction (pressure–flow studies or Whitaker test).

Contraindications

The following are relative contraindications.
1 Single functioning kidney.
2 Uncontrolled hypertension.
3 Bleeding diathesis.
In addition, there is reluctance to perform the study on both kidneys at the same sitting.

Technique

In adults antegrade pyelography is performed under local anaesthesia with the patient lying prone oblique on a fluoroscopy table. Children require sedation. A preliminary ultrasound scan of the kidney in question is extremely useful to indicate the correct site of puncture and for showing the depth of the drainage system (typically 7–8 cm in adults, 2–3 cm in infants). Alternatively, IVU may be obtained, but patients selected for antegrade studies frequently have poor or absent pyelograms. A metallic marker is placed on the proposed puncture site under fluoroscopic guidance. In the majority of cases this will lie 1–2 cm below the 12th rib in the mid-clavicular line. The skin and subcutaneous tissues at the marked site are infiltrated with 1% lignocaine. A 22 gauge spinal or Chiba needle is then passed vertically through the loin under fluoroscopic or ultrasound guidance. Further lignocaine is injected as the needle is advanced. The needle is directed towards a calyx, rather than to the renal pelvis, because the renal parenchyma provides a better seal around the needle track than the thin-walled renal pelvis. A peripheral point of entry makes the inadvertent puncture of a vessel less likely. There is a characteristic 'give' as the needle tip enters the collecting system. Correct positioning may be confirmed by the aspiration of urine and a sample can be sent at this stage for appropriate cytological, bacteriological and chemical analysis. Failure to aspirate urine at the appropriate depth indicates that the needle should be retracted and readvanced in a slightly different direction until its tip lies within the collecting system.

The correctly positioned needle is then connected to a flexible extension tube which is taped to the patient's back. Contrast medium, for example Urografin 150, is carefully and slowly injected through the needle under fluoroscopic guidance (Fig. 16.8). In the obstructed system, no more contrast medium should be injected than the aspirated volume of urine as overdistension in these circumstances is associated with a significantly higher risk of septicaemia. Appropriate radiographs are exposed once the pelvicalyceal system and ureter have been well delineated by contrast medium. The site of obstruction may be more clearly demonstrated by bringing the patient upright on the screening table. At the end of the procedure, as much contrast medium as possible is aspirated prior to withdrawal of the needle. The patient should subsequently be observed for a few hours but the procedure can be performed on an out-patient or day-case basis in suitable patients.

Modification of basic technique

Pressure–flow studies

These studies are useful in establishing the diagnosis of ureteric obstruction when non-invasive tests such as diuresis renography are equivocal. A needle or pressure-sensitive catheter is introduced into the renal pelvis and perfused at the rate of 10 ml min^{-1} with saline or dilute contrast medium. Pressure in the upper urinary tract is constantly monitored through a side-arm in the perfusion system, as is the bladder pressure via a bladder catheter. This is known as the Whitaker test (Whitaker, 1979). Any rise in renal pelvic pressure of greater than 20 cm of water above bladder pressure indicates ureteric obstruction. This technique is useful in differentiating obstructed dilated ureters from dilated but non-obstructed ureters but the result is sometimes in the equivocal range, namely a pressure rise of more than 10 cm of water and less than 20 cm water. Higher perfusion rates, for instance 20 ml min^{-1}, may be helpful in these equivocal cases.

Percutaneous nephrostomy

Insertion of a nephrostomy drainage catheter is a

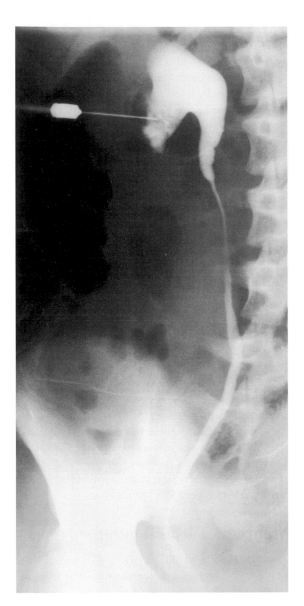

Fig. 16.8 Antegrade pyelogram demonstrating a hydronephrosis due to a stricture in the upper third of the ureter. This was caused by retroperitoneal fibrosis.

commonly performed extension of antegrade pyelography. The procedure is discussed below.

Antegrade pyelography in renal transplant

The puncture site should be lateral to the abdominal incision in order to avoid the bowel and to ensure entering the renal pelvis through the cortex. When there is significant calyceal dilatation the upper pole calyx is the preferred route.

Complications

The complication rate is exceedingly low but includes the following:

1 *Loin pain*. Pain may result from overdistension of an obstructed renal pelvis with contrast medium or from extravasation of contrast medium into the perirenal tissues.

2 *Haematuria and haemorrhage*. Microscopic haematuria is relatively common and usually transient following antegrade pyelography. Macroscopic haematuria occurs in 15% of cases. Clot obstruction and perirenal haematoma are rare complications.

3 *Septicaemia*. This may occur following overfilling of an obstructed system, particularly if the contrast medium is not aspirated at the end of the procedure. Infection is otherwise not a problem after antegrade pyelography.

4 *Miscellaneous*. Pneumothorax, urinoma and damage to other viscera are all very unusual. Seeding of a transitional cell carcinoma along the needle track is a theoretical possibility.

Relationship to other imaging modalities

Antegrade pyelography should be regarded as a preferable alternative to retrograde pyeloureterography in cases of ureteric obstruction or upper tract abnormality inadequately demonstrated by IVU. Antegrade pyelography is occasionally indicated in the newborn when ultrasound has failed to differentiate hydronephrosis from a multicystic kidney.

Percutaneous nephrostomy (PCN)

PCN is the insertion of a drainage catheter into the renal collecting system under radiological control. It has become indispensable in the diagnosis and management of many urological problems and has completely replaced surgical nephrostomy.

Indications

1 *To relieve renal or ureteric obstruction*. The technique is especially useful when ureteric obstruction is associated with renal failure or when the patient is pyrexial with loin pain, indicating upper urinary tract sepsis in association with calculus obstruction (pyonephrosis). In these cases it is a life-saving procedure.

2 *To provide access to the upper urinary tract* for supplementary procedures. These include percutaneous stone removal, nephroscopy and biopsy, ureteric stent insertion, dilatation of ureteric strictures or PUJ obstruction.

3 *To temporarily divert urine* in the presence of urinary tract leaks and fistulae, for example after surgery, so that healing may occur.

4 *To assess recoverable function* in a diseased kidney when non-invasive tests are unhelpful or equivocal. The response to PCN in this situation can decide whether nephrectomy or corrective surgery is the appropriate management.

Contraindications

An uncorrectable bleeding diathesis is the only absolute contraindication.

Technique

With informed consent, the patient is placed in a prone oblique position on a fluoroscopy table with the side to be punctured slightly elevated. Sedation and analgesia may be appropriate. Antibiotic cover is indicated in patients with proven or suspected urinary tract infection.

The kidney is usually located by ultrasound unless it has been opacified by a previous contrast examination or contains a staghorn calculus, in which case fluoroscopy is appropriate.

In order to reduce the incidence of urinary leakage, the puncture should be transparenchymal rather than directly into the renal pelvis. A lower pole calyx puncture is ideal. A local anaesthetic agent is injected down to the renal capsule, with the approach preferably below the 12th rib. If the renal collecting system is grossly distended then direct puncture with a needle–catheter system may be possible. This consists of a needle within a preshaped pig-tail catheter. When the puncture is successful the needle is withdrawn, leaving the pig-tail catheter *in situ* (Fig. 16.9).

Alternatively, a modified Seldinger technique is used. The unopacified renal collecting system is initially punctured under ultrasound control and an antegrade pyelogram performed, opacifying the collecting system by injecting contrast medium, for instance Urografin 150, using a 22 gauge Chiba needle. The appropriate calyx is then punctured with a sheathed needle under fluoroscopic control. The needle is removed and a J-wire inserted into the collecting system via the sheath. A 6–9F nephrostomy catheter is then passed into the collecting system. If pus is encountered, a larger nephrostomy catheter must be used.

In experienced hands percutaneous nephrostomy is successful in over 98% of cases (Leroy, 1990) Minimally dilated systems provide a greater technical challenge.

Complications

Haematuria, usually mild and self-limiting, occurs in almost all cases. Serious complications are unusual but include colonic perforation, pneumothorax, pleural effusions and retroperitoneal haematoma. Septicaemia is associated with drainage of a pyonephrosis. Major vascular injury is recognized in about 1% of cases. The most common complication is displacement of the catheter. This is minimized by secure skin attachment and the use of self-retaining nephrostomy catheters.

Percutaneous nephrolithotomy (PCNL)

Percutaneous nephrolithotomy is an alternative to open renal surgery for stone disease. Extracorporeal lithotripsy is nowadays the technique of choice in the management of most calculous disease. As lithotripsy facilities became widely available, there has been a decrease in the use of PCNL.

Indications

1 *Failed lithotripsy.* If the patient has undergone several sessions of lithotripsy and the stones have not passed, PCNL may be indicated. Cystine stones in particular are not fragmented by lithotripsy.

2 *Large stone bulk.* Stones more than 2 cm in diameter may be more appropriately managed by PCNL.

pelviureteric obstruction, the stone removal may be combined with ureteric balloon dilatation or endopyelotomy, respectively.

Technique

PCNL is performed under general anaesthesia. It is usually a combined technique carried out by a urologist and radiologist. A catheter is initially placed in the renal pelvis or upper ureter by means of cystoscopy. A bladder catheter is also inserted to drain away irrigation fluid during the procedure. The patient is then turned prone oblique, with the kidney to be punctured uppermost. The collecting system is opacified and distended by dilute contrast medium via the retrograde catheter. The addition of 2 ml of methylene blue to the contrast medium makes it easy to determine whether the collecting system has been punctured.

The puncture is carried out with a sheathed needle, aiming at a posterior lower pole calyx. The position of puncture is crucial to the success of the technique. Whilst a renal pelvis stone is approached via a lower calyx, stones in other calyces and in calyceal diverticula must be approached by direct puncture of the appropriate calyx or diverticulum. An Amplatz-type stiff guide wire is inserted through the sheath and directed down the ureter so that a long length of wire is within the collecting system and displacement of the wire does not occur during the procedure. The wire may be directed down the ureter by the use of a preshaped catheter, such as a cobra head. A track is then dilated by passing serial dilators over the guide wire. The dilators may either be polyethylene, which are available in disposable kits, or a telescopic metal dilator which is reusable and results in continuous track tamponade during dilatation, thus minimizing bleeding. When the track is dilated to 30F, an Amplatz sheath is inserted over the dilators and the dilators removed. A nephroscope may then be inserted through the sheath to localize and retrieve the stone. Stones of larger dimensions than the sheath have to be disintegrated before removal by passing down the nephroscope ultrasonic or electrohy-draulic probes which fragment the stone on direct contract.

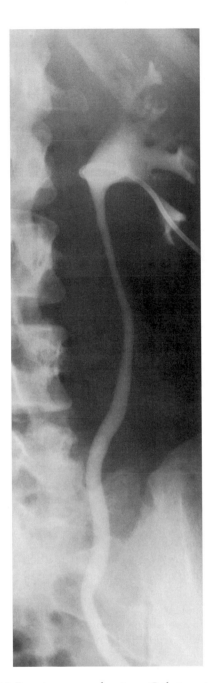

Fig. 16.9 Percutaneous nephrostomy. Catheter enters the renal pelvis via a lower calyx with a transparenchymal puncture.

3 *Staghorn calculus.* Most staghorn calculi are treated by initial debulking followed by lithotripsy. When the stone is associated with ureteric stricture or

Complications

Although dilatation of the track through the kidney is by displacement of tissues rather than cutting, haemorrhage is the commonest complication. A drain in the track, establishing tamponade following the procedure, reduces the need for transfusion to around 5% of patients.

Septicaemia is possible when there is renal infection, so antibiotic cover is given in all cases. The collecting system may be ruptured but this heals spontaneously if a nephrostomy tube is placed at the end of the procedure.

Other techniques associated with PCN

Ureteric stent insertion

Indications

In ureteric obstruction, a ureteric stent may provide relief without the need for an external drainage catheter and bag (Lang, 1984). Damage to the ureter by trauma, surgical or otherwise, may be treated by stent insertion. Stents may be inserted prior to lithotripsy when there is fear that the stone fragments may cause ureteric obstruction. This normally occurs with stones more than 2 cm in diameter.

The stents have a double pig-tail and are available in sets which include a guide wire and a pusher for stent placement. In most cases they are inserted retrogradely via the bladder. When this fails, for example in the presence of a bladder neoplasm occluding the ureteric orifice, or when there is a PCN already *in situ*, the stents are passed antegradely down the ureter under fluoroscopic control. Following nephrostomy, a wire is passed down the ureter through an obstructing lesion if present. The stent is loaded onto the wire, advanced as far as possible by hand, and then the upper end is pushed into the kidney using the pusher provided. The guide wire is then removed.

The antegrade technique is successful in over 90% of cases, does not require general anaesthesia and enables ureteric healing following trauma or limitation of renal damage in cases of obstruction.

If the stent is in position for many months it may become encrusted and obstruct. It may also become displaced either downwards into the bladder, mak-

ing it ineffective, or upwards into the ureter making removal difficult.

Metallic stents are now being evaluated in the ureter.

Percutaneous stone dissolution

Chemolysis of renal calculi via the nephrostomy catheter may be appropriate complementary therapy with PCNL or lithotripsy. Both cystine and uric acid calculi may be dissolved in this way.

Endopyelotomy for PUJ obstruction

The cause of PUJ obstruction is not understood in all cases but a motility disturbance at the PUJ or an aberrant renal artery causing extrinsic compression are possible causes. Recently, minimally invasive techniques have been introduced in the treatment of this condition (Lee *et al.*, 1988).

Endopyelotomy is carried out by incising the PUJ under direct vision via a nephroscope following PCN. Alternatively, balloon dilatation may be employed either antegradely following PCN or retrogradely via the bladder, thus splitting the PUJ and allowing healing around a temporary wide ureteric stent. These techniques are successful in about 75% of cases and do not hinder subsequent open surgery if necessary.

Ureteric stricture dilatation (Fig. 16.10)

Benign post-surgical ureteric strictures respond favourably to balloon dilatation in up to 84% of cases, success decreasing with increasing length of stricture (Beckman *et al.*, 1989). This technique is particularly advantageous in the stenosis of the transplant kidney ureteroneocystostomy when surgery is technically difficult and hazardous.

Renal biopsy

Medical renal disease

Indications

Biopsy of the kidney in medical renal disease is performed under ultrasound guidance. Non-urological

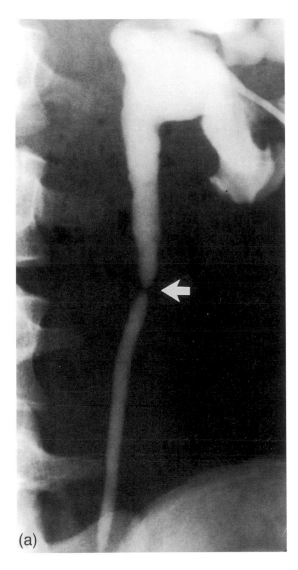

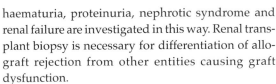

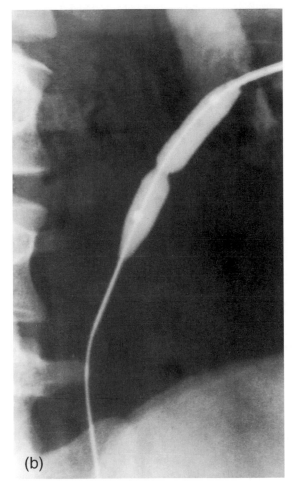

Fig. 16.10 (a) Stricture of the upper third of the ureter (arrow). (b) Antegrade dilatation by balloon catheter.

haematuria, proteinuria, nephrotic syndrome and renal failure are investigated in this way. Renal transplant biopsy is necessary for differentiation of allograft rejection from other entities causing graft dysfunction.

Techniques

The ideal site for a renal biopsy is the lower pole of either kidney, well away from major vessels. The procedure is carried out under local anesthesia after informed consent. A clotting disorder should be excluded and corrected if present.

Following localization of the lower pole by ultrasound, deep infiltration with lignocaine 1% is performed. An 18 gauge Tru-cut needle is appropriate, preferably fired by a Biopty-type gun as this seems to provide better sample cores. The biopsy needle should be visualized on its path to the renal capsule. With the tip at the renal capsule and the patient breath-holding, at least two biopsies are taken. When the biopsy is taken, the tip of the needle advances up to 2 cm so that a good core of renal cortex is obtained. Failing to see the needle adequately is due to faulty technique. The kidneys may be difficult to visualize when small and echogenic.

Biopsy of the transplant kidney, which is usually subcutaneous in position and does not move with respiration, is technically easier than the native kidney.

Contraindications

Bleeding disorders are a contraindication or should be corrected. Biopsy of small kidneys, less than 7 cm in length, usually has no therapeutic consequence and should not be undertaken. They are endstage kidneys with no recoverable function.

Biopsy of a single kidney should be carefully considered in view of the small but significant incidence of complications. This does not apply in the transplant kidney where biopsy is crucial in patient management.

Complications

The only significant complications are haematuria, arteriovenous fistula and perirenal haematoma. These complications occur in about 1% of cases and can often be managed by selective transcatheter embolization of the lesion.

Renal mass biopsy

The vast majority of solid renal lesions are primary renal malignancies and biopsy is unnecessary before surgery. Ultrasound can differentiate cysts from solid tumours and CT can reliably diagnose a fat-containing benign angiomyolipoma.

In a few cases, the masses may be indeterminate, either on imaging criteria or on clinical grounds. For example, a solid renal mass in a patient with a known primary elsewhere may be a secondary deposit or a further primary. Percutaneous renal mass biopsy is undertaken in such cases.

Method

In most cases of indeterminate solid lesions, a fine-needle aspiration of the mass by a Chiba needle is initially performed and sent for cytological analysis. This technique minimizes the risk of tumour seeding, which is well recognized with transitional cell carcinoma. When cytology is also indeterminate, as

is often the case, and a crucial patient management decision depends on the renal pathology, then a core biopsy will be obtained as previously described for medical renal disease.

Ascending urethrography

This is the anatomical demonstration of the male urethra by the retrograde injection of contrast medium.

Indications

There are two main indications for ascending urethrography: (i) diagnosis and assessment of *urethral stricture*; and (ii) evaluation of suspected *urethral trauma*. Urethral trauma includes injuries sustained, for example, in road traffic accidents as well as the complications of difficult urethral instrumentation, such as false passages, periurethral sepsis and fistulae.

Urethrography is also occasionally helpful in the following circumstances.
1 Diagnosis of *urethral tumours*. Tumours are well shown by this technique but in practice are very rare.
2 Diagnosis of *congenital abnormalities* of the urethra, for example hypospadias, epispadias, double urethra.

Contraindications

1 *Urinary tract infection*. Active urethritis must be treated with appropriate antibiotics before urethrography is performed.
2 *Recent urethral instrumentation*. Urethrography should be postponed for 1 week following urethral instrumentation, as there is invariably some mucosal damage and an increased risk of intravasation of contrast medium.
3 *Hypersensitivity to contrast medium*. This is a relative contraindication as an allergic reaction may be provoked if there is intravasation of contrast medium.

Technique

The patient empties his bladder immediately prior to the examination. Urethrography is carried out under sterile conditions. The prepuce is retracted, the glans cleaned with a mild antiseptic solution and lignocaine gel is inserted into the external meatus. The procedure is most commonly performed by inserting a small Foley catheter into the navicular fossa. A size 8 catheter is usually appropriate (Fig. 16.11). The catheter is filled with contrast medium to eliminate air bubbles, and its tip is inserted into the distal portion of the penile urethra. The balloon is then gently filled with 1–2 ml of saline. If it is correctly positioned in the navicular fossa, the balloon will now be well anchored and feel a tight fit. The patient will find inflation of the balloon very uncomfortable if it is not in the navicular fossa. If this is the case, the balloon is deflated and the catheter is replaced until a satisfactory position is achieved Conventional water-soluble contrast media are appropriate for urethrography, for example Conray 280 or Urografin 290. Contrast medium is injected under fluoroscopic control and spot radiographs are exposed in supine PA and oblique projections (right and left anterior oblique views with abduction of the contralateral leg and flexion of the knee) to delineate the whole length of the urethra and the bladder base (Fig. 16.12). While the anterior urethra is well demonstrated by ascending urethrography, a voiding study may be necessary for adequate distension of the posterior urethra. In this case the bladder is filled with contrast medium via the catheter and further radiographs are taken of the posterior urethra as the patient micturates into a bottle. Even better distension of the posterior urethra may be seen during arrested micturition.

An alternative method for performing ascending urethrography uses the Knuttson penile clamp (Fig. 16.13). The adjustable clamp holds the penis just behind the glans. Attached to it is a metal cannula which has a rubber nozzle at one end. The nozzle is covered with lignocaine gel and inserted into the external meatus. The clamp is then engaged to hold the nozzle in place and contrast medium is injected under fluoroscopic guidance. The Knuttson clamp cannot be used in cases of phimosis or hypospadias. The Foley catheter technique, on the other hand, is applicable in most cases of phimosis and the radiologist's hands are more likely to be kept out the X-ray beam than with the clamp method.

Complications

In general, complications after ascending urethrography are infrequent and of little clinical significance, but the following problems may occur.

1 *Urethral trauma and bleeding per urethram*. Bleeding is usually minor and stops spontaneously after a few minutes.

2 *Intravasation of contrast medium* (Fig. 16.14). Predisposing factors include excessive injection pressure in the presence of a stricture, recent urethral instrumentation and active urethral inflammation. Intravasation has been recorded in 5.5% of urethrograms. It is prudent to terminate the examination should intravasation be apparent on fluoroscopy. After significant intravasation, some urethral bleeding is often seen at the end of the procedure but this is self-limiting.

3 *Urinary tract infection*.

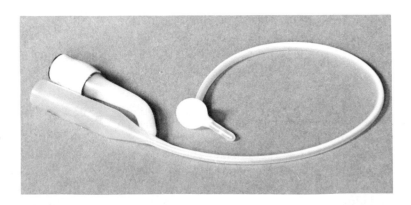

Fig. 16.11 A size 8 Foley catheter for retrograde urethrography.

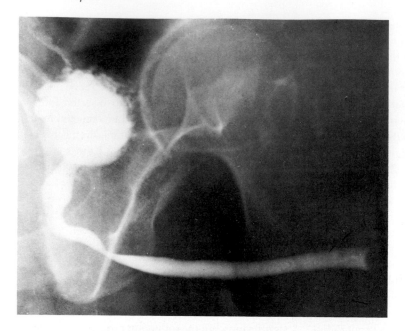

Fig. 16.12 Retrograde urethrogram using a Foley catheter. Stricture of the membranous urethra. Filling of the bladder is occurring. There is thickening of the bladder wall.

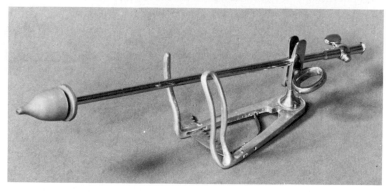

Fig. 16.13 The Knuttson penile clamp for retrograde urethrography.

Relationship to other imaging modalities

MCU and urodynamic studies are applied in some patients with urethral disease and provide a functional as well as anatomical assessment of the urethra.

Ultrasound has recently been used in the assessment of urethral strictures (Gluck *et al.*, 1988; Merckle *et al.*, 1988; Bearcroft & Berman, 1994). A Foley catheter is inserted into the external meatus, as for an ascending urethrogram, and the balloon is inflated in the navicular fossa. Saline is injected through the catheter in order to distend the urethra and ultrasound imaging is performed using a high-frequency probe (5–7 mHz). A Zipser penile clamp may be used to augment urethral distension. A transpenile approach allows examination of the distal urethra, while a transscrotal or transperineal approach is necessary to study the proximal urethra. The technique appears to be a promising alternative to radiographic studies in patients with urethral stricture but it is unlikely to replace ascending urethrography.

Magnetic resonance imaging (MRI) of the perineum provides excellent anatomical detail of the periurethral soft tissues. This information is helpful in the management of urethral trauma, particularly

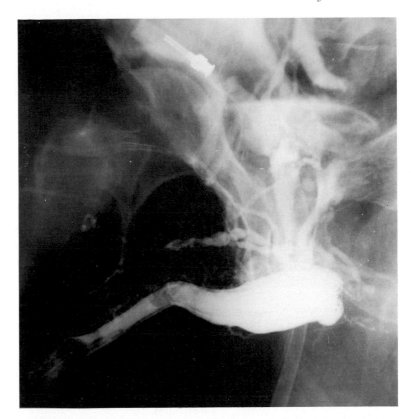

Fig. 16.14 Marked venous intravasation during retrograde urethrography.

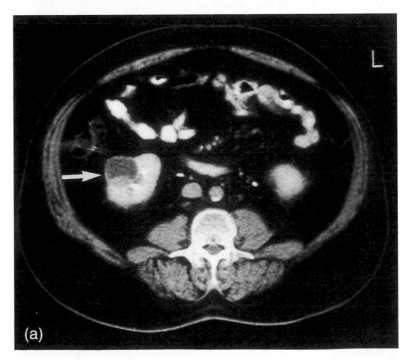

Fig. 16.15 Cyst puncture. (a) Computed tomography scan which, like an ultrasound scan in this patient, showed a complex cyst (arrow) with a soft-tissue density within it.

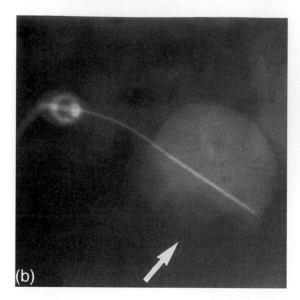

(b)

Fig. 16.15 *Continued.* (b) Cyst puncture confirmed a filling defect (arrow) within the cyst, proven to be adenocarcinoma.

injuries involving the posterior urethra (Dixon *et al.*, 1992; Narumi *et al.*, 1993). In this context MRI has a complementary role to ascending urethrography and information from both studies influences the surgical management in these patients.

Renal cyst puncture

Renal cysts are often detected incidentally during abdominal ultrasound and CT scanning. In fact, up to half the elderly population have renal cysts. Ultrasound and CT quite confidently confirm the simple nature of the cyst in well over 96% of cases, no other investigation being required. On ultrasound, criteria of benignity include a rounded echo-free mass with through transmission of sound. At CT, the mass will have a Hounsfield number approximating water with no enhancement after i.v. contrast medium.

The current *indications* for cyst puncture include the following.

1 Indeterminate nature at ultrasound and CT; for example septation, calcification or intermediate density (Fig. 16.15).

2 Loin pain possibly caused by the cyst.

3 Fever possibly due to an infected cyst.

4 Haematuria for which no possible cause other than a cyst can be found.

Contraindications

Bleeding diathesis and hydatid disease are contraindications.

Method

The procedure may be peformed on an out-patient or day-care basis. The patient lies in the prone position. Ultrasound guidance is now preferred to i.v. contrast medium. Aseptic precautions are taken and the puncture site is infiltrated with lignocaine 1%. An infracostal approach is preferred.

A 22 gauge Chiba or an 18 gauge sheathed needle in inserted into the cyst under suspended respiration and continuous guidance by ultrasound. Straw-coloured fluid is aspirated from a simple cyst. This in itself is reassuring, but the fluid may be sent for cytology, biochemistry and bacteriological analysis. A cystic tumour may contain blood, malignant cells and high levels of fat protein and lactic dehydrogenase (Fig. 16.15).

The cyst should not be completely aspirated and the fluid withdrawn should be replaced by an equal volume of contrast medium (Urografin 150) and air if there is a question of a tumour within the cyst. Radiographs of all parts of the cyst wall may then be obtained in double contrast.

Modification of basic technique

Simple cysts recur after aspiration. Sclerosants have been injected at the time of puncture, for example tetracycline. Their efficacy is questionable. Multiple cysts are sometimes aspirated in patients with adult polycystic disease when the voluminous kidneys cause abdominal discomfort and distension.

Complications

These are very few, and the procedure is now usually performed on an out-patient basis.

Significantly haemorrhage is unusual, microhaematuria is common. Other complications are rare.

Relationship to other modalities

It must be emphasized that almost all renal cysts can be evaluated non-invasively by ultrasound and CT. A small number, perhaps only 1–2%, may require cyst puncture.

Renal arteriography

Renal arteriography is now usually performed using a digital subtraction technique (DSA), following either i.v. or i.a. injection. A digital image of the renal areas is acquired immediately prior to injection of contrast medium and then subtracted from the post-contrast image series, removing unwanted structures such as bones and bowel gas shadows.

Intravenous DSA (i.v. DSA) is carried out by the rapid bolus injection of 50 ml of non-ionic contrast medium (350 or 370 mg iodine ml^{-1}) via a catheter passed from a vein in the antecubital fossa into the superior vena cava. If the patient has a good cardiac output then the main renal arteries are adequately visualized in over 92% of cases, although superimposition of other abdominal vessels can be a problem. Intrarenal vessels are poorly delineated. This is an out-patient procedure.

Intra-arterial DSA (i.a. DSA) is more invasive than i.v. DSA but results in much improved visualization of the renal arteries. The use of 4 and 5F catheters means that the technique is increasingly performed on a day-case or out-patient basis. A pig-tail catheter is passed from the femoral artery into the abdominal aorta at L1/L2 level. An aortogram is initially obtained by injection of 20–30 ml of non-ionic contrast, 300 mg ml^{-1} at 10–15 ml s^{-1}, much less than for conventional radiographic angiography. An aortogram is a mandatory first step in renal artery evaluation because multiple arteries are present in 20–30% of cases. If this does not provide sufficient information, then oblique views or selective renal artery catheterization may be necessary (see Chapter 8). The selective study is performed by exchanging the pig-tail for a preshaped cobra-head catheter. Unless there is a stenosis at the ostium, the renal arteries are easy to catheterize. The injection of 8–10 ml of contrast medium over 1–2 s will demonstrate the main renal artery, together with segmental and interlobar arteries.

The *indications* for renal arteriography include the following.

1 Suspected renal artery stenosis, in association with either renal failure or hypertension.
2 Evaluation prior to a live donor transplant, to determine the number of renal arteries — a preoperative vascular map.
3 Renal trauma, especially bleeding after renal biopsy.
4 Haematuria of unknown origin, for example when bleeding from a ureteric orifice is seen at cystoscopy but no renal cause for bleeding is shown by other imaging techniques.
5 Prior to embolization or renal artery thrombolysis.
6 Suspected arteritis, for example polyarteritis nodosa.
7 To plan surgery in a solitary kidney, for example prior to partial nephrectomy for tumour.

Complications

The morbidity from renal arteriography is very low in experienced hands, hence the trend to perform it as an out-patient procedure.

1 At the puncture site: haematoma, thrombosis and arteriovenous fistula.
2 Renal artery damage caused by dissection during selective catheterization.
3 Contrast medium-related complications. Proteinuria is common after selective renal arteriography, implying a degree of nephrotoxicity. This is usually mild and self-limiting, but it is appropriate to use the least amount of contrast medium consistent with obtaining the relevant diagnostic information.

Relationship to other techniques

The number of renal angiograms performed has declined significantly in the past two decades, primarily owing to the development of ultrasound, CT, nuclear medicine and percutaneous biopsy. Renal masses are rarely evaluated by angiography and currently the most common indication for arteriography is the investigation of hypertension in selected patients.

Renal venography

Venography for the detection of tumour thrombus in the renal veins is no longer necessary as the relevant information is available on ultrasound, CT or MRI. Renal vein thrombosis from other causes, such as nephrotic syndrome, may similarly be detected.

In the few cases where the examination is indicated, images of the renal veins may be obtained *directly* via femoral vein catheterization, performing a cavogram followed by selective renal vein catheterization, or *indirectly* by taking late images after selective renal arterial injection of contrast medium.

Renal angioplasty (Fig. 16.16)

The prevalence of renovascular hypertension is only 1–5%. Most hypertensive patients do not require any investigation. The selection of patients for angiography and possible angioplasty from the general hypertensive population remains controversial. The IVU has been abandoned because it has a sensitivity of only 74%. Isotope renography has a similar sensitivity. The Captopril renogram has a sensitivity and specificity of around 90%, although it is not as sensitive when there is renal dysfunction. Evaluation of the renal arteries by duplex Doppler ultrasound is possible in 95% of right and 82% of left renal arteries, but the procedure is technically challenging and time-consuming.

Magnetic resonance angiography has a sensitivity of around 86–100% with a specificity of 92–94%. Spiral CT is promising in its ability to demonstrate the renal arteries non-invasively. In essence, there is no good screening test for the detection of renal artery stenosis in all hypertensive patients. Clinical criteria are applied to select patients for further investigation:

1 Patients with severe or sudden worsening of hypertension.
2 Inappropriate age of onset, for instance in the very young or very old with no family history.
3 Poor control on drug therapy.

4 Hypertension and renal insufficiency, especially with evidence of arterial disease elsewhere.

These selected patients undergo i.a. DSA using small-bore catheters on an out-patient or day-case basis.

Technique

An aortogram is initially performed to demonstrate main renal arteries and any accessory vessels. Oblique views may be necessary to demonstrate the ostia. When a stenotic lesion is identified, the pigtail catheter is exchanged for a cobra-head or shepherd's-crook catheter and the abnormal vessel is selectively catheterized. A floppy-tipped wire is used to cross the stenosis, followed by the diagnostic catheter. The floppy-tipped wire is then exchanged for a more rigid one, the diagnostic catheter is removed and a balloon dilatation catheter is passed through the stenosis. The diameter of the balloon is the same as the estimated size of the renal artery on the angiogram. In general, a 5 or 6 mm diameter balloon is used. In some centres heparin is administered during and after the procedure. Aspirin or dipyridamole are prescribed for a few months subsequently.

Complications

Complication rates are between 5 and 10%. These include renal artery dissection, perforation or thrombosis, and reversible renal insufficiency.

Results

In a recent review, hypertension secondary to atheromatous disease was cured in 19% and improved in 51%, with no improvement in 30%. In fibromuscular disease 46% were cured and 45% improved, with a failure rate of 9%. Most published series report a 15–20% incidence of restenosis related to (i) atheromatous disease; (ii) inadequate dilatation; and (iii) intimal fibrous proliferation at the site of angioplasty.

Newer techniques now being tried in renal artery stenosis include renal artery stenting in patients whose stenoses recur following angioplasty (Granor, 1994).

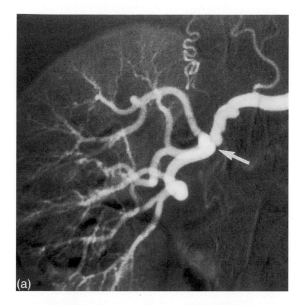

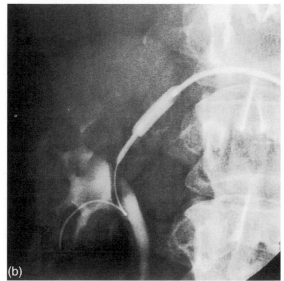

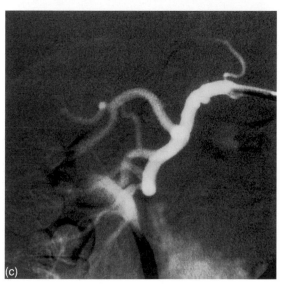

Fig. 16.16 (a) A segment of fibromuscular disease of the main renal artery with a localized right stenosis (arrow). (b) Angioplasty catheter and guide wire across the stenosis. (c) Post-angioplasty appearance. The stenosis has been satisfactorily dilated.

Embolization in the urinary tract

Indications include the following:
1 Renal tract carcinoma — preoperative and palliative.
2 Trauma with bleeding — blunt and penetrating, including after percutaneous biopsy.
3 Renal arteriovenous fistulae.
4 Bladder embolization — haemorrhage from neoplasm, following radiation or arteriovenous malformation.

5 Priapism.
6 Varicocoele embolization.
   Embolic materials available include:
1 Particulate material:
   (a) Gelfoam, Sterispon: these provide temporary vascular occlusion but may be combined with other materials for permanent occlusion;
   (b) Polyvinyl alcohol sponge (Ivalon): this is introduced by catheter in a similar way to Gelfoam but produces permanent occlusion.

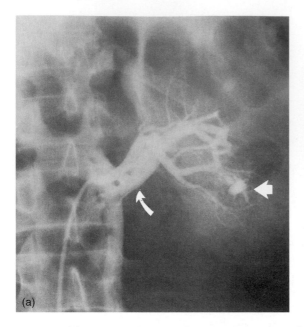
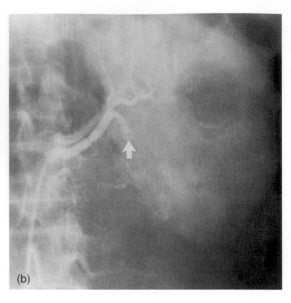

Fig. 16.17 (a) Arteriovenous fistula following biopsy (straight arrow) with early venous filling (curved arrow). There was also a calyceal connection causing gross haematuria and shock. (b) Appearance after embolization. Note coil (arrow) in a branch of the renal artery. The lower pole is avascular.

2 Coils (Gianturco). These steel coils have wool fibres attached to encourage thrombosis. The coils are pushed through a selectively placed catheter using a guide wire. Multiple coils may be necessary for complete occlusion. They are often used in association with particulate material to provide complete vascular occlusion.

3 Balloons. Detachable balloons cause permanent occlusion and are ideal large vessel occluders, for example for arteriovenous malformations or arteriovenous fistulae.

4 Liquid emboli. This group includes absolute alcohol, boiling saline or contrast medium and superglue (isobutyl-2-cyanoacrylate). All provide permanent occlusion.

Preoperative embolization of renal carcinomas is no longer routinely performed. Embolization of renal tumours is now confined to the control of bleeding and pain from large inoperable lesions.

Embolization is the method of choice in the control of haematuria following trauma or biopsy (Fig. 16.17). If the exact site of bleeding is identified then selective catheterization and occlusion with Gelfoam,

with or without coils, can conserve a large amount of normal renal tissue.

Embolization of the anterior division of the internal iliac artery is effective in the control of haemorrhage from inoperable bladder lesions and postradiation cystitis. It is usually necessary to embolize both sides for haemorrhage control because of abundant collaterals within the pelvis.

In priapism, the occlusion of the internal pudendal arteries by temporary agents such as Gelfoam can reduce arterial inflow, allowing resolution of symptoms and can allow the return of normal sexual function.

In the presence of pain or associated infertility, treatment of varicocoeles may be necessary. Surgical ligation has been replaced by embolization. A transfemoral approach is used. Most varicocoeles are left sided. The left renal vein is initially entered by a cobra-head catheter and then the gonadal vein is cannulated. A spermatic venogram is obtained. There are single or double veins but not multiple veins, embolization is performed using coils. Results and recurrence rates of 15% are similar to surgery.

Complications

The major complication is the inadvertent embolization of other organs. In addition patients experience pain, fever, leucocytosis, vomiting and ileus: the so-called post-infarction syndrome. These symptoms resolve in 24–48 hours.

References

Bagg, M.N.J., Horwitz, T.A. & Bester, L. (1986) Comparison of patient responsiveness to high and low osmolality contrast agents injected intravenously. *AJR*, **147**, 185–9.

Bearcroft, P.W.P. & Berman, L.H. (1994) Sonography in the evaluation of the male anterior urethra. *Clin. Radiol.*, **49**, 621–6.

Beckman, C.F., Roth, R.A. & Bihrle, W. (1989) Dilatation of benign ureteral strictures. *Radiology*, **172**, 437–41.

Caro, J.J., Trindale, E. & McGregor, M. (1991) Risks of death and of severe non-fatal reactions with high versus low osmolality contrast medium: a meta-analysis. *AJR*, **56**, 825–32.

Dawson, P. & Sidhu, P.S. (1993) Is there a role for corticosteroid prophylaxis in patients at risk of adverse reaction to intravascular contrast medium? *Clin. Radiol.*, **48**, 225–6.

Dixon, C.M., Hricak, H. & McAninch, J.M. (1992) Magnetic resonance imaging of traumatic posterior urethral defects and pelvic crush injuries. *J. Urol.*, **148**, 1162–5.

Evans, C. (1987) Renal failure radiology. *Clin. Radiol.*, **38**, 457–62.

Gavant, M.L., Ellis, J.V. & Klesges, L.M. (1992) Maximizing opacification during excretory urography: effect of low osmolality contrast medium. *J. Can. Assoc. Radiol.*, **43**, 111–15.

George, C.D., Vinnicombe, S.J., Balkisson, A.R.A. & Heron, C.W. (1993) Bowel preparation before intravenous urography. Is it necessary? *Br. J. Radiol.*, **66**, 17–19.

Gluck, C.D., Bundy, A.L., Fine, C. *et al.* (1988) Sonographic urethrogram: comparison to roentgenographic techniques in 22 patients. *J. Urol.*, **140**, 1404–8.

Grainger, R.G. & Dawson, P. (1990) Low osmolar contrast media: an appraisal. *Clin. Radiol.*, **42**, 1–5.

Granor, R.A. (1994) New techniques for percutaneous renal revascularization: atherectomy and stenting. *Urol. Clin. N. Am.*, **21**, 245–53.

Haddad, M.C., Sharif, H.S., Shahed, H.S. *et al.* (1992) Renal colic diagnosis and outcome. *Radiology*, **184**, 83–8.

Katayama, H., Yamaguchi, K., Kozuka, T. *et al.* (1990) Adverse reactions to ionic and non-ionic contrast media: a report from the Japanese Committee on the Safety of Contrast Media. *Radiology*, **175**, 621–8.

Lang, E.K. (1984) Antegrade ureteral stenting for dehiscence, strictures and fistulae. *AJR*, **143**, 795–801.

Lasser, E.C., Berry, C.C., Talner, L.B. *et al.* (1987) Pretreatment with corticosteroids to alleviate reactions to intravenous contrast material. *New Engl. J. Med.*, **317**, 845–9.

Lee, W.J., Badlan, G.H., Karlin, G.S. & Smith, A.D. (1988) Treatment of ureteropelvic strictures with percutaneous pyelography: experience in 62 patients. *AJR*, **151**, 515–18.

Leroy, A.J. (1990) Percutaneous nephrostomy: techniques and instrumentation. *In* Pollock, H.M. (ed.) *Clinical Urology*, pp. 272–6. WB Saunders, Philadelphia.

Libertine, J.A. & Beckman, C.F. (1994) Surgery and percutaneous angioplasty in the management of renovascular hypertension. *Urol. Clin. N. Am.*, **21**, 235–43.

Mawhinney, R.R. & Gregson, R.H.S. (1987) Is ureteric compression still necessary? *Clin. Radiol.*, **38**, 178–80.

Merkle, W. & Wagner, W. (1988) Sonography of the distal male urethra: a new diagnostic procedure for urethral strictures — results of a retrospective study. *J. Urol.*, **140**, 1409–11.

Narumi, Y., Hricak, H., Armenakas, N.A. *et al.* (1993) Magnetic resonance imaging of traumatic posterior urethral injury. *Radiology*, **188**, 439–44.

Palmer, F.J. (1988) The RACR survey of intravenous contrast media reactions: final report. *Austral. Radiol.*, **32**, 426–8.

Parfrey, P.S., Griffiths, S.M., Barrett, B.J. *et al.* (1989) Contrast material induced renal failure in patients with diabetes mellitus, renal insufficiency or both: a prospective study. *N. Engl. J. Med.*, **320**, 143–9.

Whitaker, R.H. (1979) The Whitaker test. *Urol. Clin. N. Am.*, **6**, 529–41.

17   Female Genital Tract

G. H. WHITEHOUSE

Hysterosalpingography (HSG)

Contrast examination of the uterine cavity was first performed by Rindfleisch (1910), when he injected bismuth emulsion through the cervical canal. A colloidal silver salt was used as an HSG contrast medium by Cary (1914) and by Rubin (1914), but this agent was soon abandoned because it was not absorbed and caused peritoneal irritation. Lipiodol was used for many years as a contrast medium but was associated with an unacceptable incidence of local and systemic complications. HSG with water-soluble contrast media is still a useful and widely employed method of investigating the female genital tract, despite the wide availability of laparoscopy and developments in ultrasound.

Indications

Infertility

HSG is generally indicated at an early stage in the investigation of infertile women. While congenital abnormalities of the uterus account for 20% of positive findings in cases of primary infertility (Pontifex *et al.*, 1972), the majority of abnormalities demonstrated on HSG in primary and especially in secondary infertility are related to tubal occlusion or peritubal adhesions from pelvic inflammatory disease or endometriosis.

After tubal surgery

HSG is used to assess the patency and length of the fallopian tubes following operations such as salpingolysis, salpingostomy, tubal resection and anastomosis, which have been performed for tubal occlusion and peritubal adhesions.

Prior to artificial insemination and in vitro fertilization techniques

Tubal patency may be evaluated by HSG before undertaking assisted reproductive techniques.

After tubal sterilization procedures

Tubal occlusion following laparoscopic sterilization may be confirmed by HSG when there has been operative difficulty or when some uncertainty remains regarding patency of the fallopian tubes.

Preoperative HSG is sometimes performed before reversal of tubal sterilization.

Following ectopic pregnancy

There is a high incidence of adhesions developing in and around the contralateral fallopian tube following a tubal pregnancy. This results from either pelvic inflammatory disease having involved both tubes or from fibrosis secondary to bleeding into the pelvic peritoneal cavity. Assessment of the contralateral fallopian tube is therefore indicated before risking another pregnancy.

Following myomectomy

HSG before myomectomy can assist in planning the surgical approach by identifying submucosal fibroids and concomitant tubal disease. After myomectomy, HSG will show residual fibroids and complications of surgery, such as synechiae and diverticula, which may affect future treatment.

Post-caesarean section

The integrity of the uterine scar following caesarean section is accurately shown by hysterography using lateral projections. The feasibility of subsequent pregnancies being delivered by the vaginal route or the need for further uterine sections is assessed from this study.

Contraindications

Pregnancy

Inadvertently performing HSG during pregnancy carries a risk of abortion as well as the teratogenic hazards of radiation. HSG during the first 2 months of pregnancy shows an enlarged, atonic and globular uterine cavity with the gestation sac as a filling defect (Fig. 17.1). Permeation of contrast medium into the thickened endometrium gives a poorly defined outline to the uterus.

Pelvic infection

A history of pelvic inflammatory disease in the previous 6 months precludes HSG unless a course of antibiotics has been given and there is complete clinical resolution of the infection. Acute vaginitis and cervicitis carry a risk of infection and should be treated before performing HSG.

Immediate pre- and postmenstrual phases

Spasm of the isthmus and cornua are least likely to occur mid-cycle. The thickened and denuded endometrium, which occurs before and after the menstrual period, respectively, increases the chance of intravasation of contrast medium and consequent obscuration of the contours of the uterus and adnexa. There is a risk of performing the investigation in the presence of an early pregnancy in the premenstrual phase.

Sensitivity to contrast medium

Susceptible subjects may have an anaphylactoid response to the contrast medium. The advisability of performing HSG and the need for antihistamine and steroid cover should be assessed in the light of sensitivity to contrast media.

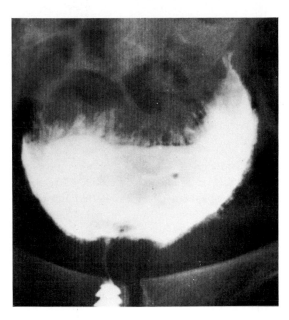

Fig. 17.1 Pregnant uterus. Large globular uterine cavity with the gestation sac seen as a filling duct. Marked endometrial thickening.

Technique

The optimal time for performing HSG is towards the end of the first week after the menstrual period. The isthmus is most easily distended at this time, tubal filling most readily occurs and there is no risk of an early pregnancy.

Preparation

Important measures for alleviating anxiety include an explanation of the procedure by the radiologist or the radiographer and a minimizing of delay between entering the radiology department and undergoing HSG (Tyrrell *et al.*, 1993). Premedication is not required in the majority of cases. HSG is most likely to be uncomfortable and painful in the anxious patient in whom it may be helpful to give 5–10 mg of diazepam 30 min beforehand or naproxen sodium 550 mg 2 hours before the examination.

Morphia and pethidine should not be given as they stimulate smooth muscle contraction, which impedes delineation of the fallopian tubes by contrast medium. General anaesthesia, or the anxiety generated by the thought of it, often precipitates tubal spasm which is unrelieved during anaesthesia.

The patient should empty her bladder immediately prior to the investigation, as a full bladder elevates the fallopian tubes and causes a spurious appearance of tubal blockage.

Method

The patient is placed in the lithotomy position on the screening table prior to a bimanual pelvic examination. A vaginal speculum is inserted and the external os is swabbed with a non-irritant antiseptic solution such as Hibitane.

If a cannula is to be inserted, topical anaesthesia such as 20% benzocaine gel can be applied to the cervix, prior to grasping the anterior lip of the cervix by tenaculum forceps. The cannula is then in-serted through the external os, followed by removal of the vaginal speculum. Cervical cannulation may be impossible in the presence of extensive cervical laceration or an abnormally small cervical canal.

The injection cannula. The Leech–Wilkinson cannula has a conical, ridged metallic end which is introduced into the cervical canal with a screwing motion (Fig. 17.2). The insertion of the cannula may be painful and contrast medium may leak back into the vagina.

The Green–Armytage cannula has a rubber acorn which is variable in position along the length of the straight metal cannula and provides a fairly watertight junction with the cervix. A plunger in the form of a screw allows controlled injection of contrast medium. Other varieties of straight or curved metal cannulae with rubber acorns are available (Fig. 17.3).

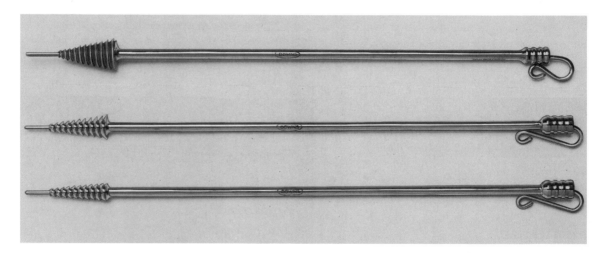

Fig. 17.2 Leech–Wilkinson cannula for hysterosalpingography. Courtesy of Downs Surgical Ltd.

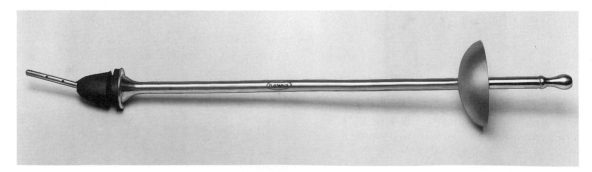

Fig. 17.3 Hayes–Provis cannula with rubber cone. Courtesy of Downs Surgical Ltd.

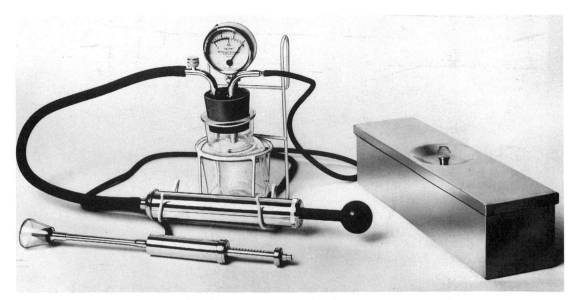

Fig. 17.4 Malstrom–Westerman cannula, with vacuum pump and syringe.

The suction cannula (Wright, 1961). A special speculum accommodates the special Malstrom–Westermann vacuum uterine cannula (Fig. 17.4) and is easily removed following insertion of the cannula. Plastic caps, which are in three sizes, fit over the external part of the cervix. An adjustable silicone rubber acorn, on a metal cannula which runs through the centre of the cup, is inserted into the cervical canal. The lumen of the cup is connected by a tube to a unit which produces a vacuum and consists of a pump, a pressure meter and a vacuum bottle. The cervix is drawn into the cup when the tip of the acorn is applied to the external os and a negative pressure of 0.2–0.3 kg cm^{-2} is established by the vacuum pump. The negative pressure is increased to 0.6 kg cm^{-2}, which draws the cannula tip into the cervical canal and applies the acorn to the external os. The injection cannula is connected via a stopcock to a syringe containing contrast medium. The stopcock is then opened to allow the injection of contrast medium.

The advantages of the vacuum method are that the potentially painful application of a tenaculum is avoided; a water-tight junction is established between the cannula and cervix; traction may be applied to the cervix; the patient may be easily rotated without dislodging the cannula; and the cervical canal is well demonstrated. The vacuum cannula cannot be applied when there is severe cervical laceration.

Catheter technique. A popular method of uterine injection involves the introduction of an 8 French (F) gauge Foley catheter into the uterine cavity (Fig. 17.5). The excessive flexibility of the Foley catheter is a disadvantage but is overcome by using catheters which have been specially modified for HSG (Sholkoff, 1987). These catheters, for instance the Sholkoff catheter,* have increased rigidity which allows them to be readily introduced through the cervical canal while being sufficiently flexible to safely follow the flexed configuration of the uterus. An alternative is to use a polypropylene filament as a flexible stiffener to an 8F Foley catheter. The balloon, having been distended by 2–3 ml of water when it lies within the uterine cavity, is then pulled downwards against the internal os prior to the injection of contrast medium. Inevitably, the cervical canal is not visualized when the balloon is inflated. However, the isthmus and cervical canal may be demonstrated by taking a radiograph while injecting contrast medium during deflation and simultaneous gentle downward withdrawal of the catheter. Catheter HSG is generally less traumatic and causes less discomfort than the cannula technique. A further advantage is that the patient may be easily rotated after catheter insertion.

* William Cook (UK) Ltd, Letchworth, Hertfordshire UK.

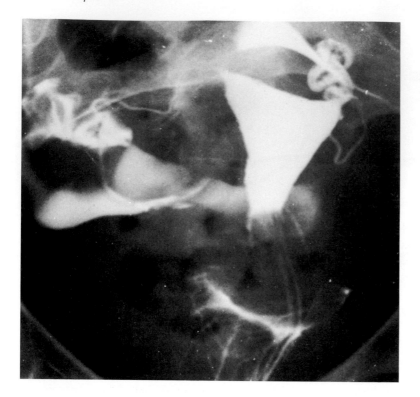

Fig. 17.5 Hysterosalpingogram with Foley catheter. Inflated balloon lies in the lower uterine segment.

The Harris uterine injector* (Fig. 17.6) is a modified balloon catheter having a curved shaft with a safety shield attached to a compression spring to prevent overinsertion. An external pilot balloon signals inflation of the intrauterine balloon.

A preliminary radiograph of the pelvic cavity is only required if some dense opacity is visible on screening. The contrast medium is warmed to body temperature and gently injected under fluoroscopic control, usually 8–12 ml being required. A lead shield protects the operator's hands. A radiograph is taken during uterine filling, before the contrast opacification becomes too dense, in order to demonstrate small uterine filling defects and deformities (Fig. 17.7). Another radiograph is exposed when the uterus and fallopian tubes are delineated and peritoneal spill is just occurring from the fimbrial ends of the tubes. A further radiograph is routinely taken 20 min later to show the pattern of peritoneal spill. While the de-

* United International Marketing Resources Inc., Canoga Park, California, USA.

layed radiograph is usually taken with the patient supine, an additional radiograph in the prone position is sometimes helpful if there is questionable loculation on the supine radiograph. All the contrast medium should have disappeared by 1 hour after the injection, but usually remains longer when there is ampullary or peritubal loculation with obstruction to free peritoneal spillage. The mean radiation dose to the ovaries during HSG is in the order of 2 mGy (van der Weiden & van Zijl, 1989). The radiographic field should be restricted as much as possible. Videotape recording during screening is a useful adjunct. The assessment of uterine retroversion and anteversion is made from the pattern of movement of the uterus during traction. Traction on the cannula, and tenaculum when present, usually allows good filling of a verted uterus and the fallopian tubes. Alternate relaxation and tension on the instruments, the 'butterfly manoeuvre', will also aid tubal filling and may overcome spasm. A disadvantage of the catheter technique is that the lack of tenaculum traction does not allow movement and straightening of the uterus.

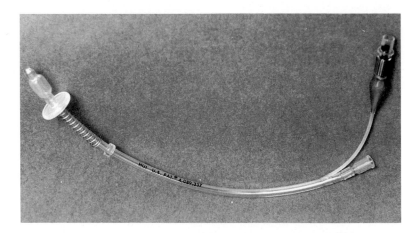

Fig. 17.6 Harris uterine injector.

Cornual spasm is often prevented by reassurance and a gentle technique. Glucagon (1 mg i.v.) is helpful in treating uterine spasm, being more reliable than atropine, trintrin or amyl nitrate. Turning the patient into a prone position has been advocated as a method of facilitating filling of the uterus and fallopian tubes by contrast medium, the fundus and cannula then being in a dependent position in an anteflexed uterus. Patients whose tubes remain undelineated after this manoeuvre may be candidates for fallopian tube catheterization.

Contrast media

Lipiodol, a stable compound of 40% iodine in poppy seed oil, was first used as a contrast medium for HSG in the 1920s. Lipiodol Ultrafluid and ethiodol, which have a lower viscosity and are ethyl esters of poppy seed oil combined with 40% and 37% iodine, respectively, have replaced Lipiodol. Unfortunately, oily contrast media carry a risk of provoking acute tubal blockage and reactivating infection, while their intravasation can cause oil embolism (Dan *et al.*, 1990; Ogihara *et al.*, 1991). There are still proponents of ethiodized poppy seed oil who claim that its application in HSG is associated with an increased pregnancy rate as well as fewer side effects (Lindequist *et al.*, 1991; Rasmussen *et al.*, 1991). Using an animal model (Moore *et al.*, 1990) chronic inflammatory changes around the ovary have been provoked by the tubal injection of ethiodol and raise further questions regarding its safety.

Water-soluble contrast media were also introduced in the 1920s but early agents tended to cause peritoneal irritation. Contrast media used in HSG must have sufficient viscosity to be retained in the uterus and fallopian tubes long enough for their radiographic demonstration, yet give a controlled spill from the ampulla without flooding the peritoneal cavity. The radiographic density of the contrast medium must be sufficient to show the uterine outline and tubal lumen without obscuring small filling defects.

Urografin 370 (10% sodium diatrizoate and 66% methylglucamine diatrizoate) is a popular contrast medium for HSG, the large molecular size and high iodine content giving it sufficient viscosity and radiographic density. Hexabrix is another contrast medium which is satisfactory in meeting these criteria.

It has been assumed that the hypertonicity of contrast media is an important factor in the causation of pain from HSG. However, low-osmolar contrast agents have little effect on reducing the overall incidence and intensity of pain when compared to high-osmolar contrast agents. However, delayed pain after HSG has a lower incidence and severity following the use of low-osmolar agents (Brokensha & Whitehouse, 1991), possibly because they cause less peritoneal irritation than high-osmolar contrast media.

Variations on basic technique

Selective catheterization of the fallopian tubes was developed by Thurmond *et al.* (1987) as a method of evaluating and treating proximal tubal obstructions. Access is gained via a vacuum cup HSG device. Un-

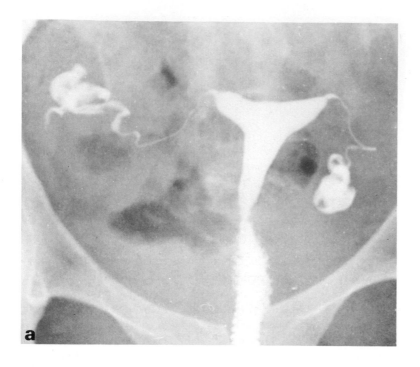

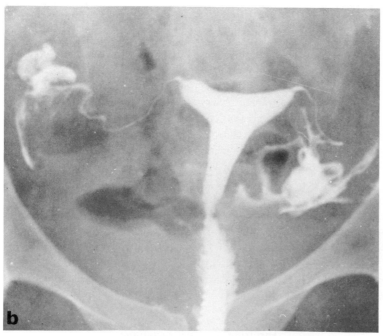

Fig. 17.7 Normal hysterosalpingogram. (a) The uterus is opacified by contrast medium and the fallopian tubes are delineated to the ampullae. (b) Slightly later, there is fuller delineation of both fallopian tubes with early peritoneal spill of contrast medium.

der fluoroscopic guidance and the application of guide wires, a 5.5F catheter is initially placed into the tubal ostium, followed by placement of a 3F catheter into the interstitial or isthmic portion of the fallopian tube. Correct catheter placement is confirmed by a selective injection of contrast medium. This selective

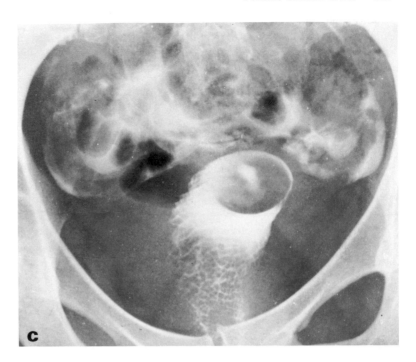

Fig. 17.7 *Continued* (c) Fifteen minutes after withdrawal of the cannula. Contrast medium delineates the pelvic peritoneum with no evidence of loculation.

salpingogram will also demonstrate the condition of the rest of the fallopian tube. Technical success rates for overcoming and visualizing distal tubal anatomy range from 76 to 95% (Thurmond, 1991). Subsequent pregnancy rates vary between 7 and 31% overall, but there is an ectopic pregnancy rate of up to 10%.

A variation of this technique uses a coaxial balloon catheter to dilate proximal tubal occlusions (Gleicher *et al.*, 1993). This method gives similar results to the Thurmond techniques but may reduce tubal reocclusion in the long term.

The technique of selective salpingography has therapeutic applications: the direct introduction of gametes and embryos into the fallopian tubes (MRI *et al.*, 1990) and the treatment of ectopic pregnancy by methotrexate infusion into the tubal lumen (Risquez *et al.*, 1992). The measurement of perfusion pressures during selective salpingography gives further information on tubal patency (Gleicher *et al.*, 1992).

Complications

Pain

Insertion of the injection cannula may result in tran-

sient lower abdominal discomfort. Distension of the uterus and fallopian tubes by contrast medium may cause lower abdominal pain, especially in those who are apprehensive or have a low pain threshold, but usually subsides within 10 min. A rapid injection of contrast medium also provokes this pain.

Tubal spasm or organic tubal obstruction is also associated with pain, which is sometimes severe and is situated lateral to the mid-line in the lower abdomen.

Some pain often occurs on peritoneal spillage of contrast media, usually lasting for 1 hour and relieved by mild analgesics. The pain is thought to result from peritoneal irritation due to hyperosmolarity of the contrast medium.

Pain occasionally commences within 1 or 2 hours of the procedure, usually disappearing within 24 hours but occasionally persisting for several days. This type of pain is more frequent and more severe with high rather than low-osmolar agents. Pelvic irritation may be the cause of this delayed pain, which must be differentiated from the pain caused by an exacerbation of pelvic inflammation.

A balloon catheter produces less pain than a standard cannula during HSG, but significantly more discomfort later in the examination day and the following day (Varpula, 1989). Stretching of the cervix and myometrium, possibly with tearing of the endometrium or endocervical mucosa, may be responsible for the pain associated with balloon catheters.

Miscellaneous

Pelvic infection. There is a reported 0.25–3% incidence of pelvic infection after HSG, usually as an acute exacerbation of a pre-existing infection but sometimes occurring *de novo.* Pelvic infection is most likely to occur in the presence of pre-existing tubal damage.

Haemorrhage. Application of the tenaculum to the cervix commonly results in slight spotting of blood. Bleeding from the uterine cavity after HSG suggests the presence of an endometrial polyp or carcinoma. The use of a cannula whose lip extends well beyond the acorn may cause endometrial bleeding.

Uterine perforation. A long cannula tip can also predispose to uterine perforation. Rough application of the cannula may cause cervical laceration.

Allergic phenomena. Urticaria, asthma and laryngeal oedema may occur as hypersensitivity reactions in susceptible subjects.

Vasovagal attacks. These occur, sometimes with syncope, in a small proportion of cases.

Venous intravasation. Intravasation of contrast medium into the venous system of the uterus shows as a fine, interlacing network of veins adjacent to the borders of the opacified uterine cavity (Fig. 17.8). Large superficial uterine veins and those which run along the broad ligament into the iliac veins and pampiniform plexuses are also seen. The reported incidence of venous intravasion is 0.6–3.7%.

Often no cause is found, but there are several predisposing causes of venous intravasation. These include (i) direct trauma to the endometrium from the tip of the injection cannula; and (ii) uterine abnormalities including hypoplasia, fibroids, carcinoma, tuberculosis and tubal occlusion, which leads to a high pressure of contrast medium in the uterine cavity.

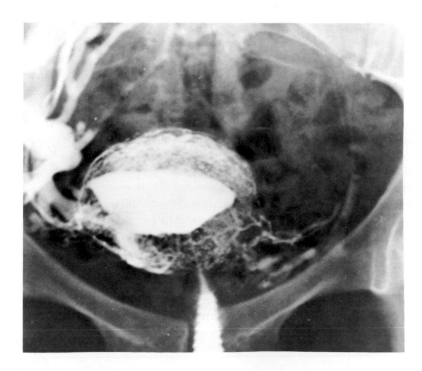

Fig. 17.8 Gross venous intravasation of contrast medium. Opacification of the veins of the uterine wall and pelvic cavity.

Relation to other techniques

Comparative studies of laparoscopy and HSG in sterility cases have found 70–96% concordance between these two methods in the assessment of tubal patency. The major discrepancy between the procedures concerns the identification of peritubal adhesions, with HSG having a high incidence of false positives (Karasick & Goldfarb, 1989). HSG is less accurate than laparoscopy in assessing extrinsic tubal adhesions, although HSG is more reliable in demonstrating uterine and intraluminal tubular pathology.

Hysteroscopy, a fibreoptic microendoscopic method for evaluating the uterine cavity after gaseous distension, is particularly useful in evaluating abnormal uterine bleeding, infertility, genital carcinoma and lost intrauterine contraceptive devices. Submucosal fibroids, uterine septa and intrauterine adhesions may be resected under direct vision.

Hysteroscopy is superior to endovaginal ultrasound in evaluating uterine abnormalities.

Salpingoscopy is the direct microendoscopic viewing of the fallopian tubes. This procedure can follow hysteroscopy, using a coaxial system, or may be performed using a linear everting catheter that does not require laparoscopic guidance.

Transvaginal ultrasound gives more detail concerning the myometrium than does HSG. The injection of normal saline or some other physiological solution into the uterine cavity and its subsequent passage along the fallopian tubes has been evaluated by ultrasound. Ultrasonic HSG is considered in some quarters to be an alternative procedure to radiographic HSG in determining tubal patency or occlusion, and has given results which are comparable to laparoscopy with dye injection (Stern *et al.*, 1992). Colour flow Doppler is preferred to grey scale imaging (Deichert *et al.*, 1992). Sonographic contrast

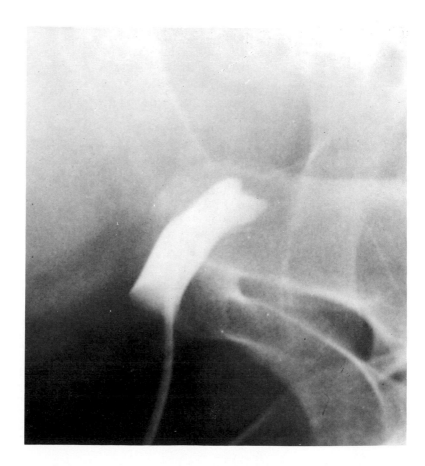

Fig. 17.9 Normal vaginogram. Contrast medium has been injected into the vagina via a balloon catheter. The balloon provided a water-tight junction in the lower part of the vagina.

media are currently being evaluated as adjuncts to ultrasonic HSG (Venezia & Zangara, 1991).

Magnetic resonance imaging is a highly accurate method of evaluating uterine anomalies (Pellerito *et al.*, 1992).

A high degree of accuracy has been claimed for radionuclide imaging in the evaluation of tubal patency, following the injection of ^{99m}Tc-labelled human albumin microspheres into the uterine cavity (Gurgan *et al.*, 1991). This method is associated with a high radiation dose to the ovaries (van der Weiden & van Zijl, 1990).

Vaginography

Indications

Vaginography is used to demonstrate the following.
1 Fistulae from the vagina to the ureter, bladder, intestine or rectum.
2 Congenital or acquired abnormalities of the vagina, such as diverticula.
3 Reflux of contrast medium up a vaginal ectopic ureter.

Contraindications

1 Acute vaginitis.
2 Imperforate hymen or vaginal atresia.

Technique

A Foley catheter is inserted into the vagina and its 30 ml balloon is distended with air. It is imperative that the inflated balloon fits snugly into the lower part of the vagina. Gentle traction is then applied to the catheter to ensure that the inflated balloon fits securely above the introitus. Water-soluble contrast medium, for instance Conray 280 or Urografin 290, is injected through the catheter after a watertight junction has been established between the balloon and the vagina. Usually 20–30 ml of contrast medium is required and spot radiographs are then taken in the anterolateral, lateral and sometimes oblique positions (Fig. 17.9). Steady traction is maintained on the catheter during the injection of contrast medium.

References

Brokensha, C. & Whitehouse, G.H. (1991) A comparison between iotrolan, a non-ionic dimer, and a hyperosmolar contrast medium, Urografin, in hysterosalpingography. *Br. J. Radiol.*, **64**, 587–90.

Cary, W.H. (1914) Note on determination of patency of fallopian tubes by the use of collargol and X-ray shadow. *Am. J. Obstet.*, **69**, 452–64.

Dan, U., Oelsner, G., Gruberg, L. *et al.*, (1990) Cerebral embolization and coma after hysterosalpingography with oil-soluble contrast medium. *Fertil. Steril.*, **53**, 939–40.

Deichert, U., Schlief, R., van de Sandt, M. & Daumet, P. (1992) Transvaginal hysterosalpingo-contrast sonography for the assessment of tubal patency with grey scale imaging and additional use of pulsed wave Doppler. *Fertil. Steril.*, **57**, 62–7.

Gleicher, N., Confino, E., Corfmann, R. et al. (1993) The multi-centre transcervical balloon tuboplasty study: conclusions and comparison of alternative technologies. *Hum. Reprod.*, **8**, 1264–71.

Gleicher, N., Parrilli, M., Redding, L. *et al.* (1992) Standardisation of hysterosalpingography and selective salpingography: a valuable adjunct to simple opacification studies. *Fertil. Steril.*, **58**, 1136–41.

Gurgan, T., Kisnisci, H.A., Yarali, H. *et al.* (1991) Radionuclide hysterosalpingography. A simple and potentially useful method of evaluating tubal patency. *J. Reprod. Med.*, **36**, 789–92.

Karasick, S. & Goldfarb, A.F. (1989) Peritubal adhesions in infertile women: diagnosis with hysterosalpingography. *AJR*, **152**, 777–9.

Lindequist, S., Justesen, P., Larsen, C. & Rasmussen, F. (1991) Diagnostic quality and complications of hysterosalpingography: oil versus water soluble contrast media — a randomised prospective study. *Radiology*, **179**, 69–74.

Moore, D.E., Segars, J.H., Winfield, A.C. *et al.* (1990) Effects of contrast agents on the fallopian tube in a rabbit model. *Radiology*, **170**, 721–4.

MRI (Medical Research International) and the Society for Assisted Reproductive Technology and The American Fertility Society. *In vitro* fertilisation–embryo transfer in the United States: 1988. Results from the IVF-ET registry. *Fertil. Steril.*, **53**, 13–20.

Ogihara, T., Miyao H., Katoh, H. *et al.* (1991) Adverse reactions to Lipiodol ultrafluid: report of an accidental case. *Keio J. Med.*, **40**, 94–6.

Pellerito, J.S., McCarthy, S.M., Doyle, M.B. *et al.* (1992) Diagnosis of uterine anomalies; relative accuracy of MR imaging, endovaginal sonography and hysterosalpingography. *Radiology*, **183**, 795–800.

Pontifex, G., Trichopoulos, D. & Karpathios, S. (1972) Hysterosalpingography in the diagnosis of infertility (statistical analysis of 3437 cases). *Fertil. Steril.*, **23**, 829–33.

Rasmussen, F., Lindequist, S., Larsen, C. & Justesen, P. (1991)

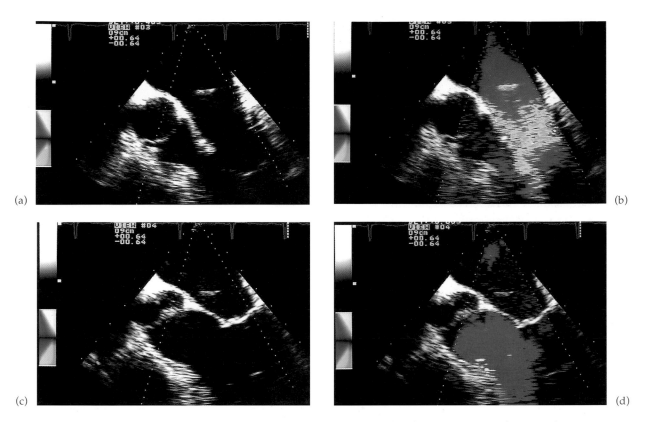

Plate 10.1 (a) Transoesophageal image of the mitral valve opening in diastole. The left atrium is at the top of the image nearest to the transducer. (b) Colour flow mapping of (a) showing normal flow through the mitral valve encoded in blue. The ligher hues of blue show slight acceleration of flow through the valve orifice. (c) Transoesophageal image of the mitral valve in systole. The left ventricle is in the lower part of the image with the aortic valve to the left. (d) Colour flow mapping of (c) showing normal flow towards the aortic valve encoded in red.

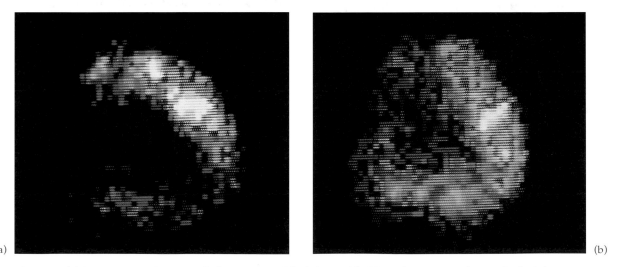

Plate 10.2 (a) A post-exercise long axis thallium image of the left ventricle. Normal activity can be seen in the left ventricular free wall but there is little tracer uptake in the apex and the inferior wall indicating ischaemia. (b) A subsequent identical resting image in the same patient demonstrating almost normal activity in the inferior wall of the left ventricle indicating the ischaemia is reversible.

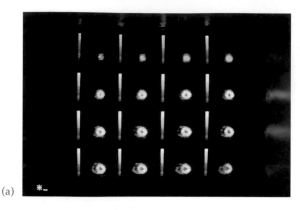
(a)

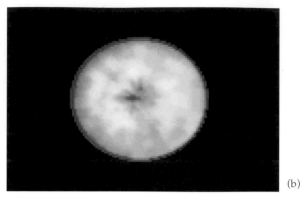
(b)

Plate 10.3 Both (a) single photon emission computed tomography (short axis views in this example) and (b) bull's-eye images (which are the equivalent of the three-dimensional left ventricle being laid flat into a two-dimensional plot) are frequently used for the detection of areas of ischaemia in myocardial perfusion imaging.

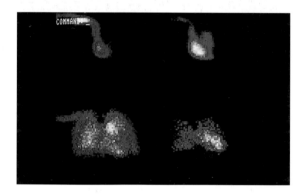

Plate 10.4 The four images show a bolus of radiopharmaceutical passing from the superior vena cava and right atrium (top left), right ventricle (top right), pulmonary vasculature (bottom left) and left ventricle (bottom right) in this patient without a shunt.

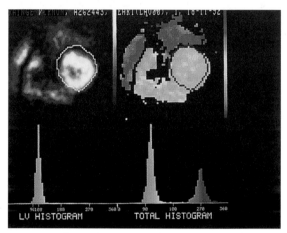

Plate 10.5 These parametric images show maximum change in activity (top left) and phase of contraction (top right). The first image (amplitude) shows the major change over the ventricles and phase images showing different colours for the atria (red) and then the ventricles (green). In this normal patient uniform green colour indicates synchronous ventricular contraction.

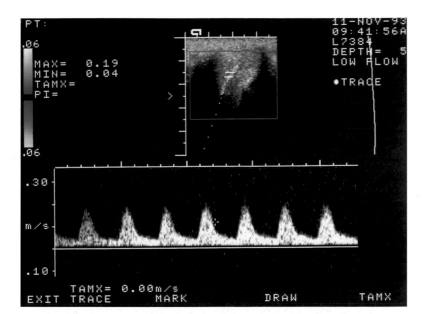

Plate 18.1 Colour Doppler of a cavernosal artery in a patient with arterial insufficiency. The maximum flow rate in systole is 19 cm s⁻¹.

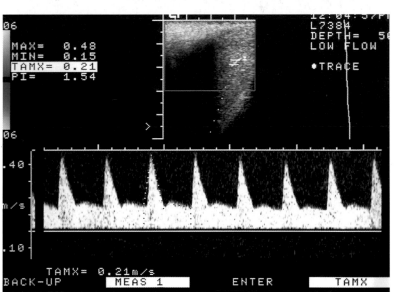

Plate 18.2 Colour Doppler in a patient with a venous leak. The maximum flow rates in systole are 48 cm s⁻¹, but the flow rates in diastole are also high at 15 cm s⁻¹.

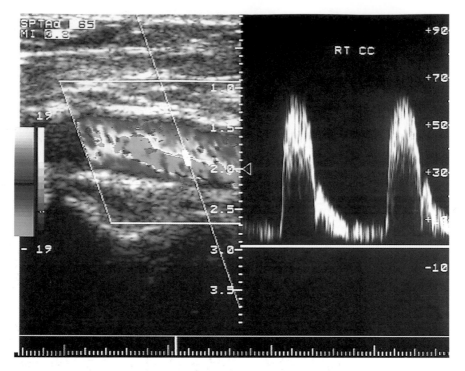

Plate 26.1 A duplex scan of the right common carotid artery. On the left-hand side of the image, flow is shown within the common carotid artery by filling in with colour. A Doppler line has been placed through the image with the small rectangular Doppler box placed within the common carotid artery. On the right-hand side of the image, the spectral trace from this sample box is visualized.

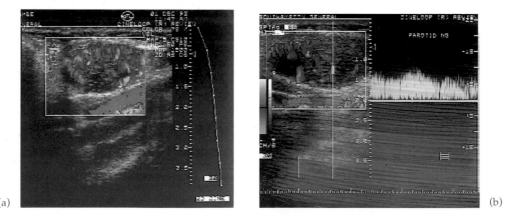

(a) (b)

Plate 26.2 (a) Colour Doppler traces through a tumour in the parotid gland. This shows marked increase in vascularity with a rather bizarre vessel pattern typical of malignancy. (b) The Doppler box has been placed in one of the bizarre vessels and the spectral trace shows high diastolic flow.

Therapeutic effect of hysterosalpingography: oil versus water-soluble contrast media — a randomised prospective study. *Radiology*, **179**, 75–8.

Rindfleisch, W. (1910) Derstellung der cavum uteri. *Berlin Klin. Wschr.*, **47**, 780–2.

Risquez, F., Forman, R., Maleika, F. *et al.* (1992) Transcervical cannulation of the fallopian tube for the management of ectopic pregnancies: prospective multicentre study. *Fertil. Steril.*, **58**, 1131–5.

Rubin, I.C. (1914) Roentgen diagnostik der uterus tumoren mit hilfe von intrauterinen collargolinjectionen. *Zbl. Gynäk.*, **38**, 658.

Sholkoff, S.D. (1987) Balloon hysterosalpingography catheter. *AJR*, **149**, 995–6.

Stern, J., Peters, A. J., & Coulam, C.B. (1992) Color Doppler ultrasonography assessment of tubal patency: a comparison study with traditional techniques. *Fertil. Steril.*, **58**, 897–900.

Thurmond, A.S. (1991) Selective salpingography and fallopian tube recanalisation. *AJR*, **156**, 33–8.

Thurmond, A.S., Novy, M., Uchida, B.T. & Rosch, J. (1987) Fallopian tube obstruction: selective salpingography and recanalisation. *Radiology*, **163**, 511–40.

Tyrrell, P.N.M., McHugo, J.M. & Hale, M. Patient perception of the hysterosalpingogram: the initial stages of the audit cycle. *Br. J. Radiol.*, **66**, 103–7.

van der Weiden, R.M. & van Zijl, J. (1989) Radiation exposure of the ovaries during hysterosalpingography. Is radionuclide hysterosalpingography justified? *Br. J. Obstet. Gynaecol.*, **96**, 471–2.

Varpula, M. (1989) Hysterosalpingography with a balloon catheter versus a cannula: evaluation of patient pain. *Radiology*, **172**, 745–7.

Venezia, R. & Zangara, C. (1991) Echohysterosalpingography: new diagnostic possibilities with S HU 450 Echovist. *Acta. Eur. Fertil.*, **22**, 279–82.

Wright, J.T. (1961) A new method of hysterosalpingography. *Br. J. Radiol.*, **34**, 465–7.

18   Male Genital Tract

D. RICKARDS

Radiological investigation of impotence

Impotence is a common problem, affecting 10% of males over the age of 40 years. Vasculogenic impotence is one of the many causes of impotence. The investigation of vasculogenic impotence should not be performed until all other causes, for instance psychological and hormonal, have been excluded. The investigation into vasculogenic impotence attempts to determine whether there is:

1 Arterial disease and poor blood supply to the corpora cavernosa.
2 A venous leak.
3 A combination of arterial insufficiency and a venous leak.
4 Normal penile vasculature.

All investigations into vasculogenic impotence should be performed after the administration of a vasoactive (smooth muscle relaxant) agent into the corpora cavernosa. The most commonly used is papaverine hydrochloride, but prostaglandin E_1 is now readily available, carries fewer complications and is now the agent of choice, although more expensive. A dose of 20 µg prostaglandin E_1 is adequate in all patients. Should papaverine be used, 40 mg should be administered into the corpora. Arterial disease should be investigated by colour Doppler and venous disease by cavernosometry.

Colour Doppler imaging

The steps involved are as follows:
1 Scan the flaccid penis. Identify the cavernosal arteries at the base of the corpora. Identify any areas of fibrosis or Peyronie's disease.
2 Inject the smooth muscle relaxant into the base of the corpora whilst holding the corpora between the thumb and forefinger.

3 Scan the cavernosal arteries at the base of the corpora bilaterally every 3 min for 15 min. The following parameters should be identified:
   (a) maximal end flow velocity (Q_{max}),
   (b) lowest end diastolic velocity (EDV),
   (c) erectile grade,
   (d) diameter of the cavernosal arteries.

Following the injection of a muscle relaxant agent there is a reduction in vascular resistance leading to an increased velocity of flow in both systole and diastole. As the intracorporeal pressure rises, the flow in diastole decreases and, in full erection, retrograde flow will occur in systole. A 75% increase in the diameter of the vessel is also considered to be within normal limits and indicates good vessel compliance.

Criteria for the diagnosis of arterial insufficiency

1 Q_{max} of less than 35 cm s^{-1} (Plate 18.1, between p. 310 and p. 311).
2 A difference between left and right cavernosal arteries of more than 12 cm s^{-1}.
3 A poor degree of tumescence.
4 Local stenoses demonstrated on colour Doppler.

Criteria for the diagnosis of venous insufficiency

1 Q_{max} greater than 35 cm s^{-1}.
2 EDV greater than 7 cm s^{-1} (Plate 18.2, between p. 310 and p. 311).
3 Poor erectile grade.

Complications

1 *Haemorrhage*. Some degree of bruising is to be expected at the needle site. This is likely to be more severe in patients in whom normal tumescence is achieved.

2 *Priapism.* This is a serious complication because, if left untreated, it will itself result in impotence. The patient must be warned that if his erection should not subside within 2 hours, or becomes painful, he must return to hospital so that detumescence can be performed. Each patient should be given a post-procedural sheet that describes possible complications and what to do in their event.

3 *Haematuria.* This is only likely to occur if the needles have been inadvertently misplaced into the urethra. No treatment is usually required.

Cavernosometry

Cavernosometry should be performed only when a colour Doppler has demonstrated that there is normal arterial end flow. It directly investigates the competence of the veno-occlusive mechanism of erection. The steps involved are as follows.

A 21 gauge butterfly needle is inserted into each corpus, just proximal to the glans penis (Fig. 18.1). Placing needles in the base of the corpora in the presence of an erecting penis will allow the needle to migrate out of the corpora, causing significant complications. Confirm that the needles are in the correct place by injecting a small amount of contrast medium under fluoroscopic control. If within the corpora, contrast medium will flow away from the needle tips without pain. If misplaced, injection will be associated with pain and contrast medium will accumulate at the needle tip.

One needle is connected to a pressure transducer, flushed through and zeroed. The other needle is connected to a pressure pump that is capable of rates from 1–100 ml min^{-1}. Modern urodynamic equipment used in the investigation of lower urinary tract abnormalities usually includes software specifically dedicated to cavernosonography and cavernosometry.

The muscle relaxant agent is injected through one of the needles. Pressure changes resulting from the injection of this muscle relaxant are monitored. Once the pressure starts to increase, it can be concluded that muscle relaxation is occurring.

Dilute contrast medium (Omnipaque 150) is then injected at a rate of 100 ml min^{-1}. Pressure changes due to the injection are monitored. A pressure rise within the corpora of 100 mmHg should be achieved with this rate of injection, assuming that the vasoactivator has been injected into the correct place. Once this pressure of 100 mmHg has been achieved, the pump flow is decreased to the rate required to maintain a pressure within the corpora of 100 mmHg. Spot radiographs of the base of the corpora should be taken (Fig. 18.2).

The injection of contrast medium is stopped and the fall is pressure within the corpora is measured over the next 30 s. Blood is then allowed to drain out

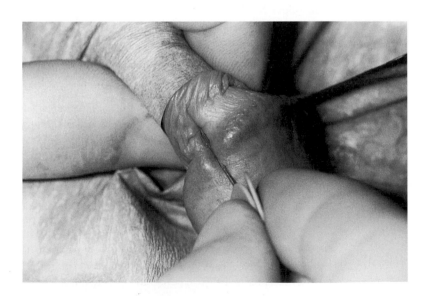

Fig. 18.1 A 21 gauge butterfly needle is inserted into the corpus just proximal to the glans penis.

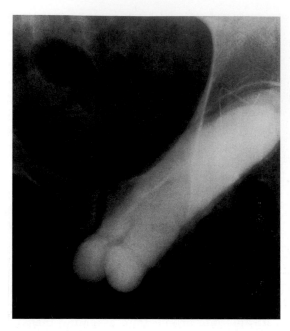

Fig. 18.2 Normal cavernogram. The two needles can be seen in the corpora. There is normal tumescence and no draining veins are seen.

of the corpora through the needles until detumescence has fully occurred.

The following parameters should be documented.
1 Erectile grade in response to both the injection of prostaglandin E_1 and the injection of contrast medium.
2 The maintenance flow rate required to maintain an intracorporeal pressure of 100 mmHg.
3 The pressure loss that occurs once injection of contrast medium has been stopped.
4 Spot radiographs of the corporeal and venous anatomy.

Criteria for a venous leak

1 Poor tumescence in response to prostaglandin E_1.
2 A maintenance flow rate of more than 20 ml min^{-1}.
3 A pressure loss of more than 50 mmHg in the first 30 s.

Complications

1 All patients should be warned to expect some bruising at the needle insertion points. This will be signifi-

cantly reduced if the patient is allowed to detumesce through the needles prior to removing them.
2 Priapism. This serious complication is significantly reduced by the administration of prostaglandin E_1 rather than the administration of papaverine hydrochloride. Patients must be warned that if they have an erection which lasts for more than 2 hours or becomes painful, to return to the hospital so that the priapism can be reversed either by aspiration or the administration of vascoconstrictor drugs.

Penile angiography

Indications

1 Sudden onset of impotence that might be due to a stenosis of the common iliac or internal iliac artery.
2 Following pelvic trauma in young men in whom revascularization of the corpora might be considered.

Technique

The femoral arteries are punctured using the Seldinger technique. Flush aortography is performed to visualize the distal aorta, common iliac and internal iliac arteries to exclude significant disease. 5 French (F) cobra catheters are inserted and placed in the contralateral internal pudendal artery. Selective angiography is then performed with the patient lying partially oblique (20°). A vasoactive agent is then injected directly into the corpora or through the catheter. A further selective angiogram is then performed (Fig. 18.3).

Complications

1 Haematoma formation at the puncture sites.
2 Arterial injury during selective catheterization.
3 Priapism.

Radiological investigation of infertility

Male infertility has many causes, ranging from disorders of spermatogenesis to obstruction in the genital tract. The role of the radiologist is to assist the andrologist in defining the level and cause of obstruction within the genital tract and identifying conditions that could alter spermatogenesis, for instance

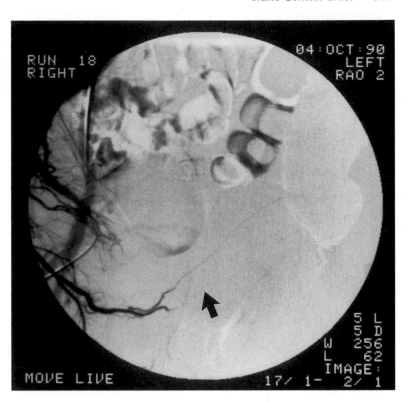

Fig. 18.3 A normal penile angiogram. The cavernosal artery is seen (arrow).

varicocoele or cryptorchism. Scrotal ultrasound is the modality of choice in the later. Vasography and antegrade percutaneous seminal vesiculography are indicated in obstructive lesions.

Vasography

At surgery, the distal vasa within the scrotum are identified and cannulated. Spot radiographs are taken during the injection of contrast medium, usually with portable equipment in theatre. This procedure is essentially a surgical one, the radiologist's role being confined to interpreting the films.

Antegrade seminal vesiculography

The lower genital tract is well demonstrated on transrectal ultrasound (TRUS). Using linear and curved array sharply focused probes, the seminal vesicles, distal vas deferens and ejaculatory ducts can be defined (Fig. 18.4). Dilatation of the seminal vesicles and/or ejaculatory ducts suggests that they are ob-

structed but dilatation is not diagnostic of obstruction. Antegrade seminal vesiculography is performed to differentiate unobstructed and dilated structures from dilated and obstructed structures.

Technique

A diagnostic TRUS is performed. The perineum is cleaned, using an antiseptic solution such as Betadine. Under continuous TRUS control, a 22 gauge needle is inserted through the perineum and local anaesthetic is injected. The needle is then advanced through the prostate and into the dilated seminal vesicle or ejaculatory duct (Fig. 18.5). Sterile water, which has been agitated within the syringe to induce air bubbles in it, is injected under continuous TRUS control (Fig. 18.6). Obstruction is unlikely if interfaces are seen to be passing through the bladder neck into the bladder. Contrast medium can be injected through the same needle and spot radiographs taken. If obstruction is surmised by further dilatation of the seminal vesicle or duct and an absence of interfaces

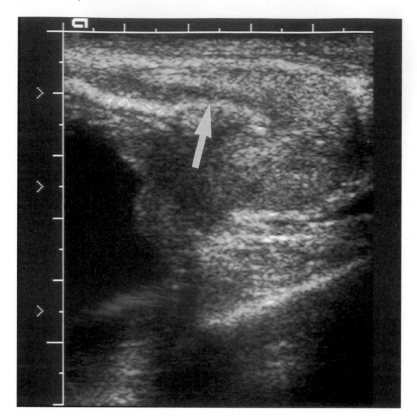

Fig. 18.4 A sagittal section of the prostate gland. The normal ejaculatory duct is seen.

entering the bladder, decompressing aspiration is performed. Finally, the needle is withdrawn.

Complications

1 *Infection.* A sterile technique is essential. If obstruction is proven, prophylactic antibiotics should be prescribed.
2 *Haemospermia.* This is likely if no obstruction exists, is temporary and needs no treatment.

Prostate biopsy

Prostate cancer is the most common genitourinary malignancy in men. Diagnosis is made either by digital rectal examination (DRE), prostate-specific antigen (PSA) evaluation or TRUS and biopsy. DRE is not specific and is operator-dependent. Cancer is suspected with elevated PSA levels (above 5 μg litre^{-1}), but the PSA can also be raised in benign disease. Abnormalities seen on TRUS can suggest malignancy, but again this is not specific enough as 80% of peripherally located echo-poor lesions will be due to benign conditions. The definitive diagnosis of prostate cancer requires biopsy.

Indications

1 Palpable abnormality on DRE.
2 Raised PSA levels.
3 Abnormality seen on TRUS when either the DRE or the PSA is abnormal. Abnormalities found on TRUS in the absence of any abnormality on DRE and normal PSA levels is not an indication to biopsy.
4 Follow-up after therapy for prostate cancer.

Contraindications

1 Anticoagulant therapy.
2 Untreated acute prostatitis or prostate abscess.

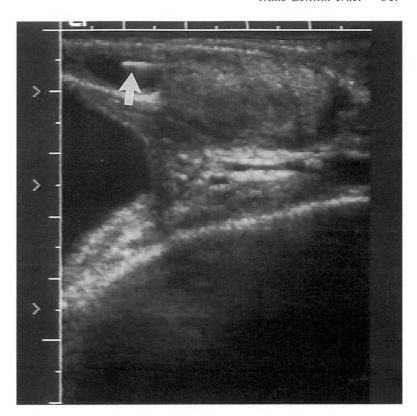

Fig. 18.5 Using a perineal approach, a 22 gauge needle has been inserted under transrectal ultrasound control into a dilated seminal vesicle (arrow).

Technique

Biopsy of the prostate gland can be performed through the rectal route or through the transperineal route. Aspiration cytology has been replaced by core biopsy using 18 gauge needles and an automatic triggering device that produces a core of tissue 2 cm long. Biopsies should be placed in formaldehyde solution and labelled individually, indicating their site within the prostate.

Transrectal biopsy

The development of forward-looking end-fire transrectal probes makes biopsy of all parts of the prostate gland easy and relatively painless.

Prophylactic antibiotics should be administered prior to biopsy: 80 mg of gentamicin is appropriate. The patient is placed in the left lateral decubitus position. A cleansing enema should be performed if the colon is found to be loaded on DRE.

A diagnostic TRUS is performed to identify any abnormal areas within the prostate (Fig. 18.7) and to measure gland volume. The biopsy transducer with guide is inserted into the rectum and computer software is used to produce a biopsy guideline (Fig. 18.8). Under continuous TRUS control, a biopsy needle is placed through the biopsy guide and anterior rectal wall. Once through the anterior rectal wall, the patient is warned to expect some discomfort and the biopsy is taken (Fig. 18.9). It is appropriate to take at least five biopsies of the prostate gland, irrespective of the DRE and TRUS findings. Biopsy of the left and right peripheral zones, the left and right central parts of the gland and of the apex of the gland to one side of the mid-line should be performed.

Following biopsy, a 500 mg Flagyl suppository should be placed within the rectum and the patient given oral antibiotics, such as Ciproxin 250 mg twice a day for 2 days.

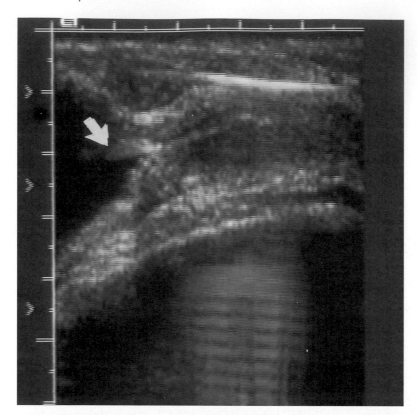

Fig. 18.6 Following puncture of a dilated seminal vesicle, sterile water mixed with air has been injected and can be seen passing through the bladder neck into the bladder (arrow).

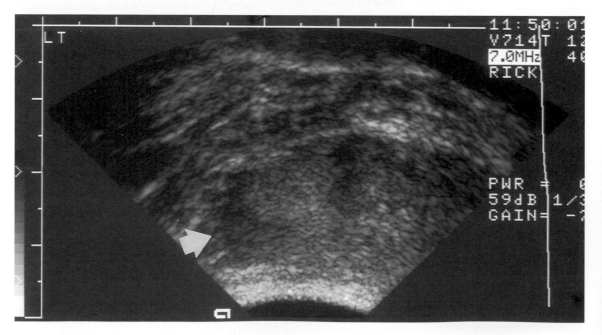

Fig. 18.7 Transverse axial transrectal ultrasound showing an echo-poor lesion in the right peripheral zone of the gland (arrow).

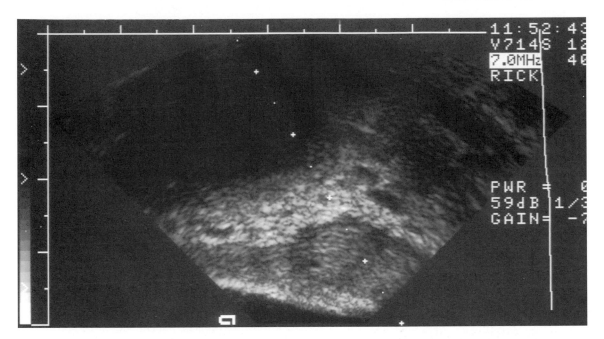

Fig. 18.8 Using a forward-looking probe, a sagittal image of the prostate is obtained and the biopsy cursor displayed passing through the abnormal area.

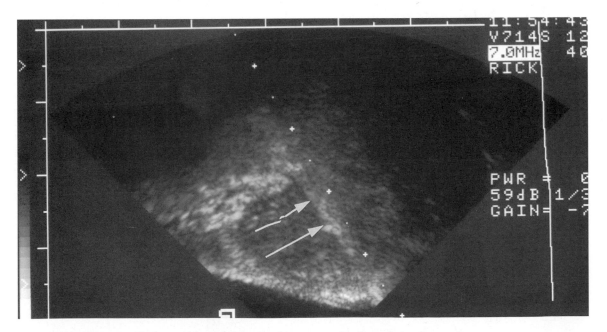

Fig. 18.9 The biopsy needle (arrows) has been fired and is seen passing through the abnormal area.

Complications

1 The patient should be warned to expect blood in the urine, ejaculate or faeces. He should be warned that this should not be heavy and should not last for more than 24 hours.

2 Infection. Prophylactic antibiotics will significantly reduce the possibility of infection. The most serious complication of prostate biopsy is septicaemia. Infective processes within the prostate itself, for instance prostatic abscess, can also occur. Again, these complications will be reduced by prophylactic antibiotics. All patients must be warned that subsequent fever must be instantly reported to the general practitioner or to the hospital.

Patients should be given a fact sheet after biopsy, describing these complications and advising on what to do should they occur.

Transperineal biopsy

To biopsy the prostate transperineally requires a linear array probe so that the advance of the needle can be continuously watched under TRUS control. Modern TRUS units do not produce such a probe, so transperineal biopsy is becoming rare. Transperineal biopsy is ideal in patients who are more likely to have benign prostatic disease, such as prostatitis.

Technique

The patient is placed in the left lateral decubitus position. A diagnostic TRUS is performed in both transverse axial and sagittal sections (Fig. 18.10). The linear array probe is inserted in to the rectum. The perineum is cleaned with an antiseptic solution, such as Betadine. Prophylactic antibiotics are not required. Local anaesthetic (15 ml of 1% lignocaine) is instilled via a 25 gauge needle, into the skin and subcutaneous tissues down to the capsule of the prostate gland. Once at the capsule, the local anaesthetic will track round the prostate. It is not necessary to redirect the needle into various aspects of the gland. The local anaesthetic needle is retracted but left *in situ* within the entry point in the perineum.

The biopsy needle is then inserted through the skin and advanced under continuous ultrasound control to a position just caudal to the lesion under suspicion (Fig. 18.11). The patient should be warned to expect some discomfort while the biopsy is taken. With experience, biopsies from all parts of the prostate can be quickly taken with this technique.

Complications

1 The patient should be warned to expect haematuria and haemospermia.

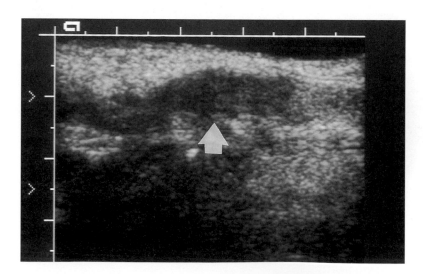

Fig. 18.10 A sagittal section of the prostate showing an echo-poor lesion at the base of the gland in the peripheral zone (arrow).

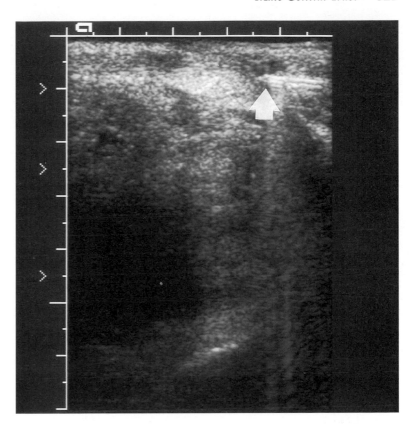

Fig. 18.11 The biopsy needle is advanced down to the capsule of the gland and placed just proximal to the abnormal area. The biopsy an then be taken.

2 Despite good antiseptic technique, infection may rarely occur. Some administer a broad spectrum antibiotic, e.g. two Septrin tablets twice a day for 2 days following a perineal biopsy.

Further reading

Burkholder, G.V. & Kaufman, I.I. (1966) Local implantation of carcinoma of the prostate with percutaneous needle biopsy. *J. Urol.*, **95**, 801–4.

Catalona, W.J. & Scott, W.W. (1986) Carcinoma of the prostate. *In* Walsh, P.C., Gittes, R.F., Perlmutter, A.D. & Stamey, T.A. (eds) *Campbell's Urology*, 5th edn, pp. 1463–534. WB Saunders, Philadelphia.

Grayhack, J.T. & Bockrath, J.M. (1981) Diagnosis of carcinoma of prostate. Urology, 17 (Suppl.), 54–60.

Rifkin, M.D. (1988) *Ultrasound of the Prostate*. Raven Press, New York.

Rifkin, M.D., Alexander, A.A., Pisarchick & Matteucci, T. (1991) Palpable masses in the prostate: superior accuracy of US-guided biopsy compared with accuracy of digitally guided biopsy. *Radiology*, **179**, 41–2.

Rifkin, M.D. & Choi, H. (1988) Endorectal prostate ultrasound: implications of the small peripheral lesions in hypechoic endorectal US of the prostate. *Radiology*, **106**, 619–22.

Rifkin, M.D. Dahnert, W. & Kurtz, A.B. (1990) State of the art: endorectal sonography of the prostate gland. *AJR*, **154**, 691–700.

Section 5
Central Nervous System

19 Brain

B. S. WORTHINGTON

Great developments have occurred in neuroradiology during the last 25 years, particularly in the field of new technology. The introduction of computed tomography (CT), digital vascular imaging and latterly magnetic resonance imaging (MRI), coupled with the availability of safer contrast media, has advanced the goal of obtaining more diagnostic information whilst reducing risk and discomfort to the patient.

The advent and subsequent refinement of CT transformed the practice of neuroradiology. This non-invasive and safe method of investigation revealed a wealth of information about intracranial and intraorbital structures. It became the only procedure required for patient management in many cases of congenital malformations, degenerative disorders, intracranial suppuration and craniocerebral trauma. CT also became the initial procedure of choice in the evaluation of patients suspected of harbouring an intracranial tumour. However, angiography still had a role in demonstrating the anatomy of intrinsic vascular disorders and in the differential diagnosis of lesions which give similar CT appearances. Furthermore, the development of interventional procedures following on a superselective angiogram has now extended its applications. The intrathecal injection of contrast medium or air as an adjunct to CT allowed the diagnosis of small tumours which encroach on the basal cisterns. In addition, direct coronal scans and reformatted sagittal and coronal images from multiple contiguous transverse scans provided a much needed multiplanar facility in CT. These developments led to the total abandonment of pneumoencephalography and ventriculography in centres where a modern CT scanner is available and, when such equipment is universally available throughout the world, these procedures will be of historical interest only.

MRI was shown at the outset to have a number of advantages over CT for the examination of the nervous system (Hawkes *et al.*, 1980). It has no planar restriction, allowing direct sagittal and coronal imaging in addition to the conventional transverse axial plane; obtrusive artefacts from bone and air-containing structures adjacent to brain are eliminated; the contrast between different tissues can be manipulated by altering the applied pulse sequence; and it avoids completely the use of ionizing radiation. Comparative clinical studies have shown that MRI is more sensitive than CT to the presence of intracranial pathology and its multiplanar facility permits the better evaluation of the topographical relationships of structural lesions prior to surgery. The introduction of gadolinium diethylenetriamine penta-acetic acid (GdDTPA), an intravascular contrast agent, has further increased the sensitivity of the technique in several contexts, such as the detection of small acoustic neuromas and the demonstration of pathology involving the meninges. The recent development of magnetic resonance angiography (Dumoulin & Hart, 1986) is based on techniques which create a difference in the signal returned from stationary structures and flowing blood within a volume of tissue. By subtracting out the former one can derive a dataset which depicts vascular structures. Studies of the extracranial and intracranial arterial or venous system can be displayed in a variety of formats, some of which resemble conventional angiograms (Fig. 19.1). It must always be remembered that magnetic resonance angiograms map flow rather than underlying vessel morphology.

If MRI were freely available, it would be preferred to CT as the initial investigation for almost all intracranial pathology. While its availability is limited, MRI is applied with greatest benefit to those clinical situations where it has been shown to have a clear superiority over CT, for example in the evaluation of suspected pathology in the posterior fossa.

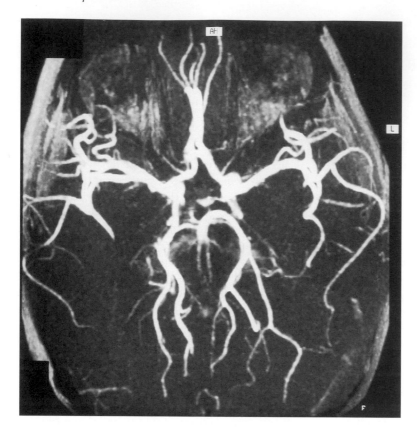

Fig. 19.1 Magnetic resonance angiogram showing the vessels comprising the circle of Willis and their branches.

CT is, however, currently superior to conventional MRI for the detection of subarachnoid blood. CT frequently assists in the characterization of lesions, particularly through the demonstration of the presence and pattern of calcification. The better rendering of bone detail on CT makes it the preferred technique in the evaluation of craniofacial trauma and study of temporal bone anatomy.

Cerebral angiography

Indications

The introduction of CT in 1972 by Hounsfield led to a reappraisal of the indications for cerebral angiography. At the present time the potential impact of magnetic resonance angiography is being assessed. Both CT and MRI can provide useful information in intrinsic disease of the blood vessels, including aneurysm, arteriovenous malformation

and venous thrombosis, particularly about their sequelae. Whilst MRI can be used to screen for aneurysms and provides useful information in vascular malformations, angiography is usually necessary to define the precise morphology of the underlying lesion and its connection to cerebral vessels. In the management of patients with cerebrovascular disease, ultrasound examination of the carotid bifurcation may be used to screen for significant stenoses or atheromatous plaques. Colour flow Doppler studies provide information on flow velocity and direction as well as the presence of turbulence. Magnetic resonance angiography is becoming increasingly competitive in providing similar information. Angiography, although relegated to a secondary role, is required to demonstrate related extracranial and intracranial vascular occlusions, stenoses and ulcerated atheromatous plaques. The examination also shows patterns of collateral blood supply when main vessels have been compromised. Angiography may also be required to confirm a suspected diagnosis of vasculitis. While CT or MRI alone may provide sufficient information in tumour cases to determine further management, there are many instances where angiography assists the differential diagnosis and provides information about vascular anatomy useful to the surgeon. CT has replaced angiography in the management of craniocerebral trauma, except where associated vascular damage such as carotid dissection is suspected.

Contraindications

1 Where there is a contraindication to arterial puncture itself. This includes patients with bleeding disorders or severe hypertension.
2 Although the age of the patient is no bar to cerebral angiography, due regard must be taken of the increasing prevalence of atherosclerotic changes with advancing age which will render the procedure potentially more hazardous. Evidence of reduced cerebral perfusion also increases the risk of the procedure.
3 In patients with known sensitivity to contrast media, it is clearly preferable to avoid angiography if possible. Appropriate precautions must be taken when it is deemed necessary to carry out the procedure.

Technical aspects

Arteriography began in 1927 when Egan Moniz reported the radiographic visualization of cerebral vessels by the injection of 25% sodium iodide solution into the surgically exposed carotid artery. The original name of 'arterial encephalography' applied to the technique has been replaced by 'cerebral angiography'. Continuous improvements in contrast media and X-ray equipment have increased the diagnostic quality of the examination whilst reducing the risk to the patient.

Contrast media

Until recently, all contrast media used for cerebral angiography were ionic salts of tri-iodinated substituted benzoic acid, the meglumine salts having a lower toxicity than sodium salts. A typical contrast medium was Conray 280 (60% w/v meglumine iothalamate) with an iodine concentration of 280 mg ml^{-1}. The introduction of the non-ionic contrast media, such as iohexol and iopamidol, represents a significant advance. They cause far less pain on intra-arterial injection, with considerably less endothelial damage and decrease in permeability of the blood–brain barrier than previous contrast media, and a consequent reduction in neurotoxicity.

X-ray equipment

Biplane serial angiography is a basic necessity for making a precise analysis of intracranial vascular anatomy and to obtain information about regional contrast flow rates. This requirement was foreseen by Moniz himself, but it was not until 1952 that Fredzell introduced a rapid cut-film changer suitable for cerebral angiography and which could expose as many as 30 radiographs at rates of up to 3 s^{-1}. Fluoroscopy and a high-quality image intensifier are required for catheter studies, coupled with a table which has a movable top capable of a wide range of excursions to follow catheter manipulations. For magnification studies, an X-ray tube with a small focal spot (0.1–0.3 mm) and a three-phase generator are essential.

Techniques

Whilst cerebral angiography can be carried out by direct puncture or by retrograde filling from injection of a remote vessel, the majority of studies are now carried out by catheterization of individual vessels.

Catheter techniques

Direct catheterization of the four major vessels is usually carried out by the femoral route although, when this is precluded, the axillary route is an alternative. The percutaneous introduction of a catheter into the femoral artery and the general conduct of a catheterization procedure are described in Chapter 8.

Whilst most studies in adults may be carried out under local anaesthesia with basal sedation, a case can be made for general anaesthesia despite the additional cost. Through the use of muscle relaxants and controlled ventilation, the arterial P_{CO_2} can be controlled so as to obtain optimum visualization of intracranial vessels while the elimination of all patient movement facilitates satisfactory subtraction studies. A variety of suitable end-hole catheters is commercially available for cerebral angiography, personal preferences and experience dictating which is selected. Some radiologists prefer to make their own catheters from soft, thin-walled 5 French (F) polythene tubing. A simple hook configuration is sufficient in the majority of cases. Preformed headhunter catheters of more complex shape, especially when formed of stiffer material to provide better torque control, are suitable when tortuous ectatic main vessels are encountered.

Under fluoroscopic control, the catheter is advanced into the ascending arch of the aorta and is then rotated until the tip is pointing in a cranial direction. The orifice of a main vessel can then be engaged by advancing and withdrawing the catheter. The position of the catheter is then confirmed by a small test injection of contrast medium. The guide wire is reinserted and advanced carefully for approximately 5 cm into the vessel, after which the catheter is advanced over the wire and finally the latter is withdrawn. Further catheter advancement, for example in superselective studies, can be achieved with the use of a guide wire. Definitive injections are made after confirming a correct catheter position by a small test injection of contrast medium. Iopamidol or iohexol (8 ml), in concentrations of 240 mg iodine ml^{-1}, is suitable for common carotid angiography while a smaller volume (6 ml) is adequate for vertebral angiography, the amount being tailored to the size of the vessel (Fig. 19.2). The catheter is removed after completing the study. Sufficient pressure is maintained on the puncture site for 10–20 min to prevent haematoma formation.

Carotid arteriography by direct puncture

Although percutaneous puncture of the carotid artery can be carried out under local anaesthesia, general anaesthesia is required for children and patients unable to provide the necessary degree of cooperation because of anxiety or neurological disturbance. A puncture site is chosen in the lower part of the neck, where the common carotid artery can be palpated medial to the sternomastoid muscle. If the vessel lies very medial, it may be necessary to displace it laterally before attempting puncture. A variety of needles and cannulae have been used. The author prefers a simple 18-gauge needle, with short bevel, mounted in a plastic hub which is continuous with a short length of plastic tubing. The skin and superficial fascia are perforated with a hypodermic needle. A 10 ml glass syringe and a simple two-way tap are connected to the needle assembly and the whole is filled with saline. The index and middle finger palpate the artery with the head slightly extended, the needle then being advanced down to the artery at an angle of approximately 60°. An assistant now disconnects the saline-filled tubing from the tap and the artery is transfixed with a quick thrust. The needle is then slowly withdrawn, applying pressure on its undersurface so that a definite click is felt as it passes through the posterior arterial wall. When blood is seen to flow freely into the tubing, it is connected to the tap. The hub of the needle is depressed and the latter stabilized by draping several moistened swabs over it. The needle is intermittently flushed with saline during the procedure. The tap should be turned off whilst saline is still flowing to ensure that there is no backflow of blood into the needle. Serial injections of 8 ml of contrast medium are then made by hand, calling for the exposure to be made close to the end of the injection. As with catheter angiography, intermittent pressure must be maintained over the puncture site for 10 min to avoid haematoma formation. Instructions are given to the ward to observe the patient for further bleeding or swelling of the neck which, if bilateral, can cause tracheal compression.

Variations on the basic technique

Compression studies

By compressing the opposite carotid artery during the injection of contrast medium, filling of the contralateral intracranial vessels is achieved to a degree which depends on the patency of the anterior communicating artery (Fig. 19.3). This manoeuvre is valuable when main-vessel ligation is being considered as an option to aneurysm surgery.

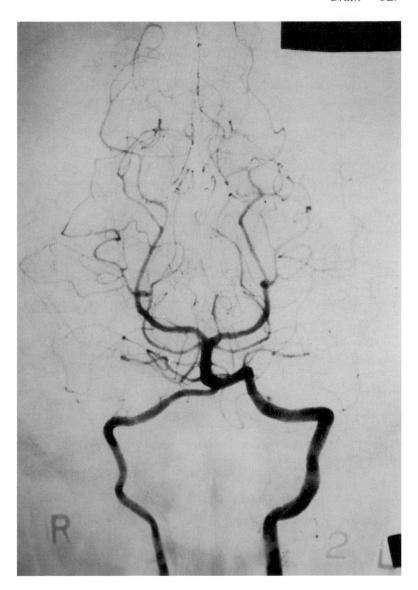

Fig. 19.2 Subtraction angiogram of the arterial phase of a normal vertebral angiogram.

Trickle arteriography

Elegant studies of pathology involving the posterior wall of the carotid artery are achieved by taking radiographs after the slow injection of 5 ml of contrast medium at 2 s intervals for 8 s. This contrast medium enters the slowly moving sleeve of fluid in the artery, permitting the identification of small thrombi and pathological stasis associated with atheromatous plaques (Hugh, 1970) (Fig. 19.4).

Vertebral arteriography

Needles such as that introduced by Sheldon in 1956 with a blocked tip and a small proximal side-hole are preferred to those with an open bevel because of the small lumen of the vertebral artery. With the head slightly extended and the carotid artery displaced laterally, the needle is directed upwards and laterally between the lateral border of the vertebral bodies and medial to the palpable anterior tubercle of

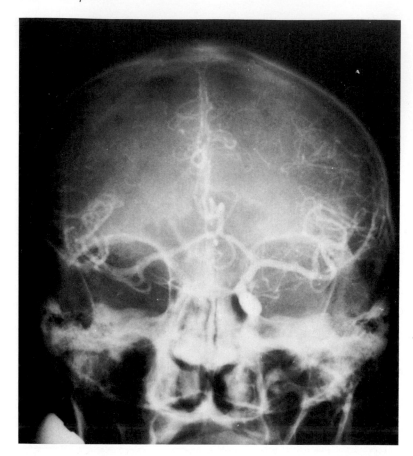

Fig. 19.3 Cross-circulation arteriographic study. The left common carotid artery has been injected with simultaneous compression of the right carotid. The anterior cerebral arteries are elevated by a suprasellar mass.

the transverse processes. The object is to puncture the vessel in the mid-cervical region as it passes between adjacent transverse foramina. Hypoplasia of the vertebral artery, which is more frequent on the right, precludes successful puncture. An injection of 5–6 ml of contrast medium is made slowly by hand. Injection of one vertebral artery normally results in sufficient filling of the distal segment of the opposite vertebral artery to outline the posterior inferior cerebellar artery.

Radiographic procedure

Routine views of the intracranial circulation are obtained in at least two projections: the lateral and the anteroposterior (AP). For the latter, the central ray is inclined 15° to the orbitomeatal line to superimpose the superior rim of the orbit and the petrous ridges in carotid studies. The angulation should be increased to 25° in vertebral angiography so that the

principal vessels are not superimposed on the skull base. A variety of oblique projections are used principally to clarify the relationship of aneurysms to their parent and adjacent arteries. Delayed radiographs (4–10 s) in the half-axial oblique position after carotid injection are valuable for demonstrating the anatomy of the principal venous sinuses. Evaluation of the extracranial carotid vessels requires coned views in the lateral and AP projections. Magnification angiography using an X-ray tube with a fine focal spot gives an improved demonstration of pathological vessel changes, as in tumours of small arteriovenous malformations. If the plane of the vessels to be studied is 4.5 cm from the tube, with a 0.3 mm focal spot and a focus film distance of 100 cm, a magnification factor of 2.25 then allows vessels as small as 120 µm to be shown.

Photographic subtraction was introduced by Ziedes de Plantes in 1934 and is a valuable adjunct to angiography, particularly in areas where contrast-

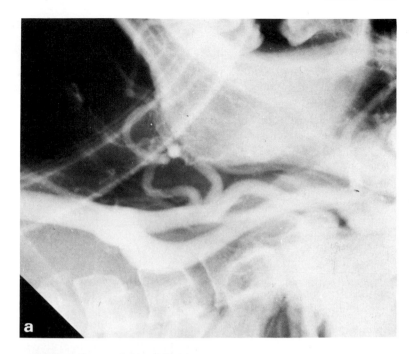

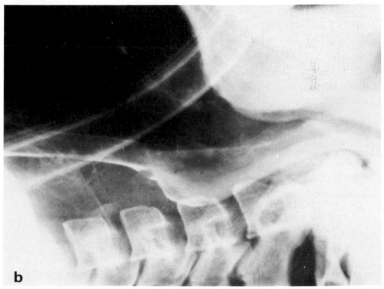

Fig. 19.4 (a) Lateral projection of an arteriographic study to show the carotid vessels in the neck. A rapid injection of contrast medium has been made. (b) Trickle arteriogram in the same patient. The contrast layer on the posterior wall outlines thrombus at the carotid bifurcation.

delineated vessels are superimposed over dense portions of the skull. A standard sequence of radiographs, which allows visualization of the intracranial vessels from the arterial phase through to the late venous phase, is two radiographs s⁻¹ for 3 s followed by one radiograph s⁻¹ for 4–6 s. Where there is rapid regional blood flow, as in arteriovenous malformations, a faster sequence may be required, whereas

delayed radiographs are necessary for studying the venous anatomy in sinus thrombosis. Only single radiographs are required for the oblique projections when studying aneurysm. Stereoscopic angiography has few advocates but is of value in defining the mutual topographical relationships of the vascular components in arteriovenous malformations and clarifying the relationship of aneurysms to parent and adjacent vessels.

Complications

Cerebral angiography is not without risk, but the most experienced angiographer will have a serious complication rate of less than 0.5% (Mani & Eisenberg, 1978). These authors stress the importance of an experienced operator, finding that a neuroradiologist is twice as safe as a general radiologist and nine times safer than a trainee. The level of experience can be translated into a shorter procedure time and the use of a smaller amount of contrast medium to complete a study, both factors contributing to a reduced morbidity. The local complications associated with femoral catheterization are discussed in Chapter 8 and only specific complications are discussed here.

Damage to the arterial wall

Improper placement of the needle tip in direct puncture procedures may lead to the injection of contrast medium beneath a flap of intima, which can lead to partial or even complete arterial occlusion. This may be followed by permanent neurological deficit when the intracranial collateral pathways are poor. The use of glass syringes allows the operator to feel the transmitted arterial pulsation in addition to seeing a free backflow of blood into the tubing, both criteria being necessary to ensure correct needle placement. Intimal damage can also follow the forcible advancement of a catheter, particularly if it is made of a rigid material.

Embolization

Both the puncturing needle and the intravascular catheter can dislodge fragments of atheroma, particularly after prolonged catheter manipulations in the aortic arch of elderly subjects. Both intravascular needles and catheters form a nidus for thrombus formation, especially in prolonged examinations. The catheter and needle system should be irrigated at frequent intervals with heparinized saline, employing a double-flush technique, that is, withdrawing into one syringe and flushing with a second.

Contrast medium toxicity

Complications, which are more frequent and severe with conventional ionic agents than with low-osmolar contrast media, are thought to be due to alteration in the permeability of the blood–brain barrier. This can cause an increase in cerebral oedema in patients with a cerebral tumour, leading to subsequent clinical deterioration. Sodium salts are more toxic in this regard than meglumine salts. Transient cortical blindness, which has been described following vertebral angiography, is thought to be due to a direct toxic effect of contrast medium on the occipital cortex. Care must be taken to avoid complete occlusion of small vertebral vessels by the catheter, which would prevent adequate wash-out of contrast medium.

Current developments

Superselective angiographic examination of smaller branches of the extracranial and intracranial vessels has allowed the development of a variety of occlusion procedures, including detachable balloons and particulate embolization. These have been used to close arteriovenous fistulae, to obliterate vascular malformations, and to reduce the blood supply to vascular lesions prior to surgery. Digital vascular imaging is based on real-time electronic subtraction of a mask from image-intensifier images following injections of contrast medium. The computer enhancement of the digital-intensifier image gives a great increase in low contrast detectability. This permits excellent visualization of extracranial vessels following an i.v. injection of contrast medium. Excellent images are also produced in cerebral arteriography with small amounts of contrast medium of much lower concentration than is required in conventional techniques. Its use is invaluable during the conduct of interventional procedures.

Air encephalography and ventriculography

The ventricular system was first studied by contrast radiography in 1918 when Dandy introduced air into the lateral ventricles by either a fontanelle puncture or a burr hole. It was quickly appreciated that the method was of value in studying cases of hydrocephalus and in the localization of tumours. In the following year, Dandy outlined the cerebrospinal fluid pathways by introducing air through a lumbar puncture. This approach allows the basal cisterns and ventricular system to be studied and is referred to as 'air encephalography'.

These techniques are now obsolete following the development of CT and MRI (see Whitehouse & Worthington, 1990).

Cisternography

Cisternography refers to the study of the basal cisterns with contrast medium in order to demonstrate small tumours in the cerebellopontine angle and suprasellar cisterns.

This brief account is given to illustrate the range of invasive techniques which were developed for this purpose. Within the past few years, they have all been rendered obsolete in those centres where high-quality MRI facilities are available since small basal tumours and their extension can be readily assessed by this totally non-invasive method.

Cerebellopontine angle cistern

It is widely accepted that CT with contrast enhancement becomes unreliable when tumours, such as acoustic neuromas, project less than 1 cm into the cerebellopontine angle. Introduction of contrast medium into the cerebellopontine angle cistern affords a method of detecting or excluding a very small tumour in the angle and internal auditory meatus. Myodil was the first contrast medium to be used for this purpose. An injection of 2–3 ml of Myodil is made by lumbar puncture and then screened into the cervical region with the patient prone. The patient's head is now rotated through 45° and, with the affected side down, the table is slowly tilted while the contrast medium is screened as it runs through the foramen magnum and then outlines the cerebellopontine angle cistern. Care must be taken to ensure that no contrast medium escapes through the tentorial hiatus, because it cannot be subsequently retrieved. AP and horizontal-beam lateral radiographs are then taken. After returning the oil to the cervical region, the procedure can be repeated to obtain comparative views of the other side.

CT following the intrathecal injection of non-ionic contrast medium to outline the basal cisterns is an alternative procedure.

Both methods were rendered obsolete by the introduction of CT-assisted gas cisternography (Sortland, 1979). For this, the patient lies on his or her side on the scanner table with the affected side uppermost and the shoulders elevated. In order to outline the angle cistern, 5–6 ml of air are injected by lumbar puncture. The patient may report a transient discomfort in the ear, which indicates successful filling. The patient is then moved into the scanner and sections are obtained at the level of the internal auditory meatus (Fig. 19.5). The opposite angle cistern can be studied by turning the patient prone and then on to his other side. High-resolution MRI studies of the cerebellopontine angle cistern can demonstrate the normal anatomy with remarkable clarity (Fig. 19.6) and permit the detection of small acoustic neuromas (Fig. 19.7).

Suprasellar cisterns

Investigation of pituitary and parapituitary lesions can be exacting because their clinical manifestations, including visual failure and endocrinological disturbances, may occur early when the lesion is small. Precise localization and a distinction between the different pathologies is required, so that the appropriate operative route or field size for irradiation can be chosen. It is also valuable to have follow-up studies to assess the results of treatment by radiotherapy or drugs on tumour size. After plain skull radiography, CT in the transverse axial plane is usually the next diagnostic method. Despite the high quality of CT images now available, difficulty can sometimes be experienced in assessing the precise extent of the extrasellar extension of a pituitary tumour and in diagnosing microadenomas. Air encephalography was sometimes used to confirm a suspected diagnosis of the empty sella syndrome and to determine the relationship of any mass to the optic chiasma.

An alternative technique was to opacify the suprasellar cisterns with non-ionic contrast medium and carry out CT in the transverse, axial and coronal planes (Fig. 19.8). Several authors pointed out the advantages of screening the contrast medium into the basal cisterns and taking plain radiographs supplemented by CT to show the anatomy in the sagittal plane. The contrast medium (12 ml of iopamidol 240 or iohexol 250 mg iodine ml^{-1}) is injected by lumbar

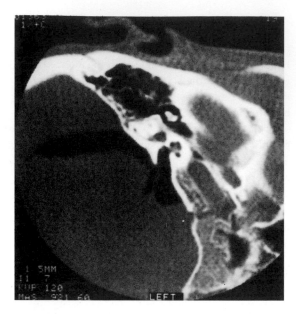

Fig. 19.5 Normal computed tomography-assisted air cisternogram.

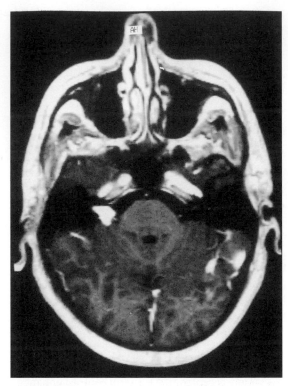

Fig. 19.7 High-resolution magnetic resonance study showing a small acoustic neuroma.

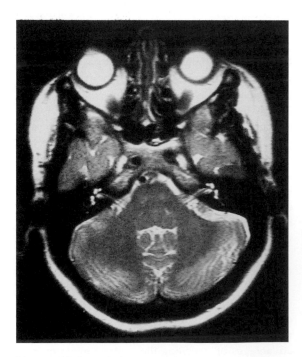

Fig. 19.6 High-resolution magnetic resonance study of the normal cerebellopontine angle cisterns.

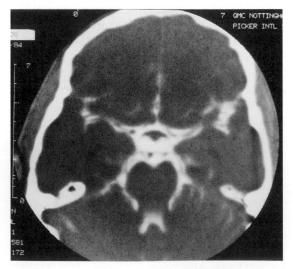

Fig. 19.8 Transverse axial computed tomography scan after intrathecal injection of water-soluble contrast medium showing normal suprasellar anatomy.

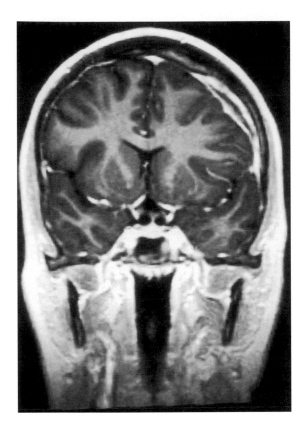

Fig. 19.9 Coronal magnetic resonance scan of the pituitary region showing normal suprasellar anatomy.

puncture and screened into the suprasellar cisterns using a lateral image intensifier. MRI now allows the anatomy of the pituitary fossa and adjacent structures to be demonstrated directly (Fig. 19.9) and is the method of choice for the investigation of suspected pituitary or parapituitary pathology.

References

Dandy, W.E. (1918) Ventriculography following the injection of air into the cerebral ventricles. *Ann. Surg.*, **68**, 5.

Dumoulin, C.L. & Hart, H.J. (1986) Magnetic resonance angiography. *Radiology*, **161**, 717–20.

Hawkes, R.C., Holland, G. N., Moore, W. S. & Worthington, B. S. (1980) NMR tomography of the brain: a preliminary clinical assessment with demonstration of pathology. *J. Comp. Assist. Tomog.*, **4**, 577.

Hugh, E.A. (1970) Trickle arteriography: demonstration of thrombi in the origin of internal carotid artery. *Br. Med. J.*, **2**, 574.

Mani, R.L. & Eisenberg, R.L. (1978) Complications of catheter cerebral angiography. *AJR*, **131**, 867.

Moniz, E. (1927) Arterial encephalography: its importance in the location of cerebral tumours. *Rev. Neurol.*, **48**, 72.

Sheldon, P. (1956) A special needle for percutaneous vertebral angiography. *Br. J. Radiol.*, 29, 231.

Sortland, O. (1979) Computer tomography combined with gas cisternography for the diagnosis of expanding lesions in the cerebellopontine angle. *Neuroradiology*, **18**, 19.

Whitehouse, G.H. & Worthington, B.S. (1990) *Techniques in Diagnostic Imaging.* Blackwell Scientific Publications, Oxford.

Ziedes de plantes, B.G. (1961) *Subtraction.* Thieme, Stuttgart.

Further reading

Anderson, C.M., Edelman, R.R. & Turski, P.A. (1993) *Clinical Magnetic Resonance Angiography.* Raven Press, New York.

Chakenes, D.W., Curtis, A. & Ford, J. (1989) Magnetic resonance imaging of pituitary and parasellar abnormalities. *Radiol. Clin. N. Am.*, **27**, 265.

Mawhinney, R., Buckley, J.H.B. & Worthington, B. S. (1986) Magnetic resonance imaging of the cerebellopontine angle. *Br. J. Radiol.*, **59**, 961.

Newton, R.H. & Potts, D.G. (eds) (1977) *Radiology of the Skull and Brain*, vol. 2, book I. *Angiography Technical Aspects*, vol. 4. *Ventricles and Cisterns.* Mosby, St Louis.

Press, G.A. & Hesselink, J.R. (1988) MR imaging of cerebellopontine angle and internal auditory canal lesions at 1.5T *Am. J. Neuroradiol.*, **9**, 241–51.

20   Orbit

G. A. S. LLOYD

Most authorities still use plain sinus radiographs to initiate the investigation of the paranasal sinuses. Since the cause of unilateral proptosis originates in the paranasal sinuses or nasopharynx in 15–20% of patients (Lloyd, 1970), plain sinus radiographs remain a useful preliminary to computed tomography (CT) or magnetic resonance imaging (MRI) in patients presenting with this sign. The cause of proptosis originating in the sinuses can almost always be identified and the type of pathology is often diagnosed. The preliminary radiographs should therefore be orientated to the sinuses and will include (i) an occipitomental projection; (ii) an occipitofrontal projection; and (iii) a lateral view. In addition an undertilted or 35° occipitomental view may be required in patients with mid-facial trauma and a suspected blow-out fracture.

Computed tomography

For the investigation of the orbit, routine axial sections should be augmented by direct scans in the coronal plane. Reformats should be reserved for sagittal or oblique imaging, or for those patients whose dental fillings make direct coronal sections difficult.

When axial scans are made, it is important that the position of the patient's head gives the optimum scanning plane through the orbit. Satisfactory axial scans should include the globes and show the lens, optic nerve and lateral and medial rectus muscles on the same section. To do this, the position of the head should be adjusted so that the scanning plane forms an angle of 16–18° caudally from the orbitomeatal line. Optimal orbital scans will be obtained if the posterior clinoids are shown on sections which also include the optic nerves and clearly show the globes on both sides. For coronal scans, the patient lies prone with elevation of the chin and suitable gantry angulation. Alternatively, a similar

scanning plane can be obtained by placing the patient supine with hyperextension of the head.

The injection of i.v. contrast medium for orbital CT should not be a routine procedure. Post-contrast scans to show tissue enhancement are to be avoided if possible, since the injection of contrast medium converts a totally non-invasive procedure into one which carries a similar morbidity and mortality to i.v. urography. In general contrast medium should only be administered to show up doubtful space-occupying lesions in better detail or when there is a suspicion of intracranial involvement. If a clearly defined lesion is shown on the unenhanced scans, the administration of contrast medium is usually unnecessary.

Magnetic resonance imaging

The role of MRI in orbital diagnosis is currently directed more towards tissue recognition than the identification of structural abnormality and mass lesions, which can readily be demonstrated by CT. However, MRI surpasses CT in its multiplanar capabilities, improved soft-tissue contrast and absence of ionizing radiation. It also has clear advantages over CT in the diagnosis of vascular and haemorrhagic lesions and in the demonstration of periorbital and orbital apex pathology.

The same scanning plane requirements pertain for MRI studies of the orbit as for CT. For the globe and more anterior structures in the orbit the best scans are obtained by use of a surface coil, but the depth limit of orbital surface coils is generally the apex of the orbit. A head coil gives a uniform signal from the entire imaging volume and is especially preferred when the orbital apex or retro-orbital structures are involved.

Gadolinium enhancement is frequently helpful in the demonstration of orbital pathology. However, gadolinium sometimes enhances the lesion to the same intensity as that of the orbital fat, thereby rendering it less conspicuous. Techniques have therefore been developed to suppress the fat signal. These include short tau inversion recovery (STIR) sequences, chemical shift techniques (Dixon, 1984) and a variation of frequency encoding gradients (Gomori, 1988). The simplest method is to use gadolinium MRI subtraction (Lloyd & Barker, 1991). The low vascularity of adipose tissue ensures almost total subtraction of the fat signal so that the extent of tumour within the orbit is optimally shown (Fig. 20.1).

Carotid angiography

The introduction of CT and MRI has rendered carotid angiography unnecessary as a routine investigation of unilateral exopthalmos. Both the intracranial and intraorbital causes of proptosis are readily demonstrated by these soft-tissue imaging techniques. Carotid angiography is only needed in selected patients, principally those with suspected vascular anomalies in either the orbit or the middle fossa, for example an infraclinoid aneurysm or arte-riovenous malformation. Arteriography may also be required preoperatively to identify the feeding vessels of a highly vascular tumour or prior to embolization.

For orbital angiography, modification of the normal technique of carotid angiography is required. Three projections are normally used for the angiogram series. These are all magnified geometrically using a an X-ray tube with a 0.3 mm focal spot.
1 A standard lateral arteriogram series and a series of lateral macroangiograms coned to the orbit.
2 An anteroposterior (AP) series. The projection is modified from that normally used in carotid angiography in that the orbitomeatal line is angled cranially 10° with the central ray at right angles to the film. This projects the ophthalmic artery through the orbit, at the same time giving adequate visualization of the internal carotid and the anterior and middle cerebral vessels.
3 A modified axial view. This provides a plan view of the ophthalmic artery and its main branches. In this projection the head and neck are extended and the tube angled cranially to make an angle of 75° to the orbitomeatal line, while the central ray is directed

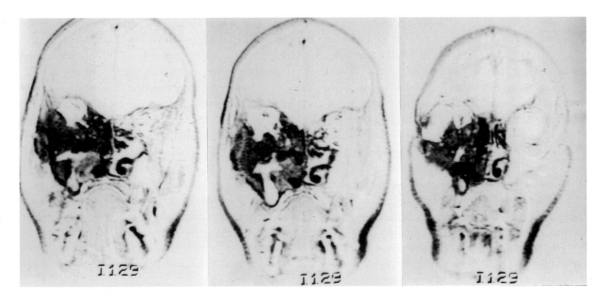

Fig. 20.1 Three subtraction coronal magnetic resonance sections showing invasion of the orbit by a squamous cell carcinoma. The low vascularity of the orbital fat gives minimal enhancement after i.v. gadolinium and is therefore removed from the final image. The exact extent of tumour invasion is shown without the obscuring fat signal present on the unsubtracted scans.

through the roof of the mouth. The position could be described as a reversed overtilted occipitomental view. Selective internal carotid injection of contrast medium is essential for a good angiogram series in this position, since filling of the external carotid circulation obscures the orbital vessels. Subtraction films should be routine.

Dacryocystography

Dacryocystography was originally described by Ewing (1909), who used bismuth subnitrate as contrast medium to outline a lacrimal sac abscess cavity. The conventional technique, derived from this method, consists of cannulation of the inferior or superior canaliculus and injection of contrast medium into the duct system. PA and lateral radiographs are taken after removal of the cannula. Campbell (1964), using this method of injection, introduced a radiographic enlargement technique and showed the advantages of the enhanced detail provided by macrodacryocystography. Iba and Hanafee (1968) described a method of distension dacryocystography, drawing attention to the advantages of making the radiographic exposure during the injection of contrast medium. The technique to be described is a combination of these two methods and, when combined with subtraction studies, is the optimum way of radiographically demonstrating the lacrimal duct system. The greater detail of the canalicular system shown by this method is of critical importance in deciding the surgical approach to abnormalities of the common canaliculus. Geometrical enlargement of the radiograph is obtained by using an X-ray tube with a 0.3 mm focal spot.

Usually two macrograms are obtained and a control exposure made prior to injection for subtraction studies, which allow bone-free visualization of the ducts. The exposure is made during the injection of the contrast medium through the catheter. Filling of the ducts is then optimal and in most instances provides an image of the contrast medium in continuity throughout the duct system. Before catheterization of the inferior canaliculus, a drop of amethocaine is instilled into the conjunctival sac and any mucus in the duct system is expressed by pressure over the inner canthus. A non-viscous contrast medium is used to allow a brisk injection through the small-bore

catheter. A dose of 2 ml of Lipiodol Ultrafluid is drawn up into a syringe which is then connected to a 30 cm i.v. catheter (outside diameter 0.63 mm) and any air bubbles are expressed. The punctum is dilated with a Nettleship dilator and the tip of the catheter is then introduced into the canaliculus. This manoeuvre is greatly facilitated if the punctum is drawn laterally and the tip of the catheter rotated between the finger and thumb during its introduction. It is essential not to advance the catheter more than 3–4 mm into the canaliculus. The catheter is held in place by sticking plaster applied to the cheek at the outer canthus. Slight pressure is applied to the loop of the catheter so that it is under tension and thereby held in place during the injection (Fig. 20.2). The lower canaliculus is usually chosen as it is the more convenient and functionally the more important. The upper canaliculus is normally outlined by reflux of contrast medium but, in special circumstances, may be catheterized and injected either individually or simultaneously.

The narrow lumen of the catheter and the viscosity of the contrast medium allow only a small positive pressure to be created, even if considerable force is applied to the syringe. In order that sufficient contrast medium circulates in the system, an interval of 3 s is allowed after starting the injection and before exposing the radiographs. The macrograms are exposed in the AP position during injection of the contrast medium. A lead–rubber screen is therefore needed to protect the operator from scattered radiation.

It is usual practice to perform simultaneously bilateral intubation macrodacryocystograms (Fig. 20.3), because of the high incidence of bilateral abnormalities (Fig. 20.4) and the useful information that can be obtained by comparison with the normal macrogram. It is wise to take a subsequent upright lateral radiograph, in order to ensure that the contrast medium has had an opportunity to reach the nasopharynx, thus confirming the patency of the system. In summary the method employs the following.

1 Intubation to produce distension of the duct system and better contrast filling, particularly of the common canaliculus.

2 Macroradiography to produce better radiographic definition.

3 Subtraction to produce bone-free visualization of the ducts, particularly the common canaliculus.

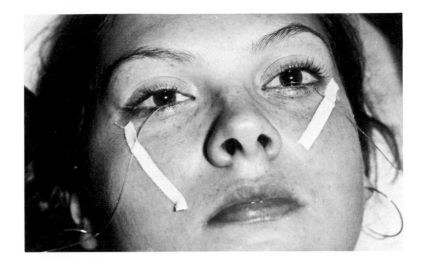

Fig. 20.2 Method of securing the catheters for intubation macrodacryocystography. Both inferior canaliculi are intubated and the catheters are kept under slight tension by fixing them to the cheek with sticking plaster.

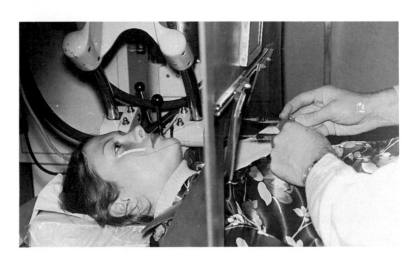

Fig. 20.3 Bilateral intubation dacryocystography is performed routinely because of the high incidence of bilateral abnormalities.

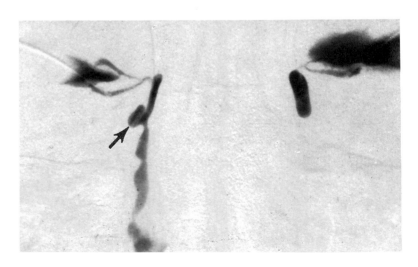

Fig. 20.4 Subtraction macrodacryocystogram showing a lacrimal sac diverticulum (arrow) and a lacrimal sac mucocoele on the left side due to duct obstruction.

Orbital venography

This technique is no longer in general use for the demonstration of orbital disease, and is now only of historic interest.

References

Campbell, W. (1964) The radiology of the lacrimal system. *Br. J. Radiol.*, **37**, 1–26.

Dixon, W.T. (1984) Simple proton spectroscopic imaging. *Radiology*, **153**, 189–94.

Ewing, A.E. (1909) Roentgen ray demonstration of the lacrymal abscess cavity. *Am. J. Ophthalmol.*, **26**, 1–4.

Gomori, J.M., Holland, G.A., Grossman, R.I., Gefter, W.B. & Lenkinski, R.E. (1988) Fat suppression by section select gradient reversal on spin echo MR imaging. *Radiology*, **168**, 493–5.

Iba, G.A. & Hanafee, W.N. (1968) Distension dacryocystography. *Radiology*, **90**, 1020–2.

Lloyd, G.A.S. (1970) The radiological investigation of proptosis. *Br. J. Radiol.*, **43**, 1–18.

Lloyd, G.A.S. & Barker, P. (1991) Subtraction magnetic resonance for tumours of the skull base and paranasal sinuses. *J. Laryngol. Otol.*, **105**, 628–32.

21   Spinal Canal

R. G. GRAINGER

In the 1970s and 1980s, oil myelography with iophendylate was completely replaced by water-soluble myelography, providing greatly improved anatomical detail and greatly reducing the major complication of chronic adhesive arachnoiditis. In the 1990s, water-soluble myelography is being rapidly replaced by magnetic resonance imaging (MRI) (an out-patient procedure, no lumbar puncture, usually no contrast medium, improved visualization in any desired anatomical plane) and to a lesser extent by computed tomography (CT), which may require intrathecal contrast injection. Within the next few years, myelography will be performed only on rare occasions (e.g. a very tortuous spine, need for erect radiographs, the presence of ferromagnetic implants or cardiac pacemakers) in the well-equipped imaging department.

Indications for myelography

The indications for myelography depend on the availability of alternate imaging facilities, especially MRI. The preceding paragraph suggests the indications for myelography when MRI is available.

There must be firm clinical indications for myelography (or radiculography), a technique which is always uncomfortable for the patient and may be followed by considerable headache. The essential consideration is that there is the definite prospect that the examination will affect the subsequent management of the patient. Myelography is virtually a procedure for preoperative assessment and will rarely be indicated if there is no possibility of surgical intervention.

The most frequent indication for lumbar myelography/radiculography is the lumbago–sciatica syndrome with suspected nerve root compression by a degenerated and prolapsed intervertebral disc. The most frequent indication for cervical myelography is the diagnosis and preoperative assessment of degenerative cervical spondylosis.

Any suspected space-occupying or other potentially operable lesions of the spinal cord, its nerve roots, meninges or the adjacent spinal canal usually merits imaging, preferably MRI but if necessary by myelography.

Contraindications for myelography

Skin sepsis over the spinal puncture site and infection of the subarachnoid space or meninges are absolute contraindications. A previous severe reaction to an intravascular injection of contrast medium is a relative contraindication to water-soluble contrast myelography, particularly of the cervical spine. If the procedure is performed, 24-hour corticosteroid prophylaxis is a strong recommendation.

In patients with a history of epilepsy, antiepileptic drugs, such as diazepam 5 mg or phenobarbitone 120 mg, should precede the myelogram and be repeated as necessary.

Myelography should preferably be deferred if there has been a lumbar puncture in the preceding 7 days, as the contrast medium may well be injected into an extradural pool of cerebrospinal fluid (CSF).

Lumbar myelography and lumbosacral radiculography (Grainger, 1975, 1979, 1981)

Contrast medium

The ideal pharmacological and technical criteria for a water-soluble myelographic agent are presented in Table 21.1. Current myelographic contrast agents are second and third generation, non-ionic, fully substituted amide derivatives of tri-iodinated benzoic acids. Ionic media, either high or low osmolar, *must*

Table 21.1 Ideal contrast medium for myelography

Pharmacology	Technical requirements
Water-soluble, miscible with CSF	Optimum radio-opacity
Iso-osmolar with CSF	Optimum viscosity
Non-ionic	Water-soluble
Highly hydrophilic	Easy delivery
Minimal brain penetrance	Acceptable price
Minimal neurotoxicity	
Minimal meningeal toxicity	
Rapid excretion from body	

Aqueous contrast medium for myelography
Iohexol (Omnipaque), Nycomed (Oslo)
Iopamidol (Niopam), Bracco (Milan)
Iotrolan (Isovist), Schering (Berlin)

never be injected into the subarachnoid space, where they may be fatal. The amount of the agents used for lumbar myelography is 2000–3000 mg of iodine, which can be injected either as 10–15 ml of the 200 mg iodine ml^{-1} strength, or 7–10 ml of the 300 mg ml^{-1} concentration. There is very little to choose between iohexol and iopamidol.

In 1987 and 1988 a new non-ionic dimer myelographic agent, iotrolan (Isovist) was introduced in some European countries. Iotrolan has six atoms of iodine attached to two benzene rings, linked in a dimeric formulation. It is an extremely hydrophilic and water-soluble non-ionic dimer, has a very high LD$_{50}$, is excreted rapidly by renal glomerular filtration, and has an osmolality of about 50% that of iohexol and iopamidol. It is iso-osmolar with CSF and plasma at 300 mg iodine ml^{-1}. Iotrolan has proved to be a very successful myelographic agent and probably causes less headache than all previous water-soluble agents (Hammer & Deisenhammer, 1985).

Premedication and patient preparation

A consent form must always be signed by the patient after the radiologist has explained the procedure, before any premedication has been given. An alert, cooperative and relaxed patient is a great asset. The patient should be well hydrated, but no food or drink is allowed for the previous 3 hours in order to reduce the possibility of vomiting. Dentures must be removed before the examination. No sedative premedication is usually necessary unless the patient

is very apprehensive, when 5 mg diazepam may be given orally or i.v.

Incompatible drugs

Drugs which reduce the epileptogenic threshold, such as phenothiazines (Hindmarsh *et al.*, 1975), may be excluded for the preceding 2 days and 2 days following the procedure. However, there is some doubt as to the importance of this drug incompatibility.

Needle

A presterilized disposable thin-walled, short-bevel, small-gauge, 22 standard wire gauge needle 9 cm long is recommended. A long-pointed bevel increases the chance of extra-arachnoid injection. Some radiologists are now using very small-calibre needles (size 24 or 25 standard wire gauge) and claim a considerable reduction in CSF leak and headache, sometimes permitting the discharge home of the patient after 6 hours of hospital observation (Harrison, 1993).

Puncture site

Lumbar puncture is recommended at the L3/L4 intervertebral space, the iliac crest usually being at the level of the L4 vertebra. Conventional frontal and lateral radiographs of the lumbosacral spine must be examined before the lumbar puncture and the puncture approach may be modified accordingly.

Local anaesthesia

Local anaesthetic is not generally recommended as its introduction is probably more painful than the skilful insertion of a 22 standard wire gauge lumbar-puncture needle. If the patient is very apprehensive, if there is difficulty in achieving a satisfactory puncture or should a larger needle be used, then 1% lignocaine can be injected to infiltrate the skin, subcutaneous tissues and distal portion of the chosen interspinous ligament.

Lumbar puncture

The procedure must be performed with strict asepsis. The radiologist must surgically scrub his or her hands, wear sterile rubber gloves with all powder removed, and use a no-touch technique.

The skin of the patient over the mid-line lumbar region is shaved as necessary and sterilized with a suitable skin antiseptic, for instance 0.05% chlorhexidine in alcohol. All excess sterilizing agent must be removed by swab.

The patient sits upright on the horizontal X-ray table with spine erect and without rotation or lateral tilt of the shoulders or iliac crests, which should be horizontal. The patient's legs hang over the side of the table and the feet rest on a chair. Immediately before the lumbar puncture, the patient is asked to flex the lumbar spine, holding a pillow into the abdomen in order to reduce the normal lumbar lordosis and to open up the lumbar interspinous spaces. It is important that the lumbar spine remains vertical when the patient curves round the pillow. A frequent error is for the patient to lean markedly forwards over the pillow instead of remaining with the lumbar spine vertical.

An alternative position for lumbar puncture is for the patient to lie in the lateral decubitus position with the spine parallel to the long axis of the horizontal X-ray table top, coronal plane perpendicular to the table top and the knees fully flexed towards the chest to induce a lumbar kyphosis. It is important for the lumbar spine to remain parallel to the long side of the X-ray table, and the coronal plane perpendicular to the table. This position permits fluoroscopy during the injection and is facilitated if the table is tilted 15° foot-down to collect the contrast in the dependent lumbosacral cul-de-sac.

The erect sitting posture is preferred for lumbar puncture because it is usually more comfortable for the patient, distends the lumbar subarachnoid space and reduces the likelihood of extra-arachnoid injection.

The lumbar puncture is made in the conventional way, preferably with the needle bevel facing laterally. CSF must flow freely, even when the needle has been rotated to vary the direction of the bevel. Five millilitres of CSF are collected for cell and protein measurement. If the needle does not enter the subarachnoid space at first attempt, it is withdrawn a little and the hub is angled towards the feet a few degrees and then advanced to puncture the dura. If this manoeuvre fails, then the next cephalad or caudal interspace may be used for the lumbar puncture. If there is any doubt that a clean lumbar puncture has been achieved, the patient should be assisted to lie down in the lateral decubitus position and the X-ray table is tilted 15° foot-down. A few drops of contrast medium are injected via a short connecting tube and will be seen on fluoroscopy to drop through the CSF into its most dependent part if the needle has been correctly placed into the subarachnoid space.

Injection of contrast medium

Fluoroscopy is not essential during the injection of contrast agent unless there is uncertainty about the adequacy of the lumbar puncture. The contrast medium is contained in a 10 ml disposable sterile syringe, which is connected to the inserted lumbar-puncture needle either directly or by a short length of sterile plastic connecting tube. The contrast medium is injected smoothly over 30–60 s. Rapid squirts of contrast agent cause turbulence in the CSF with undesirable mixing and dilution of the contrast medium. Having completed the injection, the lumbar-puncture needle is withdrawn and the skin puncture is sealed with a sterile dressing or plastic skin.

Patient movement

Jerky or rapid patient movements must be avoided throughout the procedure, so as not to disperse and dilute the injected aqueous contrast medium with CSF.

The X-ray table is tilted 20° foot-down and the patient is gently assisted to change posture from the sitting position into the prone position, always maintaining the patient's sacrum below the level of the upper lumbar spine.

X-ray table tilt

Table movement must be smooth as jerky or rapid movements disperse the contrast medium. For water-soluble myelography of any region, a head-down tilt of more than 25–30° is rarely required (Fig. 21.1).

Fluoroscopy

Fluoroscopy with an image intensifier on the frontal

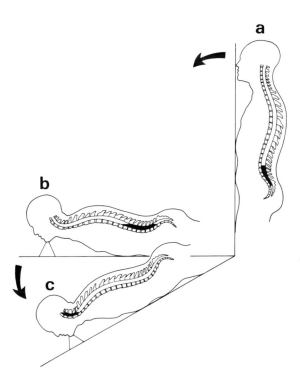

Fig. 21.1 (a) Patient erect. Contrast medium occupies lumbosacral subarachnoid cul-de-sac. (b) Patient tilted horizontal. Head and neck extended. Contrast medium in upper and mid-lumbar region prevented from entering the dorsal region by the lumbar lordosis and the dorsal kyphosis. (c) Patient tilted 20–30° head-down. Head and neck well extended, exaggerating cervical lordosis in which contrast medium collects.

tube is necessary to control the movement of the contrast medium. Lateral fluoroscopy with a horizontal tube is not necessary for lumbar or dorsal water-soluble myelography. For cervical myelography, even with a water-soluble contrast medium, lateral fluoroscopy is of considerable assistance and, some would say, essential.

Radiography

Radiography must be commenced within a few minutes of the injection as the contrast agent becomes progressively less dense due to dilution, dispersion and absorption. A low kilovoltage (70–75 kV) is advised for the frontal and oblique projections with a high milliampere and a fast film-screen combination to obtain a short exposure time and thus reduce movement blur. All exposures must be taken with either a static or a moving absorption grid and with a very well collimated X-ray beam.

Radiographic quality is considerably improved if the patient is examined with a long focus–film distance, as with an overcouch tube and an under-table image intensifier with remote fluoroscopic control.

Radiographic projections

The first radiographs are taken with the patient prone and the foot end of the table tilted 45° down. The prone oblique radiographs are taken with the patient rotating in his or her own long axis, the entire right side and then the entire left side of the patient being rotated in turn, about 15–25°, in order to align the uppermost lumbosacral nerve roots parallel to the table top (Figs 21.2 & 21.3). All these radiographs are taken under fluoroscopic control, using the frontal X-ray tube. Several radiographs with different degrees of obliquity may be necessary to show optimum detail of all the lumbosacral nerve roots and their sleeves.

A lateral view of the lower lumbar spine and lumbosacral junction is then taken in either of two ways:
1 The patient turns slowly into the lateral decubitus; the X-ray table is still tilted 45° foot-down. A true lateral radiograph is then taken under fluoroscopic control using the frontal tube (Fig. 21.4b).
2 The table is still tilted 45° foot-down. The patient lies prone and a shoot-through horizontal beam lateral film may be obtained (Fig. 21.4a) by using a

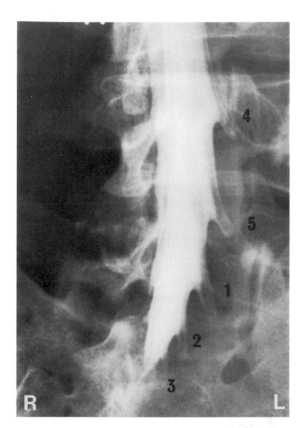

Fig. 21.2 Normal prone oblique lumbosacral water-soluble myelogram. Patient prone and rotated 20° with left side elevated. Overcouch X-ray tube. Table tilted 45° foot-down. The left lumbosacral nerve roots are enumerated (lumbar 4, 5; sacral 1, 2, 3).

second (lateral) X-ray tube or a C-arm tube shooting horizontally.

Having checked the radiographs of the lower lumbar and lumbosacral region, the X-ray table is then tilted into the horizontal with the patient still prone. This tilt of the table moves the bolus of contrast medium into the mid- and upper lumbar spine; frontal, oblique and lateral radiographs of this region are then obtained as previously described. To show the lower dorsal subarachnoid space, a head-down tilt of about 5–10° under fluoroscopic control is usually necessary and further frontal, oblique and lateral radiographs are then taken.

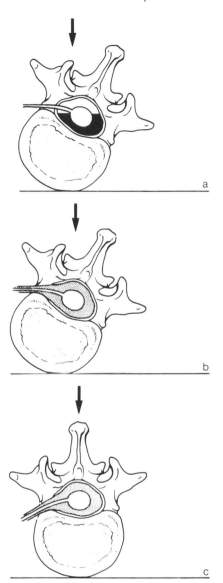

Fig. 21.3 Oblique projections to show emerging spinal nerve roots and their subarachnoid sleeves. (a) Patient rotated 20–30°. Using an *oily medium*, the nerve root sleeve parallel to the table top (the uppermost nerve root) *may not* be exposed to the contrast medium. (b) Patient rotated 20–30°. Using a *water-soluble medium*, the nerve root parallel to the table top *is* well exposed to the contrast medium and, being parallel to the film, is ideally projected. (c) With patient prone, a vertical X-ray beam will foreshorten the projection of the nerve roots and their sleeves.

Accessory radiographic projections

Lateral decubitus projections

These may be obtained with a horizontal ray from a second (lateral) X-ray tube (or a C-arm), a well-collimated beam and a stationary grid cassette. The patient is in the lateral decubitus and the water-soluable contrast medium, being heavier than CSF, concentrates on the dependent side of the subarachnoid space. This technique is therefore most appropriate when the contrast medium has been injected with the patient in the lateral decubitus position and the suspected disease side dependent.

With the patient's back towards the lateral X-ray tube and the patient's abdomen adjacent to the cassette, rotation of the patient 15° upper side towards the cassette and away from the X-ray tube, will project the *dependent nerve roots* parallel to the film (Fig. 21.5). After the diagnostic quality of the first lateral decubitus radiograph has been checked, the patient may be gently rotated through 150° about his long axis into the opposite oblique lateral decubitus and a further lateral film is taken of the lumbosacral nerve roots, which were previously uppermost but are now dependent.

As the lower lumbosacral nerve roots are usually under suspicion, the X-ray table should be tilted 15–30° foot-down for the above lateral decubitus views.

Tomography

Tomography is occasionally a useful accessory technique and is best performed on a remote-control table with an overcouch fluoroscopic tube and tomographic facilities.

Erect lateral radiographs

The table is brought gently into the vertical position and the patient is turned so that his or her coronal plane is perpendicular to the table top. Lateral exposures are made under fluoroscopic control, using the frontal tube with the patient stooping in flexion and then in full extension.

Dorsal myelography

Dorsal water-soluble myelography is a simple extension of lumbosacral myelography. The lumbosacral films are taken first. The patient is turned into the lateral decubitus position with the X-ray table horizontal. The X-ray table is then tilted very slowly head-down in 5° increments under fluoroscopic control.

The bolus of contrast medium may take a few seconds to begin to move. Once movement has started, the contrast medium moves very quickly towards the cervical region. In order to prevent the contrast medium entering the skull, the neck of the patient should be flexed *laterally* on a high pillow towards the uppermost shoulder, raising the head from the table (Fig. 21.6)

A head-down tilt of 10–15° is usually sufficient to move the contrast medium into the middle and lower dorsal regions. A deep inspiration lowers the diaphragm

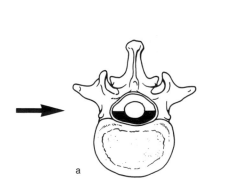
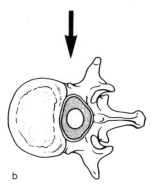

a   b

Fig. 21.4 Lateral projections during lumbar myelography. (a) Using an oily medium, the patient *must* be prone, using the lateral X-ray tube with horizontal ray. (b) Using a water-soluble medium, the lateral radiograph may be taken with a vertical ray with patient in lateral decubitus without need of a lateral X-ray tube. Alternatively position (a) may also be used. The first method is simpler and quicker and does not require a second X-ray tube.

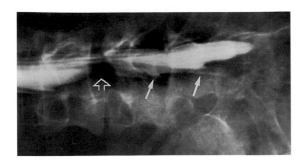

Fig. 21.5 Water-soluble myelogram. Lateral oblique decubitus position to show the dependent lumbar nerve roots. Patient's back to the X-ray tube, abdomen adjacent to the cassette, patient's upper side rotated 15° towards the cassette and away from the tube. Table tilted 30° foot-down. Horizontal-ray lateral X-ray beam. Large lateral disc prolapse (open arrow) at L4/L5 causing marked medial displacement, compression and oedema of the right L5 and S1 nerve roots (white arrows).

as the contrast medium moves cephalad and gives a much improved view. A low kilovoltage lateral radiograph is exposed from the frontal tube under fluoroscopic control with the patient in lateral decubitus. The patient is then turned slowly on his or her back, the table still being tilted 10–15° head-down with the head and neck raised off the table on the high pillow. This manoeuvre pools the bolus of contrast medium in the dorsal kyphosis and a frontal radiograph is taken on the explorator with the patient supine. The right and left film markers on the explorator need to be reversed, as the original frontal radiographs of the lumbar spine were taken with the patient prone. The above radiographs demonstrate the dorsal subarachnoid space from D5 to D12 (Fig. 21.7).

To visualize the upper dorsal subarachnoid space, the tilt of the table is increased in 5° increments head-down with the patient supine until the contrast medium reaches the upper dorsal spine. A frontal (supine) radiograph is then taken. The head of the patient must be well elevated from the table by a high pillow in order to prevent the contrast medium entering the skull. The patient is then turned slowly into an oblique lateral position and an off-lateral view is obtained of the upper dorsal spine.

Cervical myelography

Water-soluble cervical myelography should only be attempted after the radiologist has become confident in the ability to control the bolus of contrast medium during lumbosacral and dorsal myelography, or has become expert in direct cervical puncture.

Both lumbar injection and direct cervical injection have their advantages and disadvantages (Teasdale & Macpherson, 1984; Belanger *et al.*, 1990) and expertise should be developed in both methods. Both techniques are much facilitated by an X-ray tube capable of producing a horizontal beam shooting across the table top. The availability of lateral tube fluoroscopy, as on a C- or U-arm assembly, is strongly recommended.

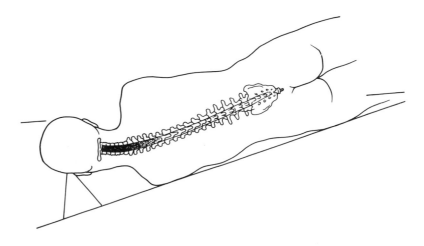

Fig. 21.6 Lateral decubitus position, head well raised on pad to create lateral curvature of the cervical spine region in which the contrast medium collects.

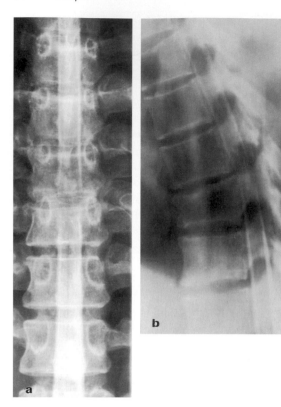

Fig. 21.7 Dorsal water-soluble myelogram. Patient horizontal and supine. Overcouch tube.
(a) Anteroposterior view. (b) Lateral view (tomogram): patient in lateral decubitus, vertical X-ray beam. Demonstrating recent fracture of dorsal vertebra with swollen damaged spinal cord. Permanent paraplegia.

Cervical myelography following lumbar injection

Contrast medium

It is important to inject contrast medium at a fairly high concentration when the cervical region is being examined following lumbar administration. Water-soluble medium (10 ml at 250–300 mg iodine ml^{-1} concentration) is advisable.

Premedication

Some radiologists prefer to give an anti-epileptic drug such as phenobarbitone sodium 120 mg or diazepam 5 mg either orally or by i.v. injection be-

fore the myelogram, particularly if the patient has an epileptic history.

Patient movement and table tilt

It is always difficult and sometimes impossible to produce diagnostic lumbar, dorsal and cervical myelographic radiographs from a single injection of aqueous contrast medium. If the cervical region is the only area of clinical interest, the contrast medium should be taken up to the cervical spine immediately after its injection.

Lateral decubitus tilt

Immediately after the lumbar puncture has been performed with the patient sitting upright on the horizontal X-ray table, the foot end of the table is tilted 30° down in order to keep the contrast bolus in the lumbosacral region. The patient is assisted in turning slowly into lateral decubitus. A thick pillow is placed under the head and neck in order to flex the head towards the uppermost side and to produce a curvature convexity downwards in the cervical spine, where the bolus of contrast medium will eventually be trapped (see Fig. 21.6).

The X-ray table is then tilted horizontal and the head end of the table is then tilted down in 5° increments with the patient in lateral decubitus. As soon as the bolus of medium begins to move, the radiologist should move the explorator, preferably using a horizontal X-ray tube, over the cervical region and fluoroscope the contrast medium which is slowly arriving and accumulating in the cervical concavity produced by the head pillow. The patient is still in lateral decubitus with head and neck strongly flexed *laterally* and raised off the table (see Fig. 21.6). Usually 15–20° of head-down tilt is adequate but, if the patient begins to slip down the table, he or she should be supported by either a previously applied harness or by a nurse steadying the shoulders. Once the bolus of contrast medium has been collected in the cervical region, the table is gently returned to the horizontal plane, the patient still lying in lateral decubitus with the neck laterally flexed towards the uppermost shoulder.

The next movement is very important for, if it is clumsily performed, the bolus of contrast medium will be dispersed and some may enter the head or run down the spine. The radiologist leaves the explorator and holds the patient's head in both hands and the patient is assisted in rotating the head and body slowly and gently into the full prone position. The patient's neck is maintained in extension throughout the procedure and a triangular radiolucent pad is placed under the chin when the prone position has been gained (Fig. 21.8a). The contrast medium is now in the concavity of the extended cervical spine. During the entire manoeuvre the head and shoulders must not be allowed to rise above the patient's trunk, to prevent loss of contrast medium into the dorsal spine. The head must not be allowed to become lower than the neck to prevent loss of contrast medium into the head.

Radiographic projections

Having collected the bolus of contrast medium in the concavity of the extended cervical spine, the degree of extension is slowly reduced and a frontal radiograph is taken, with the patient prone and the X-ray table horizontal. The radiologist then slowly turns the patient's head, neck and shoulders into a 20–30° prone oblique position, the patient following this rotation with the body. The nerve roots on the elevated side are now now parallel to the explorator (see Fig. 21.3b) and a vertical ray exposure is made in order to demonstrate these nerve roots (Fig. 21.9). Having checked these radiographs, the radiologist holds the patient's head and neck and rotates them 40–60° into the opposite 20–30° prone oblique position and a further radiograph is taken to show the nerve roots on the previously dependent but now uppermost side.

Two projections in different degrees of obliquity (20–40°) may be necessary for each side. When the radiographs have been checked, the patient is slowly returned into the prone position.

It is essential that all of these movements are executed smoothly and gently as jerky movements disperse the water-soluble contrast medium, causing much dilution and loss of radio-opacity.

The lateral cervical radiograph is then taken by an X-ray tube shooting horizontally across the table with the patient prone and with the arms and shoulders pulled well down in order to visualize the lower

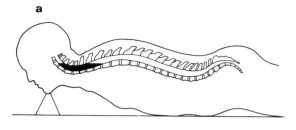

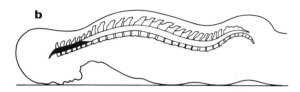

Fig. 21.8 (a) Patient returned from position in Fig. 21.1c into the horizontal position. Head and neck still well extended, maintaining contrast medium in the exaggerated cervical lordosis. Radiographs of the mid- and lower cervical spine can be taken in this position or with controlled reduction of cervical lordosis. (b) Pad removed from under patient's chin. Head and neck gradually flexed under lateral fluoroscopic control until contrast medium flows through foramen magnum to flow on to the clivus. This position is used for the frontal open-mouth occipitoatlantoaxial projection (using the frontal tube) and for the lateral cervical spine projection in flexion (using the lateral tube).

cervical spine (Fig. 21.10b). Lateral tube fluoroscopy is very helpful in coning down with the light beam diaphragm and in adjusting the degree of neck flexion accurately so that the contrast medium just reaches the foramen magnum. The C- or U-arm installation or a biplane image intensifier system is a great advantage.

Accessory projections

Extension and flexion lateral horizontal beam radiographs of the cervical spine are essential as some disc protrusions are only visible in extension. The extension radiograph is taken first, followed by the flexion radiograph.

Additional lateral radiographs with reduced neck extension and slight foot-down tilt may be required to image the lower cervical spine. A minor degree (5°) of head-down tilt of the table with fluoroscopy-

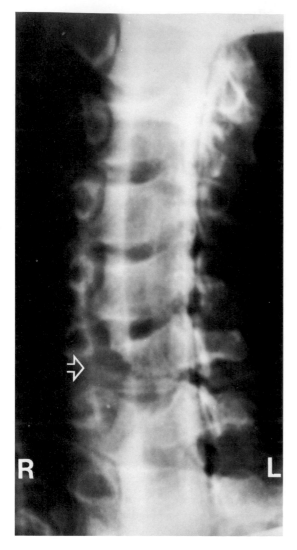

Fig. 21.9 Frontal oblique cervical water-soluble myelogram. Patient prone, right side raised 20°. Vertical X-ray beam. Demonstrates right cervical nerve roots. Large disc lesion C5/C6 right side (open arrow).

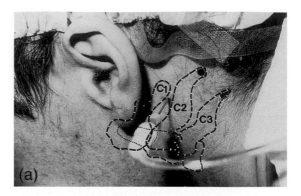

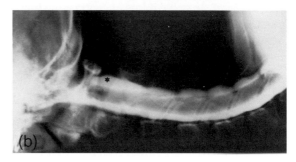

Fig. 21.10 (a) Showing ideal position of needle for lateral C1/C2 puncture with the vertebrae outlined. The head is on the left. (b) Normal cervical water-soluble myelogram. Lateral projection. Neck in slight extension, table horizontal, arms well pulled down, horizontal-ray lateral X-ray beam. Water-soluble contrast medium injected by C1/C2 lateral puncture at *. The head is on the right.

controlled flexion of the neck may be necessary to allow the contrast medium to reach the clivus, but care must be taken to prevent a large quantity floating into the head (see Fig. 21.8b). Immediately after the flexion radiograph has been taken, the neck is extended in order to retain the contrast medium in the concavity of the extended cervical spine.

Tomography. If the radiographic equipment includes a tomographic attachment on the lateral tube, mid-line lateral tomography with the patient prone is sometimes helpful as mid-line cervical disc lesions may be obscured on the conventional lateral films.

Open-mouth view of the occipitoatlantal axis region. If the conventional frontal view has not adequately demonstrated this area, a further frontal view may be obtained under fluoroscopic control with the patient prone, head gently flexed, mouth wide open and table horizontal.

Drop-arm view. In order to visualize the lower cervical and upper dorsal region in the lateral projection, the prone patient is assisted to move both arms so that they hang vertically downwards, displacing the shoulders in front of the cervicodorsal spine. In order to visualize the upper dorsal region, after cervical myelography, the myelographic table usually has to be tilted 10–15° foot-down.

Shoot-through lateral swimmer's view. This is an alternative method of obtaining a lateral projection of the lower cervical and upper dorsal spine. With the patient prone, one arm is carefully extended and stretched out parallel to the side of the head with the other arm pulled down towards the feet. The X-ray table is tilted 10–15° foot-down under fluoroscopic control to move the bolus of contrast medium down from the mid-cervical region. A 10° off-lateral radiograph is then taken with the horizontal ray lateral tube, using high kilovoltage to penetrate the upper dorsal region. A rice or water bath can be used as a filter adjacent to the neck to prevent overexposure of the cervical region.

Supine view. A supine view of the cervical spine may demonstrate better the posterior aspects of the cervical subarachnoid space and the region of the cerebellar tonsils. The patient is carefully assisted in rotating from the prone to the supine position around his or her longitudinal axis without raising the head or shoulders. A lateral view of the neck is then taken with a horizontal beam.

The myelographic examination of the cervical spine is now completed and the patient is assisted in sitting upright on the X-ray table in order to allow the contrast medium to run down into the lumbar region. The patient is then returned to the ward with the head and shoulders well propped up.

Prone position tilt

The bolus of contrast medium which has been injected into the lumbar region may be transported to the cervical area by tilting the patient head-down in the prone position (see Fig. 21.1). After the introduction of the contrast medium into the lumbar subarachnoid space, the table is tilted 30° foot-down with the patient prone in order to collect the contrast medium as a bolus in the lumbosacral region. The table is then slowly tilted head-down into the horizontal position with the patient prone and neck fully extended and supported in this position by a radiolucent triangular pad under the chin.

The table top is tilted from the horizontal in 5°head-down increments until the bolus begins to move towards the head. Once the bolus begins to move it usually moves quite quickly cephalad. Once the bolus is seen to begin to flow cephalad, the explorator, which is preferably on lateral fluoroscopy, is moved to the cervical region and the arrival and collection of the contrast medium bolus in the concavity of the extended cervical spine is awaited (see Fig. 21.1c). Usually 20–30° of tilt is adequate but more may be required if there is a prominent dorsal kyphosis, in which case the lateral decubitus technique is preferred. Once the complete bolus of contrast medium has been collected in the extended cervical region, the table is returned to the horizontal plane, the extension pad is carefully removed from the patient's chin and a lesser degree of cervical extension is maintained. Radiographs are now taken of the cervical region, exactly as described for the lateral decubitus tilt technique following lumbar injection.

Cervical water-soluble myelography by lateral C1/C2 puncture

This technique is not difficult to learn but must only be practised after the radiologist has observed an experienced operator. Lateral fluoroscopy with image intensification is essential. The technique is well described by Orrison *et al.* (1983). The objective is to insert a spinal needle at C1/C2 level, behind the cervical cord, and to inject water-soluble contrast medium directly into the cervical subarachnoid space (see Fig. 21.10).

Contrast medium

As little dilution will occur in the absence of transportation of the bolus, 6–10 ml of water-soluble contrast medium containing 200–250 mg iodine ml^{-1} is recommended.

Needle

A 20 or 22 standard wire gauge needle may be used. CSF may not drip freely through the narrower 22 gauge needle, despite a satisfactory puncture, and some radiologists prefer the 20 standard wire gauge needle. Frontal and lateral radiographs of the cervical spine must be examined before the puncture to assess any deformity or relevant disease.

Cervical spinal puncture

The patient lies prone on a thick (10 cm) radiolucent mattress on the horizontal X-ray table. The hair is shaved for a few square centimetres over and caudal to the mastoid process and any loose strands of hair are restrained by adhesive tape or a hair net. The patient's neck is gently extended with a triangular Polyfoam pad or Perspex angled support under the chin. The patient must be comfortable in this position and able to breathe easily.

The puncture site is determined by moving a metal pointer, such as the tip of another needle, just caudal to the tip of the mastoid processes so that, on lateral fluoroscopy (horizontal beam), it is projected over the interspace between C1 and C2 posterior neural arches just anterior to the bone cortex where the right and left laminae fuse. This landmark indicates the posterior boundary of the cervical subarachnoid space (see Fig. 21.10). The optimum site for puncture is usually 5–10 mm caudal and up to 5 mm anterior or posterior to the mastoid tip. This point for the puncture is marked with indelible ink (Fig. 21.10). The area around the entry point is surgically cleaned and local anaesthetic (1% lignocaine) is infiltrated into the skin, subcutaneous tissues and ligamentous tissues by a 4 cm needle. The 20 or 22 gauge spinal needle is then inserted, precisely directed parallel to the horizontal table top in the exact coronal plane of the patient, perpendicular to the long axis of the patient, pointing neither cephalad nor caudad. Intermittent lateral fluoroscopy is essential in order to maintain this exact line of approach and any necessary adjustments to the needle direction are made if the needle is not precisely in the desired line. It is most important that the needle is directed behind the spinal cord, just anterior to the posterior limit of the bony spinal canal. It is a great comfort for the patient, and a help for the operator, if a nurse, who is adequately shielded from the X-ray beam, is placed at the head of the table and uses a hand to steady the patient's head (the hand is kept well out of the X-ray beam by coning the light beam diaphragm to a very small field over the puncture site).

The dura is punctured at a depth of about 5 cm from the skin, but this varies considerably with the thickness of the neck. If the operator is concerned that the needle tip has passed beyond the mid-sagittal plane, a few seconds of frontal fluoroscopy will be very helpful. As the dura is punctured, the patient may feel a little discomfort and the radiologist also appreciates a change in resistance. The needle tip is then advanced 2 mm to clear the arachnoid, the stylet of the needle is removed and CSF should then drip slowly from the hub of the needle. The first few ml are collected for the laboratory and a sterile disposable syringe, previously loaded with 200–250 mg iodine ml^{-1} concentration water-soluble myelographic medium is connected by a short length of flexible tube to the needle. The first few drops of contrast medium are then injected under lateral fluoroscopic control and should descend through the CSF to lie against the posterior aspects of the mid-cervical vertebral bodies. Having confirmed the free entry of contrast medium into the subarachnoid space, a further 2–3 ml of contrast medium is injected under intermittent lateral fluoroscopy. Any obstructing lesion in the cervical subarachnoid space will now become evident and, if there is such an obstruction, no further contrast medium should be injected as it will probably spill into the skull.

In the absence of an obstructing lesion, a further 2–4 ml contrast medium, making a total of 6–8 ml, is injected with intermittent lateral fluoroscopic control until the entire cervical subarachnoid space is demonstrated on the fluoroscope. A slight tilt of the table top or modification of the degree of extension of the patient's neck may be necessary in order to encourage the contrast medium to outline the whole of the cervical subarachnoid space. The needle is left *in situ*, still connected by the plastic tube to the syringe. Radiography can now commence.

Radiographic projections

With the patient prone and the neck slightly extended, radiographs are exposed in the frontal, 20–30° right and left prone oblique and lateral projections as previously described (see Figs 21.9 and 21.10). All these radiographs are taken on one tube without moving the prone patient if a U- or C-arm tube is being used. Two lateral exposures, one at conventional and the other at higher penetration (kV), may be taken to visualize both the spinal cord and the subarachnoid space to best advantage. Having checked these radiographs, the needle is removed and the puncture wound is sealed by plastic skin or a sterile adhesive.

Accessory projections

Lateral radiographs of the cervical spine are taken in flexion and extension under fluoroscopic control with a horizontal ray from the laterally positioned X-ray tube. Further views, as previously described, are taken when necessary.

If the dorsal subarachnoid space is to be investigated, the patient is assisted to roll his or her body, maintained as rigid as a log, to reach the supine position without raising the shoulders. The nurse moves the undermost arm under the patient's chest and assists the patient in turning into the supine position, whilst the radiologist holds the patient's head and shoulders to prevent their elevation. It is important that the patient maintains the body in a rigid attitude during this rotation from prone to supine position and does not elevate the head, neck or shoulders.

The contrast medium will now be in the cervical region, patient supine. The table is then tilted slowly foot-down in 5° increments under fluoroscopic control until the contrast moves into the dorsal (thoracic) area. Supine frontal radiographs are then taken of the dorsal spine and the patient is then rotated again into a lateral position, when lateral radiographs of the dorsal spine are taken using a well-collimated vertical beam.

Spinal block

Kendall and Valentine (1981) described a modification of the lateral decubitus lumbar injection technique to induce some contrast medium to pass cephalad beyond an obstructing lesion, thus demonstrating its upper margin. The patient lies in the lateral decubitus position with the spine bowed so that the suspected site of the obstructing lesion is dependent, with the spine both cephalad and caudad to the lesion sloping upwards. Water-soluble contrast medium is slowly injected by lumbar puncture un-

der screen control so that the obstructing lesion and both the upper and lower margins of the lesion are almost always demonstrated. Where very little contrast medium passes an obstructing lesion, so that delineation of its upper border is poor, the necessary information is usually obtained if CT scanning can be carried out through the involved area.

CT scanning after myelography is also useful to assess the topographical relationship of pathology in the transverse axial plane, define the extent of extradural pathology and achieve a measure of tissue characterization. Where cord cavitation is suspected, scanning should be delayed several hours, when some contrast will probably have entered the cord cavity.

Postmyelographic posture and care

Immediately after lumbar or cervical water-soluble myelography, the patient is sat up, in order to run the contrast medium into the lumbosacral region, then returned to the ward by chair or trolley with the head and shoulders propped up on pillows. The patient is encouraged to remain in bed in this position for 6 hours and must be told not to lower the head during this period. The patient should be encouraged to drink fluids freely. Vomiting may be treated by metoclopramide (Maxolon). Phenothiazines such as Stemetil or Largactil should be avoided for at least 2 days.

Oil myelography

Oil myelography with iophendylate (Myodil, Pantopaque) is now very rarely practised, having been almost entirely replaced first by water-soluble myelography and then by CT and MRI. Oil myelography will therefore not be described here but full details are included in Whitehouse and Worthington (1990).

Radiographic equipment

The above descriptions refer to the use of conventional radiographic equipment which may be found in any well equipped X-ray department. An overcouch tube with undercouch image intensification and remote control fluoroscopy will provide a longer-focus film distance and considerably improved anatomical detail.

A C-or U-arm fluoroscopic system is a great advantage, as the single tube may be used for all projections. A C-arm or lateral X-ray tube with horizontal fluoroscopy and radiography is not necessary for lumbar and dorsal water-soluble myelography, but is virtually essential for cervical aqueous myelo-graphy and especially when the contrast medium is injected by cervical puncture. A head-down tilt of more than 30° is rarely required for water-soluble myelography.

Specially designed myelographic tables reduce to a minimum the rotation movements of the patient and help to retain a bolus of contrast medium. Such equipment comprises a tilting table, with rotating cradle, and an X-ray tube mounted on a U- or C-arm (Morris & Cail, 1981).

Complications

Headache, nausea, vomiting and dizziness are the most frequent adverse reactions, usually beginning 4–6 hours after the investigation and lasting another 4–6 hours. Post-myelographic headache occurs in 20–30% of patients and about 10% will have more severe and prolonged headache, especially females. The headache is usually worse when the patient assumes the erect posture and is relieved by lying down. The headache is at least partly due to escape of CSF through the puncture hole in the arachnoid. The use of a small-gauge needle, for instance 25 standard wire gauge, reduces the frequency and severity of the headache. Iotrolan may produce rather less headache than iohexol or iopamidol but this is not yet proven (Hammer & Deisenhammer, 1985). The headache is aggravated by dehydration and the patient should be encouraged to drink freely before the examination, although not in the immediately preceding 3 hours, and also 1–2 litres (but no more) after the procedure.

Lower back pain. Aggravation of pre-existing lumbago or sciatica may occur after myelography, probably related more to the loss of CSF and the disturbance of the nerve roots than to the contrast medium.

Epileptic fits. Fits are now very rare after water-soluble myelography, even of the cervical region. Some radiologists advise preoperative oral diazepam 5 mg or phenobarbitone 120 mg especially in epileptics. These drugs should also be injected i.v. immediately and repeatedly if a fit develops.

Mental reaction. Confusion, time–space disorientation and changes of mood occasionally follow cervical iohexol, iopamidol or iotrolan myelography.

Adhesive arachnoiditis. Although a recognized complication of oil myelography, this probably does not occur following myelography with modern water-soluble contrast agents.

Subdural and epidural injection of water-soluble contrast agents may occur but they are rapidly absorbed within hours and do not usually cause diagnostic problems, as it is obvious whether the CSF has been opacified by a correctly injected water-soluble agent.

Relationship to other imaging modalities

CT provides excellent imaging of the bony spinal canal, its joints and the vertebrae, and is superb in demonstrating their disease, tumours, fractures and bony spinal stenosis. CT does not provide good contrast differentiation between disc material, CSF and the spinal cord but experienced radiologists achieve a high degree of diagnostic accuracy for degenerative disc disease without the necessity for myelo-graphic contrast medium. CT information is much enhanced if there is a low concentration of water-soluble contrast medium in the subarachnoid space.

MRI can replace the whole of both myelography and radiculography. It provides any desired projection, including the cross-sectional facility of CT. It is superior to both techniques in providing information on the internal structure of the spinal cord and intervertebral discs.

References

Belanger, J.G., Blair, I.G., Elder, A.M. *et al.* (1990). Adult myelography with iohexol. *Can. Assoc. Radiol. J.*, **41**(4), 191–4.

Grainger, R.G. (1975) Water-soluble radiculography. *In* Lodge, T. & Steiner, R.E. (eds) *Recent Advances in Radiology*, vol. 5, pp. 37–50. Churchill Livingstone, Edinburgh.

Grainger, R.G. (1979) Further developments in water-soluble myelography 1974–1977. *In* Lodge, T. & Steiner, R.E. (eds) *Recent Advances in Radiology and Medical Imaging*, vol. 6, pp. 177–94. Churchill Livingstone, Edinburgh.

Grainger, R.G. (1981) The technique of lumbar myelography with metrizamide. *In* Grainger, R.G. & Lamb, J.T. (eds) *Myelographic Techniques with Metrizamide*, pp. 31–6. Nycomed (UK) Ltd, Birmingham.

Grainger, R.G., Kendall, B.E. & Wylie, I.G. (1976) Lumbar myelography with metrizamide. *Br. J. Radiol.*, **49**, 996–1003.

Harrison, P.B. (1993) The contribution of needle size and other factors to headache following myelography. *Neuroradiology*, **35**(7), 487–9.

Hammer, B. & Deisenhammer, E. (1985) Iotrol, a new water-soluble non-ionic dimeric contrast medium for intrathecal use. *Neuroradiology*, **27**, 337–41.

Hindmarsh, T., Grepe, A. & Widen, L. (1975) Metrizamide-Phenothiazine interaction. *Acta Radiol. Diagn.*, **15**, 497–507.

Kendall, B.E. & Valentine, A.R. (1981) Myelographic study of the obstructed spinal theca with water-soluble contrast medium. *Br. J. Radiol.*, **54** 408–12

Morris, J.L. & Cail, W.S. (1981) C-arm X-ray unit for use in water-soluble myelography. *In* Grainger, R.G. & Lamb, J.T. (eds) *Myelographic Techniques with Metrizamide*, pp. 79–94. Nycomed (UK) Ltd, Birmingham.

Orrison, W.W., Sacket, J.F., Amundson, P. & Eldevik, O.P. (1983) Lateral C1–C2 puncture for cervical myelography. *Radiology*, **146**(2), 395–400, 401–8.

Shapiro, R. (1984) *Myelography*, 4th edn. Year Book, Chicago.

Teasdale, E. & Macpherson, P. (1984) Guidelines for cervical myelography: lumbar versus cervical puncture techniques. *Br. J. Radiol.*, **57**, 789–93.

Whitehouse, G.H. & Worthington, B.S. (eds) (1990) *Techniques in Diagnostic Radiology*, 2nd edn. Blackwell Scientific Publications, Oxford.

Further reading

Amundsen, P. & Skalpe, I.O. (1975) Cervical myelography with metrizamide: technical aspects. *Neuroradiology*, **8**, 209–12.

Grainger, R.G. & Lamb, J.T. (eds) (1981) *Myelographic Techniques with Metrizamide*. Nycomed (UK) Ltd, Birmingham.

Lamb, J.T. (1985) Iohexol versus iopamidol for myelography. *Invest. Radiol.*, **20** (Suppl. I), 537–43.

Occleshaw, J.V. (1981) Metrizamide myelography in the lumbar region. *In* Grainger R.G. & Lamb, J.T. (eds) *Myelographic Techniques with Metrizamide*, pp. 37–52. Nycomed (UK) Ltd, Birmingham.

Skalpe, I.O. & Shortland, O. (1978) *Myelography — Textbook and Atlas*. Tanum-Notli, Oslo.

Section 6
Miscellaneous

22   Imaging of Joints

K. LAKIN, S. OSTLERE AND D. J. WILSON

During the late 1980s and early 1990s a revolution has occurred in the imaging of joints. The introduction of magnetic resonance imaging (MRI) has rendered arthrography of the knee obsolete and has demoted arthrography of other joints to a supporting role. Ultrasound has a place in the investigation of suspected abnormalities of the periarticular soft tissues, particularly the rotator cuff of the shoulder, in selected screening for developmental dysplasia of the hip and for detecting a hip effusion. Determining the appropriate test for any particular patient will depend on factors such as the availability of equipment and variations in local clinical practice.

Temporomandibular joint

MRI can provide static images of the joint with the mouth in the open and closed positions, and is usually the only investigation required. Occasionally, an arthrogram is needed as some abnormalities are only appreciated on a dynamic examination. In some centres arthroscopy has a major role in diagnosis and treatment, imaging being reserved for selected cases.

Magnetic resonance imaging

Indications

Suspected internal derangement.

Technique

T_1 weighted spin-echo sagittal oblique scans oriented at 90° to the long axis of the mandibular condyles are obtained using a small field of view surface coil or a dedicated dual surface coil which allows imaging of both joints at the same time. Images are obtained with the mouth open and closed (Fig. 22.1). Unlike arthrography, MRI is not truly dynamic and a negative result does not exclude derangement that is only observed during active movement.

Arthrography

Indications

Suspected internal derangement.

Technique

The procedure is quite painful and sedation with a short-acting benzodiazepine is beneficial. The patient lies prone with the head turned and tilted so that the joint to be examined is uppermost and projected slightly above the opposite joint. With a C-arm fluoroscopy unit, the joint can be imaged using a horizontal beam angled 20° towards the head with the patient lying in the supine position. The skin is cleaned, care being taken not to allow antiseptic solution to run into the eyes. The skin and capsule are infiltrated with local anaesthetic. A 25 gauge needle is inserted, aiming for the posterosuperior aspect of the mandibular condyle and thus entering the inferior joint space. Contrast medium (0.5–1 ml) is injected with 0.1 ml of 1 : 1000 adrenaline if delayed tomography is being considered. Occasionally, the superior joint fills due to inadvertent puncture or perforation of the meniscus and this makes interpretation more difficult. Video recording is made while screening the joint in the lateral oblique position, with the patient opening and closing the mouth. An additional frontal oblique view (Townes view with head rotated 5–10° towards side being examined) is sometimes used to demonstrate the meniscal displacement in the coronal plane. Planar tomography with the mouth in varying degrees of openness is occasionally required, particularly if the

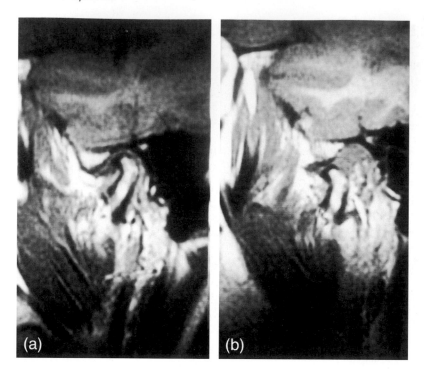

Fig. 22.1 T_1 weighted spin-echo sagittal oblique scans in (a) the mouth closed and (b) mouth open positions. The meniscus is anteriorly displaced and does not reduce on mouth-opening.

superior joint has been opacified and is obscuring the meniscus.

Complications

Transient facial nerve palsy with inhibition of the blink reflex may occur as a result of the local anaesthetic and may require temporary protection of the eye with lubricant and pad.

Shoulder

Ultrasound and MRI have replaced arthrography in most cases of suspected rotator cuff disease. MRI, MR arthrography and computed tomographic (CT) arthrography are used for assessment of instability.

Ultrasound

Indications

Suspected disorders of the rotator cuff or biceps tendon. Ultrasound is a rapid and inexpensive method of evaluating the integrity of the rotator cuff and in the best hands has a high sensitivity and specificity

for the detection of full thickness rotator cuff tears. However, the test is very operator dependent and results of studies show widely varying degrees of success with this technique (Mack *et al.*, 1985). In equivocal cases the patient may proceed to MRI or arthrography.

Technique

The operator stands behind the patient who is seated. A high frequency (e.g. 7.5 mHz) linear-array probe should be used. A large percentage of rotator cuff tears occur near the attachment of the supraspinatus tendon to the greater tuberosity. The supraspinatus tendon is best visualized with the shoulder in internal rotation and the arm behind the back (Middleton *et al.*, 1984) (Fig. 22.2). This ensures that the tendon is uncovered by the acromium and allows optimum access to the distal portion of tendon. With the arm in this position the long axis of the tendon lies close to the sagittal plane. The tendon must be carefully scanned along its long and transverse axes, giving special attention to its most anterolateral portion where small tears are common and easy to miss. The infraspinatus tendon, which inserts into the greater

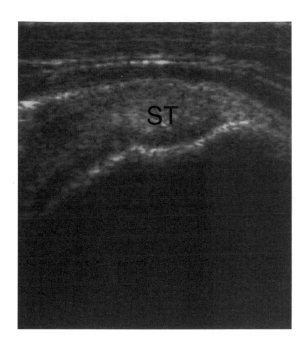

Fig. 22.2 Ultrasound examination of the distal end of the normal supraspinatus tendon (ST) with the probe orientated along the long axis of the tendon.

tuberosity directly posterior to the attachment of the supraspinatus tendon, should also be assessed although isolated tears here are rare. To visualize the bicipital groove, the patient's arm should be returned to the neutral position. The position of the biceps tendon (in cross-section) and integrity of the subscapularis tendon (in longitudinal section) can be assessed by scanning in the axial plane.

Magnetic resonance imaging

Indications

In many centres, MRI has become the first-line investigation for patients with symptoms related to the shoulder. MRI can reliably detect full thickness (Kneeland *et al.*, 1987) and partial thickness tears (Seeger, 1989) of the rotator cuff although occasionally differentiation between these two entities may be difficult. In shoulder instability plain MRI can be used to assess the state of the glenoid labrum and the capsule (Flannigan *et al.*, 1990) although MRI arthrography is more sensitive (Flannigan *et al.*,

1990). MRI is the technique of choice in patients with an unexplained painful shoulder.

Technique

The patient lies supine in the scanner with the hand held in a neutral position. The use of a surface coil is essential. For the assessment of the rotator cuff, cor-onal oblique slices along the long axis of the supraspinatus tendon are obtained (Fig. 22.3). T_1 weighted spin-echo and a T_2 weighted sequence (either spin-echo, STIR or gradient-echo) are required. Sagittal oblique images may be performed but rarely provide useful additional information. Axial images are required for patients with shoulder instability. The glenoid labrum is best visualized on gradient-echo $T_2{}^*$ weighted images (Tsai & Zlatkin, 1990). The state of the capsule may be difficult to assess without a joint effusion. Visualization of both labrum and capsule is improved with the introduction of either iodinated contrast medium (allowing confirmation of intra-articular injection on screening) or gadolinium diethylenetriaminepenta-acetic acid (GdDTPA) (0.1 ml of Gd-DTPA in 10 ml of iodinated contrast or saline) into the joint prior to scanning. If intra-articular gadolinium is used then T_1 weighted scans should be performed (Tsai & Zlatkin, 1990).

Arthrography

Indications

The preoperative assessment of patients with suspected rotator cuff disease in which ultrasound or MRI is equivocal or not available.

Technique

The patient lies in the supine position. Under screening control, the skin is marked over the middle of the glenohumeral joint at the most medial point of the humeral head. The arm is held in the neutral or externally rotated position to avoid impingement of the needle on the lesser tuberosity. A 22 gauge spinal needle is inserted into the joint and the position confirmed by the injection of a small amount of contrast medium. For the double-contrast technique

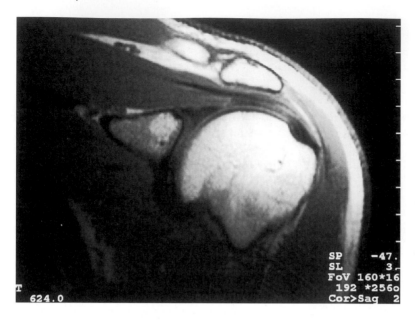

SP   -47.
SL   3.
FoV 160*16
    192 *256o
Cor>Sag   2

Fig. 22.3 T_1 weighted spin-echo coronal image of the normal supraspinatus tendon.

10 ml of contrast medium is injected followed by 10 ml of air. Non-ionic contrast medium is preferred as it is less irritant and gives fewer side effects. The shoulder is subjected to a range of passive motion to encourage contrast medium to enter small defects in the rotator cuff. The procedure may be recorded on video to identify the exact location of a rotator cuff tear before the area is obscured by contrast medium in the subacromial bursa. An AP view of the shoulder in external rotation, with a weight held in the patient's hand and with the tube angled 15° in a caudal direction, will give a good view of the underside of the supraspinatus tendon for the detection of partial tears. The presence of contrast medium in the subacromial bursa indicates a full thickness tear and will be detected on a frontal view. An inferosuperior view through the bicipital grove identifies the position of the tendon of the long head of biceps.

CT arthrography

Indications

Preoperative assessment of suspected instability.

Technique

The needle is placed within the joint as described under shoulder arthrography. Relatively dilute (3 ml of 180 mg iodine ml^{-1}) non-ionic contrast medium and approximately 15 ml of air are injected into the joint; 0.3 ml of 1 : 1000 adrenaline may be added to delay reabsorption of contrast medium. Consecutive 5-mm thick slices are obtained through the glenohumeral joint with the patient lying supine with the arm internally rotated. Additional views with the arm in external rotation may increase the sensitivity (Pennes *et al.*, 1989) Positioning the patient in the lateral oblique position to provide a double contrast view of both anterior and posterior portions of the labrum has been described (Turner *et al.*, 1994).

Elbow

Magnetic resonance imaging

Indications

Suspected loose body or cartilaginous defect including osteochondritis dissecans .

Technique

Although the role of MRI in the assessment of the elbow joint is not well established, the technique may be used as an alternative to arthrography. Examination is difficult due to positioning problems. A surface coil should be used with the patient lying in the most comfortable position that will result in good quality images. Spin-echo or gradient-echo T_2^* weighted sequences are suitable for identifying loose bodies or cartilaginous defects. T_1 weighted and STIR sequences are used to define anatomy and intramedullary abnormalities.

Arthrography

Indications

Suspected loose body or cartilaginous defect including osteochondritis dissecans.

Technique

The patient either lies prone on the screening table with the elbow flexed at 90° above the head or sits on a stool with the flexed elbow resting on the table. The elbow is positioned so that a true lateral projection is obtained when screening. A 21 gauge needle is inserted into the lateral aspect of the joint between the radial head and the capitulum. Either 6 ml of contrast medium (for a single-contrast examination), or 0.5 ml of contrast medium and 8 ml of air (for a double-contrast examination) is injected. Antero-posterior (AP) and two oblique views with the elbow extended and a lateral view with the elbow flexed are obtained. The single-contrast arthrogram may be followed by planar tomography which will improve the sensitivity of the technique. CT following a double-contrast technique using dilute contrast medium has been shown to be effective in identifying loose bodies and articular cartilage defects (Holland *et al.*, 1994).

Wrist

Fluoroscopy

Indications

Diagnosis or classification of suspected transient carpal instability.

Technique

Fluoroscopic examination of the wrist is occasionally required as instability may only be apparent during movement and plain radiographs may be normal. The patient may be aware of a click during certain wrist movements. A video recording is made of a frontal view of the wrist in the pronated position during active radial and ulnar deviation with the fist gripped and a lateral view during extension and flexion (White *et al.*, 1984). Further manoeuvres may be needed in order to record an audible click.

Magnetic resonance imaging

Indications

Chronic wrist pain, suspected osteonecrosis, carpal tunnel syndrome or occult ganglia.

Technique

Using a small surface coil, the wrist is positioned above the head with the patient lying in the prone position. If this cannot be tolerated, the patient may lie supine with the wrist positioned by his side. T_2^* weighted coronal gradient-echo images are particularly useful in the assessment of the triangular cartilage and intercarpal ligaments (Fig. 22.4). T_1 and T_2 weighted axial images are used to assess carpal tunnel syndrome and detect small ganglia.

Arthrography

Indications

Suspected tear of the triangular cartilage or intercarpal ligaments. MRI is reasonably accurate in the detection of pathology of the triangular cartilage but arthrography is still the technique of choice for assessing the integrity of the intercarpal ligaments.

Technique

The patient may lie prone with the hand above the head or sit aside the screening table with the wrist in

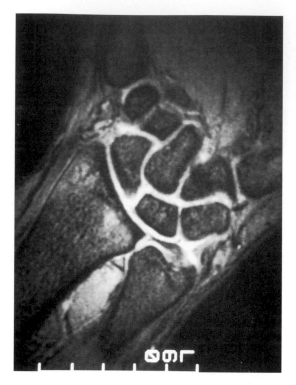

Fig. 22.4 T$_2$*weighted gradient-echo coronal image of the normal wrist. The normal triangular cartilage is well demonstrated.

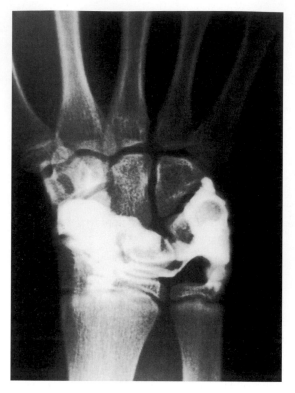

Fig. 22.5 Normal arthrogram of the wrist. Contrast medium remains confined to the wrist joint.

the prone position. The wrist is supported in a slightly flexed position. The ridge of the distal end of the radius is palpated and a 21 gauge needle is inserted into the joint at the mid point of the scaphoid. Care must be taken not to insert the needle into the scapholunate joint as this communicates with the mid-carpal joint. Approximately 2 ml of contrast medium is injected under moderate positive pressure and the wrist is exercised (Fig. 22.5). It is useful to video record the injection as it may be difficult to differentiate which of the proximal intercarpal ligaments is torn once the mid-carpal joint has been filled through a defect. Frontal, lateral and two oblique views are taken. Contrast medium in the distal radioulnar joint or the mid-carpal joint indicates rupture of the triangular cartilage or one or both of the proximal intercarpal ligaments, respectively. An improvement in the sensitivity of the examination can be achieved by performing the three-phase technique in which the wrist joint, mid-carpal and distal radioulnar joints are injected separately. Sufficient

time must be allowed for the contrast to clear between each injection (Zinberg *et al.*, 1988), although the injections can be done at the same sitting using digital subtraction. Because small tears may exhibit a ball-valve effect more defects will be detected using the three-phase technique but the clinical significance of such lesions is debatable (Wilson *et al.*, 1991).

Hip

Ultrasound

Indications

Developmental dysplasia of the hip; irritable hip.

Technique

Developmental dysplasia of the hip

Ultrasound is the investigation of choice for screening

babies under the age of 1 year for dysplastic hips. Most centres employ a selective screening service, only examining babies with certain risk factors. There are several described methods of assessing the acetabular depth and the degree of subluxation. For screening, a single coronal view with the hip flexed is adequate. Some centres use Graf's method of measuring the slope of the bony and cartilaginous roofs in the coronal plane (Graf & Schuler, 1986), while others believe equally good results may be obtained by visually assessing the degree of coverage of the femoral head without undertaking measurements (Clarke *et al.*, 1985). Dynamic stress views are also useful and are obtained by applying gentle posterolateral pressure to the flexed hip while imaging in the coronal plane (Wilson, 1988).

Irritable hip

The purpose of the examination is to detect an effusion. The anterior surface of the neck of the femur is viewed along its long axis. Comparison should be made with the asymptomatic hip as the normal capsule is of variable thickness and may mimic an effusion (Alexander *et al.*, 1989). Ultrasound may be used to guide aspiration.

Magnetic resonance imaging

Indications

Hip pain; suspected osteonecrosis.

Technique

For most indications T_1 and T_2 weighted spin-echo in the coronal plane using the body coil is sufficient (Fig. 22.6). For assessment of the acetabular labrum gradient-echo T_2^* weighted images are useful but a suitable surface coil (for example a Helmholz coil) is needed to obtain adequate images (Helms *et al.*, 1984).

Arthrography

Indications

Developmental dysplasia of the hip, articular cartilage defects and loose bodies. Loose hip prostheses.

Technique

No prosthesis

The patient lies supine and the position of the femoral

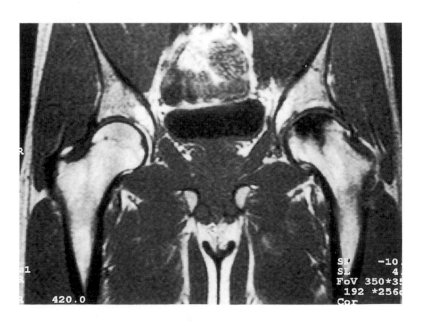

Fig. 22.6 T_1 weighted spin-echo coronal image of the hips. The subchondral low signal intensity focus in the left femoral head represents osteonecrosis.

artery is identified by palpation. A mark is made on the skin over the centre of the femoral neck. A 22 gauge needle is inserted down to the femoral neck. A small amount of contrast medium is injected to confirm the position of the needle. Minor manipulation of the needle may be required in order to enter the joint space and slight flexion of the hip may help in stubborn cases. Approximately 10 ml of contrast medium is injected (Fig. 22.7). For preoperative assessment of dysplastic hips, views of the hip in various positions are useful in determining the best-fit of the head in the acetabulum. For the detection of loose bodies, planar or computed tomography immediately following the arthrogram improves sensitivity. In babies, who will require a general anaesthetic, the needle may be inserted using the same method as that in the adult or directly onto the superolateral aspect of the femoral head, which is exposed anteriorly at this stage of development. About 2 ml of contrast medium is required in a baby. Video recording while manoeuvring the hip with the addition of spot radiographs can be used to assess stability and the presence of interposed soft tissue between the femoral head and the acetabulum. Alternatively, frontal radiographs with the hip in neutral, adduction and abduction, and a frogleg lateral view are obtained (Grech, 1972).

With hip prosthesis

Arthrography is used in patients with a hip prosthesis to assess for loosening. The patient lies supine and the position of the femoral artery is identified as this structure may overlie the hip joint if it is tortuous. AP control radiograph(s) of the entire prosthesis are performed. A 19 gauge needle is inserted down to the central point of the neck of the femoral prosthesis. Aspiration is attempted in order to obtain a sample for bacteriological examination. Contrast medium is then injected, the amount needed depending on the degree of laxity of the capsule. Radiographs are then obtained with the hip in an identical position to the control radiograph(s). Digital or subtraction techniques may be used if the patient has not moved between the two sets of radiographs and the radiographic projections are identical (Walker *et al.*, 1991). In practice, the value of arthrography in the assessment of loosening is limited as it is not infrequent to have a normal arthrogram in a proven loose prosthesis.

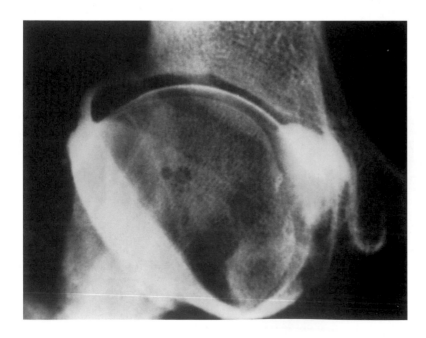

Fig. 22.7 Single-contrast arthogram showing minor dysplasia of the hip. The acetabular labrum is intact.

Knee

Magnetic resonance imaging

Indications

Suspected internal derangement; knee pain. MRI has replaced other techniques for imaging the knee in nearly all cases.

Technique

A surface coil is required. There are several different options when choosing a routine protocol but thin section (3 mm or less) T_1 weighted or proton density spin-echo images in the sagittal and coronal planes or a gradient-echo volume acquisition sequence should be included. The main use of the coronal plane is to assess the mid-portions of the menisci and the collateral ligaments. In addition a T_2^* weighted gradient-echo sagittal sequence is helpful in defining the intact anterior cruciate ligament in the presence of an effusion and in making the diagnosis of meniscocapsular separation (Fig. 22.8). Patellar maltracking can be assessed dynamically by performing single-slice axial fast gradient-echo scans (with an image acquisition time of less than 1 s) during controlled knee extension (Shellock *et al.*, 1991).

Ankle

Ultrasound

Indications

Suspected or known tendon pathology.

Technique

The Achilles' tendon is imaged using a high-frequency linear-array probe in the sagittal and axial planes with the patient in the prone position and the feet hanging over the end of the couch. To detect subtle diffuse swelling, comparison with the contralateral tendon should be performed. The assessment of the integrity of the other tendons of the ankle is technically more demanding but can be assisted by dynamic imaging with the patient repeatedly contracting the relevant muscle.

Magnetic resonance imaging

Indications

Assessment of ligamentous, tendinous and bony pathology.

Technique

The ankle is best imaged using a head or knee coil. For most indications T_1 and T_2 weighted images are obtained in one or two planes, depending on the indication. For example, axial views are best for demonstrating tendon pathology and coronal views best for detecting osteochondritis dissecans of the talus. With the foot held in plantar flexion axial images may

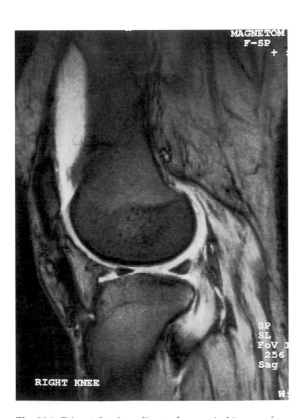

Fig. 22.8 T_2^* weighted gradient-echo saggital image of the knee. There is an effusion.

be used to assess all three components of the lateral ligament complex.

Arthrography

Indications

MRI has replaced arthrography in most instances. Arthrography with or without tomography or CT is still occasionally indicated when a loose body is suspected

Technique

With the patient lying supine a 22 gauge needle is inserted at a point overlying the medial corner of the talar dome. Approximately 8 ml of contrast medium is injected for a single-contrast examination and 1 ml of contrast medium and about 8 ml of air for a double-contrast examination. If the arthrogram is being followed by CT then diluted contrast medium or air should be used. AP, lateral and oblique views are obtained.

Peroneal tenogram

Indications

This examination is occasionally performed to assess the integrity of the calcaneofibular ligament.

Technique

The examination should be performed within 24 hours of injury as an unacceptable rate of false negative results occurs after this time due to plugging of the defect with blood clot. A 21 gauge needle is inserted into the peritoneal tendon sheath which can be palpated behind the lateral malleolus. Contrast medium is injected with the application of moderate pressure and a frontal view is taken following passive manipulation of the ankle. If the calcaneofibular ligament is disrupted then contrast medium will be seen to enter the ankle joint (Blanshard *et al.*, 1986).

References

Alexander, J.E., Seibert, J.J., Glasier, C.M. *et al.* (1989) High resolution hip ultrasound in the limping child. *J. Clin. Ultrasound*, **17**, 19–24.

Blanshard, K.S., Finlay, D.B.L. & Scott, D.J.A. (1986) A radiological analysis of lateral ligament injuries of the ankle. *Clin. Radiol.*, **37**, 247–51.

Clarke, N.M.P., Hacke, H.T., McHugh, P. *et al.* (1985) Real time ultrasound in the diagnosis of congenital dislocation and dysplasia of the hip. *J. Bone Joint Surg.*, **67**, 406–12.

Flannigan, B., Kursonoglu Brahme, S., Snyder, S., Karzel, R., Del Pizzo, W. & Resnick, D. (1990) MR arthrography of the shoulder: comparison with conventional MR imaging. *Am. J. Roentgenol.*, **155**, 829–32.

Graf, R. & Schuler, P. (1986) *Sonography of the Infant Hip: an Atlas*. Verlag Chemie, Weinheim.

Grech, P. (1972) *Hip Arthrography*. Chapman & Hall, London.

Helms, C.A., Moon, K.L., Genant, H.K. & Chafetz, N. (1984) MRI; skeletal applications. *Orthopedics*, **219**, 1429–35.

Holland, P., Davies, A.M. & Cassar-Pullicino, V.N. (1994) Computed tomography arthrography in the assessment of osteochondritis dissecans of the elbow. *Clin. Radiol.*, **49/4**, 231–5.

Kneeland, J.B., Middleton, W.D., Carrera, J.F. *et al.* (1987) Magnetic resonance imaging of the shoulder: diagnosis of rotator cuff tears. *Am. J. Roentgenol.*, **149**, 333–7.

Mack, L.A., Matsen, F.A., Kilcoyne, R.F. *et al.* (1985) Ultrasound evaluation of the rotator cuff. *Radiology*, **157**, 205–9.

Middleton, W.D., Edelstein, G.R., William, R. *et al.* (1984) Ultrasonography of the rotator cuff. *J. Ultrasound Med.*, **3** 549–51.

Pennes, D.R., Jonsson, K., Buchwalter, K., Braunstein, E., Blasier, R. & Wojtys, E. (1989) Computed arthrotomography of the shoulder: comparison of examinations made with internal and external rotation of the humerus. *Am. J. Roentgenol.*, **153**, 1017–19.

Seeger, L.L. (1989) Magnetic resonance imaging of the shoulder. *Clin. Orthoped. Rel. Res.*, **244**, 48–59.

Shellock, F.G., Foo, T.K., Deutsch, A.L. & Minck, J.H. (1991) Patellofemoral joint: evaluation during active flexion with ultrafast spoiled GRASS MR imaging. *Radiology*, **180(2)**, 581–5.

Tsai, J.C. & Zlatkin, M.B. (1990) MRI of the shoulder. *Radiol. Clin. N. Am.*, **28**, 279–91.

Turner, P.J., O'Connor, P.J., Saifuddin, A., Williams, J., Coral, A. & Butt, W.P. (1994) Prone oblique positioning for computed tomographic arthrography of the shoulder. *Br. J. Radiol.*, **801**, 835–9.

Walker, C.W., Fitzrandolph, R.L., Collins, D.N. & Dalrymple, G.V. (1991) Arthrography of painful hips following arthroplasty. Digital versus plain film subtraction. *Skel. Radiol.*, **20**, 403–7.

White, S.J., Louis, D.S., Braunstein, E.M. *et al.* (1984) Capitate–lunate instability, recognition by manipulation under fluoroscopy. *Am. J. Roentgenol.*, **143**, 361–4.

Wilson, A.J., Gilula, L.A. & Mann, F.A. (1991) Unidirectional joint communication in in wrist arthrography: an evaluation of 250 cases. *Am. J. Roentgenol.*, **157**, 105–9.

Wilson, D.J. (1988) Diagnostic ultrasound in the musculoskeletal system. *Curr. Orthop.*, **2**(1), 41–50.

Zinberg, E.M., Palmer, A.K., Coren, A.B. *et al.* (1988) The triple injection wrist arthrogram. *J. Hand Surg.*, **13**, 803–9.

23 Breast

E. J. ROEBUCK

Radiological demonstration of the breast is no different from that of many other organs in that a knowledge of the radiological anatomy and the possible radiographic projections are a fundamental prerequisite to the production of diagnostically useful images. It differs, however, in three important respects.

1 The female breast is subject to a wide spectrum of anatomical variations and is comprised of tissues which respond to a highly complex series of physiological stimuli.

2 There is a danger of radiation-induced breast cancer when using X-ray mammography. This places a responsibility upon the radiologist to reduce the radiation dose as far as is possible without prejudicing image quality. Images of the highest quality are essential for accurate diagnosis. It is therefore mandatory that radiologists must be familiar with the technical problems involved in order to achieve an optimum balance between image quality and radiation hazard.

3 Breast cancer is a potentially life-threatening disease, the fear of which affects the attitude of every woman with a breast problem. Add to this, her possibly inaccurate knowledge of the radiation hazard and then the mammographic examination is inevitably accompanied by certain degree of anxiety. It follows that each woman should be treated as an individual from a humanitarian as well as a technical point of view.

Role of the radiologist in breast imaging

Radiologists have an important role in ensuring that radiographers obtain the basic and complementary projections appropriate to the woman's problem and also that they do not repeat examinations which are perfectly adequate for interpretation. To do this, the radiologist must have an adequate knowledge of radiographic technique. In the UK, responding to the demands of the National Breast Screening Programme, the College of Radiographers has established an accreditation system for radiographers involved in mammography. This has contributed to a uniformly high standard of expertise and results in high-quality images. It is recommended that, in order to understand the technique, any radiologist wishing to become involved in a mammographic service should undertake practical work alongside an accredited radiographer.

In addition to X-ray mammography, a radiologist should be familiar with examination of the breast using ultrasound. The two techniques are complementary. The radiologist should be aware of the advantages and limitations of each in order to select the most appropriate method for each particular circumstance. These two imaging modalities are the basis of the radiologist's contribution to breast disease diagnosis and management.

Assessment of breast problems should never be performed using imaging in isolation. For each woman the imaging investigations should be chosen to integrate with clinical and pathology procedures. The accuracy of assessment of breast problems, using a combination of imaging with specialist clinical examination and percutaneous tissue diagnosis by cytology or needle histology, has firmly established triple assessment as optimal practice. It is therefore essential that radiologists involved in breast disease diagnosis and management are aware of surgical and pathology techniques and are fully equipped to collaborate with specialist colleagues and to participate in triple assessment.

Radiation-induced breast cancer

It is well established that there is an increased incidence of breast cancer associated with high-dose radiation. Studies of women receiving relatively high doses of radiation have been compared with non-irradiated women (Feig, 1979). However, there are no studies relating to low radiation doses, such as occur with mammography. The radiation dose assumes great importance when screening asymptomatic women by mammography. Although every effort must be made to reduce the radiation dose to the breast, this factor is relatively less important in women with breast symptoms.

The cancer induction rate from mammography, if it indeed exists, is extremely low. It is impossible to estimate such a low incidence relationship by epidemiological means without studying groups of irradiated and control populations, each numbering several millions. This is impracticable.

The theoretical radiation risk of mammography may be calculated from the assumptions that there is no threshold below which radiation has no effect, and that the dose–response curve remains linear for low doses. These basic assumptions will inevitably result in an overestimate of risk. The validity of assuming linearity is not confirmed by animal experiments, in which there is an exponential decrease of the low dose risk (Fig. 23.1).

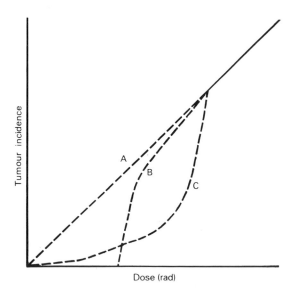

Fig. 23.1 Possibilities for the induction of human breast cancer at low doses of radiation. (–) Known linear relationship. A, Straight line extrapolation; B, extrapolation assuming a threshold dose; C, relationship found in animals.

Study of the data on the groups of irradiated women indicates that there is a latent period of the order of 15–20 years before the onset of breast cancer. An exception to this is the case of atomic bomb survivors where the latent period was between 5 and 9 years. This variation may be due to the neutron component of the atomic bomb irradiation, to the fact that a whole-body irradiation was received, or an expression of a variation in susceptibility between Japanese and Caucasian women. The duration of the radiation effect is uncertain but population studies indicate that this is at least 30 years.

One factor of importance regarding the induction of breast cancer is the increased susceptibility of younger women. The cancer induction rate with high doses of radiation in women of 20 years of age is 50% higher than in girls of 10, and more than three times that of women of 30 years of age. By the time a woman is 40, her risk is less than 10% of that of a 20 year old. It would seem therefore that it is the developing glandular tissue which is particularly at risk of being influenced by irradiation. For this reason X-ray mammography is not indicated under the age of 30 years, unless there is a specific problem which cannot be solved by other means such as ultrasound or fine-needle aspiration (FNA) for cytology.

There are four important factors regarding the risk of breast cancer induction due to diagnostic mammography.
1 If there is any increased risk then this is so small that it has never been demonstrated.
2 Even if there is no proven risk we should be cautious and act on the worst case theoretical calculations.
3 Technical advances have resulted in a reduction of the radiation dose required to give adequate mammographic demonstration.
4 It is the radiologist's responsibility to balance the assumption of risk against the anticipated benefits of any examination in each individual case.

Basic imaging system

A mammographic image requires excellent resolution and good visible contrast in the low tissue contrast ranges. The image must be easily reproducible to facilitate comparison between present, previous and future radiographs. From these requirements a series of technical possibilities arise which are constrained by two factors.

1 A low kilovoltage is mandatory because the breast consists of soft tissues and the detection of interfaces between tissues with only slightly differing absorption rates is of extreme importance. Very small calcium deposits in the breast must also be demonstrable, but, in technical terms, are much easier to visualize than the soft-tissue changes which are probably of more importance from a clinical point of view. The selected kilovoltage should be that which maximizes the small differences in absorption between adjacent soft-tissue structures in the breast. In practice this is ideally in the 28–30 kV range.

2 It is essential to employ the lowest possible dose of radiation because the breast is an organ liable to develop radiation-induced cancer.

The radiologist must determine the 'trade-off' point where a further reduction in dose will lead to a degradation of the image which will cause loss of diagnostically important detail.

Two main modalities have been used for X-ray mammography — xeromammography and film mammography. Xeromammography was popular because the edge enhancement effect which made well-defined objects more easy to visualize. The technique produced images equally as good as the non-screen 'industrial' radiographs which were used at that time. However, technical developments in high-speed, high-resolution radiographs and intensifying screens have resulted in far better images combined with a lower radiation dose. Some xeromammography machines are still in use and so a short description of the technique is given below.

Xeromammography

The production of xeromammographic images results from the partial discharge of an electrostatically charged selenium plate by the emergent X-ray beam. A powder of charged blue particles is then dusted over the plate and adheres to various areas on the plate proportional to the residual electrostatic charge. The image so produced is then transferred to paper and fixed.

The advantages of xeromammography include a very wide latitude, the chest wall and retromammary space being as well demonstrated as the skin and subcutaneous fat. An appearance of very high contrast is achieved within a small area of the xerographic image as a result of the edge enhancement effect, whilst the overall contrast is low and gives the effect of good penetration of dense glandular tissue.

The disadvantages are the higher radiation dose required, and, relative to modern film/screen mammography, an inferior image. The edge enhancement effect makes visualization of calcific particles easier but details of configuration of the individual particles is destroyed, thus removing an extremely important diagnostic feature. Demonstration of low-density structures is markedly inferior to that achieved by film/screen techniques, and the detection of small mass lesions within glandular tissue densities is rendered very difficult or impossible.

Film mammography

Non-screen, 'industrial' X-ray radiography was initially used for mammography but film/screen combinations are now used virtually exclusively. A high-speed, high-resolution film is used with a single intensifying screen placed behind. Mammographic cassettes are specifically designed to have a low attenuation front face, often constructed of carbon fibre. Manufacturers produce matched sets of high-speed, high-resolution films and intensifying screens, and processing chemistry designed for particular film emulsions. The speed of the systems is such that the requisite radiation dose is so low that antiscatter grids can now be used with confidence. The image quality resulting from these technical developments represents a vast improvement.

The use of a matched set comprising film, intensifying screen and processing chemistry cannot be recommended too highly. The processing parameters are particularly important. Even though a standard 90 s automatic processor can be used, there is no doubt that greatly improved image quality is achieved by dedicated mammographic processing with a higher temperature and longer processing cycle, both chosen to maximize the performance of the film.

X-ray beam quality

It is now accepted that a narrow spectral band optimizes the mammographic image within the low kilovoltage range essential for breast examinations. The quality of the beam is chosen to give maximal response from the preferred recording system (Hanss *et al.*, 1976).

Molybdenum is a technically convenient material for anode target construction, emitting a very narrow spectral band with characteristic radiation peaks at 17.9 and 19.5 keV. However, there is a significant emission of higher energy radiation in addition to the double peak of characteristic radiation. A 0.3 mm molybdenum filter is used to suppress the spectrum above 20 keV (Fig. 23.2). Energy of the resultant quality gives good contrast in film mammography, but requires a rather high dose for thick and dense breasts. Target materials with a higher atomic number would give a lower dose but inferior contrast.

Recently different filtration materials have been used in addition to molybdenum with the objective of reducing radiation dose, particularly in the imaging of dense breasts. Palladium was the first reported, but rhodium is now being adopted both for filtration and as a tube target material. One manufacturer offers a dual filter/dual target system for the selection of the most appropriate combination according to the breast density (Table 23.1).

Radiographic exposure times are best determined by an automatic exposure control device since premammographic assessment of breast density is virtually impossible. This is usually an ionization chamber which can be positioned, within a fairly limited area, under that part of the breast which the radiographer considers to be the most dense. Unless there is access to previous films in order to determine this with accuracy, a point some 3–5 cm above and behind the nipple should be chosen.

Operating voltages for X-ray tubes with molybdenum targets are usually in the 26–30 kV range, with 28 kV being optimal. In practice, when a denser breast is being examined, the best image results are obtained when the kilovoltage remains fixed and the milliampere level is higher. The increase in radiation risk is justified by the improved diagnostic quality.

Image quality

Geometric unsharpness is an important factor in image quality and depends upon the size and shape of the focal spot on the X-ray tube target. Also important is the ratio between the focus to object and the object to film distances. The development of microfocal spots not only gives the potential for improvement in image quality by reducing geometric unsharpness, but also makes possible the employment of magnification techniques.

Compression of the breast is a mandatory part of mammography which improves image quality by:

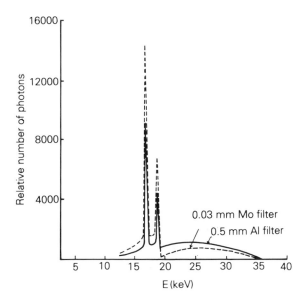

Fig. 23.2 Energy spectrum from a molybdenum anode with molybdenum (Mo) and aluminium (Al) filtration.

Table 23.1 Different X-ray tube target and filter materials for differing densities of breast

Type of breast	Tube target material	Tube filter material
Normal	Molybdenum	Molybdenum
Moderately dense	Molybdenum	Rhodium
Dense	Rhodium	Rhodium

1 Reducing geometrical insharpness.

2 Minimizing blurring due to movement.

3 Improving contrast by a reduction of scattered radiation.

4 Giving an even tissue thickness, which results in a homogenous film density with the posterior portion of the breast being as well visualized as the anterior part.

5 Reducing the overlapping projection of images by the spreading apart of intramammary structures.

6 Reducing the radiation dose.

It is necessary to compress the average breast to a thickness of about 4 cm in order to achieve these improvements.

Degradation of the final image by scattered radiation can be reduced by a collimating cone. However, this should never be so narrow as to leave a white margin on the radiograph around the image of the breast. Should there be a white margin, when the radiograph is being viewed the white light entering the eye through the white area will reduce perception of detail to a degree very considerably greater than any improvement achieved by the collimator. Scattered radiation can also be reduced by the use of a radiographic antiscatter grid between the breast and the film. This increases the dose but, by using an appropriate tube filter and modern high-speed recording systems, the resultant image is such that the dose can be justified.

It cannot be over emphasized that, whilst the radiation dose to the breast must be minimized, it is essential that each step in the production of the final image is calculated to minimize image degradation.

The application of the modulation transfer functions (MTF) allows accurate assessment of the efficiency of each part of the imaging system (Meredith & Massey, 1979). The quality of the final image depends upon the product of the MTF of each constituent part of the imaging system,

MTF (whole system) = MTF1 × MTF2 × MTF3 ... etc.

It follows that each constituent part should be chosen and adjusted to give the highest possible image quality. The poorest element in the chain does not absolutely determine the final image quality. If this were so, all the other elements need only be slightly better than the worst without having an influence on the final image quality.

The balance between image quality and a lower radiation dose is a subjective one and will always depend on the preference of the individual radiologist.

Radiological anatomy

The breast is a hemispherical structure, with a concave base applied to the chest wall and the axillary tail as a superolateral prolongation. Each breast is divided into 15–20 lobes by fibrous septa, not unlike the septa which divide an orange or a grapefruit into segments. Within each lobe are about 20 lobules of glandular tissue, each consisting of terminal lactiferous ducts with glandular out-pouches, the alveoli (Fig. 23.3). The terminal ductolobular unit (TDL) is not only the basic functional unit of breast tissue, it is also the site at which carcinoma and most benign processes have their origin. The terminal ducts join successively to form larger ducts so that each lobe is drained by a single duct to the nipple.

In the absence of pregnancy, mammary gland tissue occupies the whole of the breast for only a short time after adolescence and appears as a more or less homogeneous density. This density is comprised of individual opacities about a millimetre in diameter, each representing a TDL, superimposed so that the individual elements cannot be visualized. Breast density, as seen on a mammogram, depends upon a number of factors. These include the degree of obesity of the woman and the relative amounts of glandular and fibrous tissue within the breast. The density varies with age, but some 40% of 80 year olds have mammographically dense breasts while some 20% of 30 year olds have a fatty appearance. Mammographic evidence of involution coincides with the replacement of interlobular connective tissue and glandular elements by fat. Radiological evidence of involution commences early in the second decade of life, with clearing of glandular shadowing from the retromammary and subcutaneous regions. Involution progresses first from the inferomedial quadrant and subsequently from the superomedial and inferolateral quadrants. Last to involute is the superolateral quadrant and axillary tail.

Radiological involution is usually completed many years before the menopause, and it is not uncommon to have no visible evidence of glandular tissue on mammograms of women in the third decade.

With the onset of pregnancy, glandular tissue shadowing reappears throughout the breast including those areas which appeared involuted. There is a rapid return to the pre-pregnancy level of involution after the cessation of lactation. The process of mammographic involution may also be affected by hormone replacement therapy, with a reappearance of soft-tissue density or a halt of progressive disappearance.

Variants of normality

Some 80–90% of women show some degree of variation from the ideal 'normal' mammographic appearance. Since so many women are involved the variation cannot be regarded as abnormal, but rather as a series of variants of normality. These various patterns of mammographic variation were initially classifed by Wolfe (1967). This classification is still widely accepted, although his correlation with the degree of risk for breast cancer is not. Numerous clinical and pathological terms have been used over the years to describe various breast changes which are now recognized to be normal variants and not disease processes. Many of these terms had become associated with different entities in the minds of pathologist, clinician and radiologist. Efforts have therefore been made to discard terms such as dysplasia, mazoplasia, mastopathy and fibrocystic disease. The radiologist should restrict terminology to descriptive terms such as nodularity and density, only venturing into more specific nomenclature in instances where firm pathological correlation has been established. The acceptable nomenclature is based on the use of one of two generic terms: benign breast change (BBC) or aberrations of normal development and involution (ANDI).

It is valuable to identify the anatomical site of a radiological feature. In this way, variations from normality due to pathological or other causes may more readily be identified.

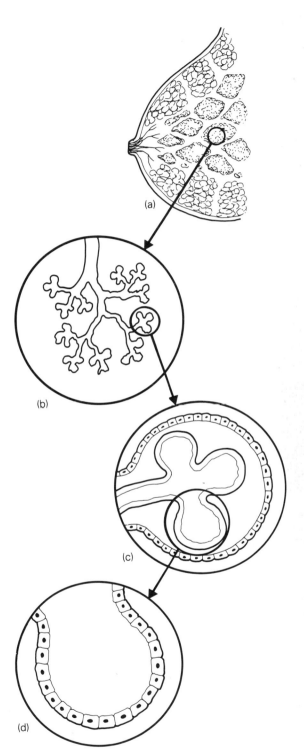

Fig. 23.3 Diagram to illustrate the microscopic structure of the breast. (a) Section of breast showing skin, fat and glandular tissue. (b) A breast lobe, with multiple lobules. (c) Terminal ductolobular unit. (d) Breast lobule, showing double layer of cells.

Subareolar ductal prominence

Subareolar ductal prominence is a common finding within the spectrum of normality, being present in some 70% of individuals. It is classified by Wolfe as parenchymal pattern P1. Histologically, it may be due to simple dilatation (duct ectasia), to dilatation resulting from internal epithelial hyperplasia, or to collagen deposition around the ducts. Duct ectasia is an aberration of involution and is more common in the fourth and fifth decades.

Deep ductal prominence

More deeply within the gland, the ductal density may become prominent due to periductal collagenosis. Duct ectasia is less common further away from the nipple. This change is classified by Wolfe as parenchymal pattern P2.

Gland level changes

This group of changes is also within the spectrum of normal. A description of fibrocystic change (but not fibrocystic disease) is an acceptable alternative term. This parenchymal pattern is referred to by Wolfe as DY. Radiologically, there are patchy ill-defined densities, which resolve as involution progresses and leaves a honeycomb-like appearance of thickened trabeculae. Histologically, the densities consist of fibrous tissue in the stroma and microcysts in the TDLs. Not infrequently, larger cysts are present and give rise to identifiable opacities. Although a variant of normality, this type of change is a not infrequent accompaniment of cyclical mastalgia.

Radiographic projections

There are two basic radiographic projections in mammography, the mediolateral oblique and the craniocaudal. These may be followed by complementary projections and supplementary techniques should an abnormality be identified on the first pair. A single oblique view is sometimes used as the basic projection in the screening of asymptomatic women. However, in many centres it is the practice when undertaking screening examinations to employ the two-view technique on a woman's first attendance and a single view on subsequent routine visits. The two-view technique is always recommended as the basic examination for women with symptoms. A summary of the projections is given below, but for details on positioning see the standard works on radiography.

Basic projections

Oblique projection

This projection was devised by Lundgren and popularized as the sole projection in a breast screening programme (Ludgren & Jackobsson, 1976). It has proved so effective that it is now universally adopted as the standard projection for all purposes, usually in combination with a craniocaudal projection. The glandular tissue in the breast lies obliquely from inferomedial to superolateral. The mediolateral oblique projection employs a central ray at right angles to this longest breast axis. Superimposition of tissue and foreshortening is thereby minimized. With meticulously careful positioning, a radiographer can demonstrate the whole of the uninvoluted part of the breast disc on one film (Fig. 23.4).

Craniocaudal projection

This is the second basic mammographic view, taken with a vertical ray in a superoinferior projection. Together with the oblique film it permits localization of intramammary abnormalities, although for accurate localization two views at right angles are required and a lateral projection is employed with the craniocaudal.

Complementary projections

An abnormality may be suspected when the basic projections have been obtained and the mammograms viewed. It may then be necessary to obtain complementary projections to elucidate the suspicious feature.

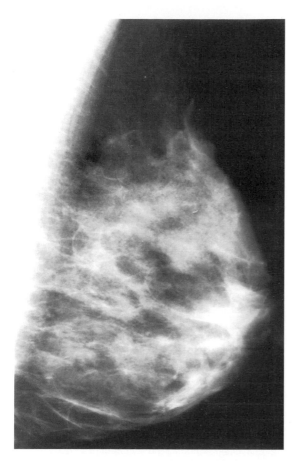

Fig. 23.4 Normal breast. Mediolateral oblique projection.

Rotated craniocaudal projections

The standard craniocaudal view projects the nipple on the mid-line axis of the radiograph. Since the posterior aspect of the breast is curved over the chest wall and the edge of the film is straight, this projection will cut off a little of the lateral and a little of the medial part of the breast. To overcome this, the patient may be slightly rotated medially to demonstrate the lateral part of the breast (the medially rotated craniocaudal) (Fig. 23.5) or laterally to demonstrate the medial part (the laterally rotated craniocaudal).

Erect lateral projection

This projection may be taken either with a mediolateral or a lateromedial technique. The former is more likely to demonstrate posterior breast structures and laterally placed lesions, whereas the latter more clearly demonstrates medially placed abnormalities. A principal advantage of this projection is that it employs a horizontal beam, and so any fluid levels will be clearly demonstrated. Breast cysts commonly contain calcium suspended as fine particles in the cyst fluid. These particles gravitate towards the bottom of the cyst and, with a horizontal ray projection, can be visualized often with 'fluid level' like interfaces between them and the radiolucent fluid — the so-called 'tea cup' sign. When present this justifies a firm diagnosis of benign cystic change.

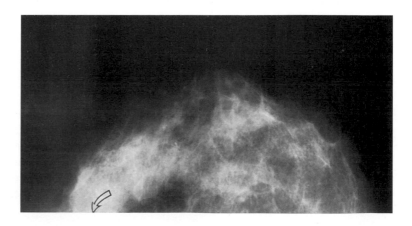

Fig. 23.5 Normal breast. Medially rotated craniocaudal projection.

Extended craniocaudal projection

This projection is utilized to elucidate suspected abnormalities in the upper outer quadrant of the breast. It is, in effect, half way between a craniocaudal and an oblique projection. From the craniocaudal position, with the arm raised and the hand behind her head, the patient turns towards the cassette table and leans backwards by about 45°. The radiographer assists the patient, spreads the breast over the cassette and applies compression ensuring that the upper outer quadrant of the breast is centrally positioned on the film. The attitude of the patient during this procedure has given rise to the description of the projection as the 'Cleopatra view'.

Supplementary techniques

Coned compression technique

If the margins of a suspect area on a basic projection are not clearly visualized, a localized view of the area may be taken using a small compression cone. This will spread the tissues more effectively and enable a distinction to be made between superimposition and a genuine irregular margin to be made. The coned compression may be applied in any direction; usually the projection in which the problem to be solved is best demonstrated on the basic examination.

Magnification technique

Radiographic magnification (Fig. 23.6) is the technique *par excellence* for demonstrating the detail of fine microcalcifications identified on a basic examination. It can be used with advantage in conjunction with a small compression cone. Magnification requires a fine focal spot X-ray tube, no larger than 0.15 mm in diameter. The shorter tube–patient distance delivers a higher dose of radiation. The longer exposure time required means that great care is necessary to avoid movement unsharpness. A grid cannot be used as the exposure time would be excessive, but the air gap between the breast and the film is sufficient to minimize image degradation due to scattered radiation.

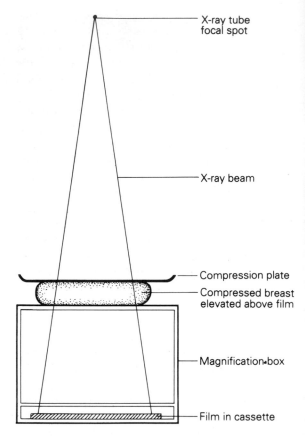

Fig. 23.6 Diagrammatic representation of a breast elevated above the film to obtain a magnified image.

Ultrasonography

Ultrasound of the breast has been practised since the early 1950s. Since that time there have been very considerable improvements in the technology. Ultrasound can produce superb images of many, if not most, of the conditions which affect the female breast. However, to consider this technique in isolation is a grave mistake.

The correct way to elucidate a breast problem, and therefore the choice of which images are likely to be useful, is to undertake the minimum number of investigations along the pathway which leads to an accurate diagnosis. A radiologist involved in breast disease diagnosis and management must be a jack of all trades and master of each.

The place of ultrasound in the breast diagnostician's armamentarium is in the field of assessment, not of primary diagnosis or detection. In breast screening, ultrasound has too many false negatives to be sufficiently accurate. One large series, typical of many, revealed an ultrasound sensitivity of 49.2% versus 93.8% for X-ray mammography alone (Rizatto *et al.*, 1992). Screening by ultrasound is certainly not cost-effective in view of the dependence upon highly skilled operators. Ultrasound is now well established as an essential technique in the assessment of symptomatic breast problems and screening detected abnormalities. Assessment using ultrasound, mammography and clinical examination (triple assessment) gives an increase in sensitivity to over 97% (Guyer & Dewbury, 1987). When applied as an assessment tool, ultrasound must be used to elucidate a problem which it is likely to solve. Thus ultrasound is frequently indicated for mass lesion problems but rarely, if ever, for the elucidation of calcifications (Fig. 23.7). An additional invaluable use is when image guidance is required for percutaneous tissue diagnosis or the marking of impalpable lesions for excision.

A major limitation to breast ultrasound examinations is the need for a high degree of expertise to perform the examination. There are also inherent limitations. Solid and cystic lesions cannot be accurately differentiated if the lesion is smaller than about 5 mm in diameter, or if the cyst content has a cheese-like or semi-solid consistency. Benign lesions cannot be differentiated from carcinomas if these are smaller than about 1 cm in diameter. Some small cancers do produce typical 'malignant' signs but many, particularly the small early lesions, can mimic exactly the features of a fibroadenoma. It is as though the ultrasonic features typical of malignancy only develop as a cancer grows to a size where secondary features develop.

The equipment used should be chosen with care. Direct A-mode systems and mechanical scanners producing multiple sections are now obsolete for breast disease diagnosis and management. Handheld, real-time equipment with transducers in the 7.5 or 12 mHz range is preferable. Linear array apparatus demonstrates a larger area of skin and subcutaneous tissue, but sector scanners with a water path give better resolution. The portable 'suitcase' type of equipment is usually inadequate for breast examination. Doppler techniques are able to demonstrate the blood supply to lesions accurately, particularly when 'contrast' media are employed. It is thus possible to suggest a diagnosis of malignancy or benignity.

It is extremely doubtful whether Doppler examination alone can ever give a sufficiently accurate preoperative diagnosis to determine definitive management, such as mastectomy, or to enable a lesion to be left *in situ* with absolute confidence. Modern practice demands triple assessment with imaging, clinical examination and percutaneous tissue diagnosis using FNA cytology or core biopsy. Thus Doppler techniques are not indicated when FNA or core biopsy are available, since these techniques can give accurate preoperative tissue diagnosis.

Radiologist techniques

The woman should have a full explanation of all mammographic procedures, of the immediate and delayed effects upon her, and just how and when she will learn the results of the investigation. It is of paramount importance to obtain the patient's cooperation for all radiologists' techniques, and for this reason it must be stressed that the radiologist should ensure that the patient is fully aware of what the procedure involves.

Needle insertion

It is necessary to insert a needle into the breast when a lesion is being aspirated for percutaneous tissue diagnosis by cytology or histology, or when an impalpable lesion is being marked prior to surgical biopsy or excision. No needle should be inserted until both the clinician and the radiologist involved in the triple assessment have completed their examinations. The technique chosen for needle insertion should be the easiest for the operator and most comfortable for the woman (Table 23.2). Ultrasound guidance is the most accurate method, since both the needle tip and the lesion can be identified on the real-time image. One can then be absolutely certain that any material aspirated actually comes from the lesion.

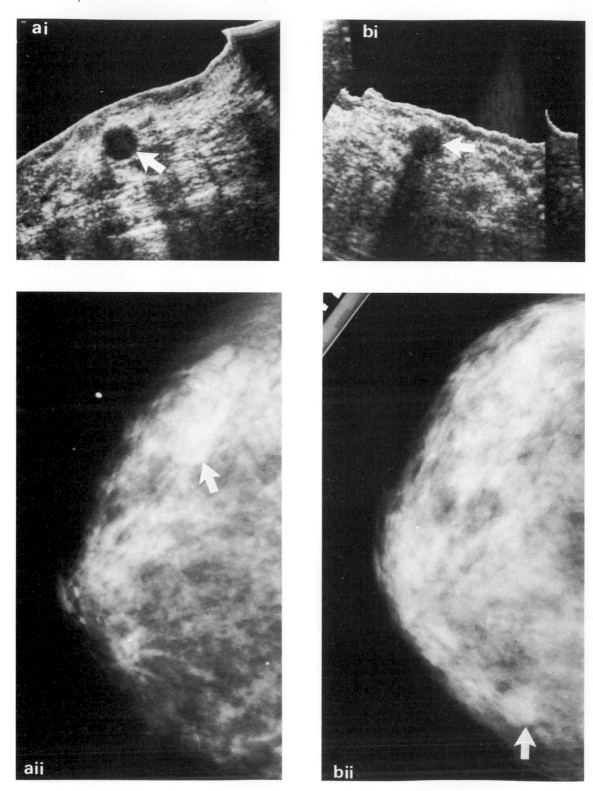

Fig. 23.7 Ultrasonography of breast lesions with corresponding mammograms: (a) cyst, (b) fibroadenoma.

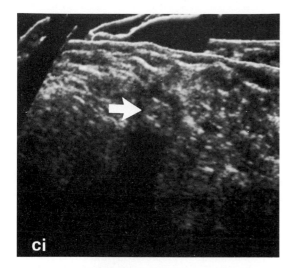

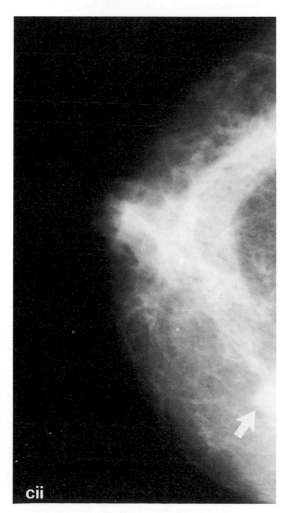

Fig. 23.7 *Continued.* (c) carcinoma.

The techniques for needle insertion are detailed on pp. 382–3.

Preoperative tissue diagnosis

Indications

Should a preoperative tissue diagnosis prove to be malignant then definitive, one-stage surgical treatment can be instituted, together with axillary surgery. This avoids the need for a preliminary excision biopsy and the inevitable wait for results which increases patient anxiety. It also avoids the dangers of relying on frozen section diagnosis. Should a diagnosis of benignity be obtained then, always provided that the woman agrees, a lesion may be safely left *in situ*, thus avoiding unnecessary surgery.

The preoperative differentiation between ductal carcinoma *in situ* (DCIS) and invasive cancer is of some importance, since in the presence of invasive disease it is common practice for axillary surgery to be undertaken to establish the prognosis by the demonstration or absence of affected lymph nodes. In some centres the axillary surgery is limited to node sampling, which has a very low morbidity rate, and in some of these centres sampling may be performed irrespective of whether invasion has been shown preoperatively or not. This avoids a second operation in those women who are subsequently shown to have areas of carcinoma with invasion. In other centres a full axillary clearance is considered necessary to establish the prognosis. This procedure carries a higher morbidity rate than simple sampling. It must be remembered that axillary surgery of any type is for prognostic and not therapeutic reasons: it does not influence the occurrence of distant metastases.

There are two procedures to establish an accurate preoperative tissue diagnosis: FNA for cytology and core biopsy. Together they are the linchpins of breast diagnosis. FNA is the aspiration of material into a fine needle for cytological examination. Core biopsy, the needle aspiration of a core of material, has the advantage of producing a specimen adequate for histological examination. The choice between the two techniques depends upon the local expertise available. To have a successful FNA service it is essential that a cytologist trained in breast cytology is a member of

Table 23.2 Indications for different methods of needle insertion

Indication	Method
A palpable lesion	Free-hand insertion
Repeat examination of a palpable lesion with an unexpected first result	Ultrasound guidance
An impalpable lesion a) visible on ultrasound b) not visible on ultrasound	Ultrasound guidance X-ray guidance

the team. If this is not the case, then it is easier for a general pathologist to interpret the histological specimen obtained by core biopsy. FNA and core biopsy are really complementary investigations. However, because of available local expertise, they have developed to become alternatives. Both techniques should be practised in the context of triple assessment.

FNA can never indicate if aspirated cancerous cells come from an area of *in situ* carcinoma or from invasive disease. Core biopsy may demonstrate invasion but when *in situ* carcinoma is found, the presence of invasive disease in areas away from the sampled site can never be excluded.

When obtaining samples by either FNA or core biopsy it should be remembered that typical cells are most likely to be obtained from the periphery of lesions. The centre of a lesion may well be necrotic or fibrotic. With expert aspiration and interpretation, accuracy rates of over 95% with less than 1% false positive rates are achievable.

In every case the pathologist should be given full information regarding the indications for the examination, otherwise it may be impossible to avoid a degree of equivocation in the subsequent report.

Factors influencing the choice between core biopsy and FNA for cytology are as follows.
1 Availability of local pathologist's expertise.
2 Mass lesions (FNA).
3 Microcalcifications (core biopsy).
4 Architectural distortions (core biopsy).

Complications of core biopsy and FNA

The patient is more likely to feel faint or experience actual syncope if the radiologist is less experienced. To avoid these problems both the radiologist and the radiographer should approach the procedure with

confidence, and the woman should have been fully informed regarding the technique to be adopted.

There is no doubt that both FNA and core biopsy do cause significant pain. This will be a less significant problem if the woman is fully informed and co-operative. Even so, it is preferable to employ local anaesthesia for both procedures. In order to minimize bruising it is preferable to use a local anaesthetic solution containing adrenaline. Pain is not uncommonly experienced as some lesions are actually being penetrated, and for core biopsy it is therefore advantageous to infiltrate down to the level of the lesion. For FNA, infiltration of the target area should be avoided if possible, otherwise local anaesthetic fluid will be aspirated at the expense of cellular material. There is little doubt that a mechanical 'gun' core biopsy apparatus causes less discomfort when it is fired than does one which is manually operated.

Both FNA and core biopsy cause bruising at the operative site. It is advantageous for a surgeon to see the woman prior to either procedure, otherwise the characteristics of the lesion are likely to be obscured by haematoma. Similarly, surgeons should be dissuaded from needling lesions prior to imaging.

Aspiration for cytology

Techniques (Table 23.2)

Freehand technique

The lesion is held firmly between the finger and thumb of one hand. A fine needle (22 or 23 gauge) is attached to a syringe. Negative pressure is applied either by means of a specially designed syringe holder or by extending the syringe plunger using the thumb. Alternatively the needle may be connected to the syringe by a plastic 'angiographic' connector tube, and the negative pressure applied by an assistant. The operator passes the needle back and forth through the lesion three or four times in one direction, rotating it as it is being advanced. The needle tip is then withdrawn to the surface of the lesion, the direction is changed by a few degrees and a further three of four passes are made. This whole procedure is repeated three or four times or until aspirated material appears in the transparent plastic adjacent to the needle. The negative pressure is then released, the needle withdrawn, and the aspirated material expressed onto a microscope slide for spreading, air drying and subsequent staining. Alternatively, depending upon the cytologist's preference, the material may be expressed into a buffered solution. Manual pressure should be applied to the puncture site in order to minimize haematoma formation.

Ultrasound guidance

Good acoustic coupling is essential and can be easily achieved by wetting the surface of the skin with antiseptic solution. If the operator or the woman desires local anaesthesia, then it is only the skin and subcutaneous tissue which should be infiltrated unless the woman complains of pain as the needle is passed more deeply. A transducer is placed above the lesion so that a satisfactory image is obtained. A fine needle (21–23 gauge) is attached by an angiographic connector to a syringe held by an assistant. The finer the needle the better the cellular harvest, but it is more difficult to manipulate a very pliable needle, particularly in the case of deep lesions which require a longer needle track. The needle is inserted adjacent to the end of the transducer and advanced obliquely along the plane of the image until the tip can be visualized adjacent to the lesion. Negative pressure is then applied, and repeated passes are made through the lesion as in the freehand technique described above. To minimize haematoma formation, manual pressure should be applied to the puncture site. The procedure may be simplified when using some machines which are equipped with a needle guide attached to the transducer.

X-ray guidance

For maximum accuracy stereotactic apparatus is desirable. Failing this, good results may be obtained using a perforated compression plate. The manufacturer's instructions should be consulted for details of operation. Several types of stereotactic apparatus are now marketed as attachments to the mammographic apparatus. They all work on the same principles.

1 Two exposures are made on one radiograph with movement of the tube and film. In one design the tube and patients are moved between the two exposures.

2 Measurements are made between a baseline marker and the target point of the lesion on each of the two images. A special viewer with cursors is supplied as part of the stereotactic set.

3 A small computer is used to undertake a mathematical computation of these measurements, knowing the distance of movement and the length of the needle to be used.

4 This computation is used to position a needle guide.

5 The depth measurement is increased sufficiently to ensure that the needle passes through to the periphery of the lesion.

6 Local anaesthetic is infiltrated into the skin and subcutaneous tissue.

7 The needle is introduced to the level of the near surface of the lesion.

8 A check stereotactic film should be taken to confirm the needle position.

9 Negative pressure is applied as described above.

10 Four or five passes are made through the lesion, or until aspirated material appears in the needle hub. The negative pressure is released, the needle withdrawn, and the aspirated material placed on a slide or in buffered solution.

11 The needle guide position is changed so that a different part of the lesion may be aspirated, and the procedure is repeated.

12 The aspiration is repeated until four or five separate needles have been used. One set of aspirations should be made through the centre of the lesion, and four from the periphery of each quadrant.

13 Manual pressure is applied to minimize haematoma formation.

Core biopsy

Indications

A core biopsy may be undertaken as an alternative to FNA, when the level of local expertise is such that this is more appropriate. It may also be indicated in specific cases where histology is required, such as in a case presenting with calcification suspected to be associated with DCIS. If DCIS is associated with invasive cancer, then the details of surgical management will differ with axillary surgery to establish the prognosis. FNA can identify cancer cells, but cannot distinguish between those which are aspirated from DCIS and those from invasive carcinoma, whereas a core biopsy may well identify invasion of cancer cells into the surrounding tissues.

If FNA has provided an acellular sample, then core biopsy may be undertaken as the next step in preference to open surgical biopsy.

Technique

Insertion of a core biopsy needle to a lesion may be achieved freehand or with ultrasound or X-ray guidance. The techniques for these are as described above.

There are a variety of special needles designed to obtain cores of tissue for histological examination. Cores obtained with finer needles tend to fragment. The larger the needle, the better core for the pathologist to examine, but the more damage to the breast and the greater the resultant haematoma. The compromise should be discussed with the pathologist.

All the different types of needle are operated on the same principles:

1 The needle is 'cocked' and inserted to the near surface of the lesion.
2 The needle is fired, either by a spring loaded trigger or manually.
3 The core is protected, sometimes automatically, sometimes by advancing a sleeve down the needle shaft.
4 The needle is withdrawn.
5 Manual pressure is applied to minimize haematoma formation.
6 When the target contains calcifications, an X-ray of the core should be taken to confirm that a representative sample has been obtained.

7 The specimen is placed into a buffered solution for subsequent fixation and staining.
8 When the procedure has been taken under ultrasound guidance, the core site can be visualized. A hard copy image of this will provide a record that the sample was obtained from the correct site.

When a mechanical biopsy gun is used, the patient should be told about the noise it will produce, otherwise she may move during the procedure.

Localization of a lesion for biopsy

Indications

All impalpable lesions which require excision or surgical biopsy.

Technique

Preoperative localization may be achieved by one of three basic methods.

1 The injection of a mixture of a radiographic contrast medium and a coloured dye into the lesion.
2 The injection of carbon granules into the lesion.
3 The passing of a marker wire into the lesion.

It is the latter method which is the most widely adopted. A variety of marker wires are in use, and the one to be used should be chosen in consultation with the surgeon who has to remove the marked specimen and the pathologist who has to remove the specimen from the marker without causing damage to the tissues.

All methods necessitate the insertion of a needle, and the techniques for this are identical to those used to insert a needle for aspiration for cytology. The marker wire should be inserted through the needle so that its tip is ideally just deep to the lesion. The needle is removed, leaving the marker wire *in situ* (Fig. 23.8). Great care is necessary in sliding the needle from over the marker wire, otherwise there is a possibility that the wire will be displaced from the chosen position.

Cyst aspiration and pneumocystography

Indications

Aspiration of simple cysts is not necessary unless

they are giving rise to problems due to the inconvenience of size or position. Some women may demand aspiration in order to satisfy themselves that the diagnosis is correct and to ensure that the cyst has disappeared. In this latter instance, it is a great advantage to aspirate the cyst under real-time ultrasound control and allow the woman to see the cyst disappear. The only medical reason for cyst aspiration is a suspicion that there is a complication such as a cyst papilloma or intracystic carcinoma. Ultrasound will usually solve this problem, but pneumocystography can also identify or exclude the presence of an intracystic lesion.

Technique

The technique of needle introduction is identical to that adopted for the insertion of a needle for any other procedure, and can be accomplished either free-hand or under ultrasound guidance. Once the needle is inserted into the lumen of the cyst, the fluid is gently aspirated to dryness. If a pneumocystogram is to be performed the needle is left *in situ*, care being taken not to change its position. A volume of air is introduced, equal to that of fluid aspirated.

Reference above has been to cyst fluid, but not frequently cyst contents are remarkably viscous, and may even be cheese-like in consistency. In these circumstances aspiration may prove difficult or even impossible. A wider bore needle should be tried as the next step should this problem be encountered. It is a waste of time to send cyst fluid for pathological examination as a matter of routine. Only if the cyst fluid contains altered blood is there any real likelihood of a positive pathological finding. Fresh blood is usually an incidental contaminant.

'Surgical' pneumocystogram

Surgical colleagues should be instructed that, should they obtain a bloody cyst aspirate, the needle should be left *in situ*, the syringe refilled with air, and a volume of air equal to that of the aspirate injected into the cyst. Mammograms taken within an hour or so will give satisfactory pneumocystogram pictures.

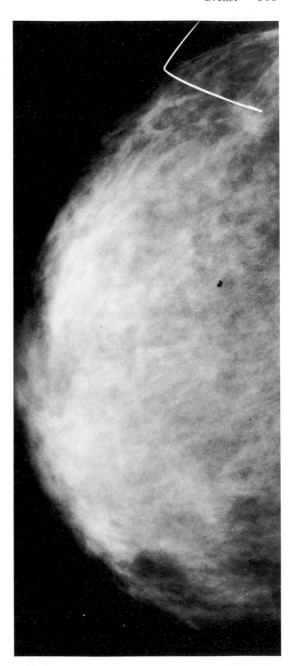

Fig. 23.8 Marker wire *in situ*.

Ductography

Indications

Demonstration of the lactiferous ducts (galactography)

is undertaken in patients with a persistent single-duct discharge of any type. It is a fallacy to believe that carcinoma is only associated with a bloody discharge: it can be serous, clear or yellow. It is the fact that the discharge is from one duct which makes a diagnosis of carcinoma possible, but not likely. In some centres ductography is no longer practised since it has been found that, in the absence of a mammographic abnormality, it is extremely unlikely to detect a carcinoma. Only one small focus of DCIS was detected in a mammographically normal group of 250 cases of single-duct discharge treated with microductectomy (Locker *et al.*, 1998). Modern high-resolution ultrasound is proving to be a non-invasive alternative for the examination of suspect ducts.

Technique

Following antiseptic cleaning of the nipple, the sus-pect duct is gently dilated with a Nettleship dilator. Between 0.5 and 1 ml of water-soluble contrast medium is slowly injected through a fine sialography or dacrocystographic cannula. Alternatively, a dacrocystogram or sialography set with plastic catheters may be used. The injection is terminated when the patient experiences a feeling of intramammary pressure or pain. The cannula is removed and immediately the duct orifice is blocked with collodium or nobecutane. Craniocaudal and lateral films are taken (Fig. 23.9). Following inspection of these complementary projections may be required.

Other modalities

Digital mammography

Digital mammography is of two types: secondary digital mammography where a standard mammo-

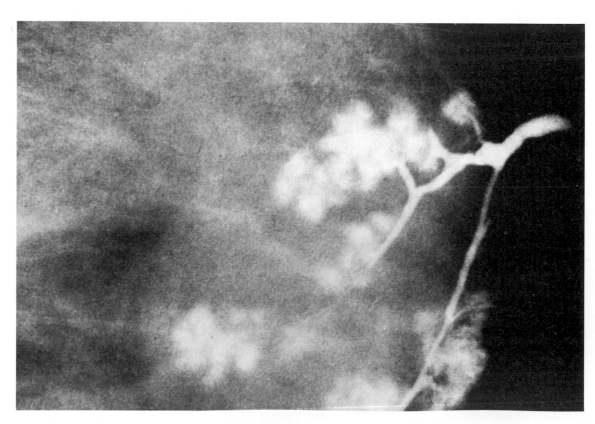

Fig. 23.9 Normal ductogram showing terminal ductolobular units.

graphic image is digitized, and primary digital mammography where there is no intermediate film image. Monitors to demonstrate the images are currently very expensive. There seems, at present, little economic value in secondary digitization in view of the cost, the extra time required to produce the images, and the increase in time taken to man-ipulate the images related to any increase in diagnostic ability which is thereby gained.

Primary digital mammography is a direct digital acquisition technique using the principle of photostimulable phosphor luminescence. An image plate of a phosphor material is exposed to X-rays using the same exposure and positioning techniques as for conventional X-ray mammography. A latent image, typically 1770 × 2370 pixels in size, with each pixel measuring 100 μm, is thereby produced on the plate. This digital image may be displayed on a monitor and/or printed onto laser hard copy. Given appropriate computer facilities the image may be manipulated to window various grey scale ranges or highlight selected features. The quality of this technique is comparable to conventional film/screen mammography in terms of both physical measurements and subjective assessment by experienced radiologists. It is a matter of cost comparison which will determine the rate at which the technique becomes adopted.

A digital mammogram has several theoretical advantages. The image may be manipulated to enhance various features, for instance, contrast in a particular area. Specific features, such as calcification, may be highlighted. Digital archive results in economy of space and rapid retrieval. The images may be transmitted 'instantaneously' over a distance, giving the possibility of remote case conference activities. Computer-assisted diagnosis may take two forms. Specific diagnostically important features may be highlighted for a trained observer. With the aid of a computer memory or neural network, diagnostically important features may be identified, classified and a diagnosis be made purely automatically. As a step towards this very remote objective, it has been suggested that mammograms be sorted into those which may be abnormal, and those which are not. The radiologist then views those designated as abnormal. The great fallacy with this approach is that the spectrum of normality is very much greater than of abnormality. The best mammographic radiologists

are those with a large experience of normal cases and who have the facility readily to recognize normality. Deprive a radiologist of the experience to develop and maintain this facility and there will be a loss of interpretative expertise.

Magnetic resonance imaging (MRI)

MRI has now an established role in breast disease diagnosis and management. It cannot yet be regarded as a primary tool, and in comparison with high quality mammography it has no place as a first investigation. However, MRI is excellent for the solution of specific problems. With gadolinium enhancement a confident differentiation can be made between postoperative fibrosis and recurrence of carcinoma. It is necessary to study the time over which gadolinium enhancement occurs and persists. Rapid enhancement indicates malignancy; slow development up to a plateau suggests a benign lesion. A further indication for MRI is in the investigation of bone — particularly spinal — lesions thought to be metastases.

The disadvantages of MRI are the cost of the apparatus and the value of the technique in other specialist fields which inevitably leads to restricted access. Moreover, specific breast coils are required to obtain high quality MRI images of the breast. It seems likely that breast MRI techniques will only become widely practised when dedicated MRI mammographic apparatus is available, which presumably will not be until manufacturers have saturated the market with expensive multipurpose machines.

References

Feig, S.A. (1979) Epidemiology of radiation related breast cancer. *In* Logan, W.W. & Muntz, E.P. (eds) *Reduced Dose Mammography*, pp. 9–19. Masson Publishing, New York.

Guyer, P.B. & Dewbury, K.C. (1987) *Sonomammography — An Atlas of Comparative Breast Ultrasound*. John Wiley, Chichester.

Hanss, A.G., Metz., C.E., Chiles, J.T. & Rossman, K. (1976) The effect of X-ray spectra from molybdenum and tungsten target tubes on image quality in mammography. *Radiology*, **118**, 705–9.

Locker, A.P., Galea, M.H., Elston, C.W. *et al.* (1988) A review of microductectomy for single duct nipple discharge. *Br. J. Clin. Prac.*, **42** (Suppl.), 77.

Lundgren, B. & Jackobsson, S. (1976) Single view mammography: a simple and efficient approach to breast screening. *Cancer*, **38**, 1124–9.

Meredith, W.J. & Massey, J.B. (1979) *Fundamental Physics of Radiology*, pp. 674–83. John Wright, Bristol.

Rizzato, G., Chersavani, R. Solbiati, L. & Derchi, L.E. (1992) High resolution sonography of breast ducts. *Radiology*, **185** (P), 378.

Wolfe, J.N. (1967) A study of breast parenchyma by mammography in the normal woman and those with benign and malignant disease. *Radiology*, **89**, 201–5.

Further reading

Aichinger, H. & Sabel, M. (1993) *X-ray Spectra and Image Quality in Mammography*. Siemens AG, Medical Engineering Group, Erlangen.

Brettle, D.S., Ward., S.C., Parkin, G.L.S. *et al.* (1994) A clinical comparison between conventional and digital mammography utilizing computed radiography. *Br. J. Radiol.*, **67**, 464–8.

Feig, S.A. (1983) Assessment of the hypothetical risk from mammography and evaluation of the potential benefit. *Radiol. Clin. N. Am.*, **21**, 173–91.

Frank, H.A., Hall. F.M. & Steer, M.L. (1976) Preoperative localisation of non-palpable breast lesions demonstrated by mammography. *N. Engl. J. Med.*, **295**, 259–60.

Gros, C.M., Quenneville, Y. & Hammel, Y. (1972) Diaphanography, in a complementary role. *J. Radiol. Electr. Med. Nucl.*, **53**, 297.

Heindsieck, R., Laurencin, G., Ponchon, A. *et al.* (1993) *Dual Target (Molybdenum/Rhodium) X-ray Tubes for Mammographic Applications: dose reduction with image quality equivalent to standard mammographic tubes*. General Electric, France.

Hickman, P.F., Moore, N.R. & Shepstone, B.J. (1994) The indeterminate breast mass: assessment using contrast enhanced magnetic resonance imaging. *Br. J. Radiol.*, **67**, 14–30.

Preece, P.E., Gravelle, I.H., Hughes, L.E. *et al.* (1977) The operative management of subclinical breast cancer. *Clin. Oncol.*, **3** 165–9.

Roebuck, E.J. (1990) *Clinical Radiology of the Breast*. Heinemann, Oxford.

Sickles, E.A. (1988) Further experience with micro-focal spot magnification in the assessment of clustered breast microcalcifications. *Radiology*, **137**, 9–14.

Tabal, L., Dean, P.B. & Penek, Z. (1983) Galactography: the diagnostic procedure of choice for nipple discharge. *Radiology*, **149**, 31–8.

Tohno, E., Cosgrove, D.O. & Sloane, J.P. (1993) *Ultrasound Diagnosis of Breast Disease*. Churchill Livingstone, London.

Wellings, S.R. & Wolfe, J.N. (1978) Correlative studies of the histological and radiographic appearance of the breast parenchyma. *Radiology*, **129**, 299–306.

24　Paediatric Radiology

R.K. LEVICK AND A. SPRIGG

General principles

Heat loss

Neonates and infants lose body heat rapidly, the risk of hypothermia being greatest in the premature baby with little subcutaneous fat. Local warmth may be obtained by special table-top heating cradles, but the most convenient way of avoiding heat loss is to maintain a room temperature of about 27°C in the X-ray room. A room thermometer is an important piece of equipment. Enhanced humidity is not normally required for the duration of an X-ray examination.

Radiation dosage

It is good practice to limit the dose of ionizing radiation to the patient as much as possible. Gonad protection is important. Image intensification and dynamic recording on videotape must be available for screening procedures. A very important principle, which may reduce the radiation dose by as much as 50%, is gridless screening. Infants under 1 year of age are always examined with the explorator grid removed, there being little scatter and no appreciable loss of detail. When fine detail such as a mucosal pattern is not required, gridless screening may be used in children up to 5 years of age.

Special X-ray equipment

Screening equipment is available which is designed specifically for the examination of infants and children. It is not always possible to accommodate older children on such apparatus. Cradle holding devices are provided which enable the infant to be rotated in relation to the table top. When this type of equipment is not available, views such as the prone shoot-through swallow for tracheo-oesophageal fistula may be obtained by using a device such as the Charteris baby holder inverted on the step of an upright adult screening table.

Sedation

Sedation may be necessary for some procedures described in this and other chapters. The timing of sedation, transport to the X-ray room and of the procedure need careful coordination. Drugs employed must be agreed with the local paediatricians and anaesthetists and are normally given after 4 hours' starvation. The child should be accompanied by a trained children's nurse. Peripheral monitoring of oxygen saturation is preferred as a further safeguard. Babies and infants under 6 months of age will often sleep after a feed and may not need sedation unless they are known to be restless, or the procedure is painful. The authors use quinalbarbitone in the dosages listed in Table 24.1.

Venous access produces less disturbance if a cannula is put in place after the area has been treated with a topical gel. Two possible areas are prepared with anaesthetic gel about 30 min before injection. Small gauge needles are used, often 25 gauge: warming of contrast medium makes injection through fine needles easier.

Upper gastrointestinal tract

Contrast study for tracheo-oesophageal fistula

Indications

To define a suspected fistula without oesophageal atresia, or a recurrent or second fistula after operation. Recurrent chest infections and air distension of the stomach and bowel may have raised the possibility of tracheo-oesophageal fistula.

Table 24.1 Dosages for quinalbarbitone mg kg^{-1}

Weight (kg)	Dose (mg)
6–<7	50
7–<10	75
10–<15	100
15–<17	150
17–<20	175
Over 20	200

Technique

Contrast medium is injected into the oesophagus with the baby positioned face down (Fig. 24.1). Screening, spot radiographs and video-recording are carried out in a prone shoot-through position. A nasogastric tube such as a 6 French (F) tube or umbilical cannula is passed to the fundus of the stomach. A rapid injection of 3 ml non-ionic low-osmolality water-soluble contrast is made whilst the catheter is withdrawn. This is observed on the VDU and recorded by spot films with video back-up (Fig. 24.2). Once contrast medium is seen in the trachea, further injections will not distinguish between a fistula and aspiration; with a clear

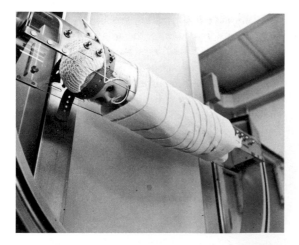

Fig. 24.1 Barium examination for tracheobronchial fistula, cradle method. The screening table is erect and the child is held face-down in the cradle after the passage of a nasogastric tube.

trachea, further injections may be made if necessary. If a safe water-soluble contrast medium is not available, a 1 : 3 dilution of non-high-density barium with water should be used. Ionic water-soluble contrast media produce pulmonary oedema if aspirated, and must not be used.

Complications

Contrast medium may be aspirated through the larynx or a fistula. Suction equipment must be available and expert resuscitation at hand. Cardiac arrest is know to have occurred during oesophageal filling and may be prevented by warming the contrast medium.

Barium swallow for reflux and hiatus hernia

Indications

Recurrent blood-stained vomiting suggests a serious oesophagitis with a risk of stricture formation.

Technique

A 1 : 3 aqueous dilution of non-high-density barium, sweetened with sucrose, is given from a normal feeding bottle and teat. The sucking and swallowing mechanisms are observed. If the feed is not taken, an 8F umbilical cannula is threaded through a flanged teat with about 1 cm catheter tip projecting (Fig. 24.3), and barium is injected slowly through the catheter. Not more than 10 ml barium is given. Oesophageal peristalsis is observed and the manner of closure at the cardia after each bolus is recorded. The baby is then turned prone oblique, left side up, and gastric emptying observed before the stomach is too full to see the pylorus through the empty fundus. If emptying is normal, the baby is turned to the opposite prone oblique position in order to pool barium in the fundus. Evidence of gastro-oesophageal reflux and/or hiatus hernia is sought during episodes of crying (Fig. 24.4), which may be produced by gentle plantar tickling, and during further swallowing of barium. Video-recording is of great help for the later slow-motion analysis and reduces screening time.

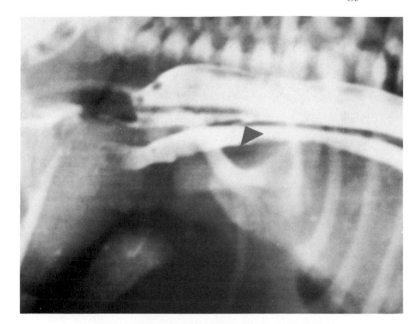

Fig. 24.2 A shoot-through spot radiograph taken during the injection of barium through a tube into the baby's oesophagus. A hairline fistula (arrow) runs upwards and anteriorly from the oesophagus to the lower cervical trachea.

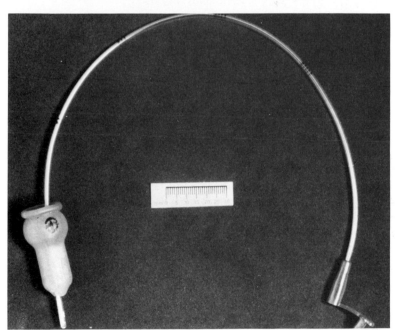

Fig. 24.3 A simple teat and catheter system for barium swallow examinations in babies. The catheter should be cemented to the teat or a wide flanged teat used to prevent the possibility of accidental swallowing of the teat.

Complications

Suction must be available in case of aspiration.

Alternative examinations

While oesophagitis is assessed by endoscopy, the barium swallow is necessary to show reflux and hia-

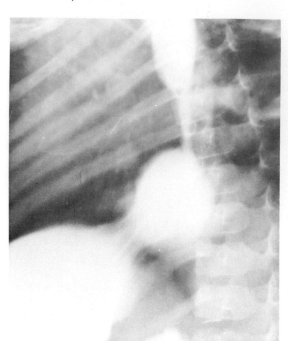

Fig. 24.4 The infant's stomach has been filled with barium. Whilst lying prone oblique, crying produces an intermittent hiatus hernia. There is gastro-oesophageal reflux and lower oesophageal spasm due to oesophagitis.

tus hernia. Isotope studies are used to show that aspiration of gastric contents is a cause of recurrent pneumonia.

Pyloric obstruction

Ultrasound examination

This is carried out with a short focus 5 MHz probe, real-time technique. The examination is performed after a feed of clear fluid which allows better definition of the antrum and of the canal length (Fig. 24.5). The Sheffield pyloric muscle index relates muscle mass to body weight and has a high discriminatory value (Carver *et al.*, 1988). The canal is measured in length and diameter; the whole pyloric image including muscle and canal is similarly measured. The total mass minus the canal volume is the muscle mass.

Alternative examinations

Barium examination is reserved for infants with a typical clinical presentation of pyloric obstruction but without a palpable tumour (Fig. 24.6).

The examination is commenced as described for reflux and hiatus hernia. It may be found that

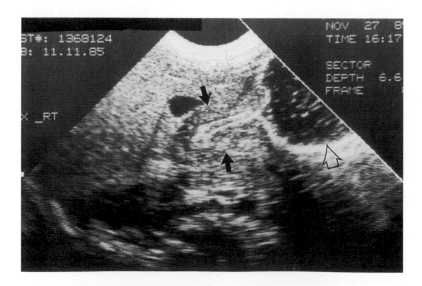

Fig. 24.5 Pyloric stenosis. Longitudinal ultrasound scan through the liver. The thickened elongated pyloric muscle (between solid arrows) is seen behind the gallbladder. The gastric antrum (open arrow) is filled with fluid residue.

emptying of the stomach is slow, especially if the baby is upset when feeding is stopped. The use of a dummy will often hasten pyloric relaxation. Glucagon, 1 μg kg⁻¹ body weight i.v., may be employed to overcome pylorospasm. The pylorus must be seen to open widely to exclude functional stenosis.

Malrotation

This is a possible cause of high small bowel obstruction and should be excluded in cases of bile-stained vomiting. It can also be partial or recurrent and produce malabsorption by partial obstruction of the venous return with bowel oedema. With the barium technique it is important to record the first bolus of barium passing through the duodenum. The duodenojejunal flexure must lie to the left of the spine in anteroposterior (AP) projection and at the level of the pylorus.

Ultrasound may be used to demonstrate the presence or absence of small-bowel malrotation (Fig. 24.7). A transverse section at pancreatic level shows the mesenteric vessels. Normally the superior me-

Use dilute barium
Keep room warm

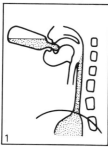

Right side down
  laterally
Lateral oesophagus
Aspiration
Nasopharynx escape

Take film 1

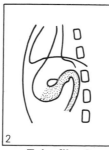

Right side down
  laterally
Gastric outlet
Duodenum 2 filled
Outlet seen through
  gas-filled fundus
Stop feeding

Take film 2

In rapid sequence

Turn baby supine
Antrum, duodenum 2 filled ⟶
D-J flexure obscured

Turn baby left side down
Barium in fundus and ⟶
duodenum 3

Turn baby supine straight
  anteroposterior
Barium in fundus and
  duodenum 3/4
D-J flexure seen through
  gas-filled antrum
  (provided baby not given
  excess barium)

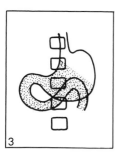

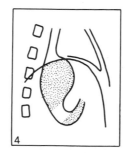

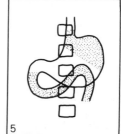

Take film 3

After the position of the D-J flexure has been determined, detailed gastric views can be taken as needed. Anteroposterior view of oesophagus (**take film 4**). Take baby off table. Give full volume barium 'feed', burp baby erect. Wait .....
Reflux: Check oesophagus is clear, check for reflux. Document level and clearing. Follow through as necessary to check small bowel or caecal position

Fig. 24.6 Paediatric barium technique.

senteric vein lies to the right of the superior mesenteric artery, but in malrotation it lies anterior or to the left of the artery. In vomiting infants ultrasound will show or exclude pyloric stenosis and malrotation or may show a non-gastrointestinal cause, for example renal.

Lower gastrointestinal tract

Contrast enema for distal bowel obstruction

Indications

Distal bowel obstruction which is not due to anorectal anomalies.

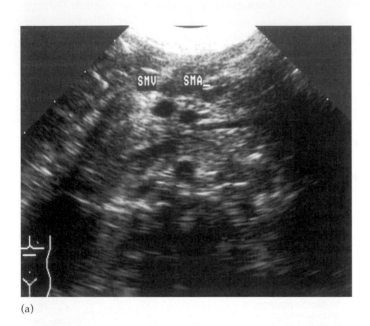

(a)

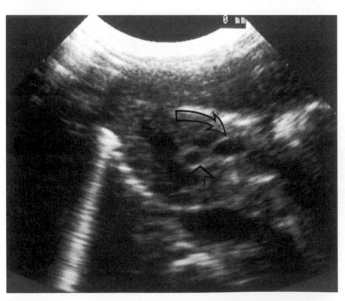

(b)

Fig. 24.7 Malrotation. Transverse ultrasound scan of the upper abdomen. (a) Normal scan. The superior mesenteric vein (SMV) lies to the right of the superior mesenteric artery (SMA). (b) Malrotation. The SMV (curved arrow) has been rotated to lie to the left of the SMA (straight arrow).

General considerations

It is important to choose the correct type of contrast medium (Levick, 1972). When there is no definite diagnosis and the level of obstruction is uncertain, a diagnostic enema may be carried out using a nearly isotonic water-soluble contrast medium such as 25% sodium diatrizoate or, alternatively, a non-ionic water-soluble contrast agent. When meconium ileus obstruction is to be relieved, a hypertonic contrast medium such as Gastrografin is needed. Finally, if Hirschprung's disease is probable, barium is used so that delayed films may be obtained at up to 24 hours.

Technique

A soft rubber catheter of about 5 mm outside diameter is passed into the rectum and retained with strapping or by a suitably protected assistant holding the buttocks together. In a diagnostic situation, a pressure head of about 30.5 cm (1 ft) is employed in case compromised bowel is present. If a firm diagnosis of meconium ileus is then reached, a hypertonic contrast medium is substituted with a pressure head of up to 1 m (3 ft). Similarly, if a corkscrew or narrow segment is seen, barium is then used for presumed Hirschsprung's disease.

Complications

Bowel perforation is always possible, so isotonic contrast and low hydrostatic pressure are used if this risk is thought to exist and an examination is still necessary. The use of hypertonic contrast medium in the relief of meconium ileus and milk inspissation is known to produce a considerable shift of tissue fluid into the bowel with a risk of serious dehydration. This type of enema should only be carried out when fluid is already being given.

Diagnostic and therapeutic barium enema for intussusception

Indications

Clinical findings, plain radiograph and ultrasound confirmation of intussusception. The length of history and the passage of blood per rectum are not contraindications provided the child's condition is satisfactory.

Contraindications

Shock, peritoneal rebound tenderness, plain radiograph findings of perforation or of small-bowel obstruction.

General considerations

The high success rate of reduction and low incidence of complication noted in various centres is mainly due to proper selection of patients. No infant who is shocked or has signs of peritoneal irritation or plain radiographic evidence of small-bowel obstruction should have an attempted enema reduction. Selection should be made by the paediatric surgeon together with the radiologist (Levick, 1970).

Technique

Relaxation is the key to good results and sedation is usually necessary before attempting hydrostatic reduction. Heavy sedation with morphine is used and does not complicate a general anaesthetic if surgical reduction is required. The enema of a 1 : 3 aqueous dilution of barium is warmed to body temperature and run in through a soft non-lubricated catheter of 5–10 mm diameter. The catheter is retained in the rectum by manual compression of the buttocks by an assistant working over a lead–rubber sheet, who may also steady the infant's legs with his other hand. The diagnosis is confirmed with a pressure head of not more than 30.5 cm (1 ft). Reduction is then attempted with a pressure of not more than 1 m (3 ft). Pressure is maintained for up to 5 min and the attempt may be repeated once or twice, provided there is no deterioration of the child's condition. Ideally, barium should be seen to enter the small bowel. It is important to obtain a post-evacuation film at about 10 min as a recurrence is occasionally found.

Barium reduction under fluoroscopic control is still the most widely practised technique (Figs 24.8 & 24.9). However, air reduction, first described by Fiorito and Cuesta in 1959, has gained some popu-

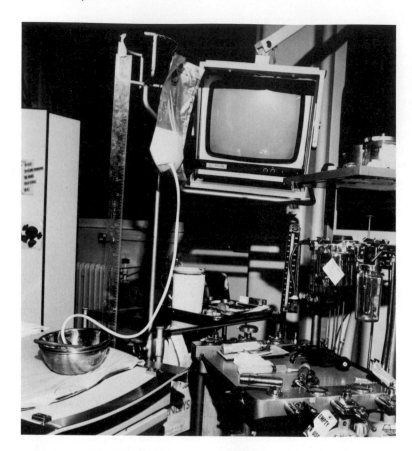

Fig. 24.8 The screening room prepared for attempted enema reduction of an intussusception. The level of barium in the reservoir is about 80 cm above the table top.

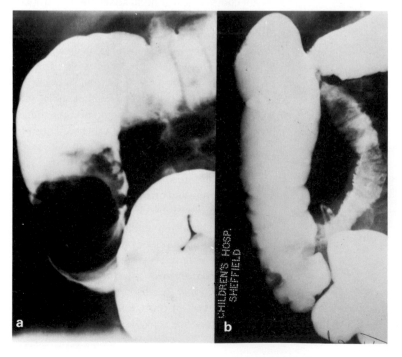

Fig. 24.9 (a) The intussusception has been reduced to the caecum, where the mass and 'coil spring' appearance is visible. (b) A few seconds later reduction is complete and barium has entered the appendix and terminal ileum.

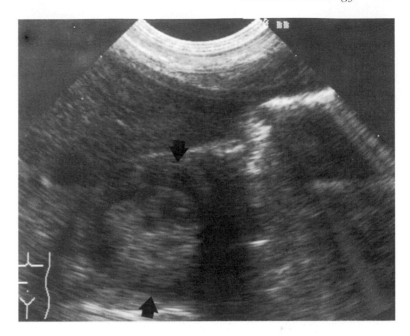

Fig. 24.10 Transverse ultrasound section of an intussusception at the hepatic flexure. It is seen as a 'doughnut' or 'target' image behind the right lobe of the liver. (between the arrrows). Intussusceptum, white; intussuscipiens, black.

larity. The success rates are little different. Neither has the advantage of ultrasound-guided reduction, which avoids radiation. Low-cost ionic contrast medium with an osmolality of about 300 mmol kg^{-1} H$_2$O is used, warmed to body temperature. Both barium and air are unsuitable as they obscure the ultrasound image. The characteristic 'doughnut' image of the intussusception is noted, which also confirms the diagnosis (Fig. 24.10). The 'doughnut' moves towards the caecal region and a streaming of contrast into the ileum is seen on reduction. The water-soluble contrast medium then enables documentation of the reduction on an abdominal radiograph.

Distal colonogram in anorectal atresia

Technique

The distal opening is identified and isotonic water-soluble contrast medium run in through a soft catheter. Lateral screening of the pelvis with a marker on the anal dimple will demonstrate the lowest point of the rectal pouch, although a distal plug of meconium may produce a temporary false higher level. Lateral and oblique views are needed to show a fis-

tula present in nearly all high lesions. If barium is used, it must be washed out to avoid subsequent concretions.

References

Bolia, A.A. (1985) Diagnosis and reduction of intussusception under ultrasound guidance: a new technique? *Clin. Radiol.*, **36**, 34.

Carver, R.A., Okorie, M., Steiner, G.M. & Dickson, J.A.S. (1988) Infantile hypertrophic pyloric stenosis diagnosis from the pyloric muscle index. *Clin. Radiol.*, **38**, 625–7.

Fiorito, E.S. & Cuestas, L.A. (1959) Diagnosis and treatment of acute intestinal intussusception with controlled inflation of air. *Paediatrics*, **42**, 241–4.

Levick, R.K. (1970) Intussusception — conservative versus surgical management. *Clin Paediat.*, **9**, 457–62.

Levick, R.K. (1972) The choice of contrast medium in neonatal obstruction. *Ann. Radiol.*, **15**, 231–6.

Contrast studies of the central nervous system

Many invasive studies of the brain and spinal cord have been replaced by magnetic resonance imaging (MRI). However, angiography and myelography are still used to road map vascular territories or when MRI facilities are limited.

Myelography in infants

Technique

General anaesthesia is advisable as the examination can be alarming. The prone approach is advised for infants under 2 years of age. The patient is laid face-down with the lumbar spine flexed over a pad (Fig. 24.11). It is important not to use too fine a needle, otherwise the dural 'give' will not be felt. A 3.8 cm (1.5 in.) 21 gauge spinal needle is suitable. The needle is screened into the spine at the 2/3 or 3/4 lumbar level and advanced until dural resistance is felt. The stylet is then withdrawn and a 2 ml syringe attached to the needle. If an attempt to aspirate cerebrospinal fluid (CSF) is unsuccessful, the needle is further advanced very slowly with aspiration until CSF is withdrawn. Dural venous blood will appear if the needle is advanced too far. It is better to postpone contrast injection for a few days if this occurs, as there will almost always be a leakage of contrast medium outside the subarachnoid space.

Having achieved a good puncture, the examination proceeds in a conventional manner. Five to eight millilitres of Niopam 200 (iopamidol, 200 mg iodine ml⁻¹) are introduced, the exact amount depending on the appearances while screening (Harwood-Nash & Fitz, 1976).

Lumbar puncture and myelography in the older child are carried out in the same way as in the adult.

Cerebral angiography in infants

Indications

Cerebrovascular malformations may require arteriography prior either to surgery or to attempted embolization. It should be noted that large lesions, such as vein of Galen 'aneurysms', can be clearly shown on contrast-enhanced computed tomography (CT) scans.

Technique

Direct puncture of the carotid or vertebral arteries is possible. A 3.8 cm (1.5 in) 21 gauge lumbar-puncture needle with a modified short bevel may be used, proprietary needles being available. However, most examinations are carried out via selective arterial catheterization. As in the adult, a straight catheter advanced from a femoral artery puncture into the dorsal aorta usually enters the left vertebral artery via the left subclavian artery. Special catheters are available in infant sizes for carotid studies. Clean femoral artery puncture is aided by a needle and stylet without an external cannula and by extending the thigh

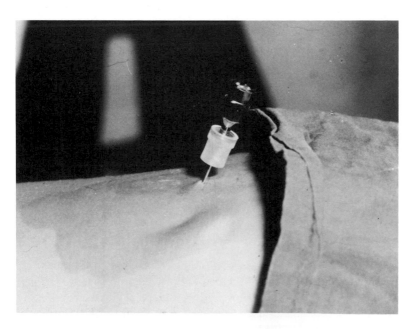

Fig. 24.11 Infant myelogram. The anaesthetized baby is placed face down over a pillow or large pad so that the lumbar spine is well flexed. Screening may used to ensure a mid-line approach.

with a pad under the buttocks to fix the rather mobile artery. Saline or local anaesthetic injected around the artery also helps to fix it in position.

Digital subtraction angiography is preferred with a reduction in contrast dose and enhanced vascular detail.

Reference

Harwood-Nash, D.C.F. & Fitz, C.R. (1976) Neurological techniques and indications in infancy and childhood. *In* Kaufman, H. (ed.) *In Progress in Paediatric Radiology*, vol. 5, pp. 49–52. Karger, Basel.

Arthrography

This investigation is usually requested for hip dysplasia in the infant. In older children, examination of the knee or shoulder is performed in the same way as in adults.

Hip arthrography in the infant

Indications

Congenital hip dislocation which does not respond to splinting, prior to operative reduction. Doubtful hip dislocations, as in infants with limited abduction, are a further indication. There is some prognostic value in Perthes' disease, but arthrography is rarely used in this condition.

Contraindications

The only major complication is septic arthritis, so that puncture should not be performed through inflamed or infected skin. Intercurrent infections in the chest or urinary tracts may increase the risk of blood-borne infection following joint puncture. Allergic reactions to contrast injection are very rare.

Technique

The examination is carried out under general anaesthesia. Adequate asepsis is essential to avoid septic arthritis. The skin is cleaned with an aqueous preparation, such as Cetavalon, and the puncture site further cleansed with iodine in spirit. The infant lies supine on the screening table with the thighs slightly abducted, flexed and externally rotated, about 10° in each direction. A short-bevel needle of 22 gauge and 3.8 cm (1.5 in.) length, with stylet, is used. Of the four different approach routes which have been described, the inferior and lateral routes have the advantage that an initial extra articular trial injection does not obscure joint detail. However, an initial trial injection of about 3 ml normal saline, after introducing the needle by any route, produces distension of the joint capsule and fluid is pushed back into the syringe when there is correct placement of the needle. The *inferior* approach is made posterior to the adductor tendon, with the needle advanced parallel to the table top. The *lateral* approach is made anterior to the greater trochanter and the needle is passed superiorly along the femoral neck. The *anterior* approach is screened directly down to the lateral border of the femoral head ossification centre. The *superior* approach is made inward and downward at 45°, screening to the same point as the anterior method. The final approach is made under screen control in all methods. Correct placement within the synovial cavity is checked with either the saline method or a small injection of contrast medium. Not more than 2 ml of water-soluble contrast medium is normally needed, the contrast agent being spread by joint movement (Fig. 24.12). Four standard spot radiographs are taken: in the neutral position, 45° abduction in both internal and external rotation, and a 'frog view' lateral. To these may be added a hyperadducted cross-over view and a 'frog view' with downward pressure on the knee. Video-recording of joint movement is of great help (Grech, 1977).

Hip ultrasound

Indications

Hip dysplasia and dislocation in the first 3 months of life. Irritable hip in the older child.

Technique

In the baby the cartilaginous margins of the acetabulum and femoral capital epiphysis are shown on scanning in the coronal plane. A linear-array probe

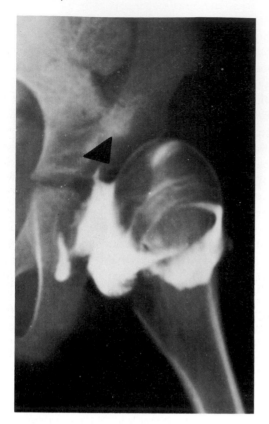

Fig. 24.12 Hip arthrogram. Unsuccessful treatment for a congenital hip dislocation. The capital epiphysis does not return to the shallow acetabulum due to the limbus (arrow).

of 5 or 7 MHz is used. Scanning over the greater trochanter with slight hip flexion is facilitated by a baby-holding device such as that designed by Graf. After 3 months, progressive ossification makes the examination difficult or impossible (Figs 24.13–24.15) (Graf & Schuler, 1986).

In the older child with a suspected irritable hip, the presence of a small effusion indicates the need for careful follow-up. The use of a 5 mHz linear-array probe positioned in the body long axis anteriorly over the femoral neck will define the curve of the femoral neck and the line of the synovial reflection. The distance between the two lines should not exceed 3 mm; a greater distance suggests an effusion.

References

Graf, R. & Schuler P. (1986) *Sonography of the Infant Hip: an*

Atlas. (Translated by T. Telger.) VCH, Weinheim.
Grech, P. (1977) Technique. *In* Grech P. (ed.) *Hip Arthrography*, pp. 15–27. Chapman & Hall, London.

Genitourinary tract

Inferior vena cavography

Indications

In the urographic examination of any intra-abdominal mass, it is good practice to combine this with an inferior vena cavogram. Opinions vary as to the value of this as a diagnostic procedure, but the small addition to normal urographic procedure is worth while.

Contraindications and complications

The risk of contrast injection are the same as those for urography, and require the usual precautions. Femoral vein puncture is not advised in infants due to the risk of septic hip arthritis.

Technique

This is usually carried out as part of the contrast injection for i.v. urography. A 21 gauge needle with flexible tube extension is inserted into a suitable ankle or foot vein and strapped in position. The system is kept open with a slow injection of normal saline. The explorator of the screening table is positioned over the pelvis and abdomen with spot radiographs in readiness. The contralateral femoral vein is compressed manually and a rapid contrast injection is made. The contrast medium is observed in the pelvic veins and inferior vena cava and spot films are then obtained. If the child is old enough, a Valsalva manoeuvre may be applied at the same time.

Cystourethrography by urethral catheterization

Indications

These include recurrent urinary tract infection and developmental abnormalities such as ectopic ureter.

Contraindications

This examination should be avoided during an acute

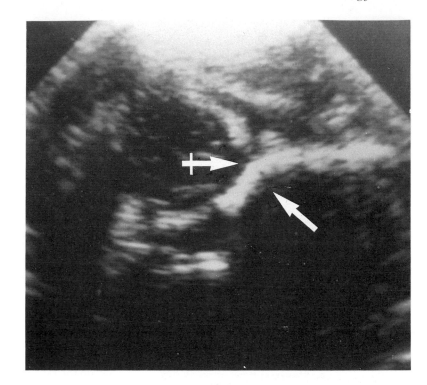

Fig. 24.13 Lateral hip scan in the neonate. There is mild dysplasia with a rounded superior bony rim of the acetabulum (arrow) and a wide cartilaginous rim (crossed arrow).

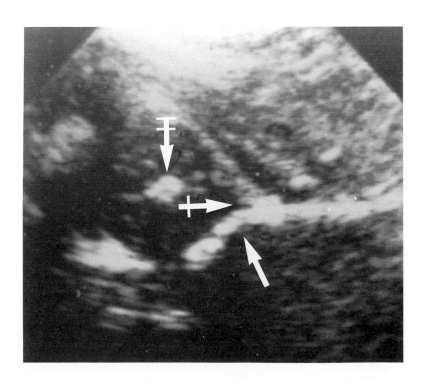

Fig. 24.14 The same infant at 2 months. The superior bony rim is now angular (arrow) and the cartilaginous rim is narrowed (crossed arrow). The appearances are now normal. Note the ossific centre in the capital epiphysis (double-crossed arrow).

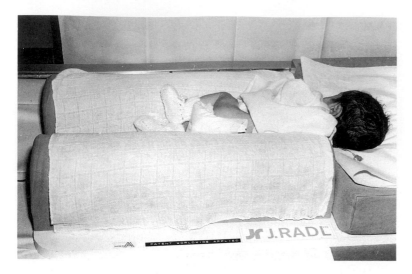

Fig. 24.15 Twin-roll baby holder designed by Graf to obtain correct position for lateral scan.

urinary infection as reflux may occur only during a cystitis.

Technique

Sedation is rarely needed. A local policy is needed in regard to antibiotic cover. The operator is scrubbed-up and gloved. The perineum and periurethral area are cleaned with a suitable aqueous antiseptic solution. A 6 or 8F umbilical feeding tube with a closed end and a side-hole is a very suitable catheter for babies. The sterile catheter is lubricated with an anaesthetic jelly prior to its introduction. Resistance due to external sphincter in boys is gently overcome, while occasionally it may be necessary to inject normal saline from a syringe whilst advancing the catheter. When the bladder has been entered, the catheter is secured with external strapping. It is good practice to obtain a urine specimen and to measure the volume of residual urine at this stage. A suitable water-soluble contrast medium is then dripped in from a container about 1 m above the table top, using a standard i.v. giving set (Fig. 24.16). Filling is continued until contrast medium begins to be passed alongside the catheter into the bladder neck and upper urethra. If the catheter is removed at this stage in infants, voiding may continue and save a long wait for spontaneous micturition. In older children, protestations of fullness may be checked by observing extension of the great toes!

Spot radiographs record the bladder shape and size, vesico–ureteric reflux if seen, and the bladder outlet and residue on voiding. The full extent of reflux should be recorded by including the top of the kidney on the radiograph to avoid missing reflux into a moiety of a duplex system. The timing of reflux, on filling, on voiding or both and the extent of reflux are of interest to the surgeon. The full extent of the urethra should be recorded in boys: anterior urethral valves or diverticula may otherwise be missed. In children with neurogenic bladders, the residue is recorded after expression. Emptying may have to be achieved by expression if cystourethrography is combined with an examination under anaesthesia.

Alternative examination

Bladder residue may be found by ultrasonography. Ureteric reflux is demonstrable by radionuclide imaging.

Cystourethrography by suprapubic puncture

Indications

This method is used when a urethral obstruction is suspected in an infant. Posterior urethral valves are usually sought in this way because urethral catheterization may temporarily fold back the membranous valve and make it difficult to visualize.

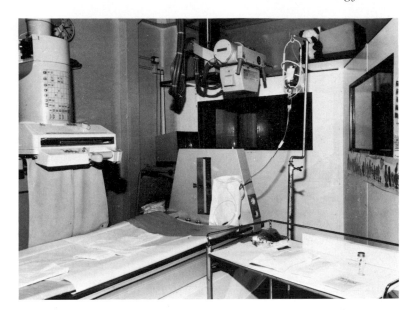

Fig. 24.16 Equipment for cystourethrography: warmed aqueous contrast medium is held in the bottle and giving set. A trolley with sterile packs is ready for the catheterization. A sterile specimen bottle is available for a urine sample.

Technique

Puncture should not be made through infected skin.

The presence of a full bladder may be confirmed by ultrasonography before examination. Skin preparation with a suitable water-soluble antiseptic is carried out over the lower abdomen. A syringe is attached to a 21 or 23 gauge short-bevel needle which is introduced in the mid-line about 1 cm above the symphysis. The needle is advanced perpendicularly, or at a slight upward angle, until urine is aspirated. When in position, a urine sample is obtained and the needle is connected to a drip-set for contrast filling. The needle may be steadied by a swab held by strapping. The examination then proceeds as previously described for the per urethral study. If pressure measurements are to be obtained, or if catheter drainage is required for some length of time, a flexible open-ended catheter may be introduced by the Seldinger technique.

Complications

Normal asepsis should prevent infection. If hydronephrosis is present, prophylactic antibiotics are given before catheterization or suprapubic puncture, if necessary by the i.v. route. Puncture of other organs, such as the bowel, or injection of contrast medium into perivesical tissues, is avoided if the bladder is full, which may be checked by ultrasonography.

Genitography for intersex problems

Indications

Ambiguous external genitalia.

Contraindications

Local infection in the perineum.

Technique

As contrast medium may spill through the fallopian tubes into the peritoneal cavity, aseptic techniques are necessary to avoid infection.

Perineal examination shows whether there is either a wide cloacal type opening or one or more small orifices. In the latter case, a catheter examination is made in the same way as a cystogram. A single large opening may be examined by the 'flush' method described by Schopfner (1964). A 10 ml syringe is filled with a water-soluble contrast medium as used for cystography. A soft rubber acorn, similar

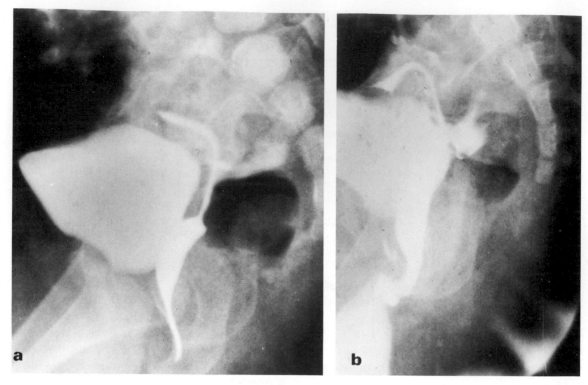

Fig. 24.17 Catheter study of a urogenital sinus in a baby with an intersex problem. (a) Filling of the urethra and bladder anteriorly. The wide vagina and narrower uterine cavity are filled with the uterus curving forward over the back of the bladder. (b) The uterine cornua are shown on a slightly oblique projection. Filling of the fallopian tubes is sometimes obtained.

to that used in the clamp for adult urethrography, is fitted to the syringe nozzle and the acorn applied with gentle pressure to the opening. An injection of 3–4 ml is made under screen control and spot radiographs obtained in AP and lateral planes (Fig. 24.17). The process may be repeated several times if necessary.

Reference

Schopfner, C.F. (1964) Genitography in intersex problems. *Radiology,* **82,** 664–74.

25   Sinography

C. I. BARTRAM

The term sinography is used to denote the catheterization and contrast examination of a cutaneous opening. If there is a communication to another mucosal surface, the examination should be called a fistulogram. However, as this is often unknown at the start of the examination, sinography is the term generally applied to all such studies. Sinography is an important examination because the findings will have a direct influence on surgical management. A good study requires care and skill.

There are three main questions to be answered by sinography:

1 Where does the track lead?
2 Is there an abscess cavity present?
3 Does it communicate with bowel or other viscus?

To answer these questions requires adequate filling of the track and radiographs taken in two planes. Some tracks may extend for a considerable distance. To fill the entire system requires significant pressure during injection into a distal part. To overcome this, the catheter should be inserted as far as possible. Alternatively, a Foley catheter is used to plug the track if this is rather wide, so that contrast medium will not simply reflux out past the catheter during the injection (Fig. 25.1). The balloon of the Foley catheter (maximum of 10 ml) should be inflated gently until it fits tightly into the track to prevent reflux of contrast.

Routine sterile precautions should be observed for the procedure. The track can be gently probed if there is doubt as to its size, patency or direction. Otherwise the catheter, held with forceps, should be inserted into the opening and fed in until resistance is felt. The catheter used will be determined by the bore of the track. A red rubber catheter — Jacques 10 French (F) gauge — is fairly atraumatic and suitable in most cases. A fine Portex catheter may be used for very narrow tracks. A Foley cath-eter is used for larger tracks, the size of the catheter reflecting the diameter of the track — usually 10–12F gauge. Water-soluble contrast medium is then injected fairly rapidly with a 20 ml syringe under screening control. Two spot radiographs at right angles, usually a supine and lateral or steep oblique, are the minimum requirement. If the bowel or a large cavity starts to fill, a radiograph should be taken immediately, otherwise the track may become obscured by contrast medium on later views. Just how much contrast medium is needed depends on the track system. If there is clinical evidence of a fistula, but one has not been demonstrated, further contrast medium should be injected until either reflux occurs or the fistula is shown.

Sometimes the fistulous track becomes intermittently occluded and the fistulous communication will not then be shown. This is the most common cause of failing to demonstrate a fistula, and, provided filling is adequate, it can only be overcome by repeating the sinogram when the fistula seems to be clinically open.

Any refluxed contrast medium should be wiped off the skin before radiographs are taken.

Complications are rare. Trauma to the track during probing or catheter insertion may lead to slight bleeding, which is rarely significant in amount. Catheter drainage should be considered if there is filling of a large abscess cavity. If this is performed, the sinogram should be repeated, injecting via the drainage catheter used for aspiration of the abscess, to show the size and extent of the residual cavity and any other loculus or fistula which was not demonstrated previously. Sinography may need repeating at intervals to monitor progress.

Sinography should precede any barium study. If there is a fistula, a contrast examination of the gastrointestinal tract may be required to assess its level and any underlying bowel condition.

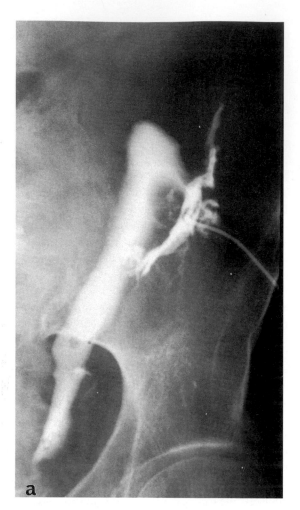 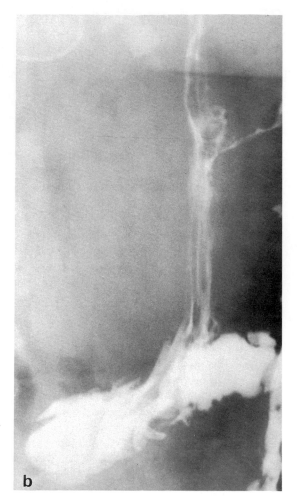

Fig. 25.1 (a) Injection into a left iliac fossa abdominal wall opening fills a short track system, but there is excess spillage of contrast onto the skin. (b) The catheter was replaced by a Foley catheter, the balloon being gently distended to occlude the lumen of the track. Further injection revealed a track extending up the left paracolic gutter, ending in a small subphrenic cavity with a communication into the stomach.

Sinography may be performed during computed tomography and may show a more extensive track system than is visible on conventional fluoroscopy.

Further reading

Alexander, E.S., Weinberg, S., Clark, R.A. & Belkin, R.D. (1982) Fistulas and sinus tracts: radiographic evaluation, management and outcome. *Gastrointest. Radiol.*, **7**, 135–40.

Alexander-Williams, J. & Irving, M. (1982) *Intestinal fistulas*. John Wright, Bristol.

Section 7
Imaging Modalities

26 Ultrasound

K. C. DEWBURY

Ultrasound is now one of the most frequently undertaken imaging investigations and is firmly established as an important soft-tissue imaging technique, producing tomographic slices of the area under examination. It can be used to quantitate the movement of structures such as cardiac valves and, when using the Doppler mode, patterns of blood flow. The soft-tissue images are produced entirely non-invasively and without the need for contrast agents. Contrast agents may be beneficial for enhancing the Doppler signal.

Ultrasound is a high-frequency mechanical vibration. It is produced by a transducer constructed of a piezoelectric material which has the property of changing thickness when a voltage is applied across it. Lead zirconate-titanate (PZT) is the most widely used material and transducers are usually cast as a thin plate with electrodes on the two surfaces. When a voltage is applied across the crystal it rings at a resonant frequency determined by its thickness. Ultrasound is transmitted from the crystal as a longitudinal wave into the tissues. Energy from the beam is lost by absorption within the tissues. Reflection is the other important tissue interaction upon which the images depend. Reflection occurs at tissue boundaries with different elasticities (acoustic impedance). This occurs in two main ways: (i) as a specular reflection of strong directional echoes from flat surfaces normal to the ultrasound beam; and (ii) as scattered reflections which are weak, non-directional echoes from small parenchymal discontinuities. The former produces 'landmark' echoes and the latter 'tissue texture', which is identified on ultrasound images. At each interface only a small proportion of the sound is reflected back towards the transducer, the remainder passing deeper into the tissues being interrogated. The conventional pulse echo ultrasound imaging process records echoes in positions that correspond to the return time

for a reflected pulse from the object to be visualized. The same principle is used in radar. In the simplest situation, only the depth of the echo-producing interface is displayed as a vertical reflection along the X-axis. This is known as the A-mode (amplitude scan). To produce a tomogram with two spatial dimensions, the ultrasound transducer is attached to a mechanical frame containing angle sensors by which the position and direction of the probe are continuously sensed. The transducer is swept across the tissue being examined and a tomogram is built up from several thousand contiguous scan lines. The brightness of the display spot corresponds to the strength of the returning echo. This is known as a B-mode (brightness modulation) or static scan. 'Grey scale' is an alternative designation because the intensity of the echo corresponds to the brightness of the final image according to a range of grey shades.

If the swept image can be repeated and displayed frequently enough, a moving picture can be produced in the same way as in cine photography. This system is called real-time scanning. There are a number of ways of producing the necessary beam scanning by either electronic or mechanical means. Real-time scanning offers major practical advantages over the old static scanning, the most obvious being the display of various kinds of tissue movement. In addition, the fact that the probe is not attached to a rigid position-sensing gantry allows the operator much greater freedom in selecting scanning planes and a far greater degree of interaction with the patient. Tissues can be 'palpated' utilizing the ultrasound image. Real-time scanning is the norm today, being simpler to perform and so more reliable and more easily learnt. A major limitation to real-time scanning is the small field of view. This may lead to a problem in interpreting and demonstrating frozen images.

Doppler

The Doppler principle is the basis of a method of assessment of movement by ultrasound. It depends on the shift in frequency produced in a sound wave, when the source moves relative to the receiver. An ultrasound wave is transmitted into the tissues and the frequency of the returning echo is compared with the original. A rise in frequency is a quantitative measure of the movement of the target towards the transducer; a fall in frequency indicates movement away from the transducer. The frequency change or 'Doppler shift' is proportional to the velocity of the moving particles and is given by the Doppler formula

$2fv \cos \theta / C$

where f = ultrasound frequency; v = velocity of movement; θ = beam vessel angle; and C = velocity of ultrasound in tissue.

Since f and c are known, the flow velocity can be calculated from the Doppler equation with a correction for the incident angle. The greatest application of Doppler ultrasound is in quantitating blood flow. Depth information can be obtained if the transmitted pulse is broken into short bursts, termed pulsed Doppler, which provides both imaging and Doppler information. Combined or so-called duplex scanners are now widely available.

Doppler signals fall within the audible range and may be played through earphones or loudspeakers. The pitch of the sound represents the blood flow velocity. In reality the flow of blood in vessels is complex, with different regions within the vessels moving at different velocities, resulting in a composite Doppler signal. This is audible as overtones superimposed on the basic frequency, giving whooshing or sighing sounds that become rough or whistling when the flow is disturbed, as in a stenosis. Display of these complex wave forms requires a spectrum analyser. This produces a grey scale tracing of frequency against time, the spectral Doppler 'tracing'. In a duplex scanner, a Doppler trace is available simultaneously with the real-time image. The Doppler sampler or gate can be positioned along the Doppler line to sample the precise vessel required. This is displayed alongside the grey scale image as a spectrogram. With pulsed Doppler systems only the small region encompassed by the range gate is sensitive to flow, so that a time-consuming and careful search must be made to map out the detail of the vascular anatomy. This was one factor that resulted in the underutilization of Doppler ultrasound for many years. With the development of colour flow mapped Doppler or 'colour Doppler', which provides flow information across the entire real-time image, there has been a dramatic resurgence of interest in Doppler ultrasound. The basic principle is the same as in conventional Doppler, but the frequency comparison between the transmitted ultrasound and the returning echoes is made along ultrasound beam lines. Each beam line is repeated several times and frequency changes indicating movement are extracted using a correlation analysis for display as a colour-coded overlay of the real-time images. Flow towards the transducer is coded in one colour and away from the transducer at the other end of the spectrum, for example red and blue. Changes of colour along the spectrum indicate velocity differences within the vessel which allows flow information to be assessed across the whole scan (or vessel), so detecting complex or turbulent flow patterns. The ability to demonstrate flow patterns over the entire image is an immense benefit when the vascular anatomy is complex. The flow information in colour Doppler is relatively crude, since only the mean velocity is measured, but for quantitative studies the colour Doppler can be used as a map to allow precise positioning of the Doppler sample for a spectral Doppler trace (see Plate 26.1, facing p. 311).

An important limit to the rate at which ultrasound information can be acquired is set by its relatively slow speed in tissue. It is necessary to wait for each pulse to have disappeared before the next is transmitted since, if the second pulse is sent too early, the last echoes from the first converge with early echoes from the second and are falsely registered in the images of superficial structures. To avoid this range ambiguity artefact, the pulse repetition rate must allow a delay of at least the time taken for the most distant echoes to return. In practice this limits the pulse repetition frequency (PRF) rate to about 1000 pulses s^{-1} (lower for deeper structures, higher for superficial). The choice of the way these pulses are distributed in time and space depends on the priorities for the particular application. They may be spread apart and the scan area restricted in order to maximize the frame rate, a solution that is appropriate for echo cardiology. However, this results in an image with a low line density. The resulting sacrifice in spatial resolution and the small image size are not ideal for general applications where image quality is paramount; here the low frame rate is generally less important, so a high line density in a wide scan is selected as the best trade-off.

The same PRF limitation has important effects in pulsed Doppler in which the frequency shift produced by flowing blood is being measured intermittently (at the PRF), instead of continuously, as in continuous wave Doppler. If the blood flow is fast, the sampling rate is unable to interpret correctly between the measured samples and the velocity ambiguity results. This is known as 'aliasing' and results in high flow rates being depicted in the reverse direction, seen in the spectral trace as peaks across the baseline and in colour Doppler as a mosaic of reverse colours.

Indications and contraindications

Ultrasound equipment is relatively inexpensive. As with much electronic equipment, the passage of time has led to its becoming more sophisticated and less expensive. Parallel to the increasing availability of ultrasound has been the expansion of its use. As a general statement, any soft-tissue structure that can be accessed can also be usefully examined with ultrasound. The areas of regular application are listed in Table 26.1.

In these areas ultrasound may range from being occasionally useful, for example in the gastrointestinal tract, to being indispensable as in obstetric practice (Fig. 26.1). As a general rule, the more the

Table 26.1 Areas in which ultrasound is regularly used

Abdominal organs	Neonatal hip
Arteries	Obstetrics
Breast	Pleura
Eye	Prostate
Gastrointestinal tract	Salivary glands
Gynaecology	Tendons
Heart	Testes
Infant brain	Thyroid
Muscles and joints	Veins

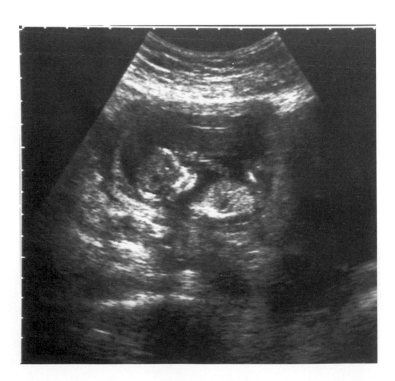

Fig. 26.1 Scan of a fetus at 12 weeks' gestation. The fetal head and body can be clearly identified. In real-time scanning, the fetal heart activity can also be identified and documented.

examination is directed at solving a specific clinical problem or answering a specific question, the more useful it will be.

There are no contraindications to ultrasound but there are limitations as to its use due to the mechanism by which sound penetrates tissue. There is total reflection at tissue–gas and tissue–bone interfaces. Gas-containing structures and bone cannot be imaged and obscure deeper lying structures. This is why ultrasound is not generally useful in the examination of the adult head, except in the presence of burr holes, or the lungs. When abdominal organs are examined, the interposition of ribs or bowel gas has to be avoided if possible; this can be achieved in the majority of situations by using appropriate acoustic windows, such as the fluid-filled bladder for the pelvis or the intercostal spaces for liver and spleen (Fig. 26.2).

Fresh wounds, dressings and drainage bags may all pose contact problems. Very ticklish patients may also be a problem to examine. These difficulties can usually be overcome with the appropriate expertise. Ultrasound is also subject to many artefactual signals which complicate interpretation. The small field of view of the real-time systems and the lack of eas-ily reproducible landmarks pose some documentation problems for ultrasound as compared to other imaging techniques.

Safety

An important feature of diagnostic ultrasound, especially in obstetric and paediatric practice, is its safety. This is evidenced by the many studies that have failed to show any damaging affect of pulsed ultrasound at diagnostic intensities when applied to intact mammals, including fetuses *in utero*. These studies include follow-ups of the growth and development of children who received obstetric scans, with particular attention being paid to the development of cataracts, hearing loss or childhood malignancy. All such follow-up tests have been negative.

There have, however, been reports of biochemical alterations to cells in suspension, including changes to DNA and in surface membrane behaviour which are obvious at high intensities but are demonstrable also, at least in some series, at diagnostic powers. It is debatable whether these are significant for the intact animal and it is notable that many of them have proved elusive when repeat studies have been

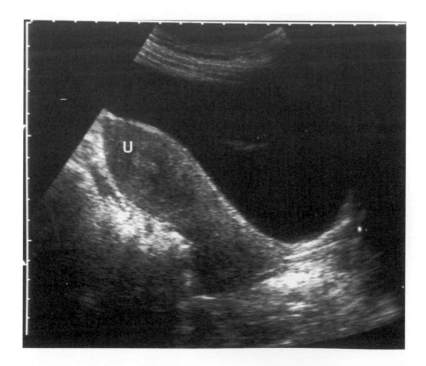

Fig. 26.2 A curved linear view of the pelvis using the window of the full bladder. This allows excellent visualization of the anteverted uterus (U).

attempted. They do, however, serve to inject a note of caution and reinforce the common-sense point that the lowest power that will give the diagnostic information required should always be used, especially in obstetrics and gynaecology where one might expect the greatest tissue sensitivity. The entire subject of safety is kept under continuous review.

Ultrasound intensity is the energy flowing across the surface; the usual units are W cm^{-2}. For pulsed ultrasound, one may take a peak or average value. Because of focusing, the energy distribution along and across the beam is non-uniform; the peak intensity at the maximum point is usually quoted. The maximum intensity level recommended by the American Institute of Ultrasound in Medicine for diagnostic use is 100 mW cm^{-2}, taken as a temporal and spatial peak.

High powers of ultrasound are clearly capable of inflicting severe damage to tissues. Most of the energy deposited appears as local heat. As with all ultrasound effects, the skin and superficial structures receive the greatest dose because of the rapid loss of energy with depth. Heating is a desired effect when ultrasound is used in physiotherapy. Not only high powers but also continuous waves are required to produce a significant rise in temperature. It is important to realize that continuous waves (as used in conventional Doppler systems) deliver at least 1000 times the dose of pulsed waves used for imaging since, with the pulsed system, energy is being transmitted for only 0.1% of the scanning time. For most of the time, the probe is in the receiving and not the transmitting mode, whereas for continous wave Doppler energy is applied continuously throughout the study.

These same factors can conspire to produce other damaging effects. The vibration of particles at high amplitudes may produce mechanical disruption of intracellular membranes and the pressure can cause fluids to flow in streaming movements. Extreme ultrasound powers can produce regions of such low pressure that dissolved gases (mainly nitrogen) can come out of solution, or water may vaporize to produce minute gas bubbles which pulsate in the sound field. This process, known as cavitation, can cause mechanical damage to the tissue and even strip off ions from atoms. Cavitation is unlikely to occur at diagnostic powers but has been demonstrated with the higher powers and continuous wave conditions used in ultrasound therapy and with continuous wave Doppler.

Examination technique

Patient

An ultrasound examination is readily accepted by patients since the procedure only requires firm pressure on the skin with the transducer. Acoustic coupling between transducer and skin is essential as sound is so strongly attenuated by air. Various oils were used with the old static scanners, but water-soluble gels of various viscosities are now standard. These can be made more acceptable to the patient by prior warming in a bottle warmer. In general, small and slim subjects are likely to be better imaged with ultrasound than large or obese patients where fatty tissue, fibrous septae and gas may scatter and attenuate the beam. The converse is true for computed tomography (CT). It follows that ultrasound is ideal for paediatric patients and for the examination of superficial organs and structures. Since ultrasound is a tomographic technique and access to particular areas and organs may require differing approaches, particularly in the abdomen, it is best used in a directed way to answer a particular clinical problem or question rather than as a screening procedure.

Most scans may be carried out in the position that is most comfortable for the patient, usually lying supine. Some scans, such as subcostal scanning for the liver, require the patient's cooperation by holding an inspiration. Moving the patient into a more advantageous position for particular anatomical problems has become an increasingly used practice. Examples of this are the right anterior oblique position to optimally display the common bile-duct, coronal views of the kidneys and retroperitoneum in the lateral decubitus position and occasionally erect views to improve access to the epigastrium, particularly for the pancreas (Fig. 26.3). Ill and immobile patients are examined in their beds, and neonates in their incubators. Toddlers may best be examined held in their mothers' arms. Patient preparation for ultrasound is minimal. A full bladder is required for obstetric and pelvic scanning and typically entails drinking 0.5 litre (1 pint) or more

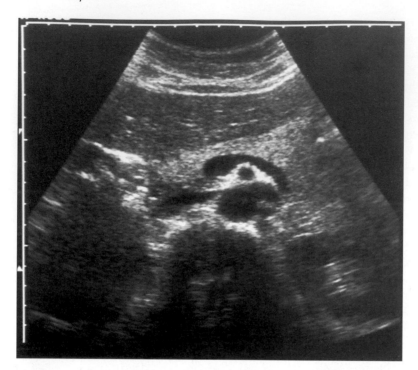

Fig. 26.3 Transverse scan of the epigastrium using a curved linear transducer. There is excellent visualization of the pancreas which stands out due to the slightly different reflectivity of the pancreas as compared with the liver. The great vessels and mesenteric vessels are clearly identified in relation to the pancreas.

of clear fluid during the hour preceding the operation. A fast of 6–8 hours is necessary for optimal gallbladder visualization. Apart from this, patients may be scanned as and when required. The most useful contrast agent in ultrasound is fluid, the full urinary bladder and gallbladder being examples of this in use. A fluid load in the stomach may also act as an acoustic window to the pancreas and lesser sac, as does the bladder for the pelvis. The use of this fluid load in the stomach may be optimized by either sitting or standing the patient erect. Using real-time scanning the movement of swallowed fluid can act as a very useful marker for the stomach, which may occasionally masquerade as a left upper quadrant mass. Similarly, in the pelvis a water enema may allow a loop of colon to be distinguished from a significant mass.

Contrast media

In addition to the use of water as an ultrasound contrast agent as described above, the general concept of contrast agents for ultrasound is not new. As early as 1968, microbubbles produced by agitating saline were used to produce contrast effects in echocardiography. The solutions tested had a very short half-life and the microbubble size was variable. The current range of contrast agents under clinical investigation are based on gas-filled microbubbles of small and uniform size. To produce systematic contrast enhancement the microbubbles must be small enough to cross the lung capillaries, which is less than 10 μm. The heart is the first organ to benefit from ultrasound contrast, where it allows improved left ventricular opacification and left ventricular border definition in the great majority of patients. Elsewhere in the body, systemic contrast injection produces a marked increase in the Doppler signal from blood vessels. In peripheral vascular disease small vessels, such as the foot vessels, are all much better seen following the use of contrast media. Another important area is in the enhancement of tumour vascularity following microbubble contrast, which may allow separation of benign from malignant tumours (see Plate 26.2, facing p. 311).

Another approach to further enhance the value of ultrasound contrast is known as harmonic imaging. This is created by tuning the contrast bubbles to resonate at twice the frequency of the transmitted pulse. Ordinarily there are no echoes at these higher frequencies from either static or moving interfaces.

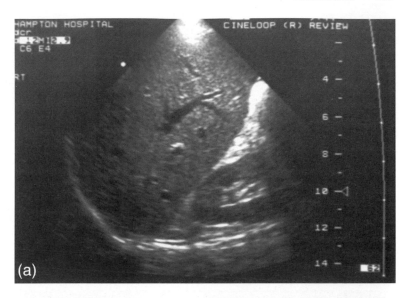

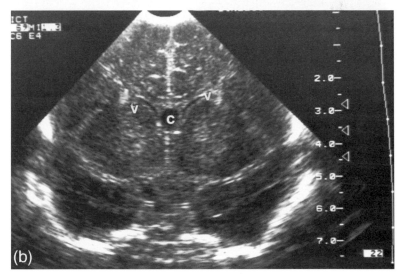

Fig. 26.4 (a) Sector scan of the right lobe of the liver taken through an intercostal space, showing detail of the liver and the upper pole of the right kidney. Note the good visualization from a small acoustic window but the relatively poor near field visualization. (b) A sector field view of the neonatal brain taken through the anterior fontanelle. In this coronal section the slit-like lateral ventricles are identified (v) and the mid-line cavum septum pellucidum (c).

Harmonic echoes are only produced when the specially tuned microbubbles are present, so that the distribution and the concentration of the contrast agent can be displayed as an overlay on the conventional image. Slower blood flow can be demonstrated with fewer artefacts.

Another emerging use for ultrasound contrast is the assessment of infertility disorders. In some centres contrast-enhanced ultrasound hysterosalpingography using a vaginal probe is replacing conventional X-ray hysterosalpingography.

Equipment

Modern real-time equipment is usually available with a choice of transducer configuration; sector, linear, curved linear and intracavity transducers will usually be offered. The sector field of view is versatile and useful for imaging the upper abdomen, the pelvis or the neonatal brain. In all these situations there is a relatively small anterior access (acoustic window) (Fig. 26.4). The linear-array transducers produce a rectangular field of view, the width of

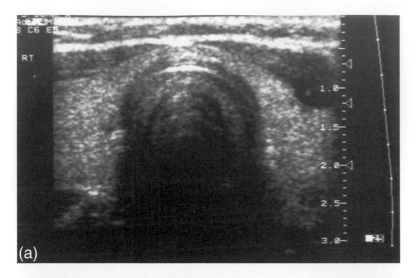

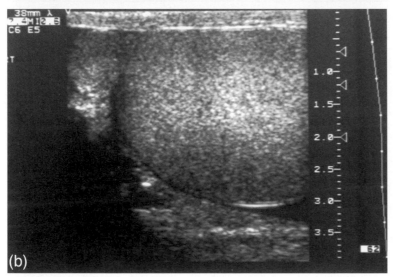

Fig. 26.5 (a) Transverse scan of the neck with a high-frequency linear-array transducer, showing both lateral lobes and the isthmus of the thyroid gland. Note the excellent near field detail. (b) A longitudinal view of testis and epididymis with a high-frequency linear array. Note the excellent resolution of these structures.

which corresponds to the length of the transducer face. This field of view may be preferred in the mid-abdomen for obstetric scanning. It is also particularly valuable for superficial scanning as it optimizes near field detail (Fig. 26.5). This is a feature very apparent in clinical practice. The curved linear transducer is a more recent development that combines the advantages of both the sector and the linear transducers. These curved transducers produce a good area of contact at the surface at the widening field of view deeper within the patient.

The larger reflected field of view of the image allows easier orientation with preservation of detailed resolution throughout the image. These transducers provide a particularly good compromise and are becoming the most widely used for many applications (Fig. 26.6).

Transducer frequency is one of the important determinants of spatial resolution of ultrasound, higher frequency producing a better resolution. Absorption is also highly dependent on ultrasound frequency, higher frequencies being more strongly

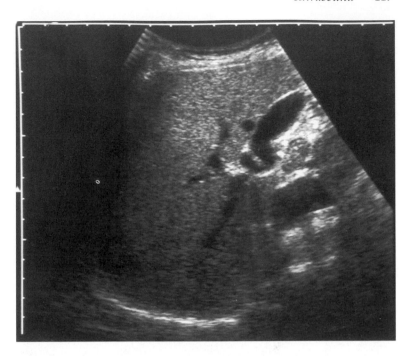

Fig. 26.6 A curved linear-array view of the right lobe of the liver and the gallbladder. Note both good near field detail and wide far field of view.

absorbed than lower frequencies. These factors must be taken into consideration when deciding which transducer to use for a particular examination. In general, the highest frequency that will penetrate the area of interest is chosen. On average, a frequency of 3.5 mHz is suitable for examination of the abdomen and pelvis. In children and slim adults 5 mHz is ideal, while for superficial scanning 7.5 mHz is used if this is available. For superficial scanning the very near field may be further improved by using some form of stand-off, either a water-bath or a small jelly block.

Intracavity transducers are now widely available; these include transvaginal, transrectal, urethral, oesophageal and intravascular probes. The object in all cases is to place the transducer as close as possible to the area of interest. In practice this means that higher frequency transducers may be used to produce images of greater detail and resolution. Despite being slightly more invasive than contact scanning, transvaginal ultrasound has rapidly become a routine part of gynaecological investigation (Fig. 26.7). This is now the standard procedure for infertility monitoring and egg retrieval, as well as being invaluable in assessing suspected ectopic

pregnancy. Transrectal ultrasound is now an increasingly frequent examination, findings a role not only in assessing specific clinical problems and performing guided biopsies but also as a screening procedure (Fig. 26.8).

Correct machine settings are essential for producing optimal ultrasound images. The overall gain and swept gain (slope, or time gain compensation) are the most important controls that must be adjusted. The aim is to produce an image with the organ under review showing a mid-grey reflectivity and the intensity being balanced between superficial and deep structures by use of the TGC control. This is usually straightforward. Numerous other controls may be available, including pre- and post-processing, edge enhancement, dynamic range and smoothing, to name but a few. The precise effects differ from machine to machine and, when optimized for a particular machine and type of examination, are not usually adjusted significantly from patient to patient. Misuse of the gain settings may obscure the visualization of both normal structures and pathology (Fig. 26.9).

An ultrasound study is most commonly recorded on radiographic film, using a multiformat

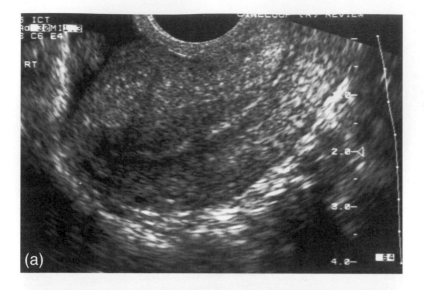

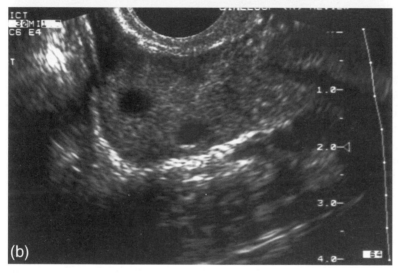

Fig. 26.7 Transvaginal scans. (a) A longitudinal view of the uterus, note the excellent anatomical detail. (b) A view of one ovary, again note the very clear textural detail visualized by this technique.

camera or a laser imager for archival storage. A representative series of images is chosen by the operator in the same way as when recording a fluoroscopic examination. A video tape recorder may be used to record the dynamic aspects of the examination. Measurements are usually made on the screen during performance of the examination rather than on the film record. Area measurement systems are available in the system microprocessor, for example to give a direct conversion of length or area to fetal age.

Interventional procedures

Real-time ultrasound is an extremely interactive process, almost providing an extension to the palpating fingers. Complex anatomy can be traced from plane to plane, allowing a truly three-dimensional understanding with rapidity. The tip of a biopsy needle or drainage catheter can be followed in real time as it is inserted into a lesion. Ultrasound is increasingly used to guide interventional procedures, being quick and readily available (Fig. 26.10).

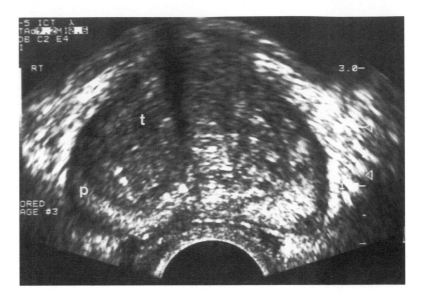

Fig. 26.8 A transrectal ultrasound of the prostate, note the excellent differentiation of the peripheral zone (p) and the transitional zone (t).

Fine-needle aspiration

Percutaneous aspiration for cytology can be applied to any organ or mass that can be identified by ultrasound. Using needles of 20–23 gauge, this is a safe procedure which is almost totally free of complications. Guidance of the needle into the lesion allows greater accuracy in diagnosis and reduces the false negative cytological results.

Abscess drainage

If an abscess can be identified with ultrasound, it can almost always be successfully drained under guidance. In regard to the detection of abscesses, ultrasound is of particular value in the subphrenic spaces and in the pelvis, but is less useful in the mid-abdomen where CT may be the imaging method of choice.

Nephrostomy

Following identification of a dilated renal collecting system with ultrasound, it is simple to use it as the initial guiding procedure for puncture of the renal calyx. This can then be opacified with contrast medium. The remainder of the procedure is often best performed under fluoroscopic control.

Interventional procedures in obstetrics and gynaecology

Ultrasound is increasingly being used in this context. Areas for which ultrasound is invaluable include oocyte recovery, chorionic villus biopsy, amniocentesis, cordocentesis and intrauterine transfusions.

Image interpretation and artefacts

Ultrasound images are often considered difficult to interpret. This is partly due to the inevitable artefacts. Recognition and understanding of these artefacts will allow a more informed process of pattern recognition.

Specular and scattered echoes

Specular echoes is the term used to describe the strong reflection from prominent smooth interfaces in the body tissues. These correspond in position and appearance to the structure that they depict but are not clearly seen if they lie parallel to the ultrasound beam, which causes some confusion (Fig. 26.11). The tissue parenchyma of an organ generates low-level scattered echoes independent of orientation. This arises when the reflectors are small

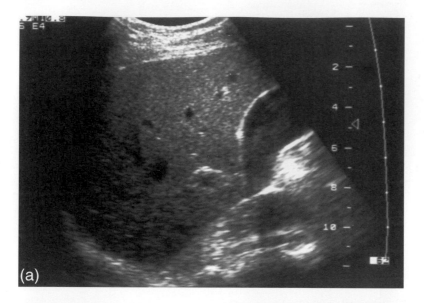

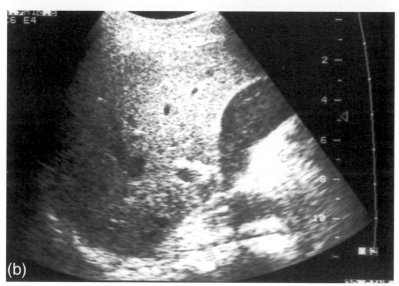

Fig. 26.9 (a) A normal reference view of the right lobe of the liver and gallbladder with correctly set gain and swept gain factors. (b) The same section with the overall gain set too high, producing rather bright image with loss of fine detail.

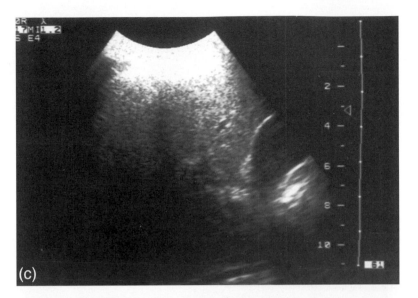

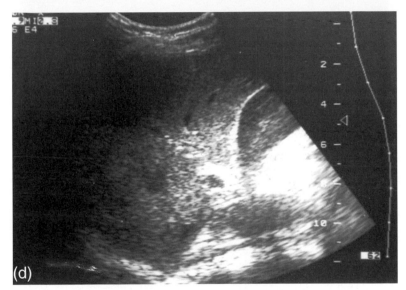

Fig. 26.9 *Continued.* (c) The same section where no swept gain has been used so there is saturation of the anteriorly placed structures with very little detail in the far field. (d) The same section with overcompensation of the swept gain in the near field obliterating detail in this area, although detail is preserved in the far field.

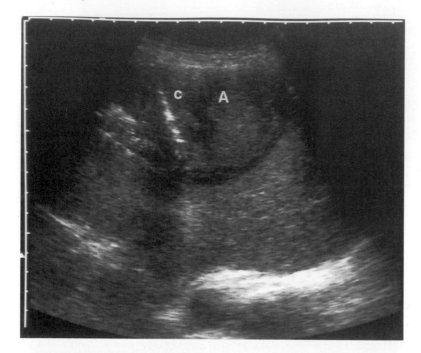

Fig. 26.10 An intercostal view of the right lobe of the liver in which a catheter is being passed into an anteriorly placed liver abscess. The high reflectivity from the catheter can be seen (c). A, abscess.

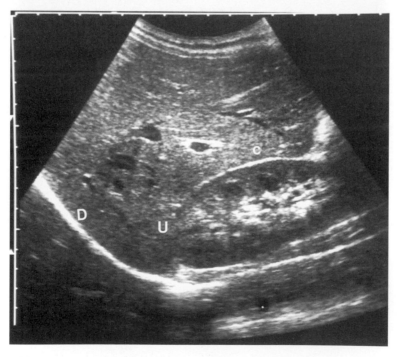

Fig. 26.11 A longitudinal curved array transducer section through the right lobe of the liver and the right kidney. The scatters are the small grey dots making up the textural pattern of the liver. The specular reflectors are the strong reflections from the diaphragm (D) and the capsule of the kidney (c). Note that the upper pole of the kidney (U) appears to have no capsule. This is because the capsule lies nearly parallel to the beam at this point and so is not clearly imaged as a specular reflector.

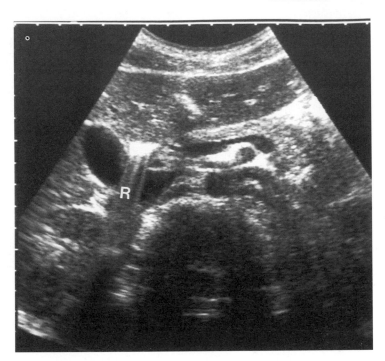

Fig. 26.12 Transverse scan through the epigastrium showing the pancreas and gallbladder. Gas in the duodenum is producing quite a marked reverberation artefact (R). Note the ring down artefact due to reflection from the transducer face.

and of the same order of size as the ultrasound wavelength. The echoes are radiated in all directions. In practice they are only detected when several wavelets from adjacent reflectors are superimposed to produce an additive effect. This final pattern is therefore an interference pattern and not a representation of the histological reality. This explains why tissues of different structures such as liver and spleen have an almost identical parenchymal pattern on ultrasound images.

Reverberation

Ultrasound travels freely in soft tissue. Where fluid is present it appears free from echoes, and therefore black, because there is no interface for reflection. Specular and scattered echoes, as described above, are generated from tissue interfaces. When a particularly strong specular reflector lies normal to the ultrasound beam, the returning reflection may be so strong as to be re-reflected from the transducer face and back again in multiple repeated images. In practice this occurs as soft tissue–gas and soft tissue–bone interfaces (Fig. 26.12). These artefacts cause the loss of clarity and shadowing in deeper

structures which so often reduces the diagnostic yield of an ultrasound examination. A rather more curious re-reflection can occur at the diaphragm, giving apparent images of liver or spleen in the lower zone of the chest. The diaphragm here acts like a parabolic mirror.

Shadowing and enhancement

Acoustic shadowing and enhancement are artefacts that arise because of the swept gain characteristics. Swept gain compensation is always set appropriate for the average through the tissue in question, to match front and back echoes. If the ultrasound beam encounters an area of higher than average attenuation, the compensation area will cause all tissues deeper to appear with a falsely low intensity — an acoustic shadow. A region of low attenuation, such as a cyst, will give rise to a band of high intensity or enhancement beyond it. Both shadows and enhancement are more marked at high ultrasound frequencies. While both these artefacts may obscure detail, in practice they are important diagnostic clues to the nature of the tissue causing them. The echo-free or echo-poor lesion should not be designated as a cyst unless clear

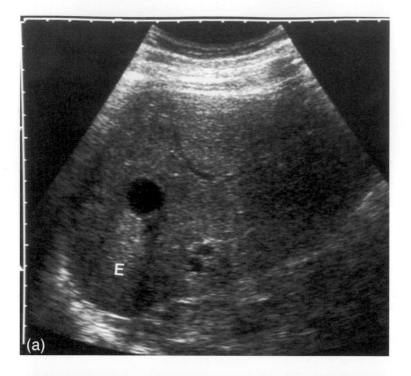

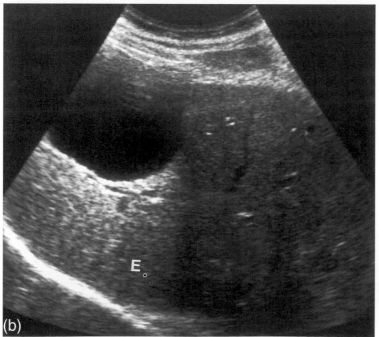

Fig. 26.13 Liver cysts. (a) Small 1.5 cm cyst in the right lobe of the liver with clear-cut margins and acoustic enhancement seen beyond the cyst. (b) Larger liver cyst in which the acoustic enhancement beyond the cyst is much more marked. E, enhancement.

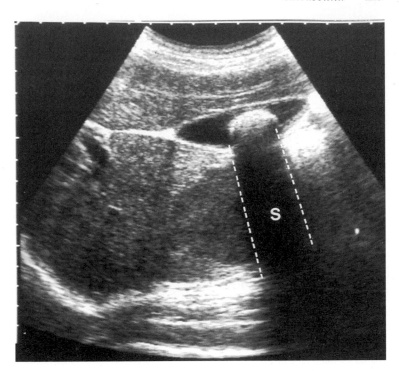

Fig. 26.14 Longitudinal scan through the gallbladder which contains a single large calculus. Note the marked acoustic shadowing seen beyond this (S).

enhancement is shown beyond it (Fig. 26.13). If acoustic shadowing is shown beyond high-level echoes, it is very likely to be caused by calcification (Fig. 26.14).

Relationship to other techniques

Ultrasound has no real competitors in obstetric practice. There are usually other possibilities elsewhere in the body, the most common overlap being with computed tomography and to some degree with magnetic resonance imaging (MRI). Since ultrasound is simple, quicker and much cheaper, it should almost always be performed first, only proceeding to CT or MRI when sufficient information is not obtained.

Further reading

Callen, P. (1994) *Ultrasonography in Obstetrics and Gynaecology*. WB Saunders, Philadelphia.

Cosgrove, D., Meire, H. & Dewbury, K. (1993) *Abdominal and General Ultrasound*, vols I & II. Churchill Livingstone, Edinburgh.

Kremkau, F.W. (1980) *Diagnostic Ultrasound Physical Principles and Exercises*. Grune & Stratton, New York.

McDicken, W.N. (1981) *Diagnostic Ultrasonics, Principles and Use of Instruments*, 2nd edn. Wiley, New York.

Meire, H.B. & Farrant, P. (1982) *Basic Clinical Ultrasound*. British Institute of Radiology, London.

Merrit, C.R.B. (1992) *Clinics in Diagnostic Ultrasound*, vol. 27. *Doppler Colour Imaging*. Churchill Livingstone, New York.

Williams, A.R. (1988) *Ultrasound: Biological Effects and Potential Hazards*. Academic Press, Oxford.

27   Isotope Imaging

M. V. MERRICK

Radioisotope imaging differs from other radiological techniques in providing regional biochemical or physiological, rather than anatomical, data. It is frequently necessary to correlate this with anatomical information, for example by viewing the isotope images in conjunction with appropriate radiographs or superimposing radioisotope tomograms on images from computed tomography (CT) or magnetic resonance imaging (MRI). It is never possible to interpret nuclear medicine images meaningfully without a full understanding of their functional significance, in anatomical terms alone.

Bone

The tracers employed demonstrate regional differences in bone turnover rate, for example in metastatic deposits, osteomyelitis or healing fractures. This usually precedes any alteration in radiographic appearance. Conversely, radiographic changes depend on the net balance between osteoblastic and osteoclastic processes, which may never become clinically manifest. Radiotracer uptake is unrelated to the quantity of bone present. The most common indications for bone scintigraphy are:

1 Staging patients with a primary tumour which carries a high risk of occult metastastis to bone, especially in carcinoma of the breast, prostate and lung.

2 When treatment may be modified if occult metastases can be demonstrated, for example avoiding cystectomy in patients with carcinoma of the bladder.

3 Identification of radiologically occult metastases in patients with known malignancy and unexplained pain of skeletal origin.

4 Restaging patients with breast and prostate cancer prior to treatment for recurrence.

5 Where fracture is suspected, but not confirmed by conventional radiography.

6 Suspicion of osteomyelitis, especially if the symptoms are not sufficiently clear-cut and typical to justify surgical decompression.

7 Some centres advocate bone scintigraphy in children suspected of physical abuse.

There are many other valid but less common indications.

Radiopharmaceuticals

A number of phosphate or phosphonate derivatives are available in kit form ready for labelling with ^{99m}Tc. Those most commonly employed are methyldiphosphonate (MDP), ethylhydroxydiphosphonate (EHDP) and methylhydroxydiphosphonate (MHDP). There is little to choose between them. Dimethyl-aminodiphosphonate (DMAD) has a slightly higher detection rate of metastatic deposits but is not commercially available. The normal administered activity in the adult is 500 MBq. If osteomyelitis in an upper limb is suspected, the injection should be given into a lower limb vein. Higher activities (up to 1000 MBq) may be required in occasional patients who are not able to tolerate the usual duration of imaging or when the interval after injection is substantially longer (18–24 hours) than normal, for example to allow clearance of residual activity in an ileal loop or other urinary diversion, which otherwise obscures skeletal structures. Skeletal uptake approaches a plateau within 30 min. The longer delay required between injection and imaging is determined by the rate of clearance of activity from soft tissues, which has considerable intersubject variability. Good images can often be obtained within 2 hours, but contrast between bone and soft tissue continues to increase for several hours. Activity remains in the skeleton and imaging can be performed up to 24 hours after injection, limited only by the reduced count rate resulting from radioactive decay.

Technique (Fig. 27.1)

A gamma camera with a field of view not less than 40 cm diameter fitted with a low-energy general purpose or preferably a high-resolution collimator, should be employed. Scanning attachments enable the entire skeleton to be displayed on a single image but the collimator face is inevitably distant from the patient, with consequent degradation in image quality.

If infection is suspected, a dynamic study at 2 frames s^{-1}, starting immediately before injection, should be obtained for not less than 2 min. Limbs should be placed symmetrically to facilitate comparison. When imaging the whole body between 2 and 6 hours after injection, a 1 million count image is collected from the posterior thorax. Sufficient other projections are then acquired to include the entire trunk and proximal thirds of the humeri and femora for the same time as the posterior thorax. The number of projections will depend on the field of view of the camera. The patient must micturate immediately before the images of the pelvis. If the camera is set for a fixed number of counts (instead of time), images of the pelvis may contain an unacceptably low count density from the skeleton, due to residual activity in the urinary tract. If imaging is performed at 24 hours, half a million counts is adequate. Noise in lower count density images can conceal low-contrast lesions. With most tumours, isolated deposits in the skull and periphery are extremely rare. There is no indication for routinely imaging the skull or distal to the mid-thigh in asymptomatic patients. The entire skeleton must be included when determining the distribution of Paget's disease and when there is a specific clinical indication.

Data processing

Data should be collected in a 128 × 128 matrix. Filtration facilitates interpretation of low-count images, for example from restless patients who cannot be restrained, but only partially compensates for the loss of information. Images should be displayed without background subtraction, employing a display which indicates when any pixel is over range. It is permissible to overrange activity in the urinary tract and bladder, but not in any part of the skeleton. In abnormalities which have very high uptake, for example Paget's disease, it may not be possible to display both high and low count rate areas simultaneously in monochrome. Colour displays have a wider dynamic range but tend to draw attention to changes which may not be of clinical significance.

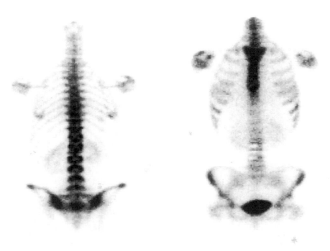

Fig. 27.1 Normal bone scintigraphy — the trunk. The image on the left is the posterior view. Note that in the normal subject uptake in the shafts of the long bone is so faint that it may not reproduce. The right-hand image is the anterior projection. Note artefacts over the 2nd and 3rd lumbar vertebrae due to a metal belt on the patient's clothing. Note here also that although the joints are well seen the shafts of the long bones are almost invisible.

Sources of error

Abnormalities may be concealed by patient movement, poor positioning and inadequate quality hard copy if images are over range, too dark or too light. Limbs must be positioned symmetrically. A full bladder conceals much of the pelvis and even a small residual volume disguises abnormalities in the pubis. The inferior angle of the scapula may conceal rib lesions.

Interpretation

The majority of abnormalities present as focal areas of increased uptake, when compared with the contralateral side or adjacent levels in mid-line structures. Some abnormalities are photon-deficient. There is no evidence that high-resolution collimators have any advantage for the detection of high count rate abnormalities, but they probably facilitate detection of photon-deficient lesions.

Bone scintigraphy is an extremely sensitive but non-specific technique for detecting focal areas of abnormal bone turnover. The significance of an abnormality is only determined by correlation with the clinical history and current radiographs. In patients with metastatic disease, radiographic changes should correspond to at least one of the scintigraphic abnormalities. If there is no radiographic confirmation at any site on plain radiographs, CT of selected sites should be performed. Under no circumstances should a solitary scintigraphic abnormality be regarded as metastatic in the absence of confirmatory evidence or in a patient without other confirmation of malignancy. Osteomyelitis treated early rarely gives radiographic confirmation. Reporting 'hot spots' without radiographic correlation is of no clinical value.

Lung

Five aspects of lung function can be investigated; (i) the distribution, wash-in and wash-out of inhaled gases, (ventilation scintigraphy); (ii) right ventricular output (perfusion scintigraphy); (iii) the rate of absorption of peripheral inhaled soluble aerosols (alveolar permeability); (iv) removal of centrally deposited non-diffusible aerosols (ciliary function); and (v) interstitial or intra-alveolar leakage of large intravascular molecules such as plasma proteins (lung capillary permeability).

Indications

The only common indication for lung ventilation and perfusion scintigraphy is the detection of suspected pulmonary emboli. Lung ventilation scintigraphy alone has a limited use in the assessment of regional severity of obstructive airways disease and segmental lung function, for example in congenital lobar emphysema and bronchiectasis.

Lung ventilation scintigraphy

Radiopharmaceuticals

^{133}Xe is used most commonly. ^{127}Xe has a higher γ-ray energy than ^{99m}Tc and can follow perfusion scintigraphy, whereas ^{133}Xe must precede it. ^{81m}Kr has a limited application because the short half-life of the generator precludes its general availability. Aerosols are sometimes used as an alternative (see below). Instillation of 70 MBq of either ^{127}Xe or ^{133}Xe is adequate, provided that a computer with good image filtration software is available, using a gamma camera with a field of view greater than 35 cm diameter and fitted with a general-purpose low-energy collimator. A high-energy collimator is required for ^{127}Xe. Inhalation of 700 MBq of either isotope is required for analogue imaging. Acquisition is started *just before* the first breath of the gas. The first breath is the most important part of the examination. Timing is critical.

A closed breathing circuit with one-way valves which direct air-flow, either a shielded spirometer or a single-use unit, is required. Exhaled air passes via a soda–lime filled chamber (to absorb carbon dioxide) into a reservoir of not less than 10 litres capacity, previously half-filled with oxygen. Oxygen–air mixture from the reservoir passes to the input valve at the mouthpiece. The patient wears a nose clip to ensure mouth breathing and a snorkel-type mouthpiece held between the teeth, with a flange between the teeth and the gums to ensure a gas-tight fit with minimum dead space. A face mask may be used by patients unable to manage the mouthpiece, but it is virtually impossible to achieve a gas-tight fit.

Xenon is introduced at the start of inspiration, for example via a 23 gauge needle inserted obliquely through the plastic of the mouthpiece. Frames are acquired at 12 per minute for the first 2 min and 2 per minute for a further 15 min. It is often possible to terminate the study after 6 min, but in patients with severe obstructive airway disease the wash-out phase may be prolonged. It is essential to start data collection *just before* xenon is injected into the system, to ensure that the whole of the ventilation phase is collected. Failure to do so invalidates the study.

Data processing

Because of the limited duration of the ventilation phase, the number of counts collected is restricted.

Filtration of the images is essential to extract the maximum information from an unavoidably noisy study.

Interpretation

All three phases must be compared (Fig. 27.2). The initial (first breath) image shows the distribution of ventilation. By 4 min the xenon has mixed completely with the air in the lungs in most subjects, with the exception of those with severe obstructive airways disease; count rate is proportional to lung volume. The third (wash-out) phase shows air trapping.

In the normal erect subject there is a smoothly reducing gradient of ventilation from base to apex. The distribution of ventilation is also proportional to regional lung volume. The first breath and equilibrium phases should be identical and wash-out complete in less than 90 s. In subjects with obstructive airways disease there is delayed wash-in; defects in the ven-

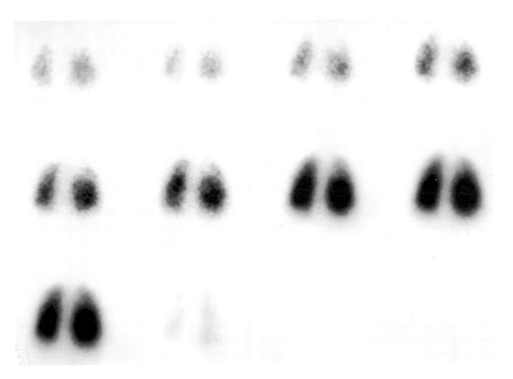

Fig. 27.2 Lung ventilation series. Sequence of views during a lung ventilation study with ¹³³Xe. The first frame on the top left represents the distribution of ventilation. Subsequent frames represent the progressive wash-in and mixture with air in the lung. The left hand frame on the bottom row is at equilibrium when gas is fully mixed with the air in the lung. In the normal subject, apart from the better count rate, the distribution is similar to that in the first breath. Subsequent frames show wash-out which in the normal case is symmetrical and rapid. If there is air trapping wash-out is slower from some regions of lung than others.

tilation image filling in at equilibrium. Delayed wash-out and regional variations in the ratio of ventilation to lung volume occur in obstructive airways disease. There may be ventilation defects in regions with no perfusion abnormality (reverse mismatch).

Sources of error

Failure to time the administration of xenon correctly, so that it is dispersed into the circuit and not inhaled as a bolus, gives an unacceptably low count rate for the first breath. Failure to obtain equilibrium due to a poor gas-tight seal between the circuit and the patient may invalidate the lung volume and wash-out phases. Because the ventilation study with ^{133}Xe must be performed before the perfusion study with ^{99m}Tc microaggregated albumin (MAA), the optimum projection is not known. It is preferable to perform the first breath, but not the full study, in three projections (posterior and both posterior oblique projections), limiting equilibrium and wash-out to the posterior.

Aerosols

A number of commercially available aerosol generators are alternatives to xenon. The characteristics and properties of an aerosol depend on several factors. It is not possible to identify obstructive airways disease with aerosols and the uniformity of deposition of aerosols depends critically on non-turbulent flow in the airways, a condition which is not fulfilled in obstructive airways disease. Depending on their size, electrical charge, surface properties and the speed and turbulence of airflow in the larger and middle order airways, particles may distribute peripherally into the alveoli or may be deposited more centrally in the bronchi. Usually both occur, in variable proportions. Once deposited, their subsequent fate depends on the nature of the radiopharmaceutical. Pertechnetate or diethylenetriamine pentaacetic acid (DTPA) are rapidly absorbed through the alveolar membrane and can be used to measure alveolar permeability. Insoluble particles deposited in the alveoli are cleared slowly by macrophages whilst particles of any type deposited in airways are cleared by ciliary action. As technetium is used both for the aerosol and for the perfusion study an interval of 6–24 hours is necessary, delaying diagnosis. Aerosol generators have an efficiency of less than 10%, leaving large amounts of ^{99m}Tc-contamination on equipment.

Lung perfusion scintigraphy

Indications

Suspected pulmonary embolism. A perfusion study in isolation is permissible only if the chest X-ray is *completely* normal and there is no history of obstructive airways disease.

Radiopharmaceuticals

75 MBq ^{99m}Tc MAA or human serum albumin microspheres (not fewer than 100 000 and not more than 500 000 particles) are administered by clean i.v. injection. Denatured protein is digested and not absorbed in usable form if the injection is extravasated. If the number of particles is too low there may be uneven distribution in the lungs; if too high there is danger from systemic embolization should there be a right to left shunt, or of exacerbating severe pre-existing pulmonary hypertension. Neither hazard is significant if the number and size of particles is within these limits. The particles now used are rapidly digested *in vivo*. Imaging should therefore start immediately after injection. If imaging is delayed, free activity in background, the thyroid and gastric mucosa may complicate interpretation.

Diagnostic studies can be obtained with 250 000 counts in each of at least six projections (posterior, anterior, both posterior and both anterior obliques), using a gamma camera with a field of view greater than 35 cm, equipped with a general-purpose low-energy collimator. Interpretation of lateral projections is complicated by shine-through from the contralateral lung. No background subtraction and no enhancement is necessary. The entire range of count rate in the field of view should be presented as good quality monochrome images.

Sources of error

Aggregation of particles may occur if blood is withdrawn and there is subsequently a delay before injection, for example because of difficulty in finding a suitable vein. This may render the study non-diagnostic. Faulty preparations containing free pertechnetate may result in visualization of thyroid and gastric mucosa, but this appearance is more commonly due to an excessive delay between administration of the radiopharmaceutical and starting imaging. Incorrect positioning, resulting in superimposition of the lungs, may give rise to difficulties when interpreting oblique projections.

Interpretation

The distribution of particles represents right ventricular output at the time of injection, with no subsequent redistribution (Fig. 27.3). The normal subject at rest has a gravity-dependent greater perfusion of the lower lobes than the upper. If injected supine, the most posterior segments are better perfused.

Most radiological abnormalities, including consolidation or collapse, are associated with abnormalities of perfusion. The ventilation and perfusion images must always be correlated with a chest radiograph taken within 12 hours. Two or more *segmental* perfusion defects in association with a normal ventilation study and a normal chest radiograph are characteristic of recent pulmonary embolism. A uniform distribution of ventilation and perfusion associated with a normal chest radiograph virtually rules out a recent pulmonary embolus. Non-segmental perfusion defects and perfusion defects with matching ventilation defects, even in the absence of radiographic consolidation, are indeterminate as are small areas of atelectasis on the chest radiograph in association with normal ventilation and perfusion. It is conventional to report in terms of high, intermediate or low probability of recent pulmonary embolism.

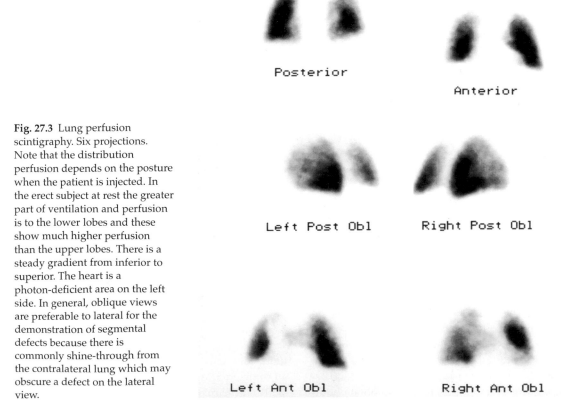

Fig. 27.3 Lung perfusion scintigraphy. Six projections. Note that the distribution perfusion depends on the posture when the patient is injected. In the erect subject at rest the greater part of ventilation and perfusion is to the lower lobes and these show much higher perfusion than the upper lobes. There is a steady gradient from inferior to superior. The heart is a photon-deficient area on the left side. In general, oblique views are preferable to lateral for the demonstration of segmental defects because there is commonly shine-through from the contralateral lung which may obscure a defect on the lateral view.

Thyroid

Scintigraphy of the thyroid was the first radioisotope investigation to be employed clinically.

Indications

These include differentiation of Graves' disease from toxic nodular goitre, and identification of ectopic or residual thyroid tissue. Fine-needle aspiration is the primary investigation in patients with palpable thyroid nodules and is used to distinguish benign nodules from malignant. Scintigraphy has a role only if there is clinical suspicion of a functioning or toxic nodule.

Radiopharmaceuticals

The pertechnetate ion has a similar ionic radius to iodide and is trapped by tissues which trap iodide. It is not organified. For most purposes 75 MBq ^{99m}Tc sodium pertechnetate is adequate. It is occasionally necessary to resort to iodine isotopes, preferably 25 MBq ^{123}I or failing this 10 MBq ^{131}I. Both pertechnetate and iodide are absorbed following oral administration but the rate is slow and erratic. There is good absorption from an extravasation. Imaging with a gamma camera equipped with a pinhole collimator may be started 15 min after injection of sodium pertechnetate. It is possible to image with sodium iodide but at this time the images principally show trapping, contrast is low and small amounts of ectopic tissue may not be clearly visualized. When using either ^{131}I or ^{123}I it is preferable to image 18–24 hours after administration.

A minimum of two projections is required, one with the pinhole as close to the thyroid as possible, but still including the whole of the gland within the field of view, and a second with the pinhole to skin distance equal to the pinhole to crystal distance. The closer the pinhole is to the skin, the greater the magnification and the smaller the nodules which can be visualized. The latter provides a fixed magnification image which enable the size of the gland to be estimated and referred to landmarks such as the outline of the neck and hot or cold markers on the sternal notch and external acoustic meati. If nodules are being imaged it is sometimes helpful to obtain additional magnified oblique views. Statistics are poor in pinhole images. Image quality can be substantially enhanced by filtration. If this is not available, smoothed images are preferable to unsmoothed.

Sources of error

Radioactivity secreted in saliva may pool in the pharynx or oesophagus. Large retrosternal goitres may have very low uptake so that their extent is underestimated with pertechnetate. Uptake of pertechnetate into thyroid metastases is often low. Iodine is therefore necessary when evaluating a suspected retrosternal goitre or metastatic thyroid carcinoma. Uptake by thyroid is suppressed by iodine-containing preparations, thyroid replacement or antithyroid drugs.

Interpretation

The normal thyroid shows smooth uptake but is rarely symmetrical (Fig. 27.4). In the normal subject uptake of pertechnetate in the thyroid is of higher intensity than that in salivary glands. Greater uptake in salivary glands than thyroid indicates hypothyroidism. Uptake that is so high that the salivary glands are either not seen or only very faintly visualized (depending on the display) implies thyrotoxicosis.

Thyroid carcinoma

The usual treatment for thyroid carcinoma is thyroid ablation followed by hormone replacement with thyroxin (T_4). When imaging for suspected metastases, thyroxin should be replaced by tri-iodothyronine (T_3) for 4 weeks. A tracer dose of ^{131}I is administered 10–14 days after stopping T_3 and 6 weeks after stopping T_4. Thyroid replacement therapy with T_4 is reinstituted 48 hours after the tracer dose of radioiodine. Whole-body imaging should be performed 7 days later. If profile (one-dimensional) scanning is available, 40 MBq ^{131}I is adequate, but any peaks identified on the profile should be imaged, using a high-energy high-sensitivity collimator; otherwise 400 MBq ^{131}I should be administered and the whole body, including the skull and trunk, imaged using a gamma camera

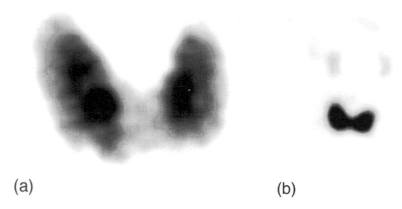

(a)   (b)

Fig. 27.4 Thyroid. (a) Magnified view of the thyroid. Uptake is slightly uneven but no clear nodules are seen. However, on this view there are no landmarks and it is not possible to determine the size of the gland. (b) Taken with a fixed pinhole to skin distance which enables the size of the gland to be related to the size of the field of view. In this case, as is normal, the salivary glands are clearly visualized and show much less uptake than the thyroid. The sternal notch can rarely be seen in the normal subject unless a marker is used.

equipped with a high-energy collimator. ^{123}I is unsuitable because contrast between deposits and background peaks at 72 hours, and excreted activity in bowel takes up to a week to clear.

Heart

The principal investigations are ventriculography, myocardial perfusion and viability, and visualization of myocardial infarcts. These are considered in Chapter 10.

Kidney

Glomerular function, tubular function, tubular mass, vesico–ureteric reflux, renal drainage and renal blood flow can be assessed.

Renography

Radiopharmaceuticals

^{99m}Tc MAG3 (mercaptoacetyltriglycine) is the agent of choice for tubular function, ^{99m}Tc DTPA for glomerular function. For most purposes MAG3 is preferable, but in renal failure MAG3 sometimes accumulates in the cortex, giving a rising curve in the absence of obstruction. The conditions under

which this occurs have not been fully defined. For this reason, DTPA is to be preferred in renal failure.

Activities of 15 MBq of ^{99m}Tc MAG3 or 150–250 MBq ^{99m}Tc DTPA are adequate for most purposes. Both must be given by clean i.v. injection. The rate of absorption of an extravasation of MAG3 is variable and unpredictable; extravasated DTPA is slowly absorbed and may give a rising curve in the absence of obstruction. If glomerular filtration rate (GFR) is measured by blood clearance, extravasation gives a falsely low value. Using a camera with at least a 35 cm field of view and a general-purpose low-energy collimator, both DTPA and MAG3 are collected as dynamic studies at 12 frames min^{-1} for 5 min, followed by 2 frames min^{-1} for up to 40 min. In normal subjects the examination can be terminated after 15 min.

Interventions

If the differential diagnosis includes pelviureteric junction obstruction, the patient should be orally hydrated with 200–500 ml of water and a diuretic (20 mg frusemide or 1 mg bumetanide i.v.) given 15 min before starting the renogram, to ensure maximal diuresis. If a rising curve is encountered during the study the patient should swallow a sip of water. If this fails to provoke contraction of the renal pelvis a similar dose of diuretic may be given. A response normally occurs 3 min after injection.

Data processing

Time–activity curves are obtained from regions of interest enclosing each kidney and renal pelvis and a 'background' region. It is sometimes useful to have a bladder curve. Images of the initial 90 s, at the peak of the renal time–activity curves and at the end of the examination after voiding are also necessary. If there is substantial persistence of activity in the renal areas, later films at 2 and 4 hours and sometimes 24 hours may be required.

The role of background subtraction is controversial. The usual practice is that time–activity curves should be corrected for counts originating from non-renal tissues around the kidney. However, all methods of background correction are crude approximations more likely to introduce artefact than increase information content. Background correction is essential for calculation of split renal function. However, it is not possible to correct accurately for differences in renal depth from a single projection. Errors due to differences in renal depth can be minimized, but not eliminated, by performing the examination supine. As gravity plays no part in drainage of urine from the normal renal pelvis this does not affect estimates of rate of drainage. Mean transit time of isotope through the kidney can be calculated by deconvolution of the renal curve with a curve obtained from a blood pool region such as the heart.

Interpretation

In the normal subject the time–activity curve peaks within 7 min then falls to less than 50% of its peak value within 15 min (Fig. 27.5). The up and down slopes are somewhat steeper with MAG3 than with DTPA, because of its higher extraction efficiency. A rising curve which falls in response to swallowing indicates a mild disturbance of contractility of the renal pelvis without obstruction. A rising curve which does not respond to swallowing, but which does respond to diuretic, indicates a hypokinetic non-obstructed kidney. A rising curve which does not respond to diuretic suggests obstruction. Obstruction should not be diagnosed on the basis of a rising curve alone. The features of obstruction are a rising curve which does not respond to diuretic, associated with a prolonged nephrographic phase and, if the obstruction has been present for more than 48 hours, impaired function. Estimates of split renal function obtained from the renogram curve are reproducible but are not accurate as there is no satisfactory method of correcting for differences in mean renal depth. Split function may be calculated by comparing the net counts in each renal area from the first arrival of activity at the kidney for the subsequent 90 s, during which time no activity can have left the kidney. These must be corrected for background, for example using a circumferential region with Goris interpolation.

Vesico–ureteric reflux

The direct method involves catheterization and instillation of 10–20 MBq of pertechnetate diluted in saline or water into the bladder. The patient voids in front of the camera, much as in a micturating cystourethrogram (MCU). Many feel that if instrumentation is to be performed the better anatomical resolution of the MCU should be obtained (see Chapter 6).

The indirect method is performed at the end of a gamma camera renogram, before dimercaptosuccinic acid (DMSA) has been given and whilst the bladder is still full. MAG3 is preferred to DTPA because the more rapid excretion gives lower background in the

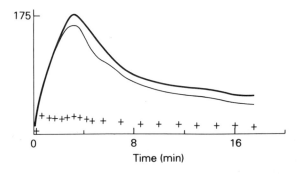

Fig. 27.5 Normal mercaptoacetyltriglycine (MAG3) renogram curve. The two solid lines are the two kidneys. The line of crosses is the background in the normal subject; the level of symmetry is such that the two curves are superimposed.

renal areas. The patient stand or sits with their back against a large field of view camera which acquires at 12 frames min^{-1} for as long as necessary. The camera should be started 30 s before the patient is instructed to void into a suitable receptacle. The frames should be filtered, viewed in cine mode to confirm that there is no patient movement, and time–activity curves obtained from the renal areas. Reflux is diagnosed if the count rate in the renal region of interest increases by more than 3 SD of the number of counts present in the first of the frames being used and in the absence of movement.

Sources of error

An extravasated injection can cause a rising curve in the absence of obstruction. A full bladder may also be associated with a rising curve. Patient movement can cause gross distortion of the curves.

Renal scintigraphy

Radiopharmaceutical

Instillation of 75 MBq ^{99m}Tc DMSA is given by clean i.v. injection. Absorption from an extravasation is poor and erratic. Imaging should be performed with a gamma camera equipped with a general-purpose or high-resolution low-energy collimator, not less than 1.5 hours after injection. Four views should be obtained: anterior, posterior and both posterior obliques. Additional anterior obliques may be required in patients with horseshoe or ectopic kidneys .In most subjects the relative function obtained at 90 min are similar to those obtained at later times. The interval should be extended in the presence of a dilated system or partial obstruction. Imaging can be performed up to 18 hours after injection.

Data processing

An accurate depth-corrected measure of relative function can be obtained using the geometric mean of the background-corrected renal counts in the anterior and posterior projections. Data should be presented as good quality monochrome images displaying the entire range of counts, with no overrange pixels.

Interpretation

In the normal subject there are photon deficiencies corresponding to the pyramids, but the cortex surrounding them should be complete (Fig. 27.6).

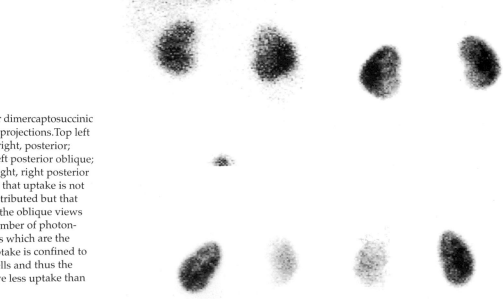

Fig. 27.6 Four dimercaptosuccinic acid (DMSA) projections.Top left anterior; top right, posterior; bottom left, left posterior oblique; and bottom right, right posterior oblique. Note that uptake is not uniformly distributed but that especially on the oblique views there are a number of photon-deficient areas which are the pyramids. Uptake is confined to the tubular cells and thus the pyramids have less uptake than the cortex.

The anatomical detail which can be obtained depends to some extent on whether the patient is breathing diaphragmatically or costally. In the case of diaphragmatic respiration there is considerable degradation in image quality.

White cell imaging

Indications

Identification of infective inflammatory foci; assessment of activity of inflammatory bowel disease.

Radiopharmaceuticals

Under sterile conditions, 50 ml of venous blood is withdrawn through a 19 gauge or larger needle into a syringe containing 8 ml of acid citrate dextrose anticoagulant. Buffy coat in plasma is separated; all cells present are labelled. Activity is preferentially retained on granulocytes, eluting fairly rapidly from the other cells. The labelled cell concentrate is reinjected. If seeking abdominal sepsis, initial imaging is performed at 20 min and repeated (and at other sites initiated) 3 hours after injection. It is occasionally helpful to perform further views at 18–24 hours. Labelled cells are concentrated in the spleen, which must be overranged to visualize abdominal and thoracic structures.

Sources of error

Because of the relatively high but variable uptake in normal marrow, osteomyelitis in the spine and marrow-containing parts of the skeleton is difficult to distinguish from normal marrow uptake. Faulty preparations with devitalized cells are associated with relatively lower uptake in the spleen. Activity eluted from cells may be excreted via the gallbladder into the gut. This makes interpretation of abdominal images more difficult as time progresses.

Interpretation

Abnormal accumulations are indicative of an active inflammatory processes. There is usually some hint on the 30-min images, which becomes more intense and easier to visualize with time. Collections separate from the gastrointestinal tract may be more clearly visualized at 24 hours, provided that the distribution of gastrointestinal activity is appreciated.

Liver

Hepatobiliary and reticuloendothelial aspects of liver function can be investigated. Reticuloendothelial function using labelled colloids was one of the earliest radioisotope investigations, principally for the detection of space-occupying lesions, but is now rarely performed having been superseded by ultrasound and other modalities. The importance of hepatobiliary imaging depends on the case mix.

Indications

Diagnosis of acute cholecystitis, bile leaks (for example following cholecystectomy) and other abnormalities of bile drainage. Other applications include the visualization of patency following biliary–enteric or entero–enteric bypasses.

Radiopharmaceuticals

For hepatobiliary imaging one of the hepatic iminodiacetic acid (HIDA) agents is employed. There is little to choose between them in subjects with normal liver function but the balance between hepatic and renal excretion is significant in jaundiced subjects, when the agent of choice is tribromo-IDA.

Technique

A dose of 50 MBq is administered by clean i.v. injection. One frame is collected per minute for 30 min. If gallbladder and small bowel are not clearly visualized at this time, further images may be taken at 30-min intervals and after 2 hours at 60 min or longer intervals, if necessary up to 24 hours. Hepatic excretion may be augmented in jaundiced subjects or those with impaired hepatic function by pretreatment with phenobarbitone at a dose of 5 mg kg^{-1} day^{-1} for 5 days.

Interpretation

Initially there is a rapid and even uptake by the whole of the liver (Fig. 27.7). The major bile-ducts should be visualized within 15 min as areas of greater concentration. The gallbladder may be visualized at this

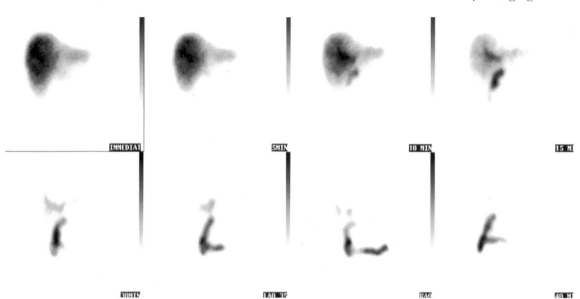

Fig. 27.7 Normal hepatobiliary scintigraphy. Sequence of frames illustrating the progressive changes. The initial frame (top left) shows uniform uptake throughout the liver. Subsequently the intrahepatic bile-ducts and common bile-duct become visualized. By the fifth frame (left-hand side second row) uptake is visible in the duodenum and the uptake subsequently passes into small bowel. In this patient the gallbladder is not visualized but it should normally be visible separate from the common bile-duct within 30 min.

time and always within 30 min. Activity is usually present in the duodenum within 30 min. If activity is in the small bowel but the gallbladder has not been identified, 2 mg of morphine may be given i.v. to provoke contraction of the sphincter of Oddi with consequent filling of the gallbladder. Visualization of the gallbladder excludes cholecystitis. However, the sensitivity of non-visualization as a sign of cholecystitis depends on the prevalence of chronic cholecystitis in the population.

Brain

The traditional brain scan, employing agents which demonstrated areas where the blood–brain barrier was disrupted, has now been almost entirely superseded by CT and MRI with contrast enhancement.

Radiopharmaceuticals

The regional distribution of blood flow can be demonstrated following the i.v. administration of one of a number of lipophilic agents including exametazime, bicisate and iodoamphetamine. It is not possible with these agents to obtain absolute

measurement of blood flow but the relative distribution is approximately proportional to blood flow. These agents have been advocated in the differential diagnosis of the dementias, but their clinical role is disputed. Injection of 500 MBq of either of the technetium agents is given i.v. and single photon emission tomographic imaging performed starting 5–10 min later.

Interpretation

Epileptic foci may appear as photon-deficient areas if the radiopharmaceutical is administered interictally and as photon-rich if given during a fit. Multi-infarct dementia may be associated with multiple randomly distributed defects, Alzheimer's disease with bilateral parietal defects and Pick's disease with bilateral frontal defects. The specificity of these signs is poor.

Further reading

Murray, I.P.C. & Ell, P.J. (1994) *Nuclear Medicine in Clinical Diagnosis and Treatment*. Churchill Livingstone, Edinburgh.

28   Computed Tomography

S. J. GOLDING

Computed tomography (CT) has become established an an essential radiological technique and one that is applicable in a wide range of clinical situations (Husband & Golding, 1982). Used correctly, CT is particularly effective in influencing clinical decisions and the management of patients (Wittenberg *et al.*, 1980).

The basic physics and instrumentation of CT are beyond the scope of this chapter and the reader is referred to Hounsfield (1973), Pullan (1979) and Berland (1986). In essence, CT is comparable to conventional radiography in that the image is a grey scale representation of the density to X-rays (attenuation) of tissues. The CT image represents a cross-section of the body and is made up of a matrix of small squares, or pixels, each representing the attenuation value of the tissues at that point. The cross-sectional display, which means that there is no superimposition of structures, together with sophisticated detector systems and computed production of the image, makes the technique superior to conventional radiography in the demonstration of structures. It is, however, important to remember that the CT image is a cross-sectional 'slice' and therefore represents only a relatively small volume of tissue.

In conventional CT, exposures are usually made separately and with the couch moving in incremental steps between exposures. In this way an examination is built up from a number of sections. In the last few years a new technique has emerged: spiral CT (Heiken *et al.*, 1993), in which the table moves continuously during a single exposure. As the exposure comes from a tube rotating in the gantry, the exposure in effect traverses helically through a volume of the patient. Axial images corresponding to those of conventional CT are then reconstructed from the volumetric data acquisition. The principal advantage of this technique is that it is possible to cover an area of the body in a very short time, characteristically about 10 s.

As in conventional radiography, the ease of distinguishing structures depends upon the difference in the attenuation or natural contrast of the tissues. In CT images of the body, much of the natural contrast is provided by fat and the technique is therefore very suitable for obese patients (Fig. 28.1a). In thin patients (Fig. 28.1b), interpretation may be much more difficult and careful technique may be critical to a successful examination. The examination techniques appropriate to specific organs or areas of the body differ considerably, depending upon the area and sometimes upon the indication for the technique. This chapter is a general account of the major indications for CT and those elements of technique, including modifications, which are common to the majority of examinations. More extensive accounts are listed in the recommended reading. CT has also become a valuable method of guiding selected interventional techniques, which are described briefly.

Indications

CT has made a major impact on the practice of radiology, completely replacing some techniques and extending diagnostic capability in other areas.

Like any other investigation, CT should be carried out only when its use is justified in a particular patient. The radiologist must select for examination only those patients whose management is most likely to be influenced by the findings. Each referral has therefore to be considered on its own merits and in the light of the clinical problem and the results of other investigations.

It is good practice to weigh the benefits of any investigation against the risks. In the case of CT the principal drawback is a high absorbed radiation

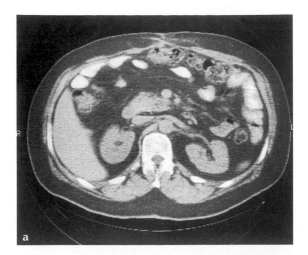

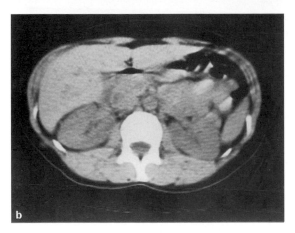

Fig. 28.1 (a) Computed tomography section at the level of the renal hila in a male patient of average weight. (b) Section at a similar level in a slim female patient.

has superseded CT in the examination of the head and neck and many areas of the musculoskeletal system, and may frequently offer a radiation-free alternative to CT in the chest, abdomen and pelvis.

Tables 28.1 and 28.2 classify the major indications for CT according to the clinical specialty generating the request. The clinical disciplines most commonly requesting CT — described in the table as 'primary user specialties' — are neurology, oncology, orthopaedics and acute medicine and surgery. Other clinical specialties do not require this level of access and may be regarded as 'secondary user specialties' (Table 28.2). It should be emphasized that this classification illustrates the relative frequency of referrals and does not imply that a request from one specialty is any more justifiable than that from another.

The tables also indicate where MRI may be considered an alternative to CT. In some of these areas, for example the brain, the superior information provided by MRI has made it the technique of choice. Where the benefits are not so clearly defined, the use of MRI is likely to depend heavily on local availability. However, MRI remains a young technique and is developing rapidly. It is probable that more clinical applications of CT will move to MRI as the latter matures and more systems become available.

Some of the major benefits of CT have been felt within radiology itself. The cross-sectional display of CT may be used to elucidate suspicious findings on conventional radiography, for example the suggestion of a mediastinal mass or area of destruction in the sacrum. This is one of the most effective uses of the technique and such examinations may often be limited to a few sections.

Examination

The CT examination is not standardized and can be varied according to the clinical problem and the circumstances of the patient. As in any other procedure, careful technique is fundamental to diagnostic success and at the start of the examination the radiologist must decide precisely how it is to be conducted. This is a good time to review the results of any other imaging studies as these may influence the choice of CT technique. Residual barium from gastrointestinal studies produces serious artefact on CT and examinations should be deferred until this has cleared.

dose. It is recognized that CT examinations, although carried out in a small number of patients, overall account for a significant proportion of the dose to the population from diagnostic radiology (Shrimpton, 1992). The technique must therefore be used responsibly, especially in young patients and those with benign disease. Where possible, techniques which do not utilize radiation should be carried out in preference. In the abdomen and pelvis, ultrasound (see Chapter 26) offers an alternative in many patients. Magnetic resonance imaging (MRI) (see Chapter 29), although not so readily available,

Table 28.1 Indications for computed tomography: primary user specialties

Neurosciences
Primary diagnosis, presurgical assessment, treatment monitoring and detection of relapse of almost all structural disease of the brain*
Diagnosis and presurgical assessment of structural lesions of the spinal cord*
Diagnosis of sensorineural hearing loss and visual disturbance*
Evaluation of head injury

Radiotherapy/oncology
Staging of almost all solid tumours, including lymphoma
Treatment monitoring and detection of relapse in tumours which are poorly demonstrated by conventional means*
Treatment planning of majority of solid tumours, including formal CT-assisted radiotherapy planning

Orthopaedics/accident services
Diagnosis and presurgical assessment of degenerative spinal and disc disease; presurgical assessment of scoliosis*
Assessment of vertebral and pelvic trauma
Diagnosis and staging of neoplasms of bone and soft tissue*
Diagnosis of instability of shoulder joint
Detection of loose bodies in the hip joint
Assessment of acetabular dysplasia*
Assessment of tarsal coalition*

Acute medicine/surgery
Diagnosis of abdominal mass
Diagnosis of neoplasms which present to these specialties, e.g. lymphoma and carcinoma of pancreas
Diagnosis and presurgical assessment of aortic aneurysm or dissection*
Assessment of abdominal trauma
Diagnosis of intra-abdominal abscess
Detection of site and cause of obstructive jaundice
Characterization of parenchymal disease of the lung

* Magnetic resonance imaging maybe an alternative.

Preparation

Most CT examinations require little preparation. If i.v. contrast media are likely to be given, patients may be starved for a few hours beforehand to reduce the incidence of contrast-induced vomiting. Patients undergoing pelvic examination should have a full bladder. A tampon is used to outline the vagina in examinations for gynaecological disease.

Table 28.2 Indications for computed tomography: secondary user specialties

Thoracic surgery
Staging of pulmonary and oesophageal neoplasms*
Diagnosis and presurgical assessment of aortic aneurysm and dissection*
Assessment of mediastinal trauma
Presurgical assessment of disease of chest wall

Urology
Differential diagnosis of renal mass where other techniques are inconclusive
Staging of carcinoma of kidney and bladder*
Assessment of renal trauma
Diagnosis of site and cause of ureteric obstruction
Assessment of renal transplant

Gynaecology
Staging of carcinoma of the cervix and ovary*
Treatment monitoring of advanced ovarian carcinoma
Pelvimetry

Ear, nose and throat surgery/ophthalmology
Diagnosis and staging of neoplasms of the sinuses, pharynx, larynx and salivary glands*
Diagnosis of middle ear disease and sensorineural hearing loss*
Evaluation of facial fractures
Evaluation of facial deformity before plastic surgery
Diagnosis of orbital masses and unilateral proptosis*

Paediatrics
Diagnosis of cerebral and spinal disease*
Staging of neoplasms, especially lymphoma, nephroblastoma and neuroblastoma*
Evaluation of congenital hip disease*

Gastroenterology
Diagnosis of pancreatic disease
Diagnosis of space-occupying lesions of the liver where other techniques are inconclusive*
Diagnosis of site and cause of obstructive jaundice

Endocrinology
Diagnosis of masses of the pituitary and adrenal glands*
Diagnosis of endocrine tumours of the pancreas
Diagnosis of parathyroid disease*

Plastic surgery
Presurgical staging of cutaneous neoplasms
Planning reconstructive surgery, especially of facial deformity

* Magnetic resonance imaging may be an alternative.

Patients should be asked to undress and a gown is provided. The radiographer should make sure that all metal items have been removed from the area of the scan as they may cause serious artefact. Patients undergoing CT may be very anxious, not only about the implications of the examination — after so many public appeals to buy CT equipment there is a general awareness that the technique is associated with malignant disease — but also because of being isolated in the examination room, surrounded by high-technology equipment. Being kept waiting tends to increase anxiety and should be avoided. Playing music in the reception area and in the examination room helps to make the atmosphere more comfortable.

No premedication is usually required but pain should be controlled. Ideally, patients should be pain-free and relaxed but able to cooperate; heavy sedation or analgesia is best avoided. An i.v. or i.m. injection of a relaxant such as diazepam is often valuable if pain is accompanied by muscle spasm.

Children present special problems (Berger *et al.*, 1981). Many children over the age of 5 can be examined with ease if they are not hungry and have not been kept waiting. It is usually valuable to ask a parent or nurse to stay with the child during the examination. Infants may sleep through the examination, particularly if they have recently been fed or are allowed to feed during the examination. However, if the child is restless and a good-quality examination is required, good sedation or general anaesthesia may be necessary. The latter has the advantage that respiration may be suspended intermittently during scanning — the anaesthetist should know beforehand if this will be required — but the disadvantage that no oral contrast medium can be given for examinations of the abdomen. General anaesthesia or strong sedation is rarely required for adults unless they are very restless or confused.

Communicating with the patient

As indicated above, patients for CT may be anxious for several reasons and a reassuring and caring approach is essential. In practice, anxiety can often be the cause of technical problems such as movement artefact or failure to suspend respiration in the correct position. It is only good practice and courtesy

for an appropriate person to explain the procedure to the patient beforehand.

Direct visual communication between the patient and operator is preferable and an intercom link with the examination room is essential. Ideally this is switched through to the examination room, except when actually being used by the radiographer, so that it is immediately obvious if the patient experiences a problem. Patients should be kept informed of the progress of their examination, especially if there are any pauses, for example while the images are being viewed.

Patients should not leave the department without being interviewed by a radiologist and being given an indication of the result of their examination. This is particularly important in oncological practice, where patients who attend for repeated examinations soon learn that the results are frequently critical to their care. Close liaison with the clinician helps to ensure that what the patient is told does not compromise the clinician's advice to the patient.

Position

Most examinations are carried out with the patient supine (Fig. 28.2). Patients with pain due to disease of the spine or retroperitoneal lymphadenopathy may find this difficult and are often helped by a support behind the knees (Fig. 28.2). A small cushion beneath the lumbar spine may also be useful. If these fail, patients may be examined prone, but a lateral decubitus position is often more comfortable. Both these positions disturb the anatomy and may make interpretation difficult (Ball *et al.*, 1980).

Patients who experience claustrophobia in the scanner are usually examined prone. Such patients also benefit from being accompanied in the examination room.

Direct coronal scans of the head and neck may be obtained with the patient either supine or prone; the prone examination is preferred as this usually extends the neck to a greater degree, making it easier to obtain sections in as near the true coronal plane as possible.

Changing the position of the patient is one of the most common manoeuvres for overcoming diagnostic problems and this is described in detail below.

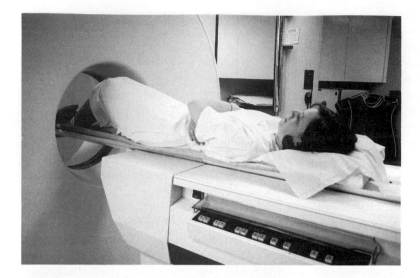

Fig. 28.2 Patient position on the examination couch, knees supported to improve comfort.

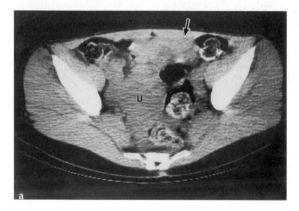
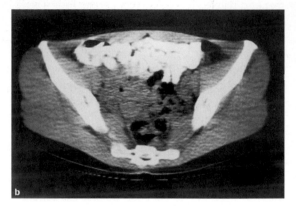

Fig. 28.3 (a) Computed tomographic (CT) section of the pelvis showing an apparent mass (arrow), lying beneath the abdominal wall and anterior to the uterus (U). (b) CT section at the same level following oral contrast medium showing that the apparent mass is due to non-opacified bowel loops. Note that the colon is identified on both sections because of characteristic appearances, although these differ on the two images.

Opacifying bowel

This is necessary in most examinations of the abdomen because the contents of the stomach and small bowel have attenuation values similar to soft tissues and may mimic pathology, especially masses (Korobkin, 1979; Kaye et al., 1980) (Fig. 28.3). In practice, the bowel 'pseudotumour' is the most important diagnostic pitfall in the abdomen.

The small bowel can be satisfactorily opacified by giving a dilute solution of aqueous contrast medium orally. The author's preference is to use Gastrografin (sodium diatrizoate 10%, meglumine diatrizoate 66%*) diluted to a 2% solution, but any similar agent is suitable. Higher concentrations should be avoided as they produce artefact.

Patients frequently find the taste of dilute contrast medium unpalatable, especially if they are already nauseated. This is sometimes improved by flavouring the solution. Dilute barium preparations are also available for CT and may be more acceptable to some patients (Hatfield *et al.*, 1980; Chambers & Best, 1984).

* Schering Health Care Ltd, Burgess Hill, West Sussex, UK.

The volume of contrast medium and the time at which it should be given before the examination depend on the area to be examined. A suitable regimen is given in Table 28.3. Oral contrast medium is not required for examinations of the kidneys or liver alone.

The proximal colon does not usually need to be opacified as the contents have a characteristic appearance on CT. However, opacification is necessary in examinations of the pelvic viscera. Although the oral route may be used, in practice it is more convenient to inject contrast medium per rectum at the start of the study: 150 ml is usually sufficient.

Reducing movement artefact

Movement is a common source of artefact in CT. Some of this, such as cardiac pulsation, is unavoidable but other forms of movement should be controlled as far as possible. Patients may move because they are anxious, in pain or confused and, as indicated above, sedation or even general anaesthesia may be necessary. Apart from this, attention is usually directed at controlling artefact due to respiration and peristalsis (Fig. 28.4).

Patients should be asked to hold their breath during the exposure in all examinations of the chest, abdomen (including the spine) and pelvic contents. Almost all patients, except those with severe dyspnoea when lying flat, can do this for the duration of scans on modern machines. However, it is tiring to hold one's breath repeatedly and if the examination is long it is often beneficial to allow the patient a short rest at intervals. Suspended respiration is not required for studies of the neck, but these

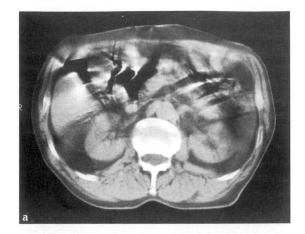

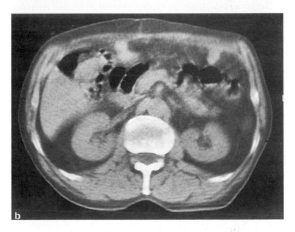

Fig. 28.4 (a) Computed tomography section of the abdomen showing severe streak artefact due to peristalsis and movement of bowel gas. The margins of the viscera are also indistinct owing to respiratory excursion. Scan duration 8 s. (b) The same section taken with a scan duration of 4 s.

Table 28.3 Regimens for opacification of bowel

Indication	Volume (ml)	Min prior to examination
Abdomen (general)	450	30
Pancreas	300	30
	150	5
Adrenal glands	150	0
Oesophagus	150	0
Pelvis	450	60
	150	15
	(+ 150 ml per rectum)	

patients should be asked not to swallow during the exposure.

When patients have difficulty holding their breath, artefact may be avoided by choosing a shorter scan duration, providing there are no compelling reasons for using long exposures (Fig. 28.4b). Alternatively, it is sometimes helpful to ask patients to hyperventilate for a short time before the exposure.

Scans may be obtained in either inspiration or expiration, but it is essential that patients hold their breath in an identical phase when examining the chest and upper abdomen. Respiratory excursion produces significant alteration in the position of organs and lesions may be overlooked if variable respiration causes them to fall between sections (Kuhns *et al.*, 1979; Krudy *et al.*, 1982). A careful radiographer will observe the images as they are processed and look for stepwise progression of the anatomy.

Artefact due to peristaltic movement of bowel gas or contrast medium may be a problem when the scan duration exceeds 5 s. An antiperistaltic agent, such as glucagon (Novo) 0.4 mg or hyoscine butylbromide (Buscopan) 20 mg, should be administered in these circumstances. As it is not necessary to abolish movement completely, but only to produce a reduction over the period of the examination, intramuscular injection is adequate.

Respiratory misregistration is much less of a problem with spiral CT, as a single body area may be covered in a single breath-hold (Fig. 28.5). Antiperistaltic agents are not required because, although the overall exposure exceeds 5 s, each level within the patient is sampled for only a fraction of this time.

Localizer view or scanogram

Almost all machines have the facility to produce a digital radiograph at the beginning of the examination. This is used to define the area and to plan and record the level of sections. It is also used to plan the degree of angulation of the gantry if this is required, for example to obtain sections at right angles to the spine (Fig. 28.6). Gantry angulation is also used in coronal sections of the head and neck if the neck cannot be extended sufficiently.

Exposure factors and radiation dose considerations

As in other forms of radiography, the exposure in CT depends upon tube potential and current, as well as the exposure time. The kilovoltage in CT is usually kept constant at about 120 kV, this being determined by the sensitivity of the detector system. Using

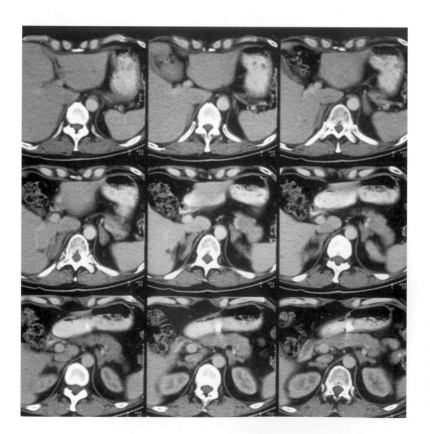

Fig. 28.5 Spiral CT. Nine images from a volume acquisition in the upper abdomen, obtained in a single breath-hold to show the adrenal glands, which are both enlarged in this patient. Note that the anatomy proceeds in contiguity between these 5 mm reconstructed sections. Courtesy of Professor A.K. Dixon, University of Cambridge.

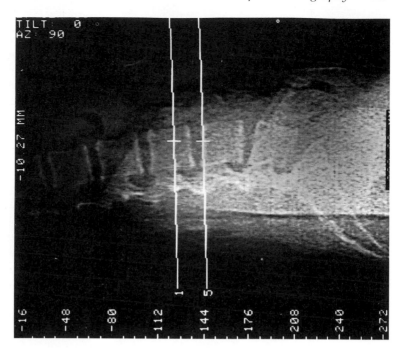

Fig. 28.6 Lateral digital radiograph of the lumbar spine showing the degree of angulation of the gantry and the first and last sections required for the examination of the L3/L4 disc space.

a higher exposure results in a better image or greater signal to noise ratio, at the cost of a higher absorbed dose. Noise in CT appears as mottle and reduces the ability to resolve small differences in attenuation (contrast resolution). Noise is also dependent on the pixel size and therefore the spatial resolution of the system, increasing as the pixel size decreases (Hounsfield, 1976).

As the pixel size is fixed for an individual system and the tube current is usually determined automatically, obtaining better contrast resolution means increasing the scan duration. As indicated above, this may increase movement artefact. Long scans are, however, necessary where good contrast resolution is necessary to diagnosis, notably in the brain and liver.

Absorbed dose is also affected by slice collimation, described below, and by slice increment, being greatest when sections are contiguous or overlap.

Slice collimation

In conventional CT, slice thickness or collimation is set as one of the exposure parameters. In spiral CT the operator chooses the thickness of section to be reconstructed from the volumetric data acquisition.

In both systems the choice of thickness depends on the organ under examination.

Sections 8 or 10 mm thick (Fig. 28.7a) are suitable for routine work, but the examination of a small organ such as the adrenal gland requires sections as thin as 5 mm or even 2 mm to avoid partial-volume averaging within the section. Thin sections are also used if the detection of lesions depends on changes of fine details in the image, such as trabeculae in fractured bone (Fig. 28.8). They are required if the image data are to be reformatted in different planes as this improves the resolution of the reformatted image.

Thin sections are subject to less partial-volume averaging and produce a crisper image. They cannot be used routinely because the exposure is smaller for a thin section and images are subject to noise (Fig. 28.7b). Thick sections are therefore important where good contrast resolution is required, as in the liver.

Slice increment

The interval between sections also depends on the area of examination and the suspected pathology. Thus 10 mm sections at 20 mm intervals, i.e. with

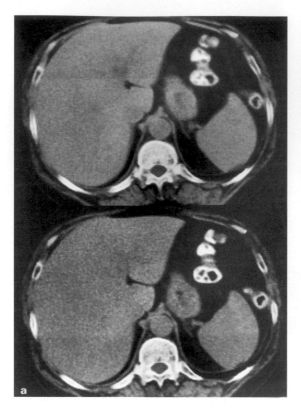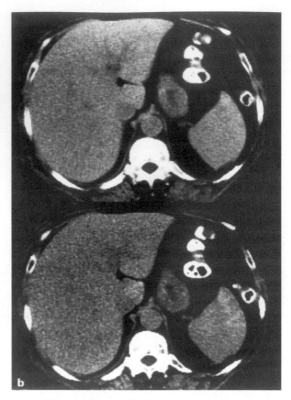

Fig. 28.7 Sections of the liver. (a) The upper image was obtained with 10 mm collimation, the lower with 5 mm collimation. The latter has a crisper appearance due to less partial-volume averaging of the margins of structures. (b) The same images viewed at appropriate window widths and levels for the liver. The image of 5 mm collimation has greater mottle due to a higher noise level.

a 10 mm interslice gap, are suitable for detecting retroperitoneal lymphadenopathy but volume acquisition or contiguous sections of the chest are needed to exclude small pulmonary metastases; these are also used if reformatted views are required.

Manipulating the image

In general, images are viewed at window widths and levels which show the anatomy to advantage. However, specific settings are required for certain situations. Areas which include a wide range of attenuation values, such as lung or bone, should be viewed at window widths of 1000 Hounsfield units (HU) or more (Fig. 28.8). The window level is usually best set between the attenuation values of normal and abnormal tissues. Lesions which differ very

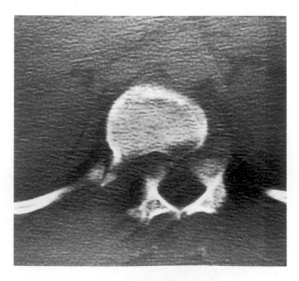

Fig. 28.8 Localized image of the spine, 5 mm collimation and high-resolution algorithm, showing a severe fracture dislocation at the thoracolumbar junction.

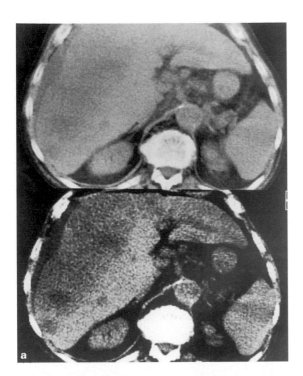

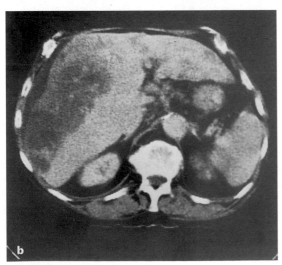

little in density from their surroundings should be viewed at narrow window widths, which increase the contrast between small differences in attenuation (Fig. 28.9).

Software algorithms are also available whereby data may be reprocessed to give a high-resolution image of a small field of view, such as the middle ear or the spine (Fig. 28.8).

High-resolution techniques are valuable where natural contrast is great. In the lung, thin sections and high-resolution algorithms may be used to show the fine lobular structure of the lung (Fig. 28.10). This technique is used to characterize disease of the pulmonary parenchyma (Muller, 1991).

The basic technique of the most common examinations is summarized in Table 28.4. More information about these and other areas will be found in the recommended reading, especially Dixon *et al.* (1983).

Supervising and modifying the examination

It should be the aim of the radiologist to ensure as far as possible that all CT examinations are successful, i.e. that they provide the information required

Fig. 28.9 Images showing a large hepatic metastasis from carcinoma of the caecum. (a) Effect of viewing settings. The upper image is set at window width and level to show the anatomy generally. The lower image is viewed with a narrow window and at a window level near that of normal hepatic tissue and shows the metastasis more clearly. (b) Image taken 60 s after an i.v. injection of contrast medium, showing better definition of the lesion.

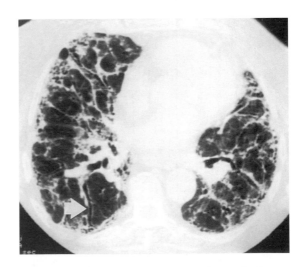

Fig. 28.10 High-resolution computed tomography in a patient with cryptogenic fibrosing alveolitis. This 1 mm section, displayed with a high-resolution algorithm, shows peripheral honeycombing and traction bronchiectasis (arrow), characteristic of this condition. Courtesy of Dr F.V. Gleeson, Churchill Hospital, Oxford.

Table 28.4 (a–d) Basic technique for common examinations

(a) *Area*	Brain	Pituitary fossa	Abdomen: mass
Preparation	None — starvation optional	None — starvation optional	None (do before barium studies)
Oral contrast	None	None	Yes
Patient position	Supine	Coronal sections, preferably prone; supine if extension of neck difficult or patient unable to lie prone	Supine
Scanogram	Not essential unless localization of sections required (e.g. for radiotherapy planning)	Lateral	Not essential
Slice thickness	4–5 mm in posterior fossa 8–10 mm above tentorium	1.5–2 mm	8–10 mm
Slice increment	Contiguous	1.5–2 mm	10 or 20 mm, depending on size of mass
Respiration	Normal	Normal	Suspended
i.v. contrast	Depending on indication; if plain scan shows a mass ?vascular lesion	Bolus or infusion	May be helpful if organ of origin not clear
Modifications		Large tumours 4–5 mm sections	Right decubitus position may be helpful
Common pitfalls	Misinterpretation of near-normal scan	Poor images due to difficulties with coronal position	Bowel pseudotumour. The larger the mass, the more difficult it is to determine the organ of origin
Variations	Enhance at start for ?metastases; high-dose enhancement for ?multiple sclerosis	Include ventricles and rest of brain	Reduce slices if answer obvious (e.g. liver with metastases); i.v. enhancement at start if ?abscess: sections from diaphragm to pelvic floor

Table 28.4 Continued.

(b) Area	Abdomen: lymph nodes	Pancreas	Pelvis
Preparation	None	Starvation	Full bladder; tampon if gynaecological disease
Oral contrast	Yes, early for pelvic studies	Yes, last glass immediately before	600 ml, plus 150 ml per rectum
Patient position	Supine	Supine	Supine
Scanogram	Not essential	Frontal	Frontal
Slice thickness	8–10 mm	8–10 mm	8–10 mm
Slice increment	20 mm in abdomen, 15 mm in pelvis	10 mm, splenic hilum to third part duodenum	15 mm, T12 to symphysis
Respiration	Suspended	Suspended — inspiration or expiration	Suspended
i.v. contrast	To distinguish vessels and nodes	Dynamic enhancement for small space-occupying lesions	Not routinely
Modifications	Intervening sections; prone sections for ?bowel loops	Right lateral decubitus position if display difficult	i.v. enhancement for ?iliac nodes / vessels (not usually required to demonstrate intravesical masses)
Common pitfalls	Unopacified bowel loops; vascular anomalies; porta hepatis nodes difficult to detect	Non-opacified bowel; failure to include inferior limit of uncinate process	Unopacified bowel; failure to distend bladder; early neoplasms may be undetectable
Variations	Wider intervals if obviously abnormal	Liver usually included if ?malignant disease; dynamic enhancement for ?endocrine tumours	No rectal contrast medium if suspected lymphadenopathy only Contiguous thin sections for T staging carcinoma of prostate

Table 28.4 *Continued.*

(c) *Area*	Lumbar spine	Shoulder joint	Hip joint/acetabulum
Preparation	None	Postarthrogram for ? instability, otherwise none	Usually none; arthrogram for intra-articular pathology
Oral contrast	None	None	None
Patient position	Supine, knees flexed	Supine — shoulder must be in scan field; arms by side (contralateral arm may be above head)	Supine
Scanogram	Lateral	Frontal	Frontal
Slice thickness	4–5 mm Soft tissue algorithm for discs	4–5 mm, soft-tissue algorithm (bone for fractures)	4–5 mm, soft-tissue algorithm for joint, bone algorithm for trauma and surgical planning
Slice increment	Contiguous, angled to individual disc spaces	Contiguous	Contiguous
Respiration	Suspended	Quiet	Normal
i.v. contrast	Not routinely	Only if vessels damaged	None
Modifications	Enhance if ?fibrosis/?disc; sagittal/coronal or 3D reformatting	Arm above head allows wide shouldered to be scanned but makes interpretation of capsular pathology difficult	Greater increment if lesion large; sagittal/coronal or 3D reformatting
Common pitfalls	Pseudodisc/partial-volume averaging	Shoulder out of range; contrast medium too dense; rotator cuff tears difficult to identify	Acetabular roof not included
Variations	Contiguous sections, vertical gantry for vertebral trauma (bone algorithm); post-myelography for nerve root/cord disease	Torsion study of humerus — arms by side, sections through shoulders and humeral epicondyles (without changing positions of arms)	Femoral torsion study — section through proximal femur/section through condyles at knees

Table 28.4 *Continued.*

(d) Area	Chest: mediastinum	Chest: lungs	Chest: HRCT	Chest: pleura/chest wall
Preparation	None	None	None	None
Oral contrast	None, unless ?oesophageal disease	None	None	None
Patient position	Supine	Supine	Supine	Supine
Scanogram	Not essential, but can be helpful	Not essential	Frontal	Frontal
Slice thickness	8–10 mm	8–10 mm	1–2 mm; high-resolution algorithm	8–10 mm
Slice increment	15 mm	8–10 mm	10–20 mm	10 mm for localized lesion otherwise 15 mm
Respiration	Suspended inspiration	Suspended inspiration	Suspended inspiration	Suspended inspiration
i.v. contrast	To distinguish vessels and nodes as required	If ?arteriovenous malformation	None	Helpful to demonstrate tissue planes
Modifications	Smaller intervals if anatomy unclear, – especially hilar regions	Prone sections to exclude atelectasis and prominent vessels	Reduced field of view to increase spatial resolution	Prone sections for ?free fluid / encysted or mass
Common pitfalls	Subcarinal / hilar nodes difficult; vascular anomalies	Benign nodules / fibrosis; partial-volume averaging	Dyspnoea; cardiac motion	Partial-volume averaging, especially where thoracic wall is curving; rib lesions difficult to define
Variations	Wider intervals if obviously abnormal; bolus + infusion enhancement for vascular disease; include liver and coeliac nodes if oesophageal neoplasm	Bolus + infusion enhancement for staging bronchial carcinoma; include liver and adrenal glands	Prone scan for ?asbestosis and to distinguish dependent density from other pathology; suspended expiration to identify air trapping	Enhanced local sections for recurrent breast carcinoma or axillary disease

Table 28.4 derives from an unpublished manual written jointly with the author's colleagues Drs A.J. Molyneux and D.J. Wilson and Professor A.K. Dixon (University of Cambridge) and is published with their kind permission. HRCT, high-resolution computed tomography.

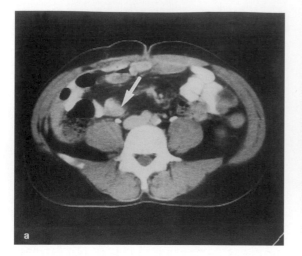 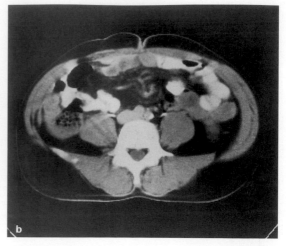

Fig. 28.11 (a) Image from an abdominal series taken for staging Hodgkin's disease, showing a possible lymph node mass on the anterior surface of the right psoas muscle (arrow). (b) Section at the same level taken 3 min later showing that the apparent mass was due to small bowel which had filled with contrast medium by peristalsis.

for clinical management. In many instances the standard technique does this, but a number of examinations need to be completed by modifying the technique. This is the principal reason why a radiologist should be present to supervise CT and to adapt the technique to the needs of the patient. CT is also subject to a number of diagnostic pitfalls, of which the radiologist must be aware.

In the simplest situation sections may fail to encompass the area or lesion. If so, it is usually sufficient to obtain more sections, either to extend the area of examination or to add more information between the sections available. There is a range of manoeuvres to choose from if this is insufficient. For example, one of the most common problems is caused by failure to opacify the small bowel uniformly, this being difficult to achieve in practice. The radiologist may choose to obtain delayed sections, when contrast medium may have moved into the area by peristalsis (Fig. 28.11). If peristalsis is sluggish, oral metoclopramide (Maxolon*) may be given. The radiologist may also move the patient into a different position to displace the bowel loops, or give an intravenous injection of contrast medium

to demonstrate the bowel wall. With practice one learns which manoeuvre will succeed in individual circumstances.

Change in patient position

Changing the position of the patient has several uses. Firstly, free collections of fluid move under the influence of gravity, allowing them to be distinguished from encapsulated collections or cysts (Fig. 28.12). Secondly, loops of non-opacified bowel change in shape when the patient moves, distinguishing them from masses, which do not (Fig. 28.13). Moving the patient in this way may also cause bowel gas or contrast medium to fill non-opacified loops and exclude a mass. Finally, the mobility of bowel allows loops overlying organs to be displaced so that the organ is clearly displayed, as may sometimes be necessary when examining the pancreas (Dixon *et al.*, 1983).

When a patient lies on his or her side, respiratory excursion tends to diminish on the dependent side and this may be used to overcome respiration artefact if other methods fail (Fig. 28.14).

Image reformatting in different planes

Most CT scanners provide the facility to reformat the

* Beecham Research, Welwyn Garden City, Hertfordshire, UK.

are useful in trauma and the assessment of complex facial lesions and it has been claimed that they may reveal pathology not otherwise evident (Hunter *et al.*, 1987).

In conventional CT both multiplanar reformatting and three-dimensional image production suffer from poor resolution in the longitudinal plane of the examination, owing to the thickness of sections. Much better images are produced from the volumetrically acquired data of spiral CT.

Enhancement

Enhancement is probably the most common modification of the examination and refers to the rise in attenuation values which takes place following injection of contrast medium, usually into a blood vessel. As in angiography, the appearances differ according to the time after injection. Immediately after an i.v. injection, contrast medium is present in veins and after about 15 s of the first circulation appears in large arteries in maximal concentration. Successive circulations produce equilibration with the blood pool in the tissues, producing a rise in their attenuation values that is largely dependent on blood flow (Ono *et al.*, 1980). Finally attenuation values fall slowly as contrast medium is excreted via the kidneys.

In the most common form of enhancement, sections are repeated during the equilibration phase. This usually emphasizes the difference between normal and abnormal tissues and is widely used in the examination of the brain, kidneys and liver (Fig. 28.9b) (Barrington & Lewtas, 1977; Moss *et al.*, 1979). In adults, 100 ml of an ionic or non-ionic contrast medium containing approximately 300 mg iodine ml^{-1} is suitable. In children the dose should be related to body weight, as in urography.

Blood vessels may also be enhanced in this way but are visualized better if the exposure is made during the first circulation, when intravascular concentration is at its highest. This technique is often loosely referred to as 'bolus enhancement'. It is sometimes used to obtain images at the same phase of enhancement but at different levels, contrast medium being injected in small increments and exposures timed accordingly. This is usually practicable for small areas only and an alternative enhancement

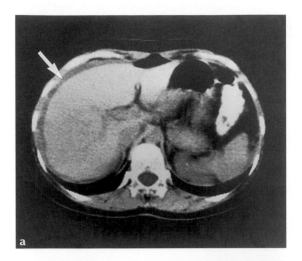
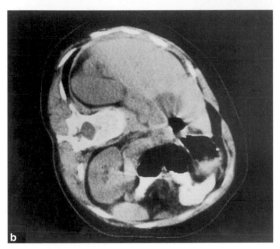

Fig. 28.12 (a) Image of the upper abdomen showing a zone of fluid over the surface of the right lobe of the liver (arrow). (b) Section at the same level in left lateral decubitus position showing that the fluid moves away from the liver and therefore represents ascites rather than a subcapsular effusion.

information from contiguous thin axial sections to produce images in different planes. Reformatted sections may be constructed in coronal, sagittal or oblique planes (Fig. 28.15a). These images are unlikely to reveal additional diagnostic information but are valuable for demonstrating complex anatomical relationships.

Programs also exist for the production of simulated three-dimensional images (Fig. 28.15b). These

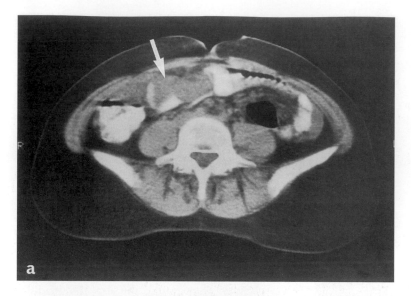

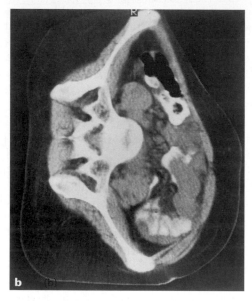

Fig. 28.13 (a) Computed tomographic section of the lower abdomen showing a possible mass related to small bowel loops (arrow). (b) Section in left lateral decubitus position. A mass is confirmed by the fact that it does not change in shape, unlike the surrounding bowel loops. Laparotomy showed peritoneal infiltration from recurrent carcinoma of the colon.

manoeuvre is necessary for more extensive examinations.

Enhancement may be used at the start of some examinations, no unenhanced sections being taken. Examples include the detection of cerebral metastases and abdominal abscesses.

Infusion techniques

Infusing a dilute solution of contrast medium, for example meglumine and sodium diatrizoate with an iodine concentration of 146 mg ml^{-1} (Urografin 150), is a convenient method of maintaining high circulating levels (Ono *et al.*, 1980). This may be used to examine blood vessels over a large area (Fig. 28.16). The author's regimen is to give an i.v. bolus injection to raise the blood level initially and then to allow the infusion to run in during the rest of the examination.

Infusion techniques are less useful for examining other organs because, although they give a high level of enhancement, the continual supply of contrast medium to the tissues may mask pathology, particularly in organs with a complex blood supply, especially the liver (Moss *et al.*, 1982).

Dynamic techniques

Dynamic CT is a means of obtaining rapidly repeated

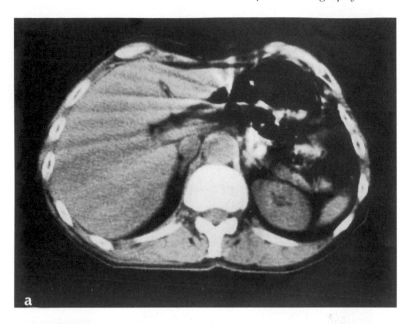

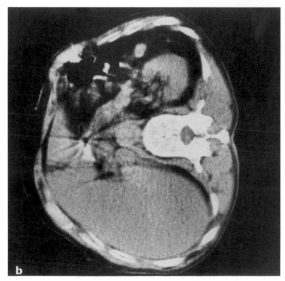

Fig. 28.14 Use of decubitus position to overcome artefact. (a) Section in supine position. Streak artefacts from bowel degrade the image of the right lobe of the liver. (b) Section in right lateral decubitus position demonstrates the liver free of artefact.

exposures (Young et al., 1980). When this is used following an injection of contrast medium, the successive phases of enhancement are demonstrated. Programs exist for expressing changes in attenuation value occurring with time (Fig. 28.17). These reflect the perfusion of tissue and may be used to assess the vascularity of a lesion prior to percutaneous biopsy or to distinguish very vascular tumours from abnormal blood vessels (Godwin & Webb, 1981; Husband & Golding, 1983). In practice, however, such precise measurements are required only rarely.

If dynamic scanning is combined with incremental table movement between exposures, it is possible to examine an area at a similar phase of enhancement. This may be used to demonstrate blood vessels and also to examine organs at an early phase of enhancement, when the difference between normal and abnormal tissues is greatest. It has been suggested that this technique may be more sensitive for detecting lesions in the liver (Moss *et al.*, 1982).

The speed with which an area of the body may be examined with spiral CT makes this a very convenient technique for examination of either blood vessels or an organ at a particular stage of enhancement. Used in conjunction with three-dimensional reconstruction, this technique has been used to produce

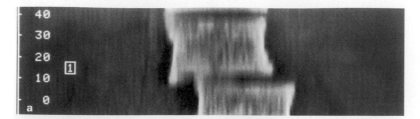

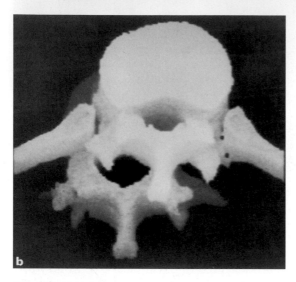

Fig. 28.15 Image reformatting to show a fracture dislocation of the spine (same patient as in Fig. 28.8). (a) Coronal reformatted image showing the degree of malalignment of the vertebral bodies. (b) Three-dimensional reformatted image (viewed from above) showing the degree of displacement of the neural arches.

impressive computed angiograms (Heiken *et al.*, 1993).

Other forms of enhancement

CT may be combined with some conventional procedures to add the benefits of cross-sectional display and superior resolution of structures. Procedures which benefit from CT assistance in this way include myelography and arthrography. Frequently, the conventional part of the study may then be curtailed, for example in arthrography of the shoulder, where CT assistance is routine in many departments.

Some early and experimental experience has been gained in using an emulsion of ethiodized oil which is taken up in the reticuloendothelial cells and pro-

duces particularly impressive enhancement of the liver and spleen (Vermess *et al.*, 1982). However, this technique is still under assessment and not generally available.

CT-guided interventional techniques

CT has proved to be a useful method of guiding percutaneous biopsy or drainage procedures when other techniques, such as ultrasound or fluoroscopy, cannot be used. This is usually when bowel gas degrades ultrasound images of the abdomen or when lesions in the chest cannot be adequately visualized on fluoroscopy, particularly masses of the mediastinum or chest wall. CT is a precise method of guidance and may be used to carry out procedures when there is a risk of damage to other structures, for example when lesions are deep in the retroperitoneum.

The principles of localization are common to both biopsy and percutaneous drainage, as well as to CT-guided coeliac ganglion neurolysis (Ferrucci & Wittenberg, 1978; Filshie *et al.*, 1983; Golding & Husband, 1984). Biopsy will be described first and the ways in which these other two procedures differ will be outlined.

Biopsy

These procedures are almost always carried out under local anaesthetic, after minimal preparation. From a diagnostic series of the area, a section is chosen which shows the lesion and an acceptable approach route, which should ideally involve only skin, muscle and fat (Fig. 28.18a).

It is usually clear which is the best point of the body surface to begin the procedure. The position of this can be confirmed by strapping a suitable marker, such as a hypodermic needle, on to the skin across the plane of the scan and obtaining a further image. Most modern CT scanners have the facility to define

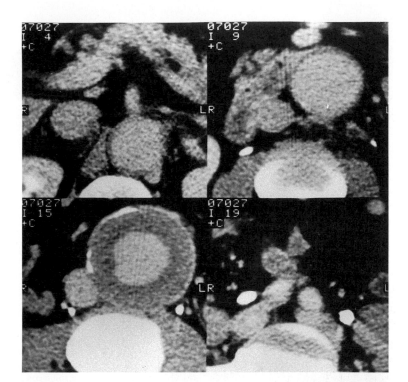

Fig. 28.16 Infusion enhancement. Four images from a study of an abdominal aortic aneurysm showing the origin of the renal vessels and superior mesenteric artery (top left), the neck of the aneurysm (top right), mural thrombus and the point of maximum diameter (bottom left) and normal iliac arteries below the aneurysm (bottom right). Using an infusion of contrast medium has allowed images to be taken at a similar phase of enhancement over a wide area.

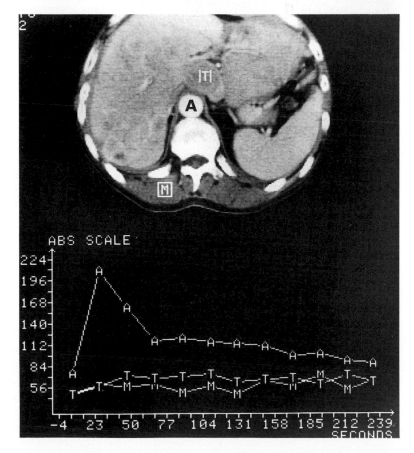

Fig. 28.17 A dynamic study in a patient with carcinoid disease to assess the vascularity of a coeliac lymph node mass prior to therapeutic embolization. Images were taken at 20-s intervals for 4 min after a bolus injection of contrast medium into a peripheral vein. The graph shows changes in attenuation value occurring in the aorta (A), resting skeletal muscle (M) and the tumour mass (T). The study indicated that the mass was poorly perfused and the tumour subsequently failed to respond to embolization.

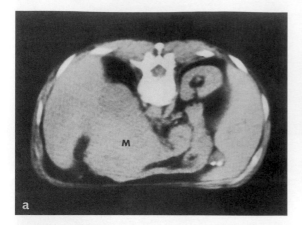

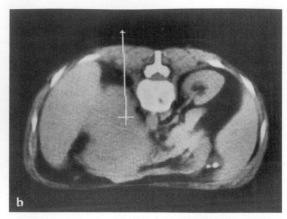

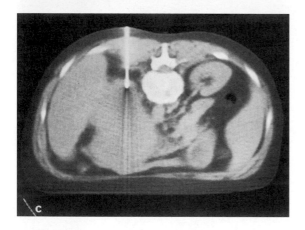

Fig. 28.18 Computed tomography-guided biopsy technique in a patient with a large upper abdominal mass due to non-Hodgkin's lymphoma. (a) Prone section showing a mass (M) lying medial to the right lobe of the liver. A satisfactory approach can be made through the skin and muscles of the back and the perirenal fat on the right side. (b) Section showing cursor measurements from a skin marker, indicating the depth and direction of the biopsy needle. (c) Image taken after insertion of a Trucut biopsy needle. When the cutting section of the needle is extended it will be at the point at which biopsy was planned in (b).

on the monitor distances and elevations from the horizontal and this is used to plan the needle route (Fig. 28.18b).

At this point, the local vessels and vascularity of the lesion are defined by obtaining a section after bolus enhancement. Vessels should be avoided when using large biopsy needles and are best avoided when using fine needles because blood from the vessel may disperse the cytology specimen.

Once a satisfactory approach plan has been defined, the skin is infiltrated with local anaesthetic and a biopsy needle inserted to the desired depth and angle. A further CT image confirms the site of the needle (Fig. 28.18c). It is usually possible to place the needle at the desired site at the first attempt, but occasionally repositioning and further sections are required. The needle should remain within the vertical plane of the section, so that its tip does not leave the image and give a misleading impression of the site

of the needle. If this occurs, sections on either side of the needle may confirm the position, otherwise it may be necessary to reposition the needle.

Insertion of the needle is usually carried out with suspended respiration. It is important that the patient should hold his or her breath in the same phase of respiration at each attempt if the imaging guidance is to be accurate. Most patients can do this satisfactorily but occasionally it helps to practise beforehand.

All types of biopsy needle can be used under CT guidance. Occasionally this is indicated specifically where a large-needle biopsy is necessary or there is a risk to other structures. The most common example is suspected lymphoma, because accurate diagnosis often requires a histology rather than cytology specimen (Husband & Golding, 1983). In other circumstances the approach route may determine the type of needle. In the abdomen it is better to use a fine needle for biopsy through the anterior abdominal wall, to reduce the risk of perforating bowel. Large needles may, however, be used when there is an entirely retroperitoneal approach route.

Care must be taken with the biopsy specimen because careless handling, in particular crushing, may make it unsuitable for diagnosis. Specimens may be preserved in a number of different ways, some of them specific to certain conditions, and it is wise to ascertain the preference of the laboratory beforehand.

Images are obtained following removal of the biopsy needle but these rarely show significant damage. Aftercare is limited to observation. Most biopsies produce no detectable effects and, after fine-needle aspiration, patients may be allowed to leave the department after a few hours of observation. Patients who have had biopsy by large cutting needles are observed in hospital until the following day as there is a greater risk of haemorrhage. Discomfort is uncommon following biopsy and, if it develops, should be regarded as a sign of local complications. The most likely complication of biopsy of the chest or upper abdomen is pneumothorax; patients should be observed for this and a chest radiograph obtained before discharge (Allison & Hemingway, 1981).

CT-guided biopsy produces a conclusive result in approximately 90% of procedures, particularly where

material has been obtained for histology. Occasionally it is necessary to repeat the procedure if the initial attempt fails. Failure sometimes occurs due to extensive necrosis of a mass but this is usually detected on initial bolus-enhanced sections.

Percutaneous drainage

This is commonly carried out for abscesses or pancreatic pseudocysts, but any localized fluid collection may be drained under CT control (Van Sonnenberg *et al.*, 1982).

The initial steps are similar to the biopsy technique, but the nature of the lesion may determine the instrument to be used in guided drainage. Simple aspiration to dryness is suitable for small fluid collections or abscesses and may be achieved using a fine needle or catheter from almost any approach. Larger collections are likely to recur, particularly in inflammatory conditions, and may require in dwelling catheter drainage.

Two options exist for catheter insertion. Either a needle and cannula can be used to position a guide wire and introducer for a catheter, in a similar way to angiographic technique, or a large needle–catheter system, such as the Ring–McLean sump drainage catheter*, can be used. This is designed to be introduced in a single manoeuvre, the central needle being withdrawn and the catheter advanced when the cavity is entered (Fig. 28.19).

The technique of localization is similar to that for biopsy. However, catheter insertion is preceded by inserting an aspirating needle to ensure that the lesion contains fluid. This allows a specimen to be taken for bacteriological or cytological examination. Care should be taken not to aspirate too much, as decompression of the cavity may make it difficult to site the drainage instrument satisfactorily.

Catheters should be secured in position and may need regular flushing if the fluid is viscous. However, most fluid collections drain with ease, even through fine catheters. Aftercare is limited to observation for complications, although these are uncommon.

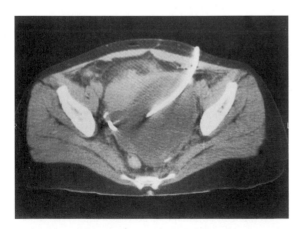

Fig. 28.19 Computed tomography-guided drainage of a cystic pelvic tumour (recurrent mucus-secreting carcinoma of the colon). Image taken after insertion of a Ring–McLean drainage catheter.

* William Cook (UK) Ltd, Letchworth, Hertfordshire, UK.

Neurolysis

In this technique for the control of severe pain, a needle is placed beside the coeliac axis or beneath the diaphragmatic crura in order to lyse respectively the coeliac ganglion or splanchnic nerves. The usual agent is concentrated alcohol, injected after a 'marker' of contrast medium has confirmed satisfactory siting of the needle. The technique carries significant risks and side effects, so that experience and care in its execution is mandatory (Filshie *et al.*, 1983). However, it is frequently very successful in that patients may become pain-free or may be able to discontinue narcotic analgesics.

References

Allison, D.J. & Hemingway, A.P. (1981) Percutaneous needle biopsy of the lung. *Br. Med. J.*, **282**, 875–8.

Ball, W.S., Wicks, J.D. & Mettler, F.A. (1980) Prone–supine change in organ position: CT demonstration. *AJR*, **135**, 815–20.

Barrington, N.A. & Lewtas, N.A. (1977) Indications for contrast medium enhancement in computed tomography of the brain. *Clin. Radiol.*, **28**, 535–7.

Berger, P.E., Kuhn, J.P. & Brusehaber, J. (1981) Techniques for computed tomography in infants and children. *Radiol. Clin. N. Am.*, **19**, 399–408.

Berland, L.L. (1986) *Practical CT — Technology and Techniques*. Raven Press, New York.

Chambers, S.E. & Best, J.K. (1984) A comparison of dilute barium and dilute water-soluble contrast in opacification of the bowel for abdominal computed tomography. *Clin. Radiol.*, **35**, 463–4.

Dixon, A.K., Stringer, D.A., Hallett, M.G. & Kelsey Fry, I. (1983) The use of the right decubitus position in computed tomography of the liver and pancreas. *Clin. Radiol.*, **32**, 113–16.

Ferrucci, J.T. & Wittenberg, J. (1978) CT biopsy of abdominal tumours: aids for lesion localization. *Radiology*, **129**, 739–44.

Filshie, J., Golding, S., Robbie, D.S. & Husband, J.E. (1983) Unilateral computerised tomography guided coeliac plexus block: a technique for pain relief. *Anaesthesia*, **38**, 498–503.

Godwin, J.D. & Webb, W.R. (1981) Dynamic computed tomography in the evaluation of vascular lung lesions. *Radiology*, **138**, 629–35.

Golding, S.J. & Husband, J.E. (1984) Percutaneous drainage of malignant cysts. *Clin. Radiol.*, **35**, 475–8.

Hatfield, K.D., Segal, S.D. & Tait, K. (1980) Barium sulfate for abdominal computer assisted tomography. *J. Comp. Assist. Tomogr.*, **4**(4), 570.

Heiken, J.P., Brink, J.A. & Vannier, M.W. (1993) Spiral (helical) CT. *Radiology*, **189**, 647–656.

Hounsfield, G.N. (1973) Computerised transverse axial scanning (tomography) 1. Description of system. *Br. J. Radiol.*, **46**, 1016–22.

Hounsfield, G.N. (1976) Picture quality of computed tomography. *AJR*, **127**, 3–9.

Hunter, J.C., Fink, I.J., Zinerich, S.J. *et al.* (1987) Three dimensional CT imaging of the lumbar spine. *In* Genant, H.K. (ed.) *Spine Update*, pp. 237–45. Radiology Research and Education Foundation, San Francisco.

Husband, J.E. & Golding, S.J. (1982) Computed tomography of the body: when should it be used? *Br. Med. J.*, **284**, 4–8.

Husband, J.E. & Golding, S.J. (1983) The role of computed tomography guided needle biopsy in an oncology service. *Clin. Radiol.*, **34**, 255–60.

Kaye, M.D., Young, S.W., Hayward, R. & Castellino, R.A. (1980) Gastric pseudotumor on CT scanning. *AJR*, **135**, 190–3.

Korobkin, M. (1979) The use of contrast material in body CT. *J. Comp. Assist. Tomogr.*, **3**(4), 556.

Krudy, A.G., Doppman, J.L. & Herdt, J.R. (1982) Failure to detect a 1.5 centimeter lung nodule by chest computed tomography. *J. Comp. Assist. Tomogr.*, **6**(6), 1178–80.

Kuhns, L.R., Thornbury, J. & Seigel, R. (1979) Variation of position of the kidneys and diaphragm in patients undergoing repeated suspension of respiratory. *J. Comp. Ass. Tomogr.*, **3**(5), 620–1.

Moss, A.A., Schrumpf, J., Schnyder, P. *et al.* (1979) Computed tomography of focal hepatic lesions: a blind clinical evaluation of the effect of contrast enhancement. *Radiology*, **131**, 427–30.

Moss, A.A., Dean, P.B., Axel, L. *et al.* (1982) Dynamic CT of hepatic masses with intravenous and intraarterial contrast material. *AJR*, **138**, 847–52.

Muller, N.L. (1991) *High Resolution CT of the Chest. Seminars in Roentenology*, vol. 26, No. 2. W.B. Saunders, Philadelphia.

Ono, N., Martinez, C.R., Fara, J.W. & Hodges, F.J. (1980) Diatrizoate distribution of dogs as a function of administration rate and time following intravenous injection. *J. Comp. Assist. Tomogr.*, **4**(2), 174–7.

Pullan, B.R. (1979) The scientific basis of computerised tomography. *In* Lodge, T. & Steiner, R.E. (eds) *Recent Advances in Radiology*, No. 6, pp. 1–15. Churchill Livingstone, Edinburgh.

Shrimpton, P.C. (1992) *Protection of the Patient in X-Ray: Computed Tomography*. Documents of the NRPB 3.4. HMSO, London.

Van Sonnenberg, E., Ferrucci, J.T., Mueller, P. R. *et al.* (1982) Percutaneous drainage of abscesses and fluid collections: technique, results and applications. *Radiology*, **142**, 1–10.

Vermess, M., Doppman, J.L., Sugarbaker, P.H. *et al.* (1982) Computed tomography of the liver and spleen with intravenous lipoid contrast material: review of 60 examinations. *AJR*, **138**, 1063–71.

Wittenberg, J., Fineberg, H.V., Ferrucci, J.T. *et al.* (1980) Clinical efficacy of computed body tomography, II. *AJR*, **134**, 1111–20.

Young, S.W., Noon, M.A., Nassi, M. & Castellino, R.A. (1980) Dynamic computed tomography body scanning. *J. Comp. Assist. Tomogr.*, **4**(2), 168–73.

Further reading

Berland, L.L. (1987) *Practical CT — Technology and Techniques.* Raven Press, New York.

Brooker, M.J. (1986) *Computed Tomography for Radiographers.* MTP Press, Lancaster.

Dixon, A.K. (1983) *Body CT: a Handbook.* Churchill Livingstone, Edinburgh.

Ellis, H., Logan, B. & Dixon, A.K. (1991) *Human Cross-sectional Anatomy; Atlas of Body Sections and CT Images.* Butterworth Heinemann, London.

Lee, J.K.T., Sagel, S.S. & Stanley, R.J. (1988) *Computed Body Tomography with MRI Correlation.* Raven Press, New York.

Webb, R.W., Brant, W.E. & Helms, C.A. (1991) *Fundamentals of Body CT.* WB Saunders, Philadelphia.

29   Magnetic Resonance Imaging

B. S. WORTHINGTON AND A.R. MOODY

Following the demonstration of the first clinical images in the early 1980s (Hawkes *et al.*, 1980) magnetic resonance imaging (MRI) has rapidly become the first line of investigation in many situations and its clinical applications are still expanding. The advantages of MRI include lack of ionizing radiation, superior tissue contrast, and multiplanar imaging. In the past, its disadvantages have included prolonged scan times in a less than ideal environment, although many of these problems have since been addressed through technical advances. Speed of data acquisition has increased by a factor of 10 000 when comparing the original spin-echo techniques with the fastest echo planar sequences available today (Mansfield, 1977). This has reduced the requirement for complex gating procedures and breath-hold abdominal studies are now available. Furthermore, three-dimensional imaging of the nervous system and musculoskeletal system has become possible within an acceptable time frame. The increased temporal resolution allows imaging of contrast medium as it perfuses tissues and dynamic imaging of joint movement. There is a future possibility of manipulating image contrast in real time and monitoring interventional procedures. The benefits of high-speed data acquisition can also be translated into improved resolution or signal to noise because of the close interrelationship of these three factors (Wehrli, 1991).

A complete description of the physics of MRI imaging is outside the scope of this chapter and the reader is referred to other sources (Smith & Ranallo, 1989; Horowitz, 1994). The MRI signal is derived from protons. Because of their polarity, alignment of protons will occur when placed in a strong external magnetic field (B_0). This situation can be disturbed by the addition of energy in the form of a radiofrequency (RF) pulse. Having been absorbed by the body tissues, this radiofrequency energy is then

given up and can be detected. However, modulation by interactions within the tissues results in unique information reflecting the tissue environment. Interactions between protons, and between protons and other macromolecules, influences the way the signal behaves, which in turn is translated into image contrast. Contrast can be altered by weighting the images to emphasize a particular characteristic of signal behaviour. Most commonly, the weighting is used to emphasize the proton–molecular interactions which can be represented by time constant T_1, or the proton–proton interactions, represented by time constant T_2. While T_1 and T_2 weighted images are the mainstay of MRI, many more techniques for enhancing image contrast have been applied and include fat suppression, chemical shift imaging, diffusion-weighted images, perfusion-weighted images, magnetization transfer contrast and contrast enhancement using exogenous contrast media.

Magnetic field gradients, generated by coils within the main magnet, are required for the isolation of one or more tissue slices during imaging and for identification of the signal source from individual tissue voxels in a given slice prior to image reconstruction. On current systems this is based on two-dimensional Fourier methods.

MRI appears complex because of the wide choice available to the radiologist in prescribing a scanning protocol, which may require several different acquisitions in multiple planes and employ a variety of pulse sequences. A simplified approach to understanding the influence of these various parameters is to consider their effects upon contrast and speed. The basic control over image contrast is provided by the repetition time (TR), echo time (TE) and flip angle (FA) of the different pulse sequences which are used, each of which consists of a different pattern of applied radiofrequency radiation which is used to generate the signal from which the image is reconstructed. More complex contrast generation is achieved by additions to these basic pulse sequence parameters, such as an inversion pulse used in fat suppression techniques; off resonance pulses used in chemical shift or magnetization transfer contrast; or preparatory pulses used for diffusion-weighted imaging.

Speed of imaging can be influenced in numerous ways, the most fundamental of which is the TR time. The number of phasing encoding steps and excitations will also limit scan speed. Improved efficiency of scanning is achieved using multislice and multiecho techniques. Subsecond imaging techniques such as fast gradient echo reduce TR to a minimum and generate contrast with preparation pulses (Haase *et al.*, 1986). Echo planer imaging is even quicker and can acquire sufficient information points for image construction using a single radiofrequency excitation (Mansfield, 1988).

The heart of the MRI scanner is the magnet, which may be either permanent or superconducting in design. Compared with permanent magnets, superconducting magnets achieve much higher field strength (B_0) but this imposes greater technical demands. Superconduction is achieved by decreasing the temperature within the magnet to near absolute zero ($4°K$), using liquid helium which requires replenishment on a regular basis.

The benefits of increased magnet strengths are reflected in increased signal to noise ratio (SNR). The interrelationship of SNR, resolution and speed can also result in magnet strength being translated into improved resolution or scan speed. Resolution improves with the square root of B_0, while the number of acquisitions to produce a given image quality is inversely proportional to the square of B_0.

Control of stray magnetic field is vital. Magnetic field straying outside the scanner can cause significant problems to nearby electrical equipment as well as posing a significant risk due to missile effects imposed upon mobile metallic objects. Stray magnetic field within the scanner will distort field homogeneity, causing loss of useful signal and image distortion. The effects can be overcome by shielding the magnet, either passively with a cage or actively by the application of magnetic shielding devices. Homogeneity of the B_0 field is paramount and is improved by either passive or active shimming of the field.

The maximum amplitude of the magnetic field gradients within the scanner has a significant effect on the minimum slice thickness and field of view, and thereby the spatial resolution which can be achieved during imaging. The rate at which the gradient can achieve the desired amplitude, known as the gradient slew rate, influences the minimum TR and TE values and thereby the minimum scan acquisition time.

A further improvement in sensitivity can be achieved using surface coils. While these may be used in both the transmit and receive modes, the SNR ratio is improved by using a small receiver coil, while a more uniform RF excitation is achieved with a larger transmit coil. Maximum SNR can be achieved by matching the size of the tissue to be imaged with that of the receiver coil (filling factor). The efficiency with which the surface coil detects the MRI signal is described as the Q (quality) factor of the coil.

Safety

The photon energy changes that are associated with nuclear excitation and relaxation are many orders of magnitude less than those associated with ionization. It is because MRI is based on a very weak radiofrequency phenomenon that there is the expectation of a very low probability of long-term ill-effect.

Static magnetic fields

Magnets will attract ferromagnetic objects with a force proportional to the strength of the applied field. While the highest fields are within the volume encompassed by the windings of the magnet in which imaging takes place, there is an extended field around the scanner that decreases as the cube of the distance. The potential hazard of objects, such as scissors or tools, in the vicinity of the magnet cannot be overstressed because they could become dangerous projectiles. Patients can be anaesthetized for MRI examinations, but the endotracheal tubes and connectors must not contain any metal parts. With resistive systems, the magnetic field can be shut down in an emergency and cardiopulmonary resuscitation equipment used in the vicinity of the scanner. For other systems, the patient can be moved on a non-ferromagnetic trolley whilst maintaining an airway and external cardiac massage if required, to outside the 5 gauss line, where full resuscitation can take place.

There have been numerous studies to assess the ferromagnetic qualities of different metallic implants, such as aneurysm clips (Shellock & Kanal 1994). Certain metallic implants and non-ferromagnetic prostheses may be safely imaged without the danger of moving the implant or prosthesis. Of greater importance is the effect of the stray magnetic field around the magnet, which could influence cardiac pacemakers that contain reed relays which are activated by magnetic fields. Certain pacemakers would be rendered inoperative in a sufficiently high field: this could be fatal in a patient with an underlying complete heart block. The most sensitive pacemaker reed relays can switch in a field of 7 gauss. Persons wearing pacemakers should not be allowed to enter a field higher than 5 gauss and prominent warning notices should be displayed outside any room or area in which the field could exceed this level.

High static magnetic fields are associated with abnormalities in the T-wave of the electrocardiogram (ECG). This is because blood is a conductor and, as it moves in relation to the magnetic field, an electric current is produced by Faraday's law of electromagnetic induction. This current is maximal when the blood moves at right angles to the field, as in the aorta in a conventional imaging system. The peak flow potential in human exposure at 2.5 T has been calculated to be 40 mV, which is the depolarization threshold for myocardial cells, but only a fraction of this potential will occur across individual cells.

Gradient magnetic fields

Spatial information in MRI is obtained by employing magnetic gradient fields. When these gradients are applied, the magnetic field is static and unchanging for typically 10 ms. As the gradient fields are switched on and off, the field rises from or falls to zero, respectively, in a period of typically 1 ms. A time-varying magnetic field is present during this 'rise time'. By Faraday's law of electromagnetic induction, electric currents will be generated in conductive loops within body tissues and could be potentially hazardous if they interfere with the normal function of nerve or muscle.

One of the best documented and most sensitive responses to rapidly changing magnetic fields is the production of magnetic phosphenes — the sensation of flashes of light caused by stimulation of the retina. There have been no reported cases of magnetophosphenes for fields of 1.95 T or less, but they have been reported in a 4 T research system in conjunction with vertigo and a metallic taste. The threshold for the effect depends not only on the rate of change of field but also on its duration and the frequency with which it is applied.

Both human nerve and muscle cells can be stimulated by rates of change of magnetic flux density which induce current densities of the order of 1.2 A m^{-2}, the threshold for stimulation frequencies being below about 100 Hz. Both can be avoided by restricting the induced current densities to a third of the value (400 mA m^{-2}) which is achievable by restricting most exposure rates to below 20 T s^{-1} (NRPB, 1991).

Radiofrequency magnetic fields

In MRI, patients are exposed to pulses of radiofrequency field that are used to excite the nuclei, although most of the power is ultimately dissipated as heat in the tissues. At the frequencies used in imaging, the magnetic component of this electromagnetic field is larger than the electrical component. The currents induced by this varying magnetic component, flowing through resistive paths in the tissues, generate heat. The wavelengths are of the order of 5 m and above: The exposure is therefore said to be 'near field' since the object lies within one wavelength. This contrasts with a wavelength of a few centimetres, where exposure occurs at a distance of several wavelengths and is therefore said to be 'far field'. In the near field exposure conditions, it is the volume of tissue exposed rather than the surface area that is important: for this reason the specific absorption rate of power deposition is measured in W kg^{-1} of tissue.

The amount of power deposited is a function of the type of pulse sequence used: in particular, the repetition rate and number of echoes in multislice techniques, the duration of the exposure and the coupling between the RF coil and the subject. The potential heating increases substantially as the field strength of the system is raised because it is related to the square of the RF frequency. The heat generated depends on the conductivity of the tissues and increases in proportion to the square of the radius of the body part being imaged, therefore being greater in larger patients. As the core temperature of the body rises, the thermoregulatory mechanism comes into operation: this leads to removal of heat which is dissipated primarily through the skin and is most efficient in a cool environment of low humidity. A normal individual can lose 2 MJ, but the tolerable heat burden may be reduced in disease, particularly in patients with an already elevated core temperature. Since the primary mechanism for removing heat from the tissue is via the circulation, there has been concern that poorly vascularized tissues in the testis and the avascular cornea may be particularly vulnerable. A rise in core temperature of up to 1°C occurs in normal subjects during light exercise. Regulations governing exposure conditions have sought to identify conditions such that a temperature rise of this order would not be exceeded. Patients with orthopaedic implants made of non-ferromagnetic stainless steel have been safely examined with MRI. Since these implants are excellent conductors, significant heating from RF exposure is unlikely. Care must be taken to ensure that all lead wires from monitoring equipment are so placed that conductive loops are not formed, since induced current may cause sufficient heating to result in thermal injury.

From the available data, the National Radiation Protection Board (NRPB, 1991) concluded that an acceptable exposure for examinations longer than 30 min, that would not result in a temperature rise exceeding 0.5°C, would be achieved if the whole-body specific absorption rate (SAR) was restricted to an average of 1 W g^{-1}. For periods less than 30 min the whole body SAR can be relaxed to an average of 2 W kg^{-1} averaged over a 15-min period.

Acoustic noise

The noise generated during MRI varies between 65 and 95 dB. Temporary or permanent hearing loss has been reported and protective devices should be offered to patients when peak noise reaches or exceeds 85 dB (Brummett *et al.*, 1988).

It would be presumptuous to assume that all possible hazards associated with MRI have been identified, particularly in the domain of high-field studies. Several million patients have now been examined worldwide and there have been several instances of missile injuries, pacemaker events and RF burns, which emphasizes the need for vigilance to eliminate all avoidable mishaps. So far, no definite long-term adverse effects of exposure have emerged.

Practical aspects of safety in MRI units

The organization of MRI units to ensure safe working practice will vary from centre to centre, but a number of important issues have to be addressed:
1 Responsibility for safety must be vested in a 'responsible person'. It may be appropriate to have a multidisciplinary safety committee which reviews procedures on a regular basis.
2 The MRI equipment will be contained within a controlled area and appropriate safety procedures established to gain entry.
3 Survey of patients before scanning to eliminate avoidable mishap.
4 Appropriate procedures must be laid down to ensure the safety of patients during scanning. These will cover communication and monitoring; requirements for anaesthesia; acoustic noise; management of contrast media reactions; and cardiac arrest.
5 Requirement for records of patients and volunteers scanned.

Contrast agents

The role of contrast agents is to discriminate between magnetically similar tissues, to increase the contrast to noise ratio of pathology by a variety of mechanisms and to permit *in vivo* functional studies. Despite a wide structural diversity, contrast agents currently in use produce their effects by altering either the proton density or relaxation times of a given tissue. In terms of the effect on the signal intensity of the tissue, some contrast agents produce a signal enhancement and some produce a signal loss. All contrast agents have sufficient magnetic activity to alter tissue signal intensity, an appropriate biodistribution, and a low toxicity with a correspondingly high margin of safety in clinical use.

Magnetic materials

These are classified in terms of their response when placed in an external magnetic field. The magnetic susceptibility is the ratio of the induced magnetization to the applied field strength. Most materials are diamagnetic and have a very weak magnetic susceptibility which arises from the motion of paired orbital electrons. Diamagnetic materials, for example kaolin and perfluoro-octylbromide, have been used as contrast agents in the bowel where they displace the normal bowel contents. Paramagnetic materials produce their own local magnetic field and this is related to the number of unpaired electrons within each atom. Superparamagnetic materials are composed of single domain crystals of small iron oxide particles (including magnetites) with properties intermediate between paramagnetic and ferromagnetic materials. Their magnetic susceptibility is much larger than paramagnetic materials but, unlike ferromagnetic materials, there is no residual magnetism when the external field is removed.

Mechanism of action

The signal intensity of tissues in MRI is largely determined by the proton density and relaxation times, varying directly with increasing T_2 values and inversely with increasing T_1 values. Effects of MRI contrast agents are indirect, being achieved through alterations induced in proton relaxation rates.

Paramagnetic contrast agents

Effective enhancement of the relaxation of water protons is achieved by paramagnetic moieties which produce their own fluctuating magnetic field. The effect on local water protons depends on complicated interactions, although the overall effect on relaxation rates is related to the size of the magnetic moment of the paramagnetic agent. Metal ions from the transition and lanthanide series of elements have large magnetic moments deriving from unpaired elecions in their outer shells. Gadolinium (Gd) has seven such unpaired electrons and its high toxicity is substantially reduced by binding it to a suitable chelating agent such as diethylenetriamine penta-acetic acid (DTPA). Such contrast agents increase the proton relaxation rates in tissues where they are distributed (Gadian *et al.*, 1985) For the same concentration of GdDTPA the reduction in T_1 or T_2 values is greater for tissues with longer values of T_1 and T_2 than shorter values. Because T_2 is smaller than T_1 for biological tissues the absolute effect on T_1 is greater than that on T_2. The effect of such contrast agents is therefore best shown on T_1 weighted images (Fig. 29.1). Various Gd complexes have been synthesized and tested. Potential criteria for their selection include relaxivity, stability, toxicity, pharmacokinetics, osmolality and cost. The overall incidence of adverse reactions is very low. Their use in the nervous system is now well established and parallels that of iodinated media in CT. There is increasing use in the cardiovascular and musculoskeletal systems. Efforts have also been made to develop hepatobiliary agents, by chelating a paramagnetic ion (Mn or Gd) to a ligand which has an affinity for hepatocytes.

Superparamagnetic contrast agents

Because local deposits of superparamagnetic particles have a greater magnetic susceptibility than the surrounding diamagnetic tissues, the magnetization induced in the particles produces a distortion in the local magnetic field. This leads to rapid spin dephasing and hence a reduction in T_2 values with a fall in signal intensity. The effect of such contrast agents is therefore best shown on T_2 weighted images. These agents have been used as a bowel marker in abdominal imaging and their uptake in cells of the reticuloendothelial system on i.v. injection has been exploited in liver imaging.

Patient preparation

The radiologist should assess all scan requests, not only ensuring that imaging is warranted but also that MRI is the imaging modality of choice. The scan sequence and planes of imaging should be prescribed in order to allow estimation of total scan time prior to booking. Because MRI is a new imaging modality, unfamiliar to most patients, it is often helpful to send an information leaflet to the patient. This may allay patient fears and allow consultation prior to scanning regarding the possibility of claustrophobia or other contraindications.

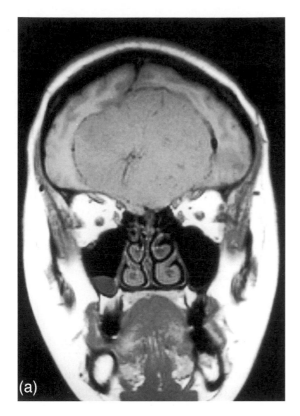 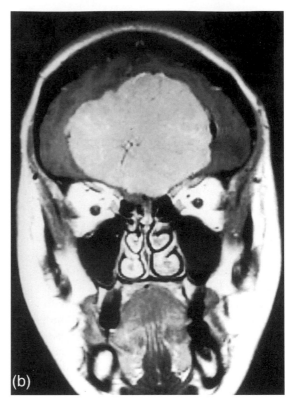

Fig. 29.1 (a) T$_1$ weighted coronal image through the anterior aspect of the head showing a large mass lesion situated in the mid-line. (b) Following i.v. contrast enhancement with gadolinium–diethylenetriaminepenta-acetic acid the tumour enhances brightly. The appearances are those of a meningioma.

On arrival, the patient should fill out a questionnaire enquiring into the possibility of any contraindications. If the patient is to be accompanied into the scan room their escort should similarly fill out a questionnaire. At this juncture the patient should be informed as to the possible use of i.v. contrast medium, which may save time when the patient is within the scanner. Although gastrointestinal contrast agents are now available, they are not routinely used at the present time. This may reflect the as yet low level of usage of MRI for general abdominal imaging.

All metal objects should be removed and locked safely away before entering the scan room. Depending on the area to be scanned, changing into a gown may be indicated. Just before entering the scan area, the patient should once again be questioned regarding the possibility of carrying any metal objects.

Metal detectors have not gained general acceptance as they may not detect all metal objects and will therefore convey a false sense of security. If there is any doubt as to the possible presence of metal prosthesis, surgical clips or fragments, plain radiography of the region of interest is indicated.

Once inside the scan area an explanation of the scanning technique is undertaken. This should include a description of the magnet tunnel, any coils that will be employed, the expected number of sequences, and the amount of noise that will be generated during the sequences. Ear plugs or ear defenders should be offered to all patients (Brummett *et al.*, 1988). While lying on the couch the patient may feel more comfortable with a support behind their knees.

Some studies will require ECG gating. Care must be taken to ensure that the ECG leads are not in contact with the patient's skin as there is a danger of generating currents within the leads during the operation of the MRI system. These currents are of sufficient magnitude to cause thermal injury to the patient. To overcome this problem, the leads should not be directly in contact with the patient's skin and the integrity of the electrical insulation of the leads should be regularly checked. Every effort should be made to ensure that the leads do not make a large loop or cross each other within the magnet bore (Shellock & Kanal, 1994). The ECG leads should be supported throughout their length in order to avoid any movement and thus generate an artefact-free trace. As the ECG trace is sensitive to patient movement, even talking, the patient should be warned to remain as still as possible during the gated acquisitions.

Imaging following an i.v. contrast medium is usually best performed after a suitable delay to allow optimum discrimination between varying tissues. However, on some occasions it will be necessary to perform a dynamic contrast enhanced study or image during slow infusion of contrast medium. This requires the siting of a line, usually within an antecubital vein, prior to imaging. A 19 or 21 gauge butterfly needle is usually sufficient, though a cannula may be used. Extension tubing allows access while the patient is within the magnet. Visualization of the butterfly tubing is still usually possible, so that the patency and positioning of the butterfly maybe checked by aspiration of blood prior to injection. However, it is not usually possible to directly monitor the needle site during contrast injection.

Some cases will require the patient to be sedated or under a full general anaesthetic. Planning is vital for the safe and smooth running of these procedures. Ideally, there should be designated anaesthetic and nursing staff familiar with the MRI environment and equipment, which is fully MRI compatible. A high level of monitoring is required, including ECG and pulse oximetry. All MRI staff should be aware of the emergency procedures for their scanner. This is becoming increasingly important as MRI is used more frequently in the investigation of acutely ill patients and those with cardiovascular disease.

Communication with the patient should be two-way. This can be achieved by an intercom system which allows the patient to talk to the radiographer.

The intercom is vital for comforting nervous patients. Regular enquiries as to the state of the patient, telling the patient the length of scan sequences and how many more sequences are to be performed will assist in relaxing the patient. Closed-circuit television allows direct visualization of the patient. The use of a buzzer system means the patient can attract the radiographer's attention in an emergency. The development of more open magnet designs should allow greater patient comfort and ease of communication. The patient should be given time to recover after the scan. The patient may be told when to expect the results to reach their doctor. While patients may ask for their results at the time of the scan this may not always be possible because of the large number of images created and the post-processing required.

Positioning and localization

As the greatest magnetic homogeneity is at the centre of the scanner, attempts should be made to position the region of interest in this area. This is achieved by positioning the patient at a certain point outside the scanner, usually using a laser marker, prior to moving them into the magnet by a set distance. The scan slices are planned from a rapidly acquired localizer image which can be acquired in any plane (Fig. 29.2). When planning the slices a wide choice is available concerning the number of slices, matrix format, field of view, number of acquisitions and interslice spacing. All of these factors will have to be weighed up when considering the speed of image acquisition, resolution and SNR. A number of saturation bands may be added to the slice prescription. These will remove movement artefact within the region of imaging. Movement artefact may be generated by flowing blood or structures such as subcutaneous fat or the larynx and cause degradation of the image. Most MRI scanning is performed with the patient in the supine position. Depending on the area to be scanned, the patient may be put into the scanner feet first. Prone positioning is unusual but may be applied when using a surface coil to image the heart or breast. When a surface coil is being employed, care should be taken to ensure the region of the body is stabilized within the coil to avoid movement.

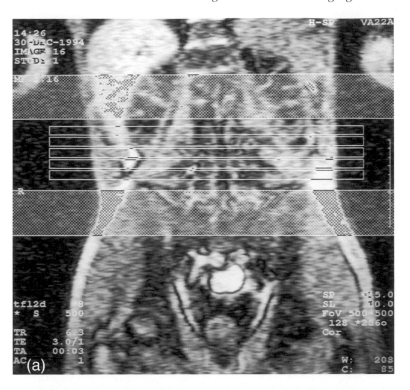

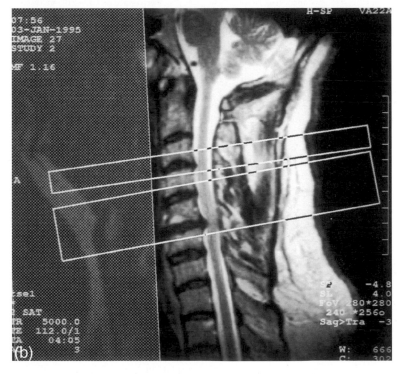

Fig. 29.2 (a) Breath-holding images of the abdomen are planned from a coronal localizer with the addition of saturation bands superiorly and inferiorly to remove unwanted vascular artefact. (b) Two transverse blocks of images are planned on a sagittal view of the cervical spine. A saturation band is placed anteriorly to remove unwanted motion artefact.

Indications

A scan should only be undertaken if its result is going to influence patient management. Possible contraindications or safety considerations should also be taken into account when arranging an MRI scan.

MRI is the first line of investigation in a number of conditions. In other situations MRI will be used when previous investigations have been unhelpful.

In reviewing the indications for MRI, the clinical signs and symptoms of the patient will provide the best guide (Tables 29.1 & 29.2).

Table 29.1 Primary indications for magnetic resonance imaging

Brain		
Adults		Raised intracranial pressure
		mass lesions
		hydrocephalus
		Focal motor or sensory neurological deficit, especially valuable in white matter disease and leptomeningeal pathology
		Epilepsy
		Acute cerebrovascular disease
		Psychiatric/degenerative orders
		dementia
		Visual disturbance
		Endocrine disturbance
		pituitary dysfunction
		Note: in trauma/acute haemorrhage computed tomography is the preferred technique
Paediatric		Perinatal
		trauma
		hypoxic brain injury
		Congenital anomalies
		Developmental delay
Spine		
Adults		Acute low back pain
		Neural compression
		benign
		malignant
		Marrow infiltration
		Acute myelitis
		infective, vascular or demyelination
		Infection
		discitis
		osteomyelitis
Paediatric		Congenital
		spinal dysraphism
		Cord compression
		benign
		malignant
Musculoskeletal		
Knee		Internal derangement
		meniscal pathology
		ligamentous injury
Shoulder		Degeneration, trauma

Table 29.1 *Continued.*

Wrist	Degeneration, trauma
Ankle	Degeneration, trauma
Mass lesions	Benign
	Malignant
Bone pain	Infection
	Inflammation
	Trauma
	Ischaemia/avascular necrosis
Chest	Apical lesions
	Pleural and pericardial lesions
	Peridiaphragmatic lesions
Pelvis	Congenital anomalies of the female genital tract
	Neoplasms — cervix and uterine body
	Endometriosis
Vascular	Cerebral venous disease
	Thoracic venous disease
	Portal venous disease

Image display and interpretation

Once the data have been acquired they are stored in a numerical matrix which represents relative signal intensity. The dynamic range of this dataset is far greater than can be encompassed in a tonal range of grey scale levels distinguishable to the human eye. To facilitate interrogation of the whole set of data, this is viewed at different grey scale window widths around a central level which can also be varied. Modern MRI systems provide increasingly greater amounts of data which can be displayed in a wide variety of formats, including 'pseudo three-dimensional' projections, cine presentations and contrast tracking techniques (Fig. 29.3). The rapid cinematic presentation of contiguous transverse axial body sections can allow information across several sections to be integrated more readily than on inspection of the individual hard copy images. Cine presentations are also now a familiar mode of display in dynamic cardiac studies.

Magnetic resonance angiography

Flowing blood can appear dark or bright on MRI images, depending on its velocity, direction and the pulse sequence. Indeed, flow effects can mimic pathology. The scientific basis of this observation has led to the development of magnetic resonance angiography, whereby vascular structures are depicted because protons in flowing blood give a high signal against a background of little or no signal from stationary tissues. In the 'time of flight' method, a series of thin slices in a selected volume is acquired using a gradient echo technique (Laub & Kaiser, 1988). During the image acquisition period this volume of tissue receives multiple RF pulses saturating the non-moving spins. The fully magnetized spins contained in flowing blood entering this volume from outside return a high signal. Both arteries and veins will be displayed, unless the vessels from which they derive outside the volume are first saturated by means of a so called presaturation band, in which case they can be selectively eliminated (Fig. 29.4). A second method of magnetic resonance angiography is referred to as phase contrast angiography (Dumoulin & Hart, 1986). In this technique, different velocity-dependent phase shifts are produced in two images. On subtracting the first image from the second stationary image, tissue

Table 29.2 Secondary indications for magnetic resonance imaging

Abdomen	Liver — neoplasia, infiltration, inflammation
	Kidney — neoplasia, infiltration, inflammation
	Pancreas — neoplasia, infiltration, inflammation
Pelvis	Bladder — neoplasia
	Prostate — neoplasia
	Ovary — neoplasia
Chest	Mediastinal disease
	Intrapulmonary masses
	Intrapulmonary nodules
	Congenital and acquired heart disease
Breast	Benign/malignant disease
Head and neck	Neck lymphadenopathy
	Pharyngeal/laryngeal malignancy
Vascular	
Brain	Cerebral arterial disease
	cerebral aneurysm
	arteriovenous malformations
	cerebral vascular occlusive disease
Neck	Carotids — stenosis, occlusion, dissection
Chest	Mediastinum
	Aorta
	dissection, aneurysm
	Pulmonary arterial disease
Abdomen	Aorta
	aneuryms (inflammatory), aortic occlusion
	Inferior vena cava
	thrombosis
	tumour extension
Pelvis	Deep venous thrombosis
Peripheral vascular disease	Arterial
	Venous

which will have the same phase shift will return a zero signal; whereas a positive signal will be returned from the moving spins in blood. The net phase shift will be determined by the flow velocity so that choice of the applied gradients allows adjustment to the particular flow velocity which is anticipated in the vessels to be imaged. With both methods vascular structures are isolated by acquiring either two- or three-dimensional image datasets. An angiogram, as usually understood, refers to a depiction of the whole or part of the vascular architecture in continuity. In conventional digital

vascular imaging this is achieved by subtraction of a mask from the series of images taken after contrast injection. In magnetic resonance angiography a special computer algorithm (maximum intensity projection) achieves the same effect by allowing selection of all the bright pixels above a threshold in contiguous sections, which are then displayed in continuity (Fig. 29.5). Problems common to all magnetic resonance angiography techniques include signal loss or regions of low signal where there is turbulent flow and difficulty in resolving small vessels.

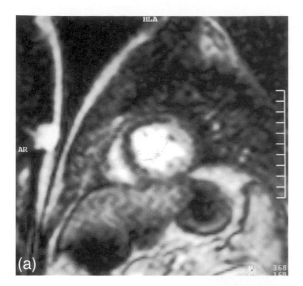

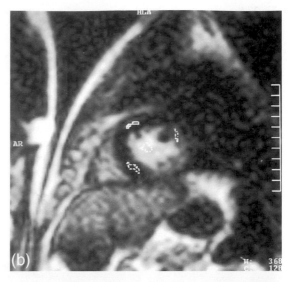

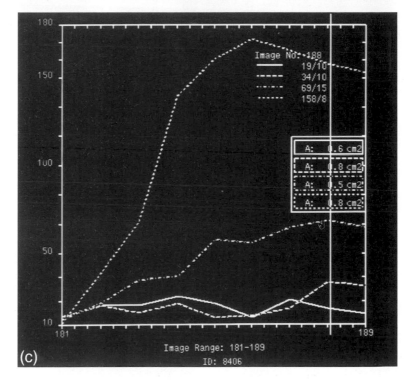

Fig. 29.3 (a & b) The dynamic contrast-enhanced image of the heart demonstrates a large anteroseptal perfusion defect in a patient with a recent myocardial infarction. (c) Quantitative data can be extracted from magnetic resonance images by plotting signal intensity versus time. The graph shows normal enhancement within the left ventricle and lateral myocardium but poor perfusion within the anteroseptal portions.

Interventional procedures

Just as computed tomography (CT) has proved to be a useful method of guiding stereotactic and needle biopsy procedures, so MRI is now being applied in the same way. Non-magnetic biopsy needles allow MRI control of these procedures. Stereotactic frames compatible with the MRI environment have been developed and allow neurosurgeons to capitalize on the

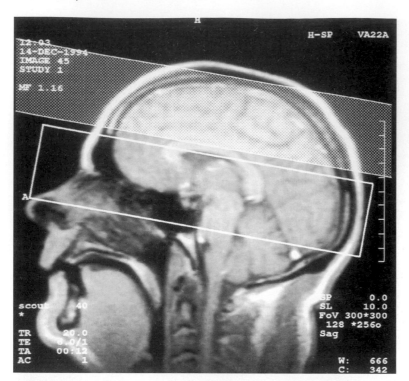

Fig. 29.4 The sagittal localizer view allows planning for magnetic resonance angiography of the circle of Willis. A saturation band (hatched) is placed superiorly to remove venous signal.

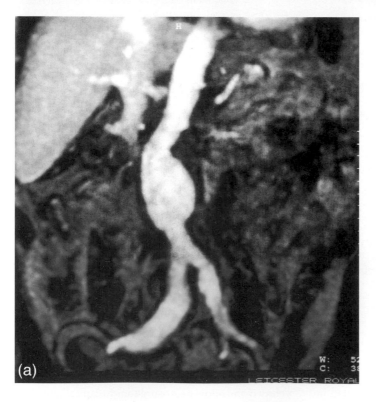

Fig. 29.5 (a) Contrast-enhanced magnetic resonance aortography allows good delineation of an abdominal aortic aneurysm and its relations to the superior and inferior aorta. The right common iliac artery is also seen to be aneurysmal.

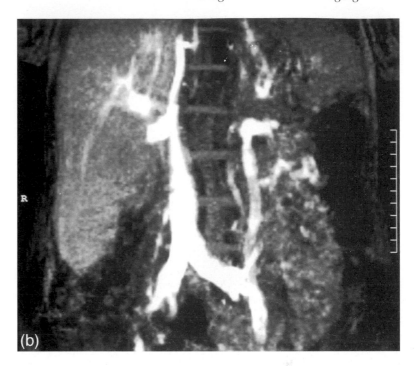

Fig. 29.5 *Continued.* (b) Magnetic resonance venography demonstrates an abnormally large vein forming a communication between the left common iliac and left renal veins. This patient had carcinoma of the pancreas with obstruction of the distal left renal vein. In addition there is complete thrombosis of the right external iliac vein and a further filling defect seen in the left external iliac vein.

superior tissue contrast of MRI compared to CT in many types of intracranial pathology. The development of open design MRI systems will faclitate the extension and refinement of biopsy procedures.

References

Brummett, R.E., Talbot, J.M. & Charuhas, P. (1988) Potential hearing loss resulting from MR imaging. *Radiology*, **169**, 539–40.

Dumoulin, C.L. & Hart, H.J. (1986) Magnetic resonance angiography. *Radiology*, **161**, 717–20.

Gadian, D., Payne, J.A., Bryant, D.J., Young, I.R., Carr, D.H. & Bydder, G.M. (1985) Gadolinium DTPA as a contrast agent in MR imaging: theoretical projections and practical observations. *J. Comput. Assist. Tomogr.*, **9**(2), L242–51.

Haase, A., Frahm, J. & Matthaei, D., (1986) Rapid NMR imaging using low flip-angle pulses. *J. Magnet. Res.*, **67**, 258–66.

Hawkes, R.C., Holland, G.N., Moore, W.S. Worthington, B.S. (1980) NMR tomography of the brain; a preliminary clinical assessment with demonstration of pathology. *J. Comput. Assist. Tomogr.*, **4**, 577–86.

Horowitz, A. (1994) *MRI Physics for Radiologists*, 2nd edn. Springer-Verlag, Berlin.

Laub, G.A. & Kaiser, W.A. (1988) MR angiography with gradient motion refocusing. *J. Comput. Assist. Tomogr.*, **12**, 377–82.

Mansfield, P. (1977) Multiplanar image formation using NMR spin echoes. *J. Phys.*, **C10**, L55–8.

Mansfield, P. (1988) Imaging by nuclear magnetic resonance. *J. Phys.*, **E21**, 18–30.

NRPB (National Radiological Protection Board) (1991) *Principles for the Protection of Patients and Volunteers During Clinical Magnetic Resonance Diagnostic Procedures.* Documents of the NRPB 2.1. HMSO, London.

Shellock, F. & Kanal, E. (1994) *Magnetic Resonance — Bioeffects, Safety and Patient Management.* Raven Press, New York.

Smith, H. & Ranallo, F. (1989) *A Non-mathematical Approach to Basic MRI.* Medical Physics Publishing Corporation, Madison.

Wehrli, F. (1991) *Fast-scan Magnetic Resonance.* Raven Press, New York.

Section 8
Other Practical Considerations

30   Water-Soluble Contrast Media

P. DAWSON

Historical development

Without the availability of good and relatively safe intravascular contrast agents, diagnostic radiology would not have come to occupy the central position it currently does in the diagnostic process. The great bulk of 'interventional radiology' would certainly have never emerged. The fact that most radiologists take them largely for granted may be seen as a tribute to the excellence of the current generation of contrast agents.

The need for intravascular contrast agents was realized very early in the history of radiology, as witnessed by the performance of angiograms on an amputated hand and on a cadaver kidney by Haschek and Lindenthal (1896) and Hicks and Addison (Burrows, 1986), respectively, both within a month of Roentgen's report of the discovery of X-rays. The radio-opaque suspensions used for these classic studies were not clinically practicable but the achievements were remarkable. In subsequent years, various agents were used to opacify the gastrointestinal tract, the bladder, ureters, renal pelvis and lymphatics by direct injection, but little progress was made with the development of agents which could be safely injected into the circulation.

Berberich and Hirsch (1923) used a strontium bromide solution for the opacification of the peripheral veins and, in the same year, Osborne *et al.* (1923) at the Mayo clinic noted opacification of the bladder in patients treated with i.v. solutions of sodium iodide for syphilis.. They had unwittingly performed the first i.v. urogram. However, the delineation of the upper urinary tract was poor and sodium iodide solutions were rather toxic for general use for urography. Enough interest was generated, however, for Brooks (1924) to try sodium iodide solutions for peripheral angiography and for Moniz, in 1927, to apply it to carotid arteriography (Moniz, 1940). Both

procedures had to be performed under general anaesthesia and Moniz was so concerned about the toxicity of sodium iodide that he diverted his activity into one of the great culs-de-sac of radiological history, namely the use of colloidal thorium dioxide ('Thorotrast') as a contrast agent (Moniz, 1940). Thorium dioxide had the great advantage of being highly radio-opaque at a time when radiographic film and equipment were much poorer than currently, and of being associated with virtually no acute side effects on injection. Unfortunately, thorium is radioactive, being an emitter of α-particles and having a half-life of 1.4×10^{10} years. It is permanently retained within the reticuloendothelial system, largely in the liver and spleen, and is associated with induction of malignancies, the first of which to be recorded in a human was a sarcoma of the liver some 20 years following its administration (MacMahon *et al.*, 1947). Other tumours described, and apparently related to the agent, include hepatoma, cholangiocarcinoma and myeloid leukaemia. Retention of Thorotrast by urothelium following retrograde pyelography has also been associated with the development of transitional cell carcinoma (Wenz, 1967), while local injections into breast and maxillary sinuses have been followed by carcinoma developing at these sites (Swarm, 1971). Perivascular extravasation of contrast is associated with local granuloma formation.

While inorganic iodide solutions were too toxic for general use, it was realized that iodine is an outstandingly good choice of element for X-ray absorption. The K-shell electron binding energy is approximately 34 KeV, which is lower than, but close to, the mean energy used in diagnostic X-ray work, thereby maximizing the cross-section for photoelectric interactions. If iodine was to be used, a suitable carrier molecule was clearly going to be necessary. The first such emerged in 1925 when Binz and Rath (Grainger, 1982) began the synthesis of a number of pyridone derivatives, for containing iodine, in the quest for a treatment of syphilis. Two compounds in this series became known as 'Selectan neutral' and 'Uroselectan'. These were used by a young American, Moses Swick, working under the supervision of, first, Lichtwitz and subsequently von Lichtenberg in Berlin, for i.v. urography in the years 1927 to 1929 (Grainger, 1982). These monoiodinated pyridone compounds (Fig. 30.1) were superseded within 3 years or so by di-iodinated pyridones of higher solubility which were also synthesized by Binz and Rath (Fig. 30.2). These became the standard contrast agents for intravascular and other applications during the next two decades or more, until they were replaced in the early 1950s by the benzene ring based compounds. In fact, as early as 1933 Swick had suggested the use of iodinated benzene ring compounds and had developed monoiodo-hippurate for this purpose. Unfortunately, the very addition of the iodine to the hippurate substantially

increased the toxicity of the compound, a point developed below. The compound was, therefore, unsuccessful in its original intention but became an important tool in renal physiology and opened the way for the eventual development of successful contrast agents of this type in the 1950s.

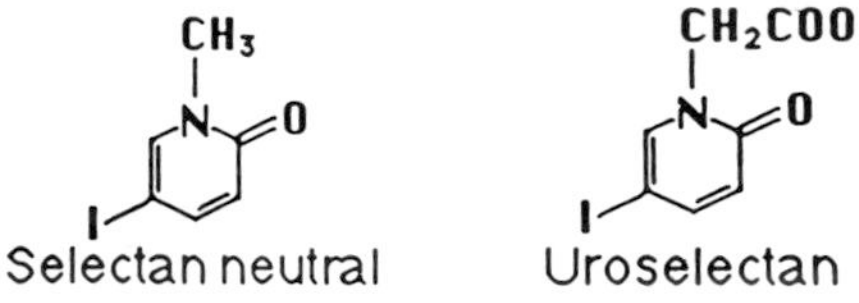

In 1952 Wallingford discovered that the introduction into the benzene ring of an amide side-chain with acetylation produced a low-toxicity compound, acetrizoic acid (Fig. 30.3) (Wallingford, 1952). Hoppe subsequently developed a doubly substituted molecule diatrizoic acid (Hoppe, 1959) and closely related compounds, such as the iothalamates and metrizoates, followed. As can be seen from Fig. 30.3, the various representatives of the type are all salts of the benzoic acids and differ only, and then in minor ways, in the substituent side-chains at the 3 and 5 positions on the benzene ring. The commercial formulations differ in being either sodium salts, meglumine salts or mixed sodium and meglumine salts, and in the concentrations available. For example, the iothalamate series is known commercially as the Conray range. Conray 280 is a pure meglumine salt at a concentration of 280 mg iodine ml^{-1} solution, whereas Conray 420 is a pure sodium salt at a concentration of 420 mg iodine ml^{-1}. The iothalamates are isomers of the diatrizoates with the NHCOCH$_3$ substituent group at position 5 merely changed to CONHCH$_3$. The diatrizoates are known as Hypaque when marketed by Winthrop* and as Urografin when marketed by Schering†. Urografin 370, for example, is a mixed sodium and meglumine salt at a concentration of 370 mg iodine ml^{-1} solution. Hypaque 270 is a pure sodium salt at a concentration of 270 mg iodine ml^{-1} solution.

The important points to consider in the choice of agent for a particular application are (i) the iodine concentration of the formulation; and (ii) the sodium and/or meglumine content. Sodium salts are more toxic to vascular endothelium and to blood–brain barrier and neural tissues and so should be avoided in venography and cerebral angiography. Meglumine salts should be used for these purposes. For cardiac work, a mixture of sodium and meglumine should be chosen (for example, Urografin 370), since both

Fig. 30.1 The contrast agents 'Selectan neutral' and 'Uroselectan'. The first generation of pyridone-based agents.

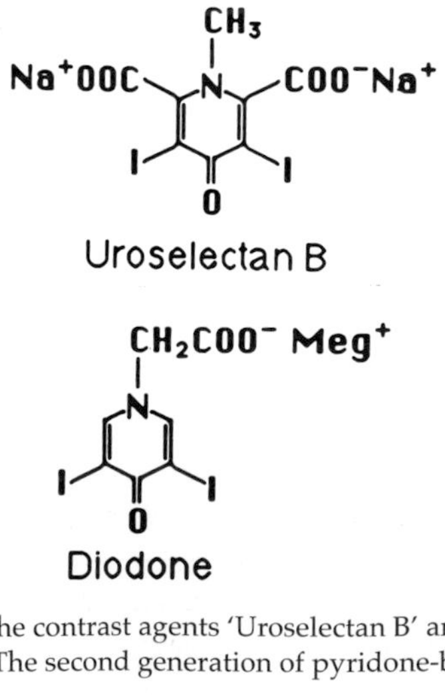

Fig. 30.2 The contrast agents 'Uroselectan B' and 'Diodine'. The second generation of pyridone-based agents.

* Winthrop, New York, USA.
† Schering AG, Berlin, Germay.

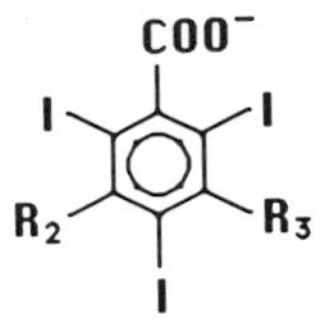

$$COO^-$$

The benzene ring structure with substituents I (three positions), R$_2$, and R$_3$.

R$_2$	R$_3$	Proper name	Commercial name
H	NHCOCH$_3$	Acetrizoate	Urokon, Diaginol
CH$_3$CONH	NHCOCH$_3$	Diatrizoate	Urografin, Hypaque
CH$_3$CONH	CONHCH$_3$	Iothalamate	Conray
CH$_3$CONH	NCOCH$_3$ / CH$_3$	Metrizoate	Isopaque, Triosil

Fig. 30.3 The structures of the benzene ring-based contrast agents.

pure sodium and pure meglumine salts are more cardiotoxic and are associated with high levels of ventricular fibrillation. Some manufacturers have made special formulations of their agents, with calcium and magnesium ions partially replacing sodium ions, in an attempt to reduce various aspects of toxicity.

Disadvantages of conventional contrast agents

At the typical iodine concentrations used in many clinical applications, 300–400 mg iodine ml^{-1}, the ionic contrast agents are substantially hyperosmolar with respect to plasma — up to seven to eight times in some cases (Grainger, 1980; Dawson *et al.*, 1983a). This hyperosmolality is associated with a number of adverse effects, both subjective and objective. Thus, when absolutely or relatively high doses of the contrast medium are injected into the circulation, as in many interventional studies or in cardiac studies in infants and small children, the osmotic load, and in some cases the sodium load, may be a threat to the patient. The effects of the hyperosmolar solutions on smooth muscle produce a generalized peripheral vasodilation with a sometimes profound fall in blood pressure followed by a reflex tachycardia, events which are poorly tolerated by some patients (Snowdon & Whitehouse, 1981). The subjective counterparts of this are the feeling of flushing and faint-

ness experienced by many patients. Other unpleasant subjective side effects, such as sensation of spontaneous bladder emptying and metallic taste, often cited by patients as most unpleasant, must be added (Grainger, 1980).

At the microscopic level there may be injury to endothelial cells which is largely, but not entirely, mediated by hyperosmolality (Raininko, 1979) and which on venous injection may lead to thrombophlebitis or frank venous thrombosis (Laerum & Holm, 1981). In arterial injections it may be a factor in the post-angiographic progression of stenosis to occlusion and to the failure, by early closure, of angioplasties. This injurious effect is of particular significance in relation to the blood–brain barrier. There is considerable experimental work demonstrating the increased permeability of the blood–brain barrier and the transfer of contrast agent into the brain and into direct contact with neurons which are very sensitive to contrast agents (Sage, 1989). Indeed, one hypothesis holds that blood–brain barrier injury and subsequent neuronal irritation is the seat of all idiosyncratic anaphylactoid adverse reactions to contrast agents.

Not only endothelial cells, but also erythrocytes, basophils and mast cells, are affected by contrast agents. Water is drawn out of erythrocytes by hyperosmolar contrast agents, so that they become shrunken and deformed and lose the flexibility essential for them to negotiate the capillary circulation (Dawson *et al.*, 1983b). The 'sludging' of rigidified erythrocytes in the microcirculation of the lungs in pulmonary angiography has been related to the (usually) transient pulmonary hypertension associated with pulmonary angiography and, in the kidney, in selective renal angiography, has been cited as a factor in contrast agent-associated nephrotoxicity.

Basophils and mast cells are induced to release histamine, which may contribute to the subjective side effects experienced by patients and perhaps, although not certainly, to anaphylactoid reactions (Assem *et al.*, 1983).

In addition to the effects on the peripheral vasculature and on the expansion of the blood volume, the hyperosmolality of contrast agents is an important component of their cardiotoxicity (Dawson, 1989).

'Low-osmolar' agents

The various important subjective and objective side effects of high-osmolar agents provided a powerful stimulus to formulate 'low-osmolar' contrast agents. The obvious way to reduce the osmolality of solutions is to dilute them, but this would also dilute the iodine concentration.

Non-ionic agents

Almen first suggested an approach to reducing the osmolality of contrast agents without diluting their iodine concentration (Almen, 1969). He pointed out that the osmolality of any solution is proportional to the number of particles in that solution and that, by definition, ionic agents dissociate into two particles, anion and cation, and thereby double their osmolality in solution. A non-ionic, non-dissociating agent theoretically should have half the osmolality at any iodine concentration of an ionic agent. The first practical result of this concept was metrizamide (Amipaque), produced by Nyegaard (now Nycomed*) in Oslo. This was a substituted amide of metrizoic acid, a choice dictated by the fact that Nyegaard were already producers of metrizoates ('Isopaque') contrast agents. The loss of solubility, inevitable on the elimination of the carboxyl group,

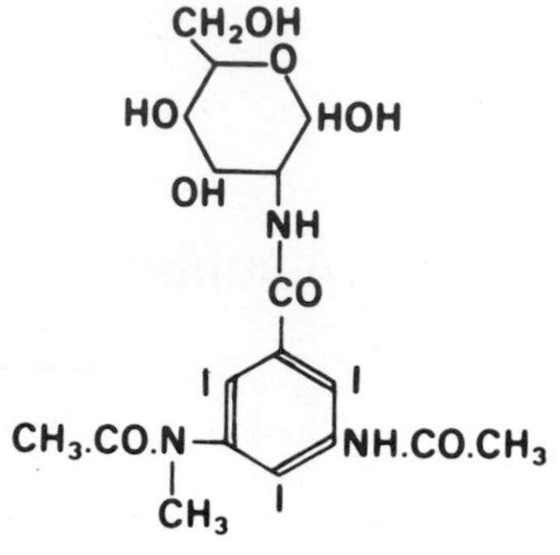

Fig. 30.4 Metrizamide (Amipaque). The first non-ionic contrast agent.

was overcome by substituting a D-glucose group which provided many hydrophilic hydroxyl groups (Fig. 30.4). Metrizamide had the serious disadvantage of being unstable at high temperatures, making its sterilization by autoclaving impossible and resulting in it having to be produced as a freeze-dried, lyophilized powder. Its instability in solution, even at room temperature, made it impossible to formulate ready to use solutions and the agent had to be made up at the time of use from a powder solute and a sterile solvent. It was therefore both expensive and inconvenient, and was not much used in intravascular applications. However, its low neurotoxicity, compared to the ionic water-soluble agents, led to a revolution in myelography.

Although they were otherwise little used in clinical practice, enough experimental and clinical work was performed to establish that such low-osmolar, non-ionic agents had considerable advantages in terms of reduced toxicity in a variety of applications, including coronary and carotid arteriography and peripheral venography. This stimulated the production of a second generation of non-ionic contrast media in ready to use formulations, of which there are now a number of representatives, including iohexol (Omnipaque, Nycomed) (Fig. 30.5), iopamidol (Niopam, Bracco*) (Fig. 30.6) and iopromide (Ultravist, Schering) (Fig. 30.7). These second-generation compounds have the convenience of being in ready to use solutions and are considerably cheaper than metrizamide, although still signifi-

---

* Nycomed AS, Oslo, Norway.

* Bracco spa, Milan, Italy.

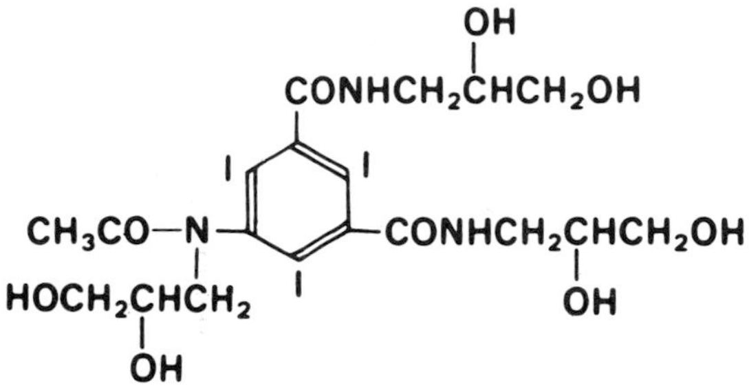

Fig. 30.5 Iohexol (Omnipaque). Second-generation non-ionic agent.

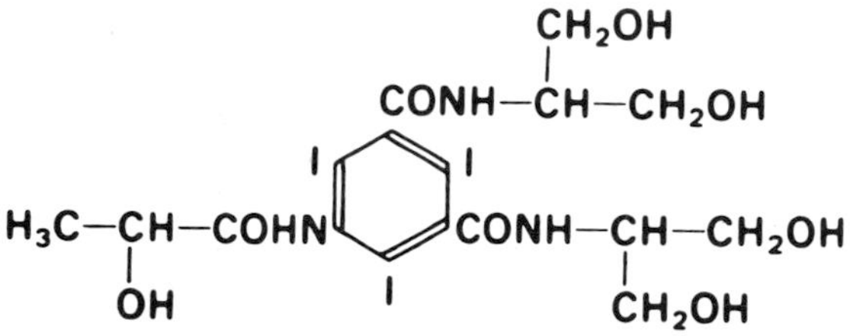

Fig. 30.6 Iopamidol (Niopam). Second-generation non-ionic agent.

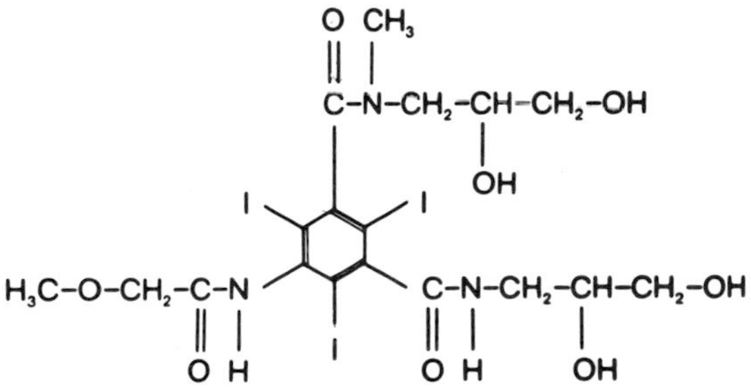

Fig. 30.7 Iopromide (Ultravist). Second-generation non-ionic agent.

cantly more expensive than the conventional ionic agents. Cost is the only factor which has militated against their replacing the conventional ionic agents completely for all applications.

A useful way in which to express the merits of any contrast agent, in terms of contrast-providing potential relative to the disadvantages in terms of osmolality, is as the ratio of iodine atoms provided per molecule (three in all cases so far considered) to the number of particles in solution derived from a molecular unit (two in the case of the ionic agents and one, the whole molecule, in the case of the non-ionic agents). Thus, the ionic agents are sometimes referred to as 3 : 2 or ratio 1.5 agents and the non-ionic variety is 3 : 1 or ratio 3 agents. The higher the ratio the better, and 3 : 1 is clearly better than 3 : 2.

Monoacid dimeric agents

If two tri-iodinated benzoic acid groups are joined by a linking bridge the result is a dimeric acid. Thus, iocarmic acid, a meglumine salt of a dimer produced by linking two iothalamic acids, was introduced as a 'Dimer X' in 1970 and used, in spite of the fact that it was ionic and relatively neurotoxic, as a myelographic agent. The ratio of number of iodine atoms to particles in solution from each molecule in this compound was 6 : 3, already an improvement on the 3 : 2 ratio associated with the conventional ionic monomeric contrast agents. Subsequently, one of the carboxyl groups of such a dicarboxylic acid has been substituted by a non-ionizing group to produce a monoacid dimer. This is ioxaglic acid (Fig. 30.8), which is produced in a commercial formulation as a mixture of sodium and meglumine salts of ioxaglic acid, as which it is known as Hexabrix*. This has a

* Laboratoire Guerbet, Paris, France.

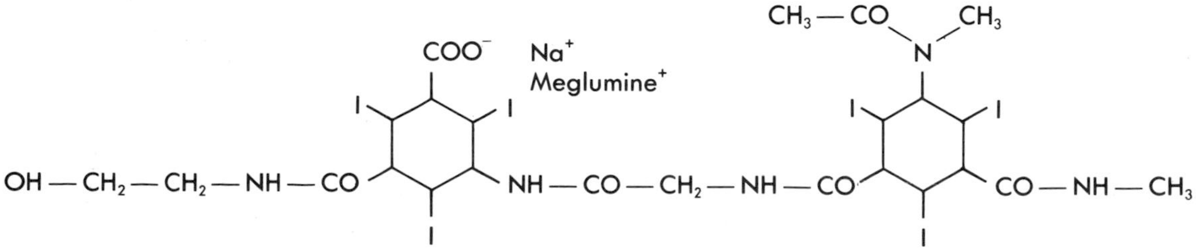

Fig. 30.8 Sodium meglumine ioxaglate (Hexabrix). A monoacid dimeric low-osmolality agent.

high iodine to particle ratio of 6 : 2 (= 3 : 1) and, while remaining an ionic agent, this compound succeeds, as do the non-ionic monomeric agents, in reducing osmolality to approximately half that of conventional ionic agents at any iodine concentration.

The osmolalities for several contrast agents, plotted as a function of iodine concentration, are shown in Fig. 30.9. Sodium iothalamate represents the conventional ionic agents in this figure. As can be seen, the reduction in osmolality, at any given iodine concentration, as compared with the conventional agent, is somewhat more than the predicted 50% for all of the agents. This is partly the result of the large size of all these molecules and partly due to a degree of molecular aggregation in solution. The differences between the osmolalities of the various new agents are real but of little clinical significance. The fact that Hexabrix has a slightly lower osmolality at any iodine concentration than any of the other agents might suggest clinical advantages, even if small. However, although Hexabrix is an acceptable arteriographic agent associated with reduced pain and discomfort, on i.v. injection it displays significantly greater toxicity than do the non-ionic agents and it should not be used for i.v. urography, i.v. digital subtraction angiography (DSA) or for enhancement of computed tomography (CT). This fact is, at first, surprising and the important reasons for it are discussed below.

Non-ionic dimeric contrast agents

One obvious next step in contrast agent development, which has been taken by both Schering and Nycomed, is to combine the dimeric approach of Hexabrix with the non-ionic concept (Dawson & Howell, 1986). This can done simply by taking a dimeric compound of the type discussed above and replacing *both* carboxyl groups by non-ionizing groups. To maintain solubility, it is now essential to substitute around the molecule a large number of hydrophilic groups. The two commercial compounds of this type now available are illustrated in Fig. 30.10. Iotrolan (Isovist, Schering) is available for myelographic and intravascular use and iodixanol (Visipaque, Nycomed) is available for intravascular use.

The osmolalities of such non-ionic dimers are lower than that of plasma at all iodine concentrations up to about 400 mg iodine ml^{-1}. This is the result of both a large molecular size and molecular aggregation producing a very high effective molecular weight and hence a lower than predicted osmo-

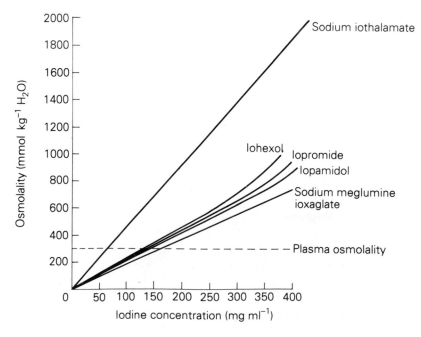

Fig. 30.9 The osmolalities of some contrast agents as a function of iodine concentration at 37°C.

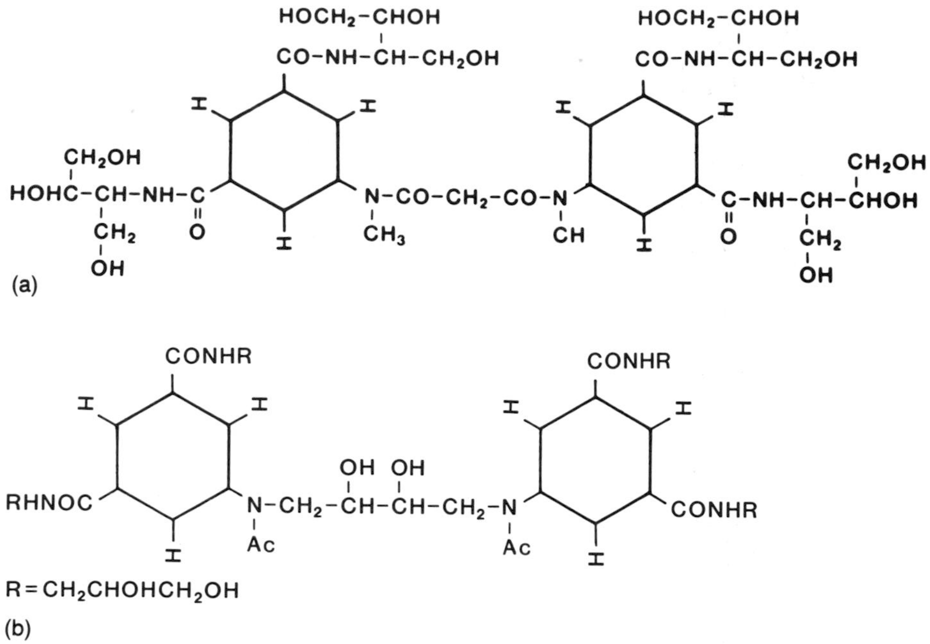

Fig. 30.10 Two non-ionic dimeric contrast agents: (a) iotrolan, and (b) iodixanol. These prepared in formulations are iso-osmolar with plasma.

lality. This problem of hypo-osmolality is a new one in the contrast agent field but is easily overcome. The addition of a little saline allows the osmolality to be adjusted upwards to become identical to that of plasma at any iodine concentration and this is done in the commercial formulations. The osmolality factor is, thereby, completely eliminated.

Such agents are more viscous than other contrast agents, largely because of their high molecular weight, but when heated to body temperature (perhaps a good manoeuvre anyway) have acceptably low viscosities for clinical use.

It has been argued that the higher viscosity, combined with the lower diffusibility of such large molecules, is advantageous in myelography.

Contrast agent toxicity

Table 30.1 shows how LD_{50} has increased (toxicity decreased) since the early 1930s. This is a very crude, but important, measure of contrast agent toxicity. It reveals an interesting fact, namely that toxicity cannot be entirely a function of osmolality. Metrizamide

and sodium meglumine ioxaglate are low-osmolality agents and, indeed, have somewhat lower osmolalities at any iodine concentration than do the second-generation non-ionic agents, and yet they have significantly lower LD_{50} (higher toxicity). Furthermore, metrizamide is a non-ionic agent. It is clear that simply to be non-ionic is not enough, to be low

Table 30.1 The LD_{50} values for a number of contrast agents from 1930 to the present day

Agent	LD_{50} (g iodine kg^{-1} mouse)
Sodium iomethamate (Uroselectan B)	2.0
Iodopyracet (Diodone)	3.2
Sodium acetrizoate (Urokon)	5.5
Sodium diatrizoate (Urografin)	8.4
Sodium meglumine ioxaglate (Hexabrix)	12.0
Metrizamide (Amipaque)	14.0
Iopamidol (Nipam)	21.0
Iohexol (Omnipaque)	24.0

osmolality is not enough, and to be low osmolality *and* non-ionic is not enough, necessarily, to achieve the lowest possible toxicity. The explanation is that contrast agents possess, by virtue of their chemical structure, an intrinsic toxicity which is sometimes labelled 'chemotoxicity' (Dawson, 1985). This toxicity is agent-specific, unlike hyperosmolality-related toxicity which is an entirely non-specific manifestation of the high concentration solutions and can be mimicked by high-concentration solutions of other materials such as glucose. A clue is that when Swick, as discussed above, substituted an iodine atom in the hippuric acid structure, a marked increase in toxicity was the result. Iodine is a highly hydrophobic atom and it has long been known that the more hydrophobic agents have a greater toxicity than the more hydrophilic ones. The relative hydrophobicity / hydrophilicity is usually measured as a 'partition coefficient' which correlates very well with various measures of toxicity. The addition of iodine to a benzene ring increases the hydrophobicity and therefore the partition coefficient.

Another parameter which correlates with the toxicity is the protein-binding capacity. None of these contrast agents possess much potential to bind to proteins but significant differences are to be found between different agents, particularly between ionic and non-ionic agents, and there is a close correlation between protein binding and toxicity. The higher binding agents are more toxic than the lower binding ones. The relationship between this observation and the partition coefficient has been explained in a synthesis of ideas as follows.

The chemotoxicity of contrast agents is mediated by non-specific weak interactions between the agents and various biological molecules. This weak binding would not be of any significance were it not that contrast agents are used at such high concentrations and total doses as compared with any other type of drug. The interaction is mediated essentially by two elements.

1 There is a Coulomb interaction in the case of the ionic agents. The absence of charge in the non-ionic agents immediately eliminates this interaction.

2 There are hydrophobic interactions between hydrophobic portions of the molecule, mainly its benzene ring / iodine core, and hydrophobic portions of the biological molecules (the hydrophilic portions of

both types of molecule being largely solvated by water molecules). The non-ionic agents have lower chemotoxicity, not only because they possess no charge, but because the many hydrophilic groups they carry, to restore the solubility lost when the carboxyl group of the ionic agent was eliminated, shield the hydrophobic core of the molecule and thus limit its availability for hydrophobic interactions.

Several concepts can now be understood from this. The addition of iodine to the molecule renders it more toxic by enhancing the hydrophobicity of the molecular core. The non-ionic agents have lower chemotoxicity, partly because they carry no charge to mediate Coulomb interactions and partly because they shield the hydrophobic core with their hydrophilic substituents. The protein-binding capacity of the molecule correlates with its toxicity because it is this binding which mediates the toxicity. The partition coefficient correlates because the more the hydrophobic core of the molecule is shielded, limiting its interaction with biological systems, the more hydrophilic the contrast agent is overall and the lower, therefore, is its partition coefficient. Conversely, the less efficiently the hydrophilic substituents shield the hydrophobic core, the more the hydrophobic interactions can take place, the more hydrophobic is the molecule and the greater the partition coefficient. Furthermore, we can now see why metrizamide has such a relatively high toxicity for a non-ionic agent. All the hydrophilic groups are carried on a glucose substituent at position 1, rather than being distributed around the molecule as is the case with the second-generation non-ionic agents. There is very little shielding of the hydrophobic core of the molecule, which therefore has a *relatively* high partition coefficient, high protein binding and high toxicity.

Figures 30.11 and 30.12 display the results of two *in vitro* studies of chemotoxic manifestations of contrast agents, namely the interactions with an enzyme and with structural proteins of platelet surfaces. The first results in an inhibition of the enzyme and the second in an inhibition of the aggregation of platelets on stimulus. As can be seen in both cases, there is a concentration-dependent effect (here expressed as iodine concentration) and there are marked differences between different agents. The same hierarchy of magnitudes is seen in both assays: the

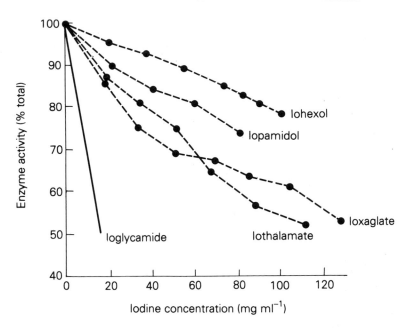

Fig. 30.11 The inhibition of the enzyme acetylcholinesterase by various contrast agents as a function of concentration.

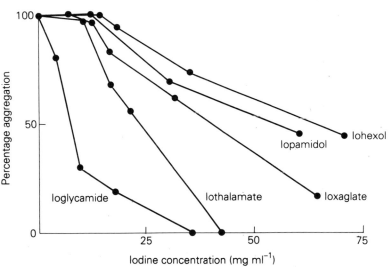

Fig. 30.12 The inhibition of platelet aggregation by various contrast agents as a function of concentration (expressed as iodine).

conventional ionic agents have the greatest effect, the non-ionic agents the least effect, and the monoacid dimeric low-osmolality ionic agent, Hexabrix, has an intermediate effect.

Although illustrations will not be given here, it may be noted that the low chemotoxicity of the non-ionic monomeric agents is shared, and perhaps shown to a greater extent, by the non-ionic dimeric agents.

The ideal contrast agent, it should be remembered,

should have no effects of any kind on biological systems. Although not quite meeting this ideal, the non-ionic agents, monomeric and dimeric, represent the closest approach so far to the ideal.

High-dose toxicity of contrast agents

While much energy has been expended on the problem of idiosyncratic/anaphylactoid reactions to contrast agents (see below), particularly with regard to the elucidation of their underlying mechanisms, their prediction and their prophylaxis and management, much less attention has been paid to the problem of the dose-dependent side effects of the agents. In terms of frequency, these are of greater importance than idiosyncratic reactions in a number of patient groups who are well represented in interventional radiology, such as those with poor cardiac reserve, impaired renal or hepatic function, and multisystem organ failure (Dawson & Hemingway, 1987). Even without such obvious underlying risk factors, many patients may be at risk from dose-dependent contrast medium toxicity, including sodium and/or osmotic overload in complex or prolonged procedures involving large total doses of contrast medium (Dawson & Hemingway 1987).

Theoretical considerations

In a typical i.v. urogram, 300 mg iodine kg^{-1} may be used. For a 70 kg man this represents 21 g iodine, which could be provided, for example, by 50 ml of sodium iothalamate containing 420 mg ml^{-1} iodine. Several rules of thumb are in use to define an upper limit for the total contrast medium dose. A maximum in a healthy adult of three times the above level, that is 1000 mg iodine kg^{-1}, is sometimes suggested. This may be compared with the measurement of 8000 mg iodine kg^{-1} for conventional contrast agents, a comparison of uncertain relevance to the clinical situation but the only guide available. There would appear to be some safety margin here, giving scope for higher doses to be used if the examination is vital and demands it. Concerning nephrotoxicity, Golman (personal communication) would support a figure in this range as being an appropriate upper limit. There is clearly a question of clinical judgement to be exercised in the context of the individual patient, the importance of the procedure, and the consequences of not proceeding with it. The time over which the total dose is to be administered is also clearly an important consideration, remembering that the half-life of contrast agents in the circulation is approximately 2 hours. One other important factor nowadays is the availability of the better low-osmolar non-ionic contrast agents. These have higher LD_{50}, present a lower

osmotic load and contain little or no sodium. Whatever arbitrary upper limit in mg iodine kg^{-1} is set for the conventional agents, it seems likely that twice this dose of a new agent can be used. Thus if 1000 mg iodine kg^{-1} may be given in the form of a conventional agent, possibly 2500 mg iodine kg^{-1} of a new agent may be given. If this is in the form of, say, Omnipaque 300 (iohexol 300 mg iodine ml^{-1}), this would mean a volume dose for a 70 kg man of $(2000 \times 70)/300 = 450$ ml.

Even higher doses may presumably be used if the contrast medium is administered over an extended period. Such high doses should never be given without serious thought but, if the procedure is vital for either diagnosis or therapy, they may then be given with caution, detailed decisions being tailored to the individual patient. A reasonable precaution, with the risk of renal function in mind, is to make sure that the patient is well hydrated at the start of the procedure (see below).

Anaphylactoid/idiosyncratic reactions

Idiosyncratic reactions may occur following the administration of any contrast agent (Ansell *et al.*, 1980). Although unpredictable, such reactions are more likely to occur in certain patient groups: (i) those that have reacted on a previous occasion to a contrast agent; (ii) those with established allergies to other drugs or agents; and (iii) asthmatic and atopic individuals. These reactions are essentially dose-independent and may even occur following subcutaneous or intradermal test doses. Occasionally, although not commonly, reactions follow non-vascular procedures such as percutaneous transhepatic cholangiography, arthrography and hysterosalpingo-graphy, presumably as a result of intravasation in these cases. It is important to realize that such reactions may be delayed up to 30 min and the patient should never be left entirely unsupervised during a procedure.

The mechanisms of these reactions remain obscure in spite of a considerable amount of study and the elaboration of a number of hypotheses. However, it has now been clarified that the non-ionic monomeric contrast agents are associated with a significantly reduced risk of such reactions, particularly in at-risk patients. This certainly is the outcome of large-scale clinical trials of ionic versus non-ionic contrast agents in Japan (Katayama *et al.*, 1990) and Australia (Palmer, 1988). It can be firmly stated, as a consequence, that non-ionic agents should be used in all cases when the patient is definably at increased risk of such a reaction.

The role of corticosteroids as prophylaxis against such reactions in at-risk patients has been the subject of considerable controversy (Dawson & Sidhu, 1993). It is widely believed that corticosteroids are effective in this regard but the evidence for it is not substantial. The paper by Lasser *et al.* (1987) describing a multicentre study in the USA is usually cited , but this paper has not been without its critics. It has been argued that even if its evidence is accepted at face value, the reduction in risk is little more than 50% whereas a 6–10-fold decrease in risk is achieved by using non-ionic contrast agents (Dawson & Sidhu, 1993).

The treatment of adverse reactions to intravascular contrast agents is summarized in Appendix 1.

Effects on coagulation

All contrast agents have antiplatelet and anticoagulant effects, a fact that has been well known, if poorly understood, by angiographers for many years. This seems a positive advantage in preventing thromboembolism from catheters and syringes. In fact, a tendency for patients to bleed following high doses of a previous generation of contrast agents was reported. There is no convincing evidence that there is any such danger, even in complex, high-dose interventional vascular procedures with the modern agents, although radiologists should be aware of the theoretical possibility.

The haematological effects of contrast agents have recently been the subject of considerable controversy, particularly in the USA. Non-ionic contrast agents have been the focus of suspicion and have been alleged to be a cause of thromboembolism and early thrombotic closure at the angioplasty site. This controversy has been extensively reviewed and only a few cardinal points will be summarized.

1 All contrast agents have concentration-dependent antiplatelet aggregation effects (see Fig. 30.12), but these effects are less pronounced with non-ionic agents than with ionic agents of high or low osmolality (Dawson *et al.*, 1986).

2 All contrast agents exhibit concentration-dependent anticoagulant effects, mediated at a number of levels in the coagulation cascade but particularly at the fibrin polymerization stage. The effects of nonionic contrast agents are less marked than those of ionic agents. A crucial point is that the hierarchy of magnitudes of effects, typical of those seen in any study of chemotoxicity, is also seen here. Any anticoagulant effect of the contrast agent is a manifestation of toxicity. When angiographers express a preference for more anticoagulant contrast agents, they are expressing a preference for more toxic contrast agents (Dawson *et al.*, 1986).

There is no evidence to justify the claim made by some authors, either openly or by implication, with the use of such words as 'thrombogenic', that nonionic contrast agents have some stimulatory effect on coagulation. The true thrombogenic influences *in vivo* are endothelial injury by contrast agents, being greater with ionic agents, or by balloon or laser injury in angioplasty; *in vitro* they are the contact of blood with the foreign surfaces of catheters and syringes. Contrast agents play a variable inhibitory role and are therefore entirely helpful in preventing thrombosis formation and subsequent thromboembolism from catheter–syringe systems.

A role for routine heparinization of the patient is widely accepted and practised in diagnostic angiocardiography and in coronary and non-coronary angioplasty. It is rarely used in routine non-cardiac diagnostic angiography. Although its use would seem reasonable, the evidence to support it is lacking and there is certainly no consensus on what doses should be used or what, if any, need there is for the monitoring of coagulation parameters during the procedure under heparinization. These are important considerations because the 'requirements' of patients for heparin vary widely.

The injection of a bolus of heparin into a diseased vessel, both before and after an angioplasty dilatation procedure, is widely sanctioned but its efficacy has not been established.

The case, therefore, for using a more anticoagulant–antiplatelet ionic contrast agent in such a vessel is, to say the least, unproven. Even if a case could be established, the advantage of a greater anticoagulant effect would have to be weighed against the fact that non-ionic contrast agents are a significantly better choice with respect to cardiotoxicity, particularly in the diseased myocardium.

Mixing of non-ionic contrast agents and heparin before injection has been suggested. There is no specific contraindication to this but, in general terms, mixing of drugs is to be avoided.

Nephrotoxicity

The nephrotoxicity of contrast agents, although an article of faith among radiologists and nephrologists, is an elusive entity. Patients thought to be its victims are often taking other nephrotoxic drugs, may be dehydrated and may be on a declining curve of renal function at the time of hospital admission. Perhaps contrast agents play the role of a non-specific co-factor (the 'last straw' hypothesis). A role has been suggested for vasopressin as a nephrotoxicity-mediating hormone in dehydrated patients. This would certainly explain the putative roles of high total dose and patient dehydration as risk factors. There is as yet no evidence to suggest that non-ionic contrast agents are less likely to be associated with these alleged nephrotoxic events than their ionic counterparts, but first principles dictate that they should be used in preference to the latter in patients with impaired renal function. All patients should, as far as possible, be well hydrated for all procedures and given the minimum dose of the chosen contrast medium compatible with a proper examination.

It should be noted that contrast agents are readily dialysable and may therefore be removed from the patient at the end of the procedure if this is thought desirable.

Appendix 1: The management of adverse reactions to intravascular contrast agents — guidelines of the Royal College of Radiologists

Symptoms and treatment

Symptoms	Treatment
Nausea/vomiting	Reassurance; retain i.v. access and observe; antiemetics rarely necessary
Mild scattered hives/urticaria	Routine treatment not necessary; retain i.v. access; observe; if troublesome, antihistamine chlorpheniramine maleate (paediatric dose 0.2 mg kg^{-1} body weight) 10–20 mg or promethazine hydrochloride 25–50 mg (max. 100 mg) by slow i.v. injection
Severe generalized urticaria	i.v. antihistamines as above
Mild wheeze	Addition of i.v. hydrocortisone 100 mg (paediatric dose 4 mg kg); 100% oxygen by Ventimask (unless evidence of chronic obstructive airways disease with hypercapnia); β_2 agonist by inhaler, e.g. salbutamol by nebulizer (5 mg in 2 ml saline). Repeat as necessary; maintain careful observation
Hypotension with bradycardia (vasovagal reaction/faint)	Raise the patient's feet; oxygen by mask 10–15 litre min^{-1}; establish 14–16 gauge i.v. cannula; i.v. fluids (preferably colloid); administer 10–15 ml kg^{-1} rapidly; administer atropine 0.6 mg i.v.; repeat at 5-min intervals up to 3 mg total (paediatric dose 0.02 mg kg^{-1} minimum 0.1 mg);

Symptoms and treatment. *Continued.*

Symptoms	Treatment
	advice of an anaesthetist *must* be requested if response is not rapid
Angio-oedema/urticaria/bronchospasm/ hypotension proceeding to anaphylactoid reaction	Give oxygen at 10–15 litres min^{-1}; establish i.v. access 14–16 gauge cannula; i.v. fluids, 10–15 ml kg^{-1}; β_2 agonist by nebulizer (5 mg in 2 ml saline); setting up may take valuable time; do not allow to delay other measures; give adrenaline 0.5–1 ml 1 : 10 000 i.v.; i.v. hydrocortisone 100 mg (paediatric dose 4 mg kg^{-1} to a maximum of 100 mg); ECG monitoring, oximetry and blood pressure monitoring should be established
Unconscious/unresponsive/pulseless/ collapsed patient	Standard cardiopulmonary resuscitation measures must be employed. Cardiac arrest team summoned. Institute standard resuscitation procedures published by the Resuscitation Council, Colchester, UK as follows: *Basic life support* • Establish airway — head tilt, chin lift • Initiate ventilation — mouth to mouth *Advanced life support* • External cardiac massage — 15 compressions every 2 breaths • Establish i.v. access 14–16 gauge cannula • Tracheal intubation • i.v. fluids established 10–15 ml kg^{-1} • Cardiac monitoring by ECG • DC defibrillation if in ventricular fibrillation (200–360 J); repeat if necessary • i.v. adrenaline — 1 mg = 10 ml 1 : 10 000 (paediatric dose 0.1 ml kg^{-1} 1 : 10 000); follow as necessary with further 1 ml aliquots • Consider administration of hydrocortisone/ antihistamines • If no i.v. access give 0.3–1 ml of 1 : 1000 adrenaline i.m. or s.c. (paediatric dose 0.01 ml kg^{-1}) • Admit patient to ICU
Seizure	May be the consequence of hypotension and primary treatment should be on above lines; 100% oxygen by MC mask; if it continues, anticonvulsant may be given, eg. diazemuls i.v. 5–10 mg, initially although much higher doses may be needed. Second-line drugs such as thiopentone may be required but by this time the patient should be intubated and ventilated

ECG, electrocardiogram; ICU, intensive care unit.

General comments

• Corticosteroids are, quite correctly, thought of as slow-acting drugs with a lag time after injection of at least 6 hours. However, there is no doubt they work very rapidly indeed when administered i.v. in severe asthma and in bronchospasm related to drug reactions and should therefore not be withheld.
• Adrenaline (i.v.) is sometimes considered a dangerous drug associated with cardiac arrhythmias. This is true and it should not be used in minor reactions but only in severe life-threatening bronchospasm and/or cardiovascular collapse, when the potential benefits greatly outweigh the risks. Doses may have to be very high and may need to be repeated.
• If i.v. access is difficult in children, intraosseous access may be considered.

General points worth reinforcing

Depending on the severity of the reaction and the length of treatment required, an i.v. cannula should be inserted as soon as is practical and drugs administered through this rather than the needle, which carries the risk of cutting out.
• Contrast agents should not be injected in an isolated clinical setting. Facilities for resuscitation should be available if required. Non-ionic contrast medium should be used if a full cardiac arrest team is not available.
• The patient should never be left alone following injection, particularly during the first 10 min. Remember serious reactions may sometimes be considerably delayed.
• Equipment and drugs routinely used in the management of medical emergencies should be immediately available. One trolley serving a unit with scattered rooms on several floors is not acceptable.

• Equipment and drugs should be regularly checked by a designated person(s) and recorded as checked.
• All persons involved in the daily running of a department should be aware of the site of resuscitation equipment.
• All personnel should attend a basic resuscitation course on a regular basis.
• Each department should have a specific protocol for dealing with various reactions, which should be updated periodically.
• The person who administers the contrast should have a basic medical history about the patient, particularly relating to previous allergies, and be adequately trained in resuscitation procedures.

Drugs

Suggested drugs for the emergency box to be placed in each room where i.v. contrast agents are used:
• chlorpheniramine maleate,
• promethazine,
• hydrocortisone,
• atropine,
• salbutamol inhaler,
• salbutamol nebulizer,
• ephedrine,
• normal saline,
• methoxamine,
• dobutamine,
• dopamine,
• adrenaline (1 : 10 000),
• adrenaline 1 : 1000, at least 10 ampoules.

The advice of the local consultant anaesthetist designated to take responsibility for anaesthetic matters within the radiology department, should be sought when formulating local policies. A plastic card, on the management of anaphylaxis, prepared by the Association of Anaesthetists, London, UK is available.

References

Almen, T. (1969) Contast agent design: some aspects of the synthesis of water soluble contast agents of low osmolality. *J. Theor. Biol.*, **24**, 216–26.
Ansell, G., Tweedie, M.C.K., West, C.R. *et al.* (1980) The current status of reaction to i.v. contrast media. *Invest. Radiol.*, **15**, 532–9.
Assem, E.S.K., Bray, K. & Dawson, P. (1983) The release of histamine from human basophils by radiological contrast agents. *Br. J. Radiol.*, **59**, 987–91.
Berberich, J. & Hirsch, S. (1923) Die Röntgenographische Darstellung der Arterien und am Lebenden. *Klin. Wschr.*, **9**, 2226–8.
Brooks, B. (1924) Intra-arterial injection of sodium iodide. *JAMA*, **82**, 1016–19.
Burrows, E.H. (1986) *Pioneers and Early Years*. Colophon Ltd, Alderney.

Dawson, P. (1985) Chemotoxicity of contrast media and clinical adverse effects. A review. *Invest. Radiol.*, **20**, 52–9.

Dawson, P. (1989) Cardiovascular effects of contrast agents. *Am. J. Cardiol.*, **64**, 2E–9.

Dawson, P., Grainger, R.G. & Pitfield, J. (1983a) The new low osmolar contrast media. A simple guide. *Clin. Radiol.*, **34**, 221–4.

Dawson, P., Harrison, J.G. & Weisblatt, E. (1983b). Effect of contrast media on red cell filtrability and morphology. *Br. J. Radiol.*, **56**, 707–10.

Dawson, P., Hewitt, P., Mackie, I.J. & Bradshaw, A. (1986) Contrast, coagulation and fibrinolysis. *Invest. Radiol.*, **21**, 248–52.

Dawson, P. & Hemingway, A.P. (1987) Contrast doses in interventional radiology. *J. Intervent. Radiol.*, **2**, 145–6.

Dawson, P. & Howell, M.J. (1986) The pharmacology of the non-ionic dimers. *Br. J. Radiol.*, **59**, 987–91.

Dawson, P. & Sidhu, P. (1993) Is there a role for corticosteroid prophylaxis in the prevention of major contrast reactions? *Clin. Radiol.*, **48**, 225–6.

Grainger, R.G. (1980) Osmolality of intravascular radiological contrast media. *Br. J. Radiol.*, **53**, 739–46.

Grainger, R.G. (1982) Intravascular contrast media — the past, the present and the future. *Br. J. Radiol.*, **55**, 1–18.

Haschek, E. & Lindenthal, T.O. (1896) Ein Beitrag zur praktischen Verwerthung der Photographie nach Roentgen. *Wien. Klin. Wschr.*, **9**, 63–4.

Hoppe, J.O. (1959) Some pharmacological aspects of radio opaque compounds. *Ann. NY Acad. Sci.*, **78**, 727–39.

Katayama, H., Yamaguchi, K., Kozuka, T. *et al.* (1990) Adverse reactions to ionic and non-ionic contrast media. *Radiology*, **175**, 621–8.

Laerum, F & Holm, H.A. (1981) Postphlebographic thrombosis. *Radiology*, **140**, 651–4.

Larsen, A.A., Moore, C., Sprague, B. *et al.* (1956) Iodinated 3, 5-diamino benzoic acid derivatives. *J. Am. Chem. Soc.*, **78**, 3210–16.

Lasser, E.C., Berry, C.C., Talner, L.B. *et al.* (1987) Pretreatment with corticosteroids to alleviate reactions to intravenous contrast material. *N. Engl. J. Med.*, **317**, 845–9.

MacMahon, H.E., Murphy, A.S. & Bates, M.I. (1947) Endothelial cell sarcoma of the liver following thorotrast injection. *Am. J. Pathol.*, **23**, 585–611.

Moniz, E. (1940) *Die Cerebrale Arteriographie und Phlebographie.* Springer-Verlag, Berlin.

Osborne, E.D., Sutherland, C.G., Scholl, A.J. & Rowntree, L.G. (1923) Roentgenography of the urinary tract during excretion of sodium iodide. *JAMA*, **80**, 368–73.

Palmer, F.J. (1988) The RACR survey of intravenous contrast media reaction. Final report. *Australas. Radiol.*, **32**, 426–8.

Raininko, R. (1979) Role of hyperosmolality: the endothelial injury caused by angiographic contrast media. *Acta Radiol.*, **20**, 410–16.

Sage, M.R. (1989) Neuroangiography. *In* Skucas, J. (ed.) *Radiographic Contrast Agents*, 2nd edn, pp. 170–88. Aspen, Rockville.

Snowdon, S.L. & Whitehouse, G.H. (1981) Blood pressure changes resulting from aortography. *J. Roy. Soc. Med.*, **74**, 419–21.

Swarm, R.L. (1971) Colloidal thorium dioxide. *In International Encyclopedia of Pharmacology and Therapeutics*, vol. 2. *Radiocontrast Agents*. Pergamon Press, Oxford.

Wallingford, V.H. (1952) Iodinated acylaminobenzoic acids as X-ray contrast media. *J. Am. Pharmacol. Assoc.*, **42**, 721–8.

Wenz, W. (1967) Tumours of the kidney following retrograde pylegraphy with colloidal thorium dioxide. *Ann. N. Y. Acad. Sci.*, **145**, 8806–10.

31   Anaesthesia and Sedation

S. L. SNOWDON

Although a large number of procedures undertaken in the X-ray department require some form of anaesthesia or analgesia, the subject has been surprisingly neglected in the past. There is the need for understanding and cooperation between the surgeon, physician, radiologist and anaesthetist in performing radiological investigations. There is also evidence that a significant number of invasive radiological procedures are requested without full justification (Macpherson *et al.*, 1980). The patient may therefore be subjected unnecessarily to the hazards of anaesthesia or heavy sedation in the radiology department.

Anaesthesia in radiological cases is often delegated to a junior anaesthetist and there are often limited and outdated anaesthetic facilities in radiology departments. Few standard texts advise on the problems that are likely to be encountered in what are often poor-risk patients (Buxton Hopkin, 1980), despite the unfavourable circumstances for anaesthesia. Radiological investigations are sometimes followed by operative intervention which requires further anaesthesia. It is therefore essential that a high standard of anaesthetic care is employed in the first instance. An experienced anaesthetist is also of assistance in the radiology department for advising on suitable analgesia, sedation, resuscitative procedures, regional blocks and clinical measurement.

Facilities required for general anaesthesia

As the hazards of anaesthetizing a patient in the X-ray department may be as great as those encountered in the main operating theatre, the facilities should be of comparable standard. There should be a separate room for induction of anaesthesia and subsequent recovery. A fully equipped anaesthetic trolley must be available and should include ventilators and a comprehensive monitoring system. Careful obser-

vation is important during anaesthesia in the X-ray department, but may be especially difficult because of the darkened conditions, awkward positioning and the need to move the patient during some procedures. There are now recommended standards of monitoring during sedation, anaesthesia and recovery set out by the Association of Anaesthetists (1988) and Joint Working Party, Royal College of Anaesthetists and Royal College of Radiologists (1992). Pulse oximeters, oxygen analysers and capnographs are 'strongly recommended', in addition to the more commonly available electrocardiograph (ECG) and blood pressure monitors.

The table provided for anaesthetizing a patient should be capable of being set at an angle and there should be facilities for obtaining a sitting position. A full range of anaesthetic drugs is required, including scheduled drugs and those drugs which are needed for resuscitation.

A patient who is anaesthetized is, of course, unable to respond or move away from a source of electrical shock and fatal electrocution has occurred in these circumstances. All equipment should therefore be rigorously checked, especially the earth leakage current from monitoring apparatus and radiological equipment.

An operating department assistant is necessary to help move and position the patient, and is also required to check all the anaesthetic and monitoring equipment within the X-ray department. It may be difficult to obtain replacement equipment should any items malfunction, especially in an isolated X-ray department.

A nurse who is trained and qualified in recovery and resuscitation skills should be available during the administration and recovery from anaesthesia. The nurse may have to manage a patient who is only semiconscious or who may have suffered other complications such as anaphylaxis or laryngospasm.

Preparation of the patient

Adequate consultation between clinician, radiologist and anaesthetist is required to avoid confusion on the ward concerning the need for anaesthesia or sedation during a radiological investigation. An appreciation of the likelihood for general anaesthesia is required so that the patient can receive correct preparation. The patient should have a full general examination and appropriate investigations.

For patients over 60 years of age, an ECG, chest radiograph, haemoglobin level, blood count and serum electrolytes are recommended on a routine basis. In younger patients, investigations may also be required where there is a specific indication; for instance, a chronic cough necessitates a chest radiograph. The primary disease requiring radiological investigation may well be linked with other disorders, such as the association of diabetes and arteriopathy, which require appropriate investigation and treatment prior to anaesthesia.

Sedation may be needed prior to the procedure and is especially important when the investigation is performed under local rather than general anaesthesia.

Choice of anaesthesia or sedation

The decision as to whether the patient should receive general or local anaesthesia seems to be arbitrary, as is exemplified by the wide variety of anaesthetic techniques used for the same radiological procedure throughout the world. The risks associated with general anaesthesia should be borne in mind when considering procedures which are diagnostic and not therapeutic, sometimes making it difficult to set any direct benefit to the patient against any potential hazard.

Having established the need for the procedure and its influence on the subsequent management of the patient, it is necessary to examine the indications and relative contraindications for general anaesthesia.

Indications for general anaesthesia

1 When the procedure is especially painful.
2 Where severe anxiety is anticipated (Finby & Kanick, 1970).

3 When the radiological procedure may produce complications which require control of the ventilation or circulation.
4 If subsequent anaesthesia is required immediately following the procedure.
5 If general anaesthesia will make the performance of the radiological procedure easier and improve the quality of a particular investigation.

Relative contraindications

1 Pre-existing disease, for example myocardial infarction, diabetes and severe respiratory embarrassment.
2 Technical anaesthetic problems, for instance an unstable neck and limited neck or jaw movement.
3 Recent ingestion of food or fluid.
4 Inadequate patient preparation for general anaesthesia, when there has not been an examination or when relevant investigations are missing.
5 A history of allergy, particularly following a previous general anaesthetic or contrast medium examination.
6 Acute or active chronic respiratory infection.
7 When coexistent disorders are of greater importance and have a higher priority for treatment than the disease about to be investigated by the radiologist.

Consideration should be given to local anaesthesia, with or without sedation, or neuroleptanaesthesia. Whilst neuroleptanaesthesia has gained popularity worldwide, it is frequently disliked by patients, who often feel disorientated and unable to express their fears fully (Morgan *et al.*, 1971). Patients have occasionally obstructed their airway during neuroleptanaesthesia. Emergency intubation and controlled ventilation are then necessary.

Equally careful preparation is required if the radiological investigation is to be performed under local anaesthesia. The confidence of the patient should be gained and the procedure carefully explained to the patient well in advance. Suitable preoperative sedation may help to relax the patient and facilitate the examination.

A wide range of hypnotics and sedatives are now available. However, it is wise to become thoroughly familiar with a few agents and to be aware of their side effects, interactions and other features. If a benzodiazepine, for example temazepam, is chosen it must be remembered that these agents are anxiolytic but not analgesic in action. Should generalized discomfort or pain be anticipated, drugs with analgesic or sedative properties should be chosen, for example papaveratum.

Preoperative medication needs to be given at the correct time prior to the procedure, if it is to be effective. Because the necessary degree of organization and coordination is difficult to achieve, i.v. sedation has become popular. The short-acting anaesthetic propofol can provide excellent control of sedation with rapid recovery in experienced hands and using a special infusion pump. Even in skilled hands, i.v. sedation can lead to unexpected degrees of respiratory depression or, less often, cardiovascular collapse. As the onset of these side effects may be delayed for several minutes following completion of injection, careful observation must be maintained throughout the procedure. The radiologist engrossed in the technical performance of an investigation is unlikely to be in the best position to give the necessary observation. When sedation is used, there must be someone immediately available who is skilled in maintaining an airway as a matter of routine and able to intubate, ventilate and treat cardiovascular collapse. To attempt i.v. sedation in the absence of such well-practised skills is probably indefensible should harm come to a patient. Special care needs to be taken in observing for respiratory depression when i.v. analgesia is used in addition to sedation, a slow injection being given over several minutes. It is also advisable to give an antiemetic agent, for instance droperidol 2 mg, prior to the opiate, as nausea and vomiting sometimes occur. The dose of sedation must of course be adjusted in elderly patients and in those with chronic respiratory disease, diminished cardiac reserve or impaired hepatic or renal function. In the absence of anaesthetic expertise, care should be taken not to deepen sedation to the point where verbal contact is lost with the patient. Local anaesthesia occasionally proves inadequate, either because of discomfort experienced by the patient or because of a technically difficult radiological procedure. General anaesthesia may then be required and the patient prepared for such an eventuality.

Anaesthetic problems associated with radiological techniques

Aortography

General anaesthesia may be required for translumbar aortography although this is an uncommon approach nowadays. However, the same general principles may be applied to a wide variety of procedures which require anaesthesia in the prone position. Intubation and controlled ventilation are indicated because of the mechanical impairment caused to spontaneous respiration by the prone position of the patient. More recently, a laryngeal mask has been used instead of tracheal intubation. Care should be taken to ensure the secure fixation of the endotracheal tube or laryngeal mask. A patient may move more than 1 m during the radiological exposure and excessive tension may then develop on the tubing attached to the anaesthetic machine. Sudden extubation in the prone position, especially in a darkened room, may lead to serious consequences because reintubation can only be undertaken with difficulty in this position. Careful positioning is also important during translumbar aortography because of the movement of the X-ray table. In particular, care must be taken to secure the arms and legs. The pelvis and chest must be raised to enable free movement of the abdomen during controlled ventilation, otherwise excessively high inflation pressures are required to ventilate the patient in this position. The patient should never be moved without first informing the anaesthetist. In order that he may observe the anaesthetic circuit connection attaching the patient to the anaesthetic machine, a ventilation alarm is of great help to the anaesthetist in ensuring satisfactory respiration.

Routine monitoring of the ECG is important because pre-existing cardiovascular disease is common and also because of the cardiovascular side effects resulting from the injection of the contrast medium. The frequency of the latter has not been fully appreciated in the past and blood pressure monitoring is advisable. It is possible to monitor blood pressure continuously, using the cannula employed for the contrast medium injection connected to a pressure transducer. Some of the contrast media employed for aortography produce a significant fall in the blood pressure immediately following their injection (Moss

& Johnson, 1981; Snowdon & Whitehouse, 1981), and sometimes cardiac dysrhythmias (Fig. 31.1). This uncontrolled hypotension is especially undesirable in patients with cardiovascular disease.

Postoperative laryngospasm is another largely unrecognized complication associated with translumbar aortography. The laryngospasm may not be immediately apparent following extubation and the first signs may only appear several minutes later. This complication is potentially life-threatening and may require urgent reintubation of the patient. It is therefore advisable that the patient remains in the recovery area under careful observation for the first 20 min. Milder forms of laryngospasm may be managed by i.v. sedation and oxygen therapy. A vicious circle may develop with the patient becoming increasingly anxious and agitated with resultant worsening of the laryngospasm. The cause of the laryngospasm is uncertain but may be related to intubation in the prone position causing irritation of the vocal cords. Inhalation of secretions, which accumulate in the nasopharynx in the prone position, may trigger the spasm. An allergic reaction to the contrast media associated with laryngeal oedema has also been implicated as a cause.

Pulmonary oedema has complicated aortography,

the first signs appearing following reversal of anaesthesia (Aps, 1975). A poor cardiac reserve and the change from positive-pressure ventilation to spontaneous respiration are precipitating factors in these cases.

Epidural anaesthesia has been used to facilitate aortography. There is a small incidence of spinal cord and nerve damage following epidural anaesthesia, which has therefore not proved to be popular because of possible ensuing medicolegal complications (Miskin *et al.*, 1973).

Carotid angiography

Patients from a neuroradiological unit may cause particular problems for an anaesthetist. Raised intracranial pressure and associated vomiting, with its consequent electrolyte disturbance, must be recognized and dealt with the anaesthetist. It is especially important to correct sodium and potassium disturbances because they may lead to potentiation of muscle relaxants and prolonged muscle relaxation. The clinical picture may then be confused with a progression of cerebral damage during the postanaesthetic period.

Anaesthesia may considerably affect the intracranial pressure (Samuel *et al.*, 1968; McDowall *et al.*,

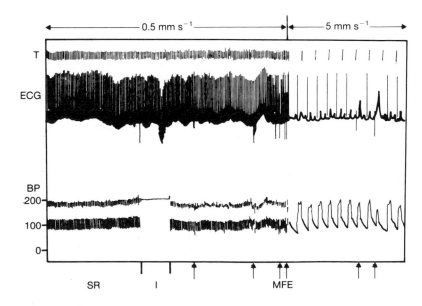

Fig. 31.1 Tracing of an electrocardiogram (ECG) and arterial pressure (BP) recorded during and following the injection of contrast medium (I), demonstrating the subsequent appearance of multifocal ectopic complexes (MFE) and fall in arterial pressure. The patient showed a stable sinus rhythm (SR) prior to injection and, as is commonly noted in patients presenting for aortography, hypotension.

1969; McDowall, 1975). Intracranial pressure is related to changes in blood gases, including oxygen and carbon dioxide blood tension (Fig. 31.2), which the anaesthetist may do much to control, aiming to keep the arterial carbon dioxide within the normal range. Control of arterial blood gas tensions may be used to alter blood vessel dilation, significantly improving radiographic demonstration of the cerebral vasculature (Dallas & Moxton, 1969). It should also be remembered that the neurosurgical patient may proceed directly to further surgery.

There is some evidence that volatile agents, especially halothane, cause a significant rise in the intracranial pressure of patients with cerebral tumours (McDowall *et al.*, 1963). Spontaneous ventilation whilst using a volatile anaesthetic agent is therefore contraindicated, intubation and controlled ventilation being used in preference. A smooth induction is desirable, avoiding coughing and straining, yet permitting maintenance of the blood pressure which will

facilitate palpation and cannulation of the carotid artery. A technique using muscle relaxants causes relaxation of the sternocleidomastoid muscle, allowing it to be displaced and thus giving an easier fixation of the artery.

It is clearly more difficult to assess the neurological state patient during general anaesthesia compared with local anaesthesia. For this reason, some anaesthetists routinely employ electroencephalographic monitoring in addition to careful monitoring of the ECG and blood pressure. If carotid angiography has been performed under general anaesthesia, a neurological examination should be undertaken during the recovery period to ensure that there has been no cerebral damage.

An intense burning sensation and severe retrobulbar pain may occasionally make it difficult for patients to remain motionless if only local anaesthetic has been used. Unexpected cardiovascular collapse may also occur during the investigation (Campkin *et al.*, 1977). The presence of an anaesthetist is therefore useful during local anaesthesia, if only to assist with resuscitation if required and to intercede if the patient finds the procedure unbearable. Prolonged apnoea has been observed following vertebral angiography (Davis & Statham, 1962), providing a further reason for using controlled ventilation during general anaesthesia.

A sudden rise in blood pressure has been noted following carotid angiography and may be associated both as a complication of the contrast media (Campkin *et al.*, 1977), especially in patients who have had a subarachnoid haemorrhage, and following the reversal of narcotics with naloxone (Cottrell & Estilo, 1981). Narcotics may, of course, be used with either local or general anaesthesia. Cottrell and Estilo (1981) have described a case where a sudden rise of arterial blood pressure to 260/140 was associated with the rupture of a cerebral aneurysm 5 min after naloxone reversal of fentanil, followed by a right hemiplegia.

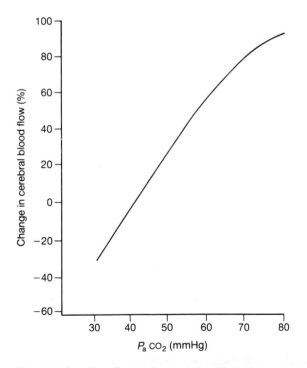

Fig. 31.2 The effect of arterial carbon dioxide tension on cerebral blood flow. Hypercarbia is frequently associated with spontaneous respiration during anaesthesia and the resulting increased cerebral blood flow may raise the intracranial pressure.

Cardiac angiography

Cardiac angiography has separate considerations in the adult and paediatric age groups.

In the adult, cardiac angiography is usually performed under local anaesthesia with the assistance of sedation. Dysrhythmias are not uncommon as a result of the direct stimulation of the heart by the catheter and following injection of the contrast medium. ECG monitoring should always be undertaken and in many centres a pacemaker is introduced prior to angiography. Left heart failure, myocardial infarction and crescendo angina have all been noticed during coronary angiography. Sedation or anaesthesia must therefore cause as little disturbance to the cardiovascular system as possible and midazolam is most commonly used for sedation. Midazolam also causes respiratory depression. This is particularly evident if a narcotic or opiate is also given, where upon profound respiratory depression may occur and require ventilatory support. Hypotension occasionally follows i.v. injection of midazolam, which should therefore be given carefully while observing the patient's respiratory pattern and blood pressure. A suitable level of sedation may be achieved by giving 1–5 mg i.v. in increments of 0.5–1 mg every 30 s until ptosis is observed.

There are two particular considerations which decide the form of anaesthesia for paediatric cardiopulmonary investigation. Firstly, the infant is usually uncooperative in the X-ray department and hence general anaesthesia may well be required regardless of any other consideration. Secondly, it is most important to maintain cardiovascular stability. While heavy sedation is employed in some centres (Nicholson & Graham, 1969; Manners, 1971), it may well result in marked respiratory depression and a considerable disturbance of the normal physiological state. Sudden cardiorespiratory failure may also occur during cardiac catheterization. If the child is already anaesthetized, he or she will have almost certainly have been intubated and will have an i.v. line. These are two vital steps in resuscitation.

The aim of the anaesthetist is to present the child for investigation with a stable circulatory state. This requires careful preoperative preparation in close conjunction with the physician and surgeon. Some children are seriously ill and present in cardiac failure as potential surgical emergencies. A muscle relaxant technique and controlled ventilation have been used to provide stable conditions. Great care must be taken to avoid hypoxaemia. It is especially important in the smaller child to maintain body temperature. Continuing therapeutic support of the cardiovascular system may be required throughout

anaesthesia and corrections may need to be made to the arterial blood gas status. Ideally, anaesthesia for such infants requires the skills of a paediatric anaesthetist in specialized centres.

Venography

Intraosseous venograms are rarely performed nowadays but may require general anaesthesia because of the discomfort to the patient. Particular care has to be taken in the preoperative assessment of patients who have experienced multiple pulmonary emboli and may have a poor cardiopulmonary reserve. The patient may well be receiving anticoagulant therapy. Trauma to the larynx and haematoma formation following intubation may cause blockage of the airway following extubation. Pulmonary function should be assessed by means of chest radiographs, isotope studies, pulmonary function tests and, most importantly, blood gas analysis following clinical assessment. Severe hypoxaemia may be found on blood gas analysis. Unfortunately, the normal homoeostatic mechanisms which maintain the distribution of blood flow and ventilation are disturbed during general anaesthesia, with a marked increase in the physiological shunt. This will lead to an increase in the severity of hypoxaemia unless suitable measures are employed, including a high inspired oxygen tension and controlled ventilation and possibly a continous positive airway pressure (CPAP).

Orthopaedic radiology

The radiological investigation of a joint under mechanical stress sometimes requires general anaesthesia. Caution must be urged in the manipulation of joints, especially if muscle relaxants are used, because considerable damage may occur to the joint which is no longer protected by the normal muscle tone.

More recently, nucleolysis of the intervertebral disc has been employed to treat prolapsed discs. Precise positioning of the needle prior to injection may cause considerable discomfort to the patient. It is also very important to have the cooperation of the patient during contrast medium injection to determine if the pain has been improved and to ensure that no damage is caused to the motor supply. A technique of light anaesthesia and neuroleptanaesthesia allows the patient to be awakened at the appropriate times, questioned as to any discomfort, and requested to move the legs. The anaesthetist must anticipate well in advance when anaesthesia is to be lightened in order that the patient may communicate coherently with the operator. For such a delicate balance of anaesthesia to be maintained, an anaesthetist must be fully familiar with the procedure. Alternatively, sedation supplemented by analgesia titrated to produce adequate pain relief without severe respiratory depression can be used. Anaphylactic reactions have occured during nucleolysis and full resuscitative facilities must be immediately available.

Computed tomography (CT)

As CT scanning may be prolonged and uncomfortable for the patient, general anaesthesia is useful on occasion. For instance, an infant is likely to require general anesthesia during CT scanning. Patients may come from the intensive care unit for a diagnostic CT scan. Again, particularly because of movement of the patient, it is important to ensure continuity of the anaesthetic breathing systems and vascular lines whilst monitoring very carefully. A CT unit should be fully equipped to deal with such critically ill patients.

Magnetic resonance imaging (MRI) and spectroscopy

Substantial technical problems are posed for the anaesthetist because of the strong magnetic field. The anaesthetist must ensure the presence of as little ferromagnetic material as possible in the anaesthetic equipment and should avoid using metal connectors and other material accessories which may interfere with the quality of the final MRI image. Furthermore, much of the standard anaesthetic monitoring equipment will malfunction when in close proximity to the magnet. Care must be taken when attaching monitoring leads to the patient in case stray electric currents are induced. Forethought and selection of suitable equipment are therefore required prior to anaesthesia or sedation in this environment (Nixon *et al.*, 1986).

A plan of action and special equipment are also

required for resuscitation. Expeditious removal of the patient from the vicinity of the magnet to a safe area prepared for resuscitation is preferred before cardiopulmonary resuscitation.

Screening of patients prior to admission for MRI investigation is necessary (Moseley, 1994). A detailed questionnaire helps to identify potential problems such as pacemakers, metal prostheses or surgical clips. Patients may well be referred from distant hospitals and advance notice of any particular medical disorders, for example epilepsy, is required so that special arrangements can be prepared to manage the patient safely.

General anaesthesia can be required, either for a prolonged investigation when the patient must remain absolutely still or because of fear of the claustrophobic environment engendered by the magnetic coil. Special anaesthetic machines, containing a minimum of ferromagnetic material, are available. The anaesthetic breathing systems must be made from plastic materials and pipeline gases should be provided in preference to cylinder gas. Plastic cannulae, rather than metal needles, should be used for intermittent injection of drugs. Pneumatic devices are available for monitoring respiration and blood pressure (Roth *et al.*, 1985, Peden, *et al.*, 1992), whilst fibreoptic-linked monitoring has been developed including, most importantly, pulse oximeters.

Light sedation or anxiolysis is helpful in keeping the patient as still as possible. Should i.v. sedation be required, respiratory monitoring and pulse oximetry at the very least is advised because of the difficulty of observing a patient inside the MRI coil.

Interventional radiology

Whilst the need for anaesthesia or heavy sedation has diminished during diagnostic radiology because of the increasing sophistication of radiological imaging techniques, interventional radiology is placing new demands on the anaesthetist.

As interventional procedures are more likely to be painful, there are greater requirements for control of autonomic reflexes and the patients are more likely to be seriously ill. This is not the area for the single-handed operator: skilled assistance must be present to monitor and care for the patient. A review of the subject has been published (Steinbrich & Goors-Fengels, 1992), providing further detail.

Resuscitation

Those responsible for i.v. sedation or anaesthesia should be skilled in resuscitation techniques. While brief guidance will be given in this section, those who need to become familiar with the subject must refer to more detailed texts (Evans, 1986).

A significant deterioration in the patient's condition requires prompt and firm action. Neither hopeful inactivity nor disorganized panic is appropriate. A named person is responsible for checking that the necessary equipment and drugs are already close at hand. It is imperative to have rehearsed a course of action. The importance of training and agreed resuscitation policies has been stressed in the Report of the Joint Working Party of the Royal Colleges of Anaesthetists and Radiologists (1992). A quick assessment must be made of both the patient's condition and any possible reason for the adverse change. Early assessment at this point may significantly affect later management. If there is cardiorespiratory failure or loss of consciousness, the following action is required:

1 Establish a clear airway.
2 Administer 100% oxygen.
3 Support ventilation if it is depressed or absent. Tracheal intubation is preferred, but do not waste precious time on unsuccessful attempts. Ventilate using a Laerdal mask if encountering difficulty. Should there be ventilatory depression following i.v. benzodiazapine, flumazenil (200 g i.v.) may well improve respiration. If an opiate has been given and is considered to be responsible for the respiratory depression, then naloxone (1 mg i.v. every 2 min up to 10 mg maximum) can be given to improve respiratory drive.
4 Assess peripheral circulation and connect an ECG monitor and blood pressure cuff. If a pulse cannot be felt, commence external cardiac massage and defibrillate if necessary. Insert an i.v. line.
5 Give appropriate drug and fluid therapy. This will depend to some extent on the earlier assessment. If anaphylactic shock is suspected, adrenaline (1 mg i.v.), an antihistamine (for example chlorpheniramine 20 mg i.v. over 1 min), steroids (for example dexamethasone 500 mg i.v.) and rapid infusion of 1–2 litres of Hartmann's solution is the recommended treatment. Following a cardiac arrest, lignocaine (100 mg i.v.), atropine (1.2 mg i.v.) and sodium bicarbonate 8.4% (100 ml i.v.) may be necessary.
6 Position the patient so that the airway is protected, aspiration of vomit is prevented and there is optimization of circulation. This will usually mean placing the patient in the lateral recovery position with a 10° head-down tilt. This action may be all that is required following a vasovagal episode. The major exception to this positioning is respiratory difficulty caused by asthma, chronic bronchitis or left ventricular failure associated with pulmonary oedema. In these circumstances, and providing there is a reasonable blood pressure, the patient should be placed in a sitting position.

The above order of action to be taken is not rigidly fixed but should be modified according to the initial assessment.

Postoperative complications and care

Special care is required during recovery from anaesthesia because the radiology department is frequently isolated from the other medical units in the hospital. An experienced nurse must be available to tend to the patient. Facilities should be provided for the patient to stay long enough to recover fully prior to the return to the ward. All too frequently an inexperienced nurse is sent to escort the patient back to the ward despite the potential risk of serious and life-endangering complications.

A surprisingly high morbidity following anaesthesia for radiological procedures has been found (Barnes & Havill, 1980). On comparing the morbidity rate per thousand procedures requiring admission to an intensive care unit after a variety of surgical procedures (Fig. 31.3), anaesthesia for radiological investigations was shown to have a morbidity second only to cardiothoracic surgery. Similar results are also mentioned in another survey on factors affecting mortality in hospital (Farrow *et al.*, 1982). A combination of factors was responsible for this relatively high morbidity, including other pre-existing conditions which predisposed to a high perioperative risk (Fowkes *et al.*, 1982), ignorance of the hazards which may arise within the radiology

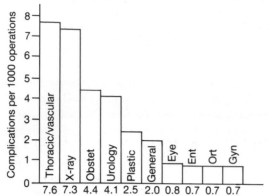

Fig. 31.3 Incidence of complications per thousand procedures requiring admission to an intensive care therapy unit in various surgical groups. Reproduced with permission from Barnes & Havill (1980).

department and the delegation of anaesthesia to junior and inexperienced staff.

The facilities provided in the recovery room should include suction and an oxygen supply. Endotracheal tubes, laryngoscopes and suitable drugs for resuscitation must be immediately available. The trolley used for patient recovery must allow the patient to be tilted head-down in case of vomiting or hypotension. An ECG and defibrillator must be available together with i.v. fluids and infusion sets. A proper assessment of the patient is frequently hampered by the poor lighting in the radiology department; the valuable sign of skin colour giving information about the patient's circulation, peripheral perfusion and the adequacy of oxygenation is therefore lost. Whilst much of the radiology department may be darkened, the recovery room should be properly illuminated with light of a neutral colour.

References

Aps, C. (1975) Pulmonary oedema following translumbar aortography. *Proc. Roy. Soc. Med.*, **68**, 996.

Association of Anaesthetists (1988) *Recommendations for Standards of Monitoring during Anaesthesia.* Association of Anaesthetists, London.

Barnes, P.J. & Havill, J.H. (1980) Anaesthetic complications requiring intensive care — a five year review. *Anaesth. Intens. Care*, **8**, 404.

Buxton Hopkin, D.A. (1980) *Hazards and Errors in Anaesthesia in Radiological Departments.* Springer Verlag, Berlin.

Campkin, T.V., Hurchings, G.M. & Philips, G. (1977) Arterial pressure studies during carotid angiography. *Br. J. Anaesth.*, **49**, 163–7.

Cottrell, J.E. & Estilo, A.E. (1981) Naloxone, hypertension and ruptured cerebral aneurysm. *Anaesthesiology*, **54**, 352.

Dallas, S.H. & Moxon, C.P. (1969) Controlled ventilation for cerebral angiography. *Br. J. Anaesth.*, **41**, 597–602.

Davis, S. & Statham, C. (1962) Prolonged apnoea following vertebral angiography. *Br. J. Anaesth.*, **34**, 119–20.

Evans, T.R. (1986) *ABC of Resuscitation.* British Medical Journal, London.

Farrow, S.C., Fawkes, F.G.R., Lunn, J.N. *et al.* (1982) Epidemiology in anaesthesia. II. Factors affecting mortality in hospitals. *Br. J. Anaesth.*, **54**, 811–17.

Finby, N. & Kanick, V. (1970) Radiology procedures and the difficult patient. *Radiology*, **94**, 101–3.

Fowkes, F.G.R., Lunn, J.N., Farrow, S.C. *et al.* (1982) Epidemiology in anaesthesia III. Mortality risk in patients with coexisting physical disease. *Br. J. Anaesth.*, **54**, 819–25.

Macpherson, D.S., James, D.C. & Bell, P.R.F. (1980) Is aortography abused in lower limb ischaemia? *Lancet*, **ii**, 80–2.

Manners, J.M. (1971) Anaesthesia for diagnostic procedures in cardiac disease. *Br. J. Anaesth.*, **43**, 276–87.

McDowall, D.G. (1975) Anaesthesia for neuroradiology. *Proc. Roy. Soc. Med.*, **68**, 765.

McDowall, D.G., Barker, W.B. & Fitch, J. (1969) Effect of anaesthesia on intracranial pressure in patients with space-occupying lesions. *Lancet*, **i**, 61–4.

McDowall, D.G., Harper, A.M. & Jacobson, I. (1963) Cerebral blood flow during halothane anaesthesia. *Br. J. Anaesth.*, **35**, 394–402.

Miskin, M.M., Baum, S. & Di Chiro, G. (1973) Emergency treatment of angiography induced paraplegia and tetraplegia. *N. Engl. J. Med.*, **288**, 1184–5.

Morgan, M., Loh, L, Singer, L. & More, P.H. (1971) Ketamine as the sole anaesthetic agent for minor surgical procedures. *Anaesthesia*, **26**(2), 158–65.

Moseley, I. (1994) Safety and magnetic resonance imaging. *Br. Med. J.*, **308**, 1181–2.

Moss, P.J. & Johnson, R.C. (1981) Case report — temporary blindness following anaesthesia after translumbar aortography. *Anaesthesia*, **36**, 954–5.

Nicholson, J.R. & Graham, G.R. (1969) Management of infants under six months of age undergoing cardiac investigation. *Br. J. Aaesth.*, **41**, 417–25.

Nixon, C., Hirsch, N.P., Ormerod, I.E.C. & Johnson, G. (1986) Nuclear magnetic resonance. *Anaesthesia*, **41**, 131–7.

Peden, C.J., Menon, D.K., Hall, A.S., Sargentoni, J. & Whitwam, J.G. (1992) Magentic resonance for the anaesthetist. *Anaesthesia*, **47**, 508–17.

Roth, J.L., Nuhent, M., Gray, J.E. *et al.* (1985) Patient monitoring during magnetic resonance imaging. *Anaesthesiology*, **62**, 80–3.

Royal Collage of Anaesthetists and Royal Collage of Radiologists (1992) *Sedation and Anaesthesia in Radiology.*

Report of a joint working party, London.

Samuel, J.R., Grange, R.A. & Hawkins, T.D. (1968) Anaesthetic technique for carotid angiography. *Anaesthesiology*, **23**(4), 543–51.

Snowdon, S.L. & Whitehouse, G.H. (1981) Blood pressure changes resulting from aortography. *J. Roy. Soc. Med.*, **74**, 419–21.

Steinbrich, W. & Goors-Fengels, W. (1992) *Interventional Radiology, Adjunctive Medication and Monitoring*. Springer-Verlag, Berlin.

32   Medical Litigation

J. O. M. C. CRAIG

Over the past few decades there has been increasing anxiety amongst medical practitioners concerning the incidence of litigation. This anxiety touches all grades of the profession from the medical student to the mature consultant. Some have argued that an awareness of the possibility of legal action has made the doctor more careful about the patient's welfare. Others have pointed out that the fear of litigation has increased the practice of defensive medicine, the increased number of radiological and laboratory tests resulting in the wasting of resources and increasing the cost of health care nationally. It is suggested that the increased incidence of litigation has had an adverse effect on the morale of the profession and has played some part in the disillusionment of the young graduate.

Some specialties, such as obstetrics and gynaecology, attract more litigation than others and litigation risk is one of the factors that has produced a decline in the recruitment of graduates into this specialty. Although there are still more applicants for places in medical schools than can be given, the numbers of those applying is declining. Doctors working in obstetrics, general surgery, orthopaedics and in the accident and emergency departments are the most liable to litigation. Radiology in the UK is not at the moment high in the list of specialties prone to litigation, but it is third in line in the USA. With the advent of interventional techniques and the enormous changes that have occurred in the practice of radiology and the advances of technology, it is likely that the trend in the UK will follow that in the USA.

At no time in the history of medicine in the UK has there been such an awareness of the vulnerability of the doctor to legal action. Doctors may find themselves liable to multiple jeopardy. Medical performance may be questioned by:

1 The coroner.
2 A hospital committee of enquiry.
3 A health service commissioner.
4 The General Medical Council.
5 Family practitioner committees.
6 Civil courts.
7 Criminal courts.

Dr Roy Palmer, Secretary of the Medical Protection Society (personal communication) has said that while he would not wish to alarm the profession, there had been an increasing number of manslaughter charges brought against medical practitioners. Even a decade ago no such criminal prosecution would have been considered.

The causes of increased medical litigation must be placed in the context of a universal trend to seek satisfaction, retribution or compensation for any mishap, imagined or real, in the secular and commercial world outside medicine. The increase in medical negligence claims may result from a number of factors. There has been more medical knowledge disseminated to the general public by all branches of the media and especially by television programmes. The advances in medical science have been remarkable and the expectations of the public from the medical profession have been raised to new heights. When these expectations are not satisfied, the patients or their relatives suspect that something may have gone wrong and search for negligence. Patients cannot distinguish between the complications of a procedure and those that result from negligence. In the present universal litigious climate there is an increased readiness to challenge those in authority and, in the case of medicine, this would include the doctor's authority or the authority that manages a hospital. It is easier at the present time to undertake litigation, with the help of the Citizens Advice Bureau, community health councils and legal aid schemes. High financial court awards make litigation inviting.

Doctors may be anxious about litigation but they are becoming increasingly aware that, as well as having a moral duty to the patient, they also carry legal responsibility for their actions and inactions. The medical profession must be mindful that where negligence does exist then compensation must be made.

Crown indemnity

Medical litigation in the UK until 1990 was dealt with by three main bodies: the Medical Protection Society, the Medical Defence Union and the Medical and Dental Defence Union of Scotland. It was a condition of employment in the UK that a doctor belonged to one of these societies. However, a Department of Health Circular (1989) effective from 1 January 1990 introduced new arrangements for dealing with negligence claims. These arrangements were that the responsibility for handling and funding existing and new claims resulting from the acts or omissions of medical or dental staff, in the course of their National Health Service employment, passed from the medical defence organizations to the health authorities. It is no longer a contractual requirement for hospital doctors working for health authorities to belong to a medical defence organization. This health circular does not apply to those doctors working in private or general practice.

This change in managing and funding medical litigation was followed by a letter in February 1991 from the National Health Service Management Executive, stating that the responsibility to pay the costs and awards in medical negligence cases now moved to the providers of health care, which were directly managed units and hospital trusts. This change has had a profound effect on the management of litigation and on the provision of health care. The National Association of Hospital Authorities and Trusts (NAHAT) reported in 1992 a concern that the cost of litigation falling on an individual unit or trust would remove finance from that available to provide a service to patients. The Association was also concerned that the costs of litigation were rising steeply. In 1989 the cost to the defence organizations was approximately £40 million. In 1990/91 the cost to the health authorities was about £53 million. It is estimated by the Department of Health (personal communication) that the cost is now greatly in excess of that figure and is still rising. Dr Duncan Murray of the Medical

Protection Society has shown that the average cost of settling a claim had risen 400% between 1976 and 1985.

Since litigation has been handled by each individual unit in the UK, there has been no central collection of statistics concerning the costs of litigation, the incidence of litigation and the specialties most often involved in litigation. The figures available to the Medical Protection Society show a remarkable increase in litigation cases since 1947. Dr Cochrane Shanks, a former President of the Medical Defence Union, published a report (1959) stating that there were 47 claims to the Union in 1947 involving all specialties and this had risen to 92 in 1957. These figures indicate the limited problem of litigation at those times. Written requests for help to the Medical Protection Society were 4800 in 1983 and 7600 in 1987, of which 4200 related to standards of care and so were possible claims. At a conference held at St Bartholomew's Hospital in July 1990, Dr Ivor Quest of the Medical Protection Society described the malpractice scene in Europe. He pointed out that the numerous routes for complaints about doctors that exist in the UK, such as family practitioner committees, hospital management committees, health service commissioners and the like, do not exist elsewhere in Europe. Social and cultural differences exist between the UK and other European Union countries. The Latin nations have fewer claims than the Anglo-Saxon nations. In Spain only 43 cases of medical litigation had been heard by the Spanish Supreme Court between 1875 and 1984, but since 1984 there had been a fourfold increase in claims. In Western Germany, as the standard of living rose, so did the claims for medical negligence. Claims in excess of 100 000 DM have increased 10-fold since 1970. A questionnaire sent to eight European countries — Spain, Greece, Italy, Hungary, Denmark, Norway, West and East Germany (prior to union) — revealed that medical negligence claims were increasing in each one.

A personal report to the Conference of Medical Royal Colleges expressing anxiety regarding litigation and its effect on the profession resulted in the Conference setting up a Litigation Working Party. This Working Party met the Chief Medical Officer who had already set up a Clinical Negligence Working Party to consider the whole problem of medical litigation, including its effect on the good practice of medicine. At the time of writing this Department of Health committee is meeting regularly and the profession must await the final outcome. It is encouraging to know that the problems that litigation poses for both profession and patient are being debated widely throughout the UK.

Medical negligence

There is considerable lack of understanding among the medical profession as to what constitutes medical negligence. Medical negligence can mean different things in different countries. The concept of medical negligence may be different in the UK from that in the USA. Indeed, it varies from one American state to another. There are numerous definitions of medical negligence in the UK, but the earliest is still the one most suitable for an understanding of the present state of affairs. This definition dates from 1838 when Chief Justice Tindal laid the foundations of the legal duties of professional people. He said:

> Any person who enters into a learned profession undertakes to bring to the exercise of it, a reasonable degree of care and skill. He does not undertake, if he is an attorney, that at all events you will gain your case, nor does a surgeon undertake that he will perform a cure, nor does he undertake to use the highest degree of skill. There may be persons, who have higher education and greater advantages than he has, but he undertakes to bring a fair reasonable and competent degree of skill.

This definition and its many implications may not apply outside the UK, and it may in future years undergo modifications. However, it does mean that the standard of care expected of an individual doctor is related to training and experience, and is judged by standards expected in his or her peers. Therefore, what is negligent in a senior surgeon is not necessarily negligent in a house surgeon. That which is negligent in a consultant radiologist is not necessarily negligent in an accident and emergency registrar. This interpretation of negligence is a great help to the profession and gives some support to the training of young doctors, when tasks must be delegated. Nevertheless there are strict criteria for delegation which will be covered later in this chapter. In practice, in a court of law, medical experts will attest as to what

may or may not be expected of a defendant at his or her stage of training.

Whether or not a doctor has failed in his or her duty to the patient is considered under the legal term of tort. The plaintiff must establish the following facts.

1 There was a duty of care owed to the patient by the named defendants.

2 The standard of care appropriate to that duty must not have been achieved and, as a result, the duty breached, either by action or inaction, advice given or failure to advise.

3 Such a breach must be shown to have caused the injury and therefore the resulting loss complained about by the patient.

4 Any loss sustained as a result of the injury and complained about by the patient must be of a kind that the courts recognize, and for which they allow compensation.

Ionizing radiation regulations

There has been a great deal of confusion regarding these regulations, which were published under the title of 'Protection of Persons Undergoing Medical Examination or Treatment' (POPUMET) in 1988. Much of the misunderstanding is found in those doctors not trained in clinical radiology. The regulations refer to 'clinically directing' and 'physically directing' a radiological examination. 'Clinically directing' is the clinical decision to effect the radiographic exposure (X-rays, γ-rays, and so on). This decision invariably rests with the radiologist who should be satisfied that the exposure to irradiation is clinically justified and that the choice of the method of exposure is the most appropriate. 'Physically directing' is the act of effecting the exposure. This is invariably the act of the radiographer. There can be times when the radiologist may be both clinically and physically directing an examination, for instance during fluoroscopy. There can be times when a non-radiologist doctor is both clinically and physically directing an examination, for example a cardiologist inserting a pacemaker. These regulations do not refer to the request for a radiological examination. Under these regulations, persons clinically or physically directing exposures to irradiation should have received 'adequate training'. Trained and training radiologists have received this training, but non-radiologists require instruction in the 'core of knowledge' relating to competence in radiological protection. A certificate of having this core of knowledge must be obtained by those not trained in radiology or radiography, before clinically or physically directing a radiological examination. A further requirement of the POPUMET regulations is that the smallest possible irradiation dose should be used to obtain a satisfactory medical result.

These regulations place a serious duty on the radiologist to ensure that each exposure to ionizing radiation does indeed have a reasonable clinical indication and that the choice of examination is that most appropriate to solve the medical problem. This is not always easy, as all requests for radiological examinations cannot be scrutinized, for instance requests for 'routine' chest radiographs. However, it is the duty of the radiologist in charge of the department to issue standing orders to cover these problems that exist when he or she is not available.

Failure to observe the ionizing radiation regulations can lead to criminal prosecution under section 15 of the Health and Safety at Work Act 1974.

Radiological cases

Before the advent of Crown Indemnity, some central collection of the types of cases involved in litigation was kept by the medical defence organizations. The analysis of 360 cases involving radiology dealt with by the Medical Protection Society was made by the author (Craig, 1989). Of these 360 cases, 78% were related to trauma. The most commonly missed fractures were those of the cervical spine, neck of the femur and of the scaphoid bone. By far the most serious cases were those in the cervical spine, and it cannot be emphasized too often that extreme care must be exercised in examining this region. A recurrent fault is to accept radiographs that are not correctly exposed or centred, and that do not show all seven cervical vertebrae. In the reported series there were eight cases concerning the cervical spine. Many of these cases were seen by accident and emergency doctors not trained in clinical radiology. If there is any clinical doubt or doubt about the interpretation of the radiographs, then a senior opinion should be

sought as soon as possible. It is always wise to obtain a radiological opinion in cases of worrying cervical spine injury. It is still surprising how often there is litigation concerning failure to diagnose a scaphoid fracture. It is clearly taught that if a scaphoid fracture is suspected then the case should be treated as a fractured scaphoid and radiographed again in approximately 10 days' time. It may be helpful in doubtful cases to obtain an isotope bone scan.

Dislocations that can be difficult to diagnose, and which need to be borne in mind in injuries involving these areas, are posterior dislocations of the shoulder and dislocations of the tarsus.

Failure to radiograph when an injury involves glass is still a problem. Glass is radio-opaque. A possible foreign body in the eye also warrants a radiograph.

Failure to radiograph was a cause for litigation in 32% of cases, and included glass foreign bodies and foreign bodies in the eye. Some of the cases also included failure to take check radiographs following manipulation of fractures and failure to radiograph for retained swabs following surgery.

In this series 22% of cases were unrelated to trauma. They included contrast reactions, barium extravasations in barium enema examinations, myelography and angiography problems, computed tomography (CT) and ultrasound errors.

The author's personal experience over the past year includes 31 cases involving radiology. The number is too few from which to draw conclusions but nonetheless the cases show an interesting pattern

Table 32.1 Author's 31 legal cases involving radiology

	No. of cases
Chest lesions	7
Fractures	7
Vascular radiology	6
Barium meals and enemas	2
Computed tomography	2
Hysterosalpingography	1
Arthrograms	1
Discography	1
Skull interpretation	1
Bone lesions	1
Intravenous urography death	1
Ultrasound	1

(classified into groups in Table 32.1). There were as many cases concerning the performance of angiography and the interpretation of chest radiographs as there were traumatic cases.

A most worrying statistic to emerge from the original series of 360 cases was that in over 30% of cases involving errors of radiological interpretation there was no radiological report. The radiological diagnosis was by junior doctors not trained in radiological interpretation. In a paper by Vincent *et al.* (1988) the ability of senior house officers in the accident and emergency department to detect radiographic abnormalities was assessed. They had an error rate of 39% for clinically significant abnormalities, when compared to a radiological report by trained radiologists. A further worrying finding was that there was no improvement in this error rate when they were reassessed after 6 months in the post. It was stated in this paper that it was unrealistic to expect junior doctors to acquire the skills necessary to interpret radiographs merely by being exposed to these radiographs over a 6-month period. On a national basis the consequences for a Health Service being subjected to this litigation risk is extremely serious. The risk could be greatly reduced by increasing the number of radiologists, placing more importance on the reporting of accident and emergency radiographs and finding some way to establish immediate reporting by trained radiologists.

Contrast media

In the UK there has been some doubt regarding the use of high- or low-osmolar contrast medium. Anxiety exists among radiologists about their medicolegal position if, while using a high-osmolar contrast medium, a mishap were to occur. Many radiologists say that they feel more comfortable when injecting low-osmolar contrast media and, by choice, would prefer to use these even in patients who have a low risk from any contrast medium. The Royal College of Radiologists felt that guidance regarding contrast agents was needed on which radiologists could base their decisions. This led to a letter written on request by Professor Ronald Grainger (1984). It was considered that low-osmolar were safer than high-osmolar contrast agents but were so much more expensive that they should not be used for all examinations, but should be used for selected cases in which the risk from contrast mechia was known to be high.

Anxiety has persisted since 1984 and the problem has been kept under review. This led to a further request from the Royal College of Radiologists, this time to both Professor Grainger and Dr Peter Dawson, to look at this issue again and to formulate guidelines (Grainger & Dawson, 1991). These were circulated by the College. In the introduction to these guidelines it is stated that a great deal of experience had been obtained concerning the new agents since 1984, and large-scale studies in Australia and Japan supported the assumption that there was greater safety in using non-ionic low-osmolar contrast agents for i.v. injections. No such data are available for ionic low-osmolar agents. It was also stated that corticosteroids administered for 12 hours or more prior to the injection of contrast media offered some prophylaxis against serious anaphylactoid reactions in patients at increased risk. This gain, which was not negligible, was apparently less than that offered by a non-ionic agent. The aim stated in this College document was to replace high-osmolar by low-osmolar media as soon as the necessary finance became available. The indications for the use of low-osmolar contrast are as follows.

1 Hexabrix (ioxaglate) may be used to best advantage in arteriography as the agent of low osmolality. Low-osmolar agents, ionic or non-ionic, should be used in all arteriography which is expected to be painful.

2 Non-ionic agents should be used in i.v. injections in all patients thought to be at higher risk of an anaphylactoid reaction, for instance in previous reactors, asthmatics, atopic patients and those allergic to other drugs or agents.

3 Non-ionic agents should be used generally in all procedures anticipated, in either absolute or relative terms, to be high-dose procedures. Patients unable to tolerate a high osmotic load, such as those in oliguric or anuric renal failure, especially if complicated by poor cardiac reserve, should be given a low-osmolar agent, ionic or non-ionic.

4 Infants and babies should be given the benefit of non-ionic agents because of the risk of 'overdose'.

5 Non-ionic agents should be used if there is difficulty in directly monitoring the patient or when

machinery makes vomiting a particular hazard, as is the case with CT scanning.

6 Patients with known haemodynamic instability or limited cardiac reserve merit the use of an agent associated with the least cardiovascular stress. Either a non-ionic agent or, in arteriography, ioxaglate should be used.

7 There is no convincing evidence that elderly patients are at significantly increased risk. However, the use of less stressful low-osmolar agents is advisable.

8 Either type of low-osmolar agent should be used in patients with sickle cell disease or trait. Ideally, they should be administered diluted approximately 1 : 2 to render them virtually iso-osmolar with respect to plasma.

9 In angioplasty low-osmolar agents should be used in order to minimize the pain of the concomitant angiography.

10 There is no evidence that clinically manifest contrast agent-associated nephrotoxicity is reduced or increased with any type of contrast agent in current use. An argument may be made that in patients with pre-existing renal impairment the most inert agent should be used, namely non-ionic, in the smallest possible dose. Dehydration should be corrected and never actively encouraged.

11 Recent concern about a possible increase in the incidence of thromboembolic phenomena in clinical angiography with non-ionic agents has probably been exaggerated. They do have less marked anticoagulant properties than ionic agents, conventional or ioxaglate, but the consequent increase in risk appears to be small in practice.

12 Adverse reactions usually begin within 10–15 min of contrast medium administration and patients should not be left unattended during that period. Major drug reactions may occasionally have a later onset.

13 No contrast agent is completely safe and full resuscitation equipment should always be close at hand whenever one is administered.

It is highly likely that if a mishap were to occur due to a contrast agent and a medicolegal case began, it would be a persuasive defence that the College guidelines had been followed.

The use of Myodil

In recent years a large number of legal claims have been made where the patient asserts that the development of arachnoiditis was due to the use of Myodil (iophendylate) to investigate spinal pathology and was aggravated by its incomplete removal following the examination. The threat posed to radiologists by these cases was substantial, as was the possible cost to the defence organizations and subsequently perhaps the health authorities. This led to the Royal College of Radiologists and the British Society of Neuroradiologists issuing a joint statement in December 1991, which gave a consensus view on the use of Myodil. It was the habit in the UK to use small quantities of Myodil, such as 6 ml, whereas considerably larger amounts, even 100 ml, were used in the USA. The questions that needed to be answered in the joint statement were whether or not the use of Myodil was justified at the time, or whether other contrast media should have been used. Should Myodil have been aspirated and what was the relevance of informed consent at the time?

The following conclusions were reached by the joint bodies.

1 Where clinical features of possible spinal pathology indicated the need for a definitive diagnosis and precise localization of a lesion, radiculography or myelography was essential.

2 In 1944–72 Myodil was the contrast medium of choice for radiculography and full myelography.

3 During the Conray/Dimer X era, the use of Myodil was still acceptable for radiculography and it remained the choice for run-up myelography.

4 Following the introduction of metrizamide, despite its advantages, a decision had to be made balancing the quality of the images against the potential severity of immediate complications. It became widely accepted as a contrast medium in the early 1980s.

5 Despite the recommendations in the data sheet that Myodil should be removed after the examination, unless it was required for a further study, it was common practice in the UK not to aspirate the relatively small volumes used here. This practice is supported by work which showed that aspiration failed to prevent the development of arachnoiditis, and non-aspiration of the contrast medium is considered to have been an acceptable practice.

6 Current practice regarding 'informed consent' did not apply in the Myodil era and, in any case, there are reports indicating that the rate of symptomatic post-Myodil arachnoiditis was not greater than 1%.

This joint statement, which was circulated to all members and Fellows of the Royal College of Radiologists contained a large number of literature references to support the opinions given.

Standing orders

All personnel working in a department of radiology should be familiar with the standing orders in that department. The standing orders are the responsibility of the consultant in charge and will usually be composed in consultation with medical, radiographic, nursing and clerical staff. These orders will include the protocol to be followed by radiographers for various radiographic examinations, for example in cervical spine, skull and sinus examinations. They will also include instructions to be followed in the care of patients having vascular or interventional procedures. The nursing and medical staff in the department, and those on the wards to which the patient is returning, should be informed of the protocol for the aftercare of the patients having these radiological investigations and treatments. Standing orders should include the protocol to deal with any large-scale emergency, such as the admission of major accident victims. Guidelines need to be given for the accepted treatment in that department to deal with contrast reactions or cardiac arrest. Everyone in the department should be familiar with the action necessary to deal with a departmental fire.

Standing orders should include the departmental policy regarding the release of unreported films and requests for films from other hospitals and medical and non-medical personnel outside the hospital.

Delegation

To delegate is to entrust or empower a colleague, medically or non-medically trained, to perform a task. Delegation is necessary for the day-to-day running of a department and also for the training of medical, nursing and radiographic staff. The need to delegate is recognized by all medical bodies, but it carries serious medicolegal responsibilities for the delegator and the delegatee. Owing to these consequences the Royal College of Radiologists issued guidelines regarding delegation in 1993. Delegation of a task may be to a medical colleague who is trained or in training in radiology. It may be to a medical colleague not trained in radiology or to a non-medically trained colleague, such as a nurse, midwife or radiographer. The General Medical Council refers to the necessity to delegate to non-medical personnel in its document 'Fitness to Practice' (1985). The policy of skill-mix encourages many tasks previously performed by medically qualified staff to be performed by non-medically trained personnel. The General Medical Council recognizes such delegations but states that it is serious professional misconduct to delegate to persons not medically qualified, tasks requiring the knowledge and skill of a medical practitioner.

Delegation may be classified as a proper or improper delegation. If a task delegated to a colleague is within the training, skill and competence of that colleague, a proper delegation has taken place. If on the other the task is outside the training and competence of the delegatee, then it is an improper delegation. If a mishap were to occur and a legal action resulted in a case where a proper delegation had been made, it is likely that the delegatee would bear the medicolegal consequences. If a mishap and a legal action were to occur concerning an improper delegation, then the delegator would carry serious legal responsibility. However, in any court case, each case is judged individually according to the existing circumstances. There is a responsibility on the part of the delegatee to state whether or not a delegated task may be outside his or her competence.

If a death were to occur from an improper delegation, the delegator could be liable to a charge of manslaughter. As stated above, there has been an increase in the number of charges of manslaughter brought against medical practitioners in recent years. Even with a proper delegation errors can occur, and if a task is delegated to a junior then the senior has a responsibility to make sure that support is available and obtainable.

In cases of skill-mix if a court case were to occur the court's attention would be directed to the training and competence of the delegatee to perform the task delegated.

Unreported radiographs

The practice of radiology has changed enormously over the past few decades and the radiological workload has surpassed the staff available. This is due in part to the increased work produced by the newer technologies of ultrasound, CT scanning and magnetic resonance imaging (MRI). The growth of vascular and interventional radiology also involves the radiologist in more time-consuming procedures. These changes have resulted in an increase in unreported radiographs in most radiological departments. This is a sad trend, but in the present circumstances an inevitable one. In the interest of the patient it may be necessary to send unreported radiographs to clinical colleagues. To do so is to delegate the immediate interpretation of the investigation to the non-radiological colleague. This carries medicolegal consequences. If the colleague acts on his or her own interpretation and a fault results in a legal action, he or she will be medicolegally responsible for that interpretation. A court might also like to know why it was necessary for the clinician to have an unreported radiograph.

Certain criteria must be followed if radiographs are to be released unreported. The hospital management should be informed that unreported radiographs are being released and the reasons for this should be stated and recorded. If radiographs are to be released unreported there must be a recognizable patient need for this. If radiographs are released to a clinic on a regular basis, this should follow an agreement between the radiologist and the relevant clinical colleague and each should understand the medicolegal consequences of this policy. The interpretation by the clinical colleague should be recorded in the patient's notes. The department of radiology must have a record of to whom the radiograph was released. The radiograph should be returned to the department of radiology for reporting as soon as possible.

Accident and emergency examinations are a particular problem, as their interpretation may be left to inexperienced junior medical staff. All departments of radiology should give priority to the reporting of accident and emergency examinations.

Ultrasound

Over the past few decades there has been an enormous increase in the number of ultrasound examinations performed in the UK. These examinations cannot all be performed by radiologists. Non-medically qualified ultrasonographers now perform ultrasound examinations as normal practice. They include radiographers, midwives, nurses and physicists. Many obstetricians perform ultrasound examinations, and surgeons and physicians are increasingly involved in cardiac and Doppler ultrasound.

In a department of radiology, the radiologist in charge can delegate examinations to radiographers and others. He or she is responsible for seeing that the delegation is a proper one, and so must be sure that it is within the training and competence of the delegatee. Obstetricians, cardiologists and other medical personnel who perform their own ultrasound examinations are medicolegally responsible for these. If they delegate to non-medical colleagues then they bear the medicolegal consequences for that delegation. If a fault by a non-medically qualified ultrasonographer were to lead to an action in court, the training and experience of the ultrasonographer and the correctness of the delegation would be examined. This would also apply to delegation to a junior doctor.

The radiologist or other consultant in charge should inform the ultrasonographer of the protocol for ultrasound examinations, which are appropriate to do and which should be referred for a medical opinion. Non-medical ultrasonographers can issue factual reports on their observations. These reports should be signed by the ultrasonographer and the status should be signified. A radiologist or other medical consultant may examine the ultrasound record and issue a report which he or she signs, but the name and status of the ultrasonographer should also appear on the report. In keeping with the General Medical Council regulations, a non-medically qualified ultrasonographer cannot give an opinion that requires the training and the skills of a medical practitioner.

The overall clinical responsibility for the patient in the ultrasound department rests with the consultant in charge.

Digital radiology

A future development in departments of radiology is the introduction of total digital imaging and the elimination of radiographs as records of the image. This development will lead to transmission of images throughout the hospital, to other hospitals and even to other counties and countries. As a result of the computerization of records, many medicolegal problems have arisen concerning confidentiality, security and disclosure. New legal issues will arise with the development of digital images, their storage and transmission.

There is no experience of these issues yet, but there are questions concerning the acceptable resolution on a visual display unit needed to obtain an accurate diagnosis, and the data compression of an image that is acceptable. What might be the legal consequences concerning digitizing films? Who is responsible for the medical problems that might follow computer breakdown? What are the legal issues of computer security? It is likely that the answers to these questions will appear over the next few years as digital departments and digital filmless hospitals become a reality. The responsibility rests with radiologists to decide what is and is not acceptable for an accurate diagnosis using digital display units, Radiologists also need to provide the lead in answering the other questions raised by these new techniques. These decisions cannot be left solely to the legal profession.

Informed consent

Many more medicolegal cases concerning consent have arisen over the past few decades. It has been said that the emphasis on consent has been detrimental to medical practice, but there is little doubt that doctors have been very lax concerning consent in the past. Anything that improves communication between doctors and patients must be encouraged.

The doctor obtaining consent to an investigation or treatment should inform the patient of all the relevant facts concerning that investigation or treatment to which a prudent patient would attach significance in arriving at a decision as to how to proceed. This is known as the 'prudent patient test'. Many doctors are anxious about how much they should or should not tell a patient about investigations or treatments. There is a concern that to state serious complications, even though they may be rare, might deter the patient from undergoing necessary investigations or treatments. If the doctor withholds these facts he or she relies on the doctrine of 'therapeutic privilege'. Lord Scarman in 1986 said that 'Medical paternalism is no longer acceptable in English law. The sovereignty of the patient has been reinstated'. He also said that 'Information of risk which the doctor judges to be significant should be given to the patient'. There appears to be room for clinical judgement here, but I suspect that the exercise of therapeutic privilege might often be difficult to defend in court. The doctor may rely on the 'professional standard test'. This is also known as the Bolam test and refers to the case of *Bolam* v. *Friern*. It states that a doctor would not be judged negligent if his or her action accorded with the practice accepted at that time by a responsible body of medical professionals (this does not mean the majority).

When is it necessary to have written consent? In clinical radiology it is difficult, and not considered essential at the present time, to obtain written consent for every radiological examination such as barium investigations, excretion urograms and the like. Oral consent may be satisfactory, but at all times the patient should be given a careful explanation of whatever procedure is to be performed, why it is necessary and what its complications are. The doctor must be prepared to answer questions about the procedure and possible alternative procedures. For complex investigations and treatments, and certainly all vascular and interventional procedures, written consent is necessary. It is now advisable to record obtaining consent in the patient's notes. If a complex procedure has been performed a record of this procedure should also be kept in the patient's notes, either separately or with the radiological report. If a patient does not wish to know the details of a procedure or its complications, then this should be recorded in the notes. If the patient refuses consent to a procedure, this should also be recorded in the notes.

Consent must at best be obtained by the doctor performing the procedure. This applies especially to complex procedures. It is recognized that difficulties may arise that make it necessary to delegate the obtaining of consent. Consent should only be delegated to someone who is completely knowledgeable about the procedure to be performed, its indications, complications and alternatives. One should not rely on junior house doctors, nurses or radiographers to obtain consent for radiological procedures that are to be performed by a radiologist.

Consent for a procedure should be obtained at a time before that procedure which allows the patient the opportunity to give it reasonable thought, and of course never after the patient has received premedication.

If a complex procedure is to be performed, the radiologist should ideally visit the patient in the ward beforehand and discuss that procedure. Unfortunately, this is not always practical but, if not, then a satisfactory alternative opportunity must be found.

There is a great need for radiologists to communicate closely with their patients. To do so will undoubtedly improve radiological practice.

Guidelines

The Royal College of Radiologists has issued guidelines concerning many aspects of radiology over the past few years. In 1989 the College published a booklet 'Making the Best Use of a Department of Radiology'. This contained guidelines concerning the 12 most frequently performed radiological examinations in National Health Service hospitals. A second edition was produced in 1993 covering, in addition, ultrasound, mammography, CT, isotope imaging and accident and emergency examinations. A further edition is being prepared at the time of writing.

Many colleges are issuing guidelines and anxiety has been expressed regarding prescriptive investigations and treatments, and what the legal position is if the guidelines have not been followed. Guidelines are subject to alteration and modification depending on local circumstances and are not legally binding. However, they are undoubtedly helpful and to have acted according to guidelines issued by the College would be a reasonable argument for the defence counsel if a legal case were to arise concerning a radiological procedure.

Conclusion

The practice of radiology has changed considerably since the discovery of X-rays by Roentgen in 1895. These changes have been most marked over the past few decades. Not only is the radiologist performing more complex investigations and treatments than previously, but he or she is also performing them at a time of increasing litigation. This is the price to be paid for such enormous advances in the specialty and for closer contact with the patient. However, this closer contact also allows better communication with the patient, and this is one of the major antagonists to litigation.

References

Craig, J.O.M.C. (1989) The Knox Lecture. Radiology and the law. *Clin. Radiol.*, **40**, 343–6.

Department of Health (1989) *Circular HC(89) 34*. HMSO, London.

General Medical Council (1985) *Professional Conduct and Discipline. Fitness to Practice*. General Medical Council, London.

Grainger, R.G. (1984) The clinical and financial implications of low osmolar contrast media. *Clin. Radiol.*, **35**, 251–52.

Grainger, R.G. & Dawson, P. (1991) Low osmolar contrast media. An appraisal. Editorial. *Clin. Radiol.*, **42**, 1–5.

National Association of Health Authorities and Trusts (1992) *Just Finance in Medical Negligence Cases*. Report.

Protection of Persons Undergoing Medical Examination and Treatment (1988) *EC(88)* **29**. HMSO, London.

Quest, I. (1992) *Standard of Excellence. Summary of the First Conference at St Bartholomew's Hospital 1990 on European Standards*.

Royal College of Radiologist (1989) *Making the Best Use of a Department of Radiology. Guidelines for Doctors* (2nd edn, 1993). Royal College of Radiologists, London.

Royal College of Radiologists (1991) *Statement on Myodil*. Royal Collage of Radiologists, London.

Royal College of Radiologists (1993) *Medico-Legal Aspects of Delegation*. Royal Collage of Radiologists, London.

Scarman (Lord) (1986) Consent, communication and responsibility. *J Roy. Soc. Med.*, **79**, 697–700.

Shanks, S.C. (1959) Medicine, radiology and the law. *J. Faculty Radiologists*, **4**, 169–74.

Tindal, Chief Justice (1838) *Lanphier* v. *Phipos*. C&P, 475.

Vincent, C.F. & Driscoll, P.A. (1988) Accuracy of detection of radiographic abnormalities by junior doctors. *Arch. Emerg. Med.*, **5**, 101–9.

Index